NEUR

DATE DUE

OC 15 '93			
NO 5 '93			
MR 11 '94			
SE 30 '94			
MR 24 '95			
OC 13 '95			
DE 7 '96			
MR 18 '97			
SE 9 '97			
FE 19 '98			
AP 12 '00			
MR 20 '01			
AP 16 '01			
AP 2 '02			
MY 10 '06			

DEMCO 38-296

CORE TEXT OF

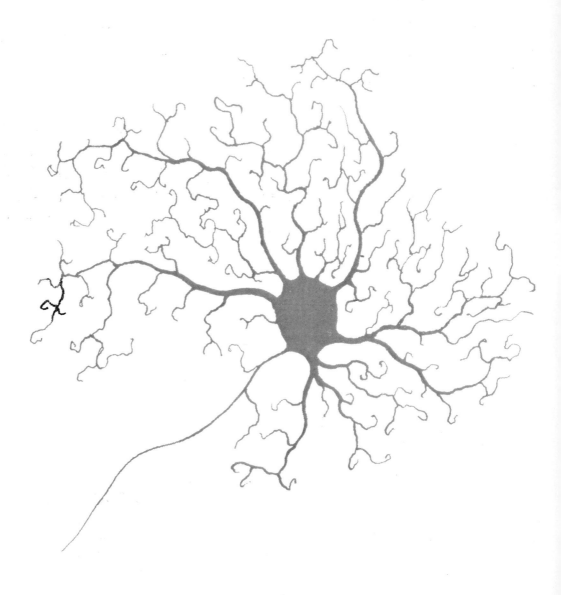

NEUROANATOMY

Fourth Edition

Malcolm B. Carpenter, A.B., M.D.

Professor and Chairman Emeritus
Department of Anatomy
F. Edward Hebert School of Medicine
Uniformed Services University of the Health Sciences
Bethesda, Maryland

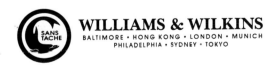

WILLIAMS & WILKINS
BALTIMORE · HONG KONG · LONDON · MUNICH
PHILADELPHIA · SYDNEY · TOKYO

Managing Editor: Victoria M. Vaughn
Copy Editor: Martha Wolf
Designer: Wilma E. Rosenberger
Illustration Planner: Ray Lowman
Production Coordinator: Adèle Boyd-Lanham

Copyright © 1991
Williams & Wilkins
428 East Preston Street
Baltimore, Maryland 21202, USA

Printed in the United States of America

First Edition, 1972
Reprinted 1972, 1973, 1974, 1975, 1976
Second Edition, 1978
Reprinted 1978, 1979, 1980, 1981, 1982, 1983, 1984
Third Edition, 1985
Reprinted 1986, 1988

Italian edition, 1976
Portuguese edition, 1979
Spanish edition, 1981
Japanese edition, 1982

Library of Congress Cataloging-in-Publication Data

Carpenter, Malcolm B.
    Core text of neuroanatomy / Malcolm B. Carpenter. -- 4th ed.
        p.   cm.
    Includes bibliographical references.
    Includes index.
    ISBN 0-683-01457-9
    1. Neuroanatomy. I. Title.
    [DNLM: 1. Nervous System--anatomy & histology. WL 101 C296c]
QM451.C37   1991
611′.8--dc20
DNLM/DLC
for Library of Congress
                                                                    90-13150
                                                                    CIP

                                                            92 93 94 95
                                            2 3 4 5 6 7 8 9 10

Preface to the Fourth Edition

From its inception, the object of this text has been to explain the functional organization of the central nervous system in a lucid and meaningful way. In the "Decade of the Brain," the explosion of information about the brain can be expected to continue at a faster pace with contributions from all basic medical sciences. In the nervous system, structural organization is central to most functional concepts. The proliferation of sophisticated new methods for exploring nearly every aspect of neural organization and function has refined old concepts, provided new insights, and opened new areas of investigation and appears likely to offer therapeutic solutions to many of the severe afflictions of the central nervous system. Information concerning putative neurotransmitters and their actions in specific neuronal systems constitutes a major advance in neuroscience. The enormous number of chemical substances in neurons is only beginning to be understood, but it is clear that this approach will lead to specific therapeutic agents that can modify and ameliorate many disease processes. The challenge presented is to synthesize this new information with the established principles of neural organization in a reasonable and understandable fashion. Serious attempts have been made to integrate the most pertinent new material with basic concepts. An attempt has been made not to duplicate material considered in depth in other disciplines. The text, with its many illustrations and schematic diagrams, provides a reasonably complete guide to the central nervous system and should meet the requirements of most medical students.

The Fourth Edition of the *Core Text of Neuroanatomy* follows the plan of prior editions but is cast in a new format with greatly improved subtitles. Reference citations have been deleted from the text, but suggested reading lists include both the newer and classical references. All chapters have been revised, shortened, and judiciously edited. Material concerning neurochemistry and neurotransmitters has been included in all chapters. Attempts have been made to balance factual material and interpretation. Sections entitled "Functional Considerations" address major anatomical, physiological, and chemical relationships and their clinical significance. Over 60 new or revised illustrations have been added, many in the form of schematic diagrams or drawings, which students have found to be helpful.

The author is grateful to his colleagues for their constructive criticisms and comments. The superb artistic skills of Robert J. Demarest of the College of Physicians and Surgeons, Columbia University, who contributed most of the drawings in all editions of this text, are evident. The success of this text over a period of years is due in large part to the artistic talents of Robert Demarest. The author is also pleased to acknowledge the expert assistance of Antonio B. Pereira over a long period of time. Mrs. Doris Lineweaver has continued to provide superb secretarial and editorial assistance, for which I am most grateful. Finally, the author is pleased to acknowledge the many courtesies, helpful suggestions, and services of the publisher. Special thanks are extended to Ms. Victoria Vaughn and Ms. Adele Boyd, who guided me through the labyrinthine pathways that lead to a finished book.

MALCOLM B. CARPENTER

Preface to the First Edition

At a time when many American medical schools have shifted to the new core curriculum, or are considering doing so, it is apparent that few of the standard textbooks are entirely appropriate. If the basic medical sciences are to be presented in one academic year, more or less, it is necessary to winnow that which is not essential, to reduce duplications and to present the basic concepts and facts so lucidly that their importance is obvious and their assimilation is possible. With these principles in mind, an attempt has been made to present a *Core Text of Neuroanatomy*.

This text is patterned after part of the material appearing in Truex and Carpenter's *Human Neuroanatomy* (6th edition) and utilizes a similar format and many of the same illustrations. Material which properly falls within the provinces of gross anatomy, histology and embryology has been left to those disciplines except where it is germane to the subject under discussion. The text deals primarily with organizations of the central nervous system. References have been kept to a minimum. While the labors of my scientific colleagues, past and present, are not always cited, they are acknowledged fully in the text of *Human Neuroanatomy*, and the interested student will have little difficulty in finding the authors who made the original contributions. The Paris Nomina Anatomica (PNA) in its amended form (1965) has been used throughout.

The author is grateful to Professor Raymond C. Truex, of Temple University School of Medicine, for his permission to use materials from Truex and Carpenter's *Human Neuroanatomy* (6th edition) and for his valued advice and encouragement. Professor Fred A. Mettler, at the College of Physicians and Surgeons, Columbia University, generously permitted the use of many superb illustrations from his *Neuroanatomy* (1948), which were made by Ivan Summers. I am indebted to both Dr. Mettler and The C. V. Mosby Company of St. Louis for permission to publish these illustrations. New illustrations were prepared by Mr. Robert J. Demarest, of the Department of Anatomy, College of Physicians and Surgeons, Columbia University. His skill and talent are acknowledged with deep appreciation. Special acknowledgment must go to Mrs. Ruth Gutmann for her excellent secretarial and editorial assistance in preparing the manuscript.

The author is especially grateful to the Publishers for their continued confidence, encouragement and numerous courtesies which have made the preparation of this book a satisfying experience.

MALCOLM B. CARPENTER

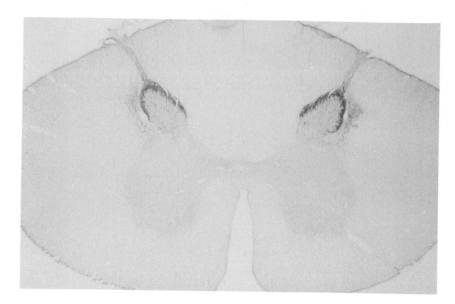

Figure 3.21 Photomicrograph of a monkey spinal cord section immunoreacted with antiserum to substance P (SP). Substance P immunoreactive fibers and terminals are present in the root entry zone and in Rexed's laminae I and II (outer part). Large numbers of smaller dorsal root ganglion cells, the source of these fibers, exhibit colocalization of SP and glutamate. See Figure 3.21 and page 75. (Courtesy of Professor Stephen Hunt, University of Cambridge.)

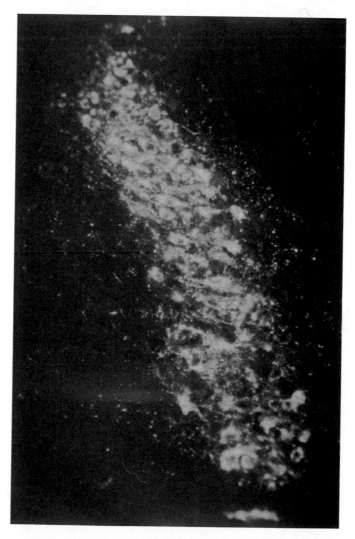

Figure 6.29 Fluoresence photomicrograph of norepinephrine-containing neurons in the locus ceruleus. Section was reacted with glyoxylic acid which gives norepinephrine in neurons a green fluoresence. Cells in the locus ceruleus distribute noradrenergic fibers widely within the brain, brain stem, cerebellum and the spinal cord. See Figures 4.15, 6.28 and 6.29. (Courtesy of Drs. Jacqueline McGinty and Floyd Bloom, Salk Institute, La Jolla, Calif.)

Contents

5/ The Medulla — 115

6/ The Pons — 151

7/ The Mesencephalon — 192

8/ The Cerebellum _____ 224

9/ The Diencephalon _____ 250

10/ The Hypothalamus _____ 297

11/ Corpus Striatum and Related Nuclei _____ 325

12/ Olfactory Pathways, Hippocampal Formation, and the Amygdala —— 361

13/ The Cerebral Cortex —————————————————— 390

14/ Blood Supply of the Central Nervous System ———————— 434

Meninges and Cerebrospinal Fluid

The brain and spinal cord are delicate semisolid structures requiring protection and support. The brain is invested by three membranes, floated in a clear fluid, and encased in a bony vault. Three membranes surround the brain. The most external membrane is a dense connective tissue envelope known as the *dura mater* or *pachymeninx*. The innermost connective tissue membrane is the *pia mater*, a thin, translucent membrane, adherent to the surface of the brain and spinal cord, which accurately follows every contour. Between these membranes is a delicate layer of reticular fibers forming a weblike membrane, the *arachnoid*. The pia mater and arachnoid have a similar structure and collectively are called the *leptomeninges*.

DURA MATER

The cranial dura consists of (1) an outer *periosteal layer* adherent to the inner surface of the cranium, which is rich in blood vessels and nerves, and (2) an inner *meningeal layer* lined with flat cells. At certain sites these layers separate and form large dural venous sinuses (Figs. 1.1, 1.2, and 1.3). The meningeal layer gives rise to several septa that divide the cranial cavity into compartments. The largest of these is the sickle-shaped *falx cerebri*, which extends in the midline from the crista galli to the internal occipital protuberance (Fig. 1.2). Posteriorly this septum is continuous with other transverse dural septa arising from the superior crest of the petrous portion of the temporal bone. These septa form the *tentorium cerebelli*, which roofs over the posterior fossa. The free borders of the tentorium form the *tentorial incisure* (Figs. 1.2 and 1.3). Thus these dural reflections divide the cranial cavity into paired lateral compartments for the cerebral hemispheres, and a single posterior compartment for the cerebellum and lower brain stem. The tentorial incisure (notch) forms the only opening between these compartments. The brain stem passes through the tentorial notch (Fig. 1.4). The occipital lobes lie on the superior surface of the tentorium. A small midsagittal septum below the tentorium forms the *falx cerebelli* (Fig. 1.2), which partially separates the cerebellar hemispheres. The *diaphragma sellae*, an extension of the dura mater that roofs over the pituitary fossa, is perforated by the infundibulum. The dural sinuses are discussed with the cerebral veins in Chapter 14.

The major blood supply for the dura is provided by the middle meningeal artery, a branch of the maxillary artery, which enters the skull via the foramen spinosum (Fig. 1.3). The ophthalmic artery gives rise to anterior meningeal branches, and the occipital and vertebral arteries provide posterior meningeal branches. Skull fractures lacerating branches of the meningeal artery produce epidural hemorrhages that separate the

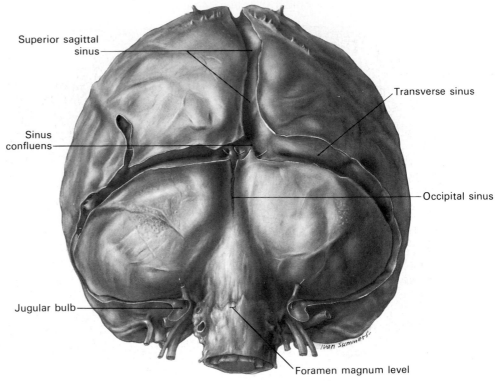

Superior sagittal sinus

Transverse sinus

Sinus confluens

Occipital sinus

Jugular bulb

Foramen magnum level

Figure 1.1. Posterior view of the dura surrounding the brain. Prominent dural sinuses have been opened. The periosteal layer of the dura has been cut at the margins of the foramen magnum. (From Mettler's *Neuroanatomy*, 1948; courtesy of The C. V. Mosby Company.)

periosteal layer of the dura from the inner table of the skull. Arterial blood in the created *epidural space* forms an expanding hematoma requiring prompt surgical intervention.

The supratentorial dura is innervated by branches of the trigeminal nerve, while the infratentorial dura is supplied by branches of the upper cervical spinal nerves and the vagus nerve.

The *spinal dura* is a tubular continuation of the meningeal layer of the cranial dura (Figs. 1.4, 1.5, and 1.6). The periosteum of successive vertebrae corresponds to the outer layer of the cranial dura. Inner and outer surfaces of the spinal dural tube are covered by a single layer of flat cells, and the dense membrane is separated from the vertebral periosteum by the *epidural space*. The spinal epidural space, containing variable amounts of loose areolar tissue (epidural fat) and the internal vertebral venous plexus, is largest at the level of the second lumbar vertebra. Injection of local anesthetic agents into the epidural space produces an extensive paravertebral nerve block, known as *epidural anesthesia. Caudal anesthesia*, used in obstetrics, is a form of epidural anesthesia in which the anesthetic agent is injected into the epidural space via the sacral canal.

The spinal dura extends as a closed tube from the margins of the foramen magnum to the level of the second sacral vertebra (Fig. 1.7). The caudal termination of the dural sac invests the filum terminale to form a thin fibrous cord, the *coccygeal ligament* (Fig. 1.7). This ligament extends caudally to the coccyx where it becomes continuous with the periosteum. The spinal cord ends at the lower border of the first lumbar vertebra. Extensions of the dura passing laterally around the spinal nerve rootlets form paired dural root sleeves (Figs. 1.5 and 1.6).

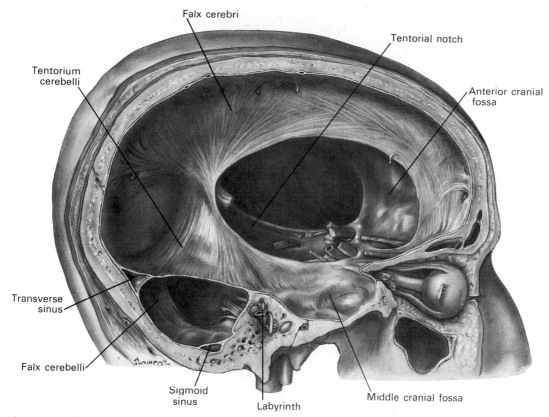

Figure 1.2.   Sagittal section of the head showing the falx cerebri, the tentorium cerebelli, and the falx cerebelli. (From Mettler's *Neuroanatomy*, 1948; courtesy of The C. V. Mosby Company.)

PIA MATER

This membrane is composed of (1) an inner membraneous layer, the *intima pia*, and (2) a more superficial *epipial layer*. The intima pia, adherent to underlying surface of nervous tissue, follows its contours closely and is composed of the fine reticular and elastic fibers. Where blood vessels enter and leave the central nervous system, the intima pia is invaginated, forming a perivascular space (Fig. 1.12). The intima pia is avascular, deriving its nutrients from the cerebrospinal fluid and underlying neural tissue. The epipial layer is formed by a meshwork of collagenous fiber bundles continuous with the arachnoid trabeculae. The blood vessels of the spinal cord lie within the epipial layer, whereas cerebral vessels lie on the surface of the intima pia anchored by arachnoid trabeculae (Fig. 1.8). Over the convex surface of the cerebral cortex the epipial layer is absent.

The spinal cord is attached to the dural tube by a series of lateral flattened bands of epipial tissue known as the *denticulate ligaments* (Figs. 1.4 and 1.5). Each triangular-shaped denticulate ligament is attached medially to the lateral surface of the spinal cord midway between the dorsal and ventral roots. The bases of these ligaments arise in the pia mater, and their apices are firmly attached to the arachnoid and the inner surface of the dura. The denticulate ligaments anchor the spinal cord to the dura and are present throughout the length of the spinal cord. In the region of the conus medullaris, epipial tissue forms a covering of the filum terminale (Fig. 1.7).

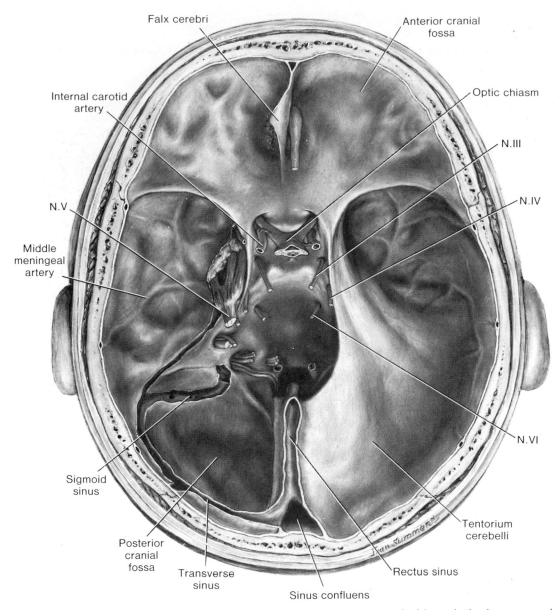

Falx cerebri

Anterior cranial fossa

Internal carotid artery

Optic chiasm

N.III

N.V

N.IV

Middle meningeal artery

N.VI

Sigmoid sinus

Tentorium cerebelli

Posterior cranial fossa

Rectus sinus

Transverse sinus

Sinus confluens

Figure 1.3. View of the base of the skull with dura mater. The falx cerebri has been removed and the tentorium cerebelli has been removed on the left to expose the posterior fossa. (From Mettler's *Neuroanatomy*, 1948; courtesy of The C. V. Mosby Company.)

The more fibrous intima pia is firmly attached to the surface of the spinal cord by the superficial glial membrane. The latter is composed of fine processes of deeply located fibrous astrocytes.

ARACHNOID

The arachnoid is a delicate nonvascular membrane between the dura and the pia mater that passes over the sulci without following their contours (Figs. 1.5 and 1.8). This membrane also extends along the proximal roots of the cranial and spinal nerves. Arachnoid trabeculae extend from the arachnoid to the pia (Figs. 1.12 and 1.13). The space between the arachnoid and the pia mater, filled with cerebrospinal fluid, is called the *subarachnoid space* (Fig. 1.9). The extent of the subarachnoid space surrounding the brain shows local variations. Over the convexity of the cerebral hemisphere this space is narrow, except in the depths of the sulci.

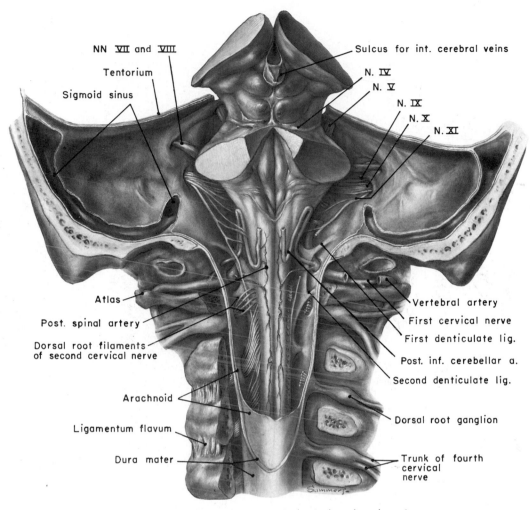

Figure 1.4. Posterior view of the brain stem, upper cervical spinal cord, and meninges. (From Mettler's *Neuroanatomy*, 1948; courtesy of The C. V. Mosby Company.)

At the base of the brain and around the brain stem the pia and the arachnoid often are widely separated, creating *subarachnoid cisterna* (Figs. 1.8 and 1.9). The largest cistern, found between the medulla and the cerebellum, is called the *cerebellomedullary cistern* (cisterna magna) (Figs. 1.8 and 1.9). Cerebrospinal fluid from the fourth ventricle passes into the cerebellomedullary cistern via the median *foramen of Magendie* and the two lateral foramina of Luschka (Figs. 1.9 and 1.10). Other cisterns of considerable size are the *pontine cistern*, the *interpeduncular cistern*, the *chiasmatic cistern*, and the *superior cistern* (Figs. 1.8 and 1.9). The superior cistern, surrounding the posterior, superior, and lateral surfaces of the midbrain, is referred to clinically as the *cisterna ambiens*. This cistern is of importance because it contains the great vein of Galen, and the posterior cerebral and superior cerebellar arteries. Most of these cisterns can be visualized in computerized tomograms and by magnetic resonance imaging technics.

The *lumbar cistern* extends from the conus medullaris (lower border of the first lumbar vertebra) to about the level of the second sacral vertebra (Fig. 1.7). It contains the filum terminale and nerve roots of the cauda equina. It is from this cistern that cerebrospinal fluid (CSF) is withdrawn most commonly for analysis (lumbar spinal tap). Withdrawal

Figure 1.5. Posterior view of part of the upper thoracic spinal cord. The dura and arachnoid have been split at the midline to expose the spinal cord and pial vessels. Above, the intact dura covers the spinal cord and spinal nerve roots. (From Mettler's *Neuroanatomy*, 1948; courtesy of The C. V. Mosby Company.)

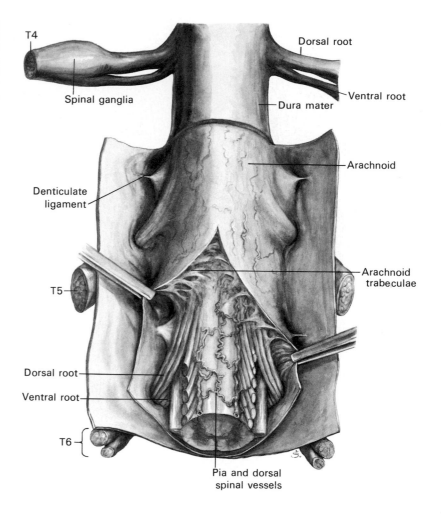

Figure 1.6. Spinal cord and its meningeal coverings in cross section. Note the continuities of the pia mater with the denticulate ligament and of the dura mater with the epineurium of the spinal nerves. (Modified from Corning, 1922; from Carpenter and Sutin, *Human Neuroanatomy*, 1983; courtesy of Williams & Wilkins.)

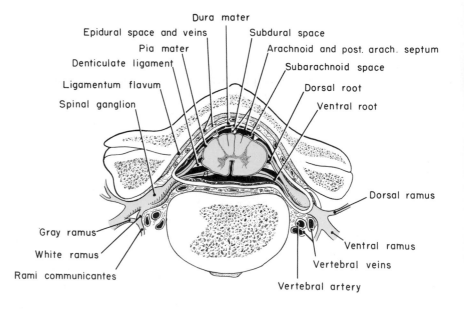

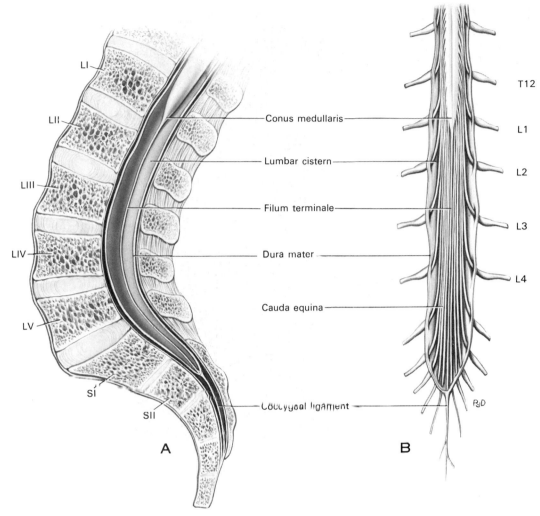

LI

LII

LIII

LIV

LV

SI

SII

A

Conus medullaris

Lumbar cistern

Filum terminale

Dura mater

Cauda equina

Coccygeal ligament

T12

L1

L2

L3

L4

B

RJD

Figure 1.7. Diagrammatic representation of the caudal part of the spinal cord and lumbar cistern. *A* is a sagittal view of the conus medullaris, lumbar cistern, and lumbosacral vertebrae. *B* is a posterior view of the cauda equina and nerve roots.

of CSF and replacement with a local anesthetic agent produces spinal anesthesia.

ARACHNOID GRANULATIONS

In regions adjacent to the superior sagittal sinus the cerebral pia-arachnoid gives rise to tufted prolongations that protrude through the meningeal layer of the dura into the superior sagittal sinus (Fig. 1.13). These granulations are variable in number and location, and each consists of numerous arachnoid villi. These villi have a thin outer limiting membrane beneath which are bundles of collagenous and elastic fibers. Cells similar to those of the pia-arachnoid are scattered among the fibers, and small oval epithelial cells cap the surface of the villi. Arachnoid granulations frequently are surrounded by venous lacunae along the margins of the superior sagittal sinus. At advanced age, the arachnoid granulations become larger, more numerous, and tend to calcify.

Arachnoid villi and granulations are considered to be a major site of transfer of CSF from the subarachnoid space to the venous system. The hydrostatic pressure of CSF is greater than venous blood in the dural sinuses, so fluid moves from the subarachnoid space into the venous

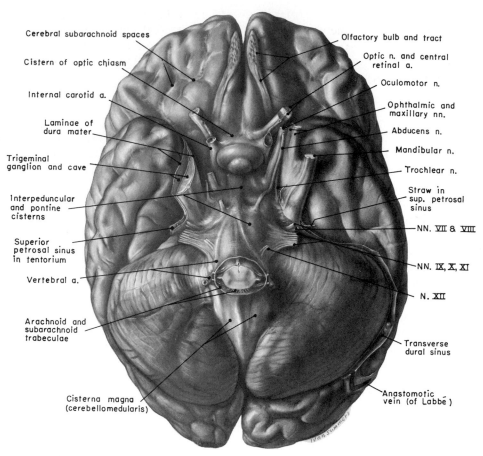

Cerebral subarachnoid spaces

Cistern of optic chiasm

Internal carotid a.

Laminae of dura mater

Trigeminal ganglion and cave

Interpeduncular and pontine cisterns

Superior petrosal sinus in tentorium

Vertebral a.

Arachnoid and subarachnoid trabeculae

Cisterna magna (cerebellomedularis)

Olfactory bulb and tract

Optic n. and central retinal a.

Oculomotor n.

Ophthalmic and maxillary nn.

Abducens n.

Mandibular n.

Trochlear n.

Straw in sup. petrosal sinus

NN. VII & VIII

NN. IX, X, XI

N. XII

Transverse dural sinus

Anastomotic vein (of Labbé)

Figure 1.8. Inferior view of brain, cranial nerves, and meninges showing locations of subarachnoid cisterns. (From Mettler's *Neuroanatomy*, 1948; courtesy of The C. V. Mosby Company.)

system. The arachnoid granulations function as pressure-dependent, one-way valves whose membranes are readily permeable. The spongy tissue of these valves contains a series of interconnecting tubules that open only when the CSF pressure exceeds venous pressure in the dural sinuses. When venous pressure exceeds that of the CSF, the tubules collapse. In the absence of pressure differences between the CSF and venous blood, the membranes of these cells are folded and have numerous microvilli. Bulk volume flow of CSF occurs through the arachnoid tubular system and between the stretched endothelial cells. Flow of CSF into the venous sinuses is proportional to the increase in CSF pressure but does not begin until it exceeds venous pressure by 3 to 6 cm of water. Even large molecular-weight substances such as plasma proteins and serum albumin can pass from the CSF to venous blood via the arachnoid granulations.

PIA-GLIA AND PERIVASCULAR SPACES

The intima pia or pia-glia is regarded as the external limiting membrane of the central nervous system (CNS). Both the intima pia and the arachnoid are of ectodermal origin. Thus the parenchyma of the CNS, neuroglia, the ependyma lining the ventricular system, and the leptomeninges arise from ectoderm. The blood vascular system and the dura mater are of mesodermal origin. As blood vessels enter and leave nervous tissue, they carry with them a sheath of arachnoid and pia-glia, which form a cuff around each vessel called the Virchow-Robins space (Fig. 1.12). It has been suggested that these spaces might permit flow of CSF into the depths of the tissue. Electron microscopic studies indicate that these two layers ultimately become continuous and there is no real space between them. At levels of the smallest veins and capillaries no adventitial elements are found, although processes of astrocytes surround the basement membranes of the capillary endothelium.

CEREBROSPINAL FLUID

The CSF is a clear, colorless liquid containing small amounts of protein, glucose, and potassium and relatively large amounts of sodium chloride. There are no substances normally found in CSF that are not also found in blood plasma. There is no cellular component in CSF, although 1 to 5 cells per cubic millimeter may be considered to be within normal limits in any CSF sample. The CSF serves to support and cushion the CNS against trauma. The buoyancy of CSF is indicated by the fact that a brain weighing 1500 g in air weighs only 50 g when immersed in CSF. This buoyancy serves to reduce the momentum and acceleration of the brain when the cranium is suddenly displaced, thereby reducing concussive damage. The CSF removes waste products of metabolism, drugs, and other substances that diffuse into the brain from the blood. As the CSF flows over the ventricular and pial surfaces of the brain it carries away solutes that pass into venous blood via the arachnoid villi. Certain drugs (penicillin) and neurotransmitters (serotonin and norepinephrine) are rapidly removed from the CSF by the choroid plexus. In addition CSF plays an important role in integrating brain and peripheral endocrine functions in that hormones, or hormone releasing factors, from the hypothalamus are secreted into the extracellular space or directly into the CSF. These hormones, which include hormone-releasing hormones, are carried via the CSF to the median eminence in the floor of the third ventricle; from this site they are transported by ependymal cells (i.e., tanycytes) into the hypophysial portal system (Figs. 10.15 and 10.16). The CSF also influences the microenvironment of neurons and glial cells because there is no diffusion barrier between the CSF and the brain at either the ependymal lining of the ventricles or the pia-glial membrane. Changes in the ionic concentrations of calcium, potassium, and magnesium in the CSF may affect blood pressure, heart rate, vasomotor reflexes, respiration, muscle tone, and the emotional state.

The CSF has been regarded as an ultra-filtrate of the blood plasma because of their resemblance, except for differences in protein concentration (plasma, 6500 mg/100 g; CSF, 25 mg/100 g). The characteristic distribution of ions and nonelectrolytes in CSF and plasma, however, is such that the CSF cannot be described as a simple filtrate, or dialysate, of the blood plasma. In general the CSF has higher Na^+, Cl^-, and Mg^{2+} concentrations and lower K^+, Ca^{2+}, and glucose concentrations than would be expected in a plasma dialysate. In addition, the osmotic pressure relationships are not sufficient to produce a virtually protein-free fluid from the blood plasma. For these reasons evidence supports the theory that the CSF is a secretory product involving active transport mechanisms controlled by enzymatic processes. Approximately 70% of the CSF is secreted by the choroid plexus located in the lateral ventricles and in the roof of the third and fourth ventricles (Figs. 1.9, 1.10, 1.11, and 2.8). The remaining 30% of the CSF is derived from metabolic water production. Estimates of metabolic water production, based on the complete oxidation of glucose, suggest a net contribution of about 12% to the CSF. Extrachoroidal sources produce the remaining 18% of the CSF, largely as a capillary ultrafiltrate. The CSF is formed under a hydrostatic pressure

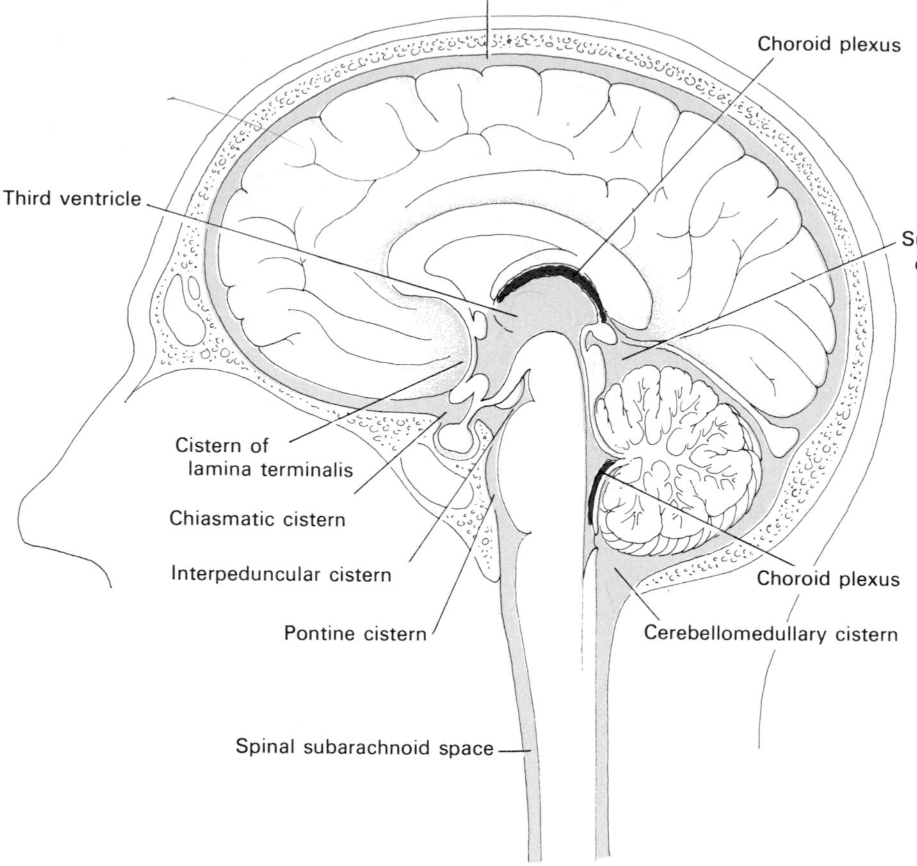

Figure 1.9.   Diagram of the subarachnoid cisterns as seen in a midsagittal view. The superior cistern is referred to clinically as the cisterna ambiens. The choroid plexus in the roof of the third ventricle and in the fourth ventricle is shown in *red*. (From Carpenter and Sutin, *Human Neuroanatomy*, 1983; courtesy of Williams & Wilkins.)

head of 15 mm of H_2O, which is sufficient to drive it through the ventricular system and into the subarachnoid space. Pulsations of the choroid plexus also contribute to the movement of CSF within the ventricular system. The total volume of the CSF in man has been estimated to be about 140 ml of which about 25 ml are contained within the ventricles. CSF is constantly being formed and removed. Net production of CSF in man has been estimated to be about 0.35 ml per minute, which indicates the formation of 400–500 ml per day.

The choroid plexus is a villous structure extending from the ventricular surface into the CSF. This plexus consists of a single layer of cuboidal epithelium with basal infoldings resting on a basement membrane enclosing an extensive capillary network embedded in a connective tissue stroma (Figs. 1.14 and 1.15). Apical microvilli of the epithelial cells are in contact with the CSF. Capillaries in the connective tissue stroma have endothelial fenestrations, but tight junctions surrounding apical regions of the epithelial cells (Figs. 1.14 and 1.15) form a barrier to the passive exchange of proteins and hydrophilic solutes between the blood and the CSF. Blood-borne horseradish peroxidase (HRP) passes through capillary fenestrations and diffuses into the connective tissue stroma but does not go beyond the tight junctions of epithelial cells. The choroid plexus regulates the production and composition of the CSF. A Na^+-K^+-exchange pump, catalyzed by Na^+-K^+-ATPase, drives Na^+ toward the

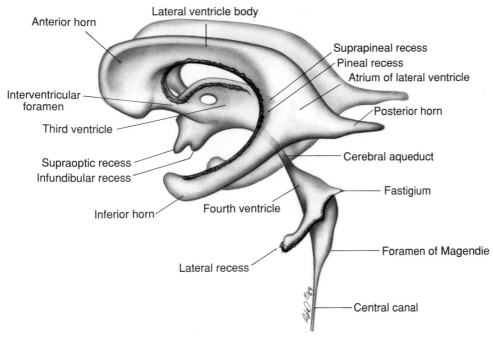

Figure 1.10. Oblique view of the midline and lateral ventricles. Choroid plexus (*red*), present in the roof of the third ventricle, passes through the interventricular foramen into the body of the lateral ventricle. The plexus follows the curvature of the lateral ventricle into the roof of the inferior horn. Choroid plexus in the roof of the posterior part of the fourth ventricle extends into the lateral recess and protrudes into the subarachnoid space (Fig. 2.7). CSF produced in the lateral ventricles by the choroid plexus flows into the third ventricle and via the cerebral aqueduct into the fourth ventricle. CSF emerges from the fourth ventricle via the paired lateral recesses (foramina of Luschka) and the midline foramen of Magendie (not illustrated).

ventricular surface of the plexus and K^+ in the opposite direction. Thus K^+ is transported out of the CSF, while Na^+ is actively transported into it. The choroid plexus also plays a role in the regulation of Mg^{2+} and Ca^{2+} in the CSF. CSF secreted by the choroid plexus contains a higher concentration of Mg^{2+} and a lower concentration of Ca^{2+} than an ultrafiltrate of the plasma. The manner in which water, the largest constituent of the CSF, moves across the choroidal epithelium is controversial. According to one theory, modifications of choroidal blood flow can increase or decrease the rate of CSF secretion. Approximately 25% of the volume of blood flowing to the choroid plexus normally is secreted as CSF. Other data suggest that water moves across the choroidal epithelium under a standing osmotic gradient established by the active transport of Na^+. This hypothesis indicates that movement of water into the CSF is coupled to the active transport of Na^+ by the choroid plexus. The formation of CSF and the movement of $24 Na^+$ are stopped when a carbonic anhydrase inhibitor is applied to the choroid plexus.

CSF formed in the lateral and third ventricles passes via the cerebral aqueduct into the fourth ventricle. The fluid enters the cerebellomedullary cistern via the median and lateral apertures of the fourth ventricle (Figs. 1.8, 1.9, 1.10, and 2.18). From this site the fluid circulates in the subarachnoid spaces surrounding both the brain and the spinal cord. The bulk of the CSF is passively returned to the venous system via the arachnoid villi (Fig. 1.13). The hydrodynamic permeability of the arachnoid villi is large compared with that of peripheral capillaries. Large protein molecules leave the CSF by passage through the arachnoid villi at roughly the same rate as smaller molecules. The exit of CSF via the arachnoid

Figure 1.11. Magnetic resonance imaging of the head in two different horizontal planes, which reveal parts of the ventricular system and other details of the brain. In *A*, a superior plane, the body and atrium of the lateral ventricle are seen. In *B*, at a lower plane, the anterior and posterior horns of the lateral ventricles and the third ventricle are imaged with other deep structures. In both *A* and *B*, CSF in the ventricles appears white. (Courtesy of John Sherman, M.D., Washington, D.C.)

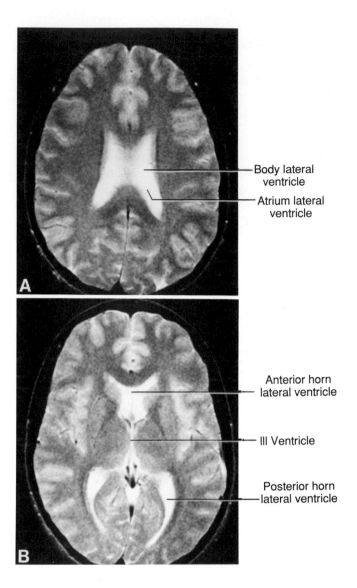

Body lateral ventricle

Atrium lateral ventricle

Anterior horn lateral ventricle

III Ventricle

Posterior horn lateral ventricle

villi is pressure dependent and begins when the CSF pressure exceeds venous pressure by 3 to 6 mm of water. The arachnoid villi serve as one-way valves. If the CSF pressure is greater than venous pressure, the tubelike valves open and CSF enters the dural venous sinuses. When venous pressure exceeds CSF pressure, the valves close and blood cannot enter the CSF. Small amounts of CSF may be taken up by the ependyma, arachnoid capillaries, and lymphatics of the meninges and perivascular tissues.

In the recumbent position, the CSF pressure measured at the lumbar cistern normally is about 100 to 150 mm of H_2O; in the sitting position, the pressure measured at the same site varies between 200 and 300 mm of H_2O. Because the brain is nearly incompressible within the cranium, the combined volumes of brain, CSF, and blood must be maintained at a constant level. A volume increase in any one of these components can only be at the expense of one or both of the others. Thus a space-occupying lesion, such as a tumor or hematoma, usually results in an increase in CSF pressure.

Excessive CSF produces an elevated pressure and in infants can cause hydrocephalus with enlargement of the ventricles, damage to neural tissue, and changes in the neural cranium. Such increases in CSF may result from an overproduction of fluid, an obstruction to its flow, or inadequate absorption. In most instances hydrocephalus results from obstruction within the ventricular system. Hydrocephalus that develops in the absence of a demonstrated blockage in the ventricular system is referred to as a communicating hydrocephalus. Removal of the choroid plexus from one lateral ventricle usually causes that ventricle to collapse, while obstruction of one interventricular foramen causes dilatation of the ipsilateral lateral ventricle.

An extensive plexus of serotonin axons exists in supra- and subependymal systems in the walls of the ventricles and in the arachnoid sheath around major cerebral blood vessels. The raphe nuclei in the pons are considered to be the source of axons forming these plexuses. It has been suggested that serotonergic axons in ventricular and pial surfaces

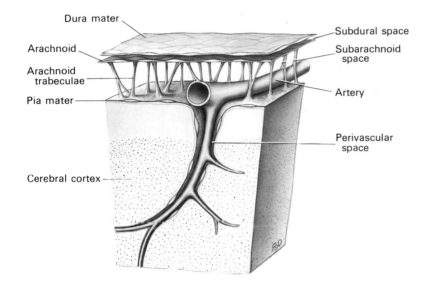

Figure 1.12. Diagram of the meninges showing relationships of the membranes to the subarachnoid and perivascular spaces. (From Carpenter and Sutin, *Human Neuroanatomy*, 1983; courtesy of Williams & Wilkins.)

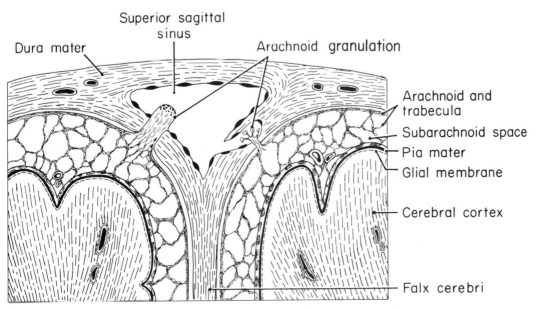

Figure 1.13. Diagram of meningeal-cortical relationships. Arachnoid granulations may penetrate dural sinus or terminate in a lateral lacuna of a sinus. The pia is firmly anchored to cortex by the glial membrane. (From Carpenter and Sutin, *Human Neuroanatomy*, 1983; courtesy of Williams & Wilkins.)

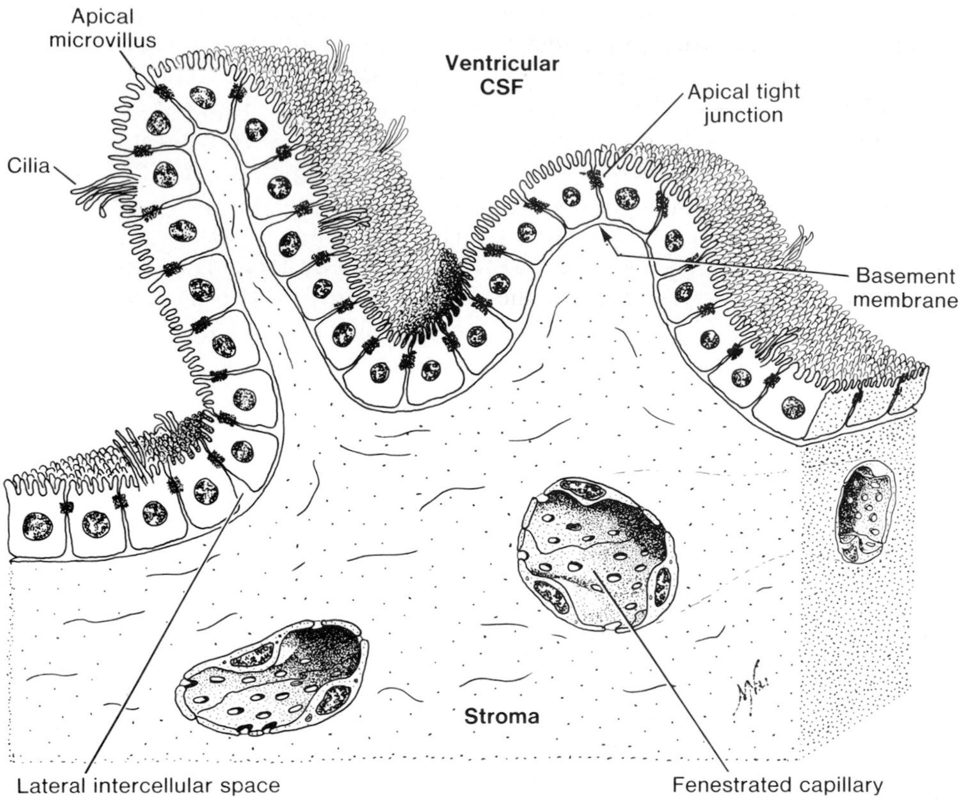

Figure 1.14. Diagram of a choroid plexus villus covered by a single layer of cuboidal epithelium with apical microvilli protruding into the ventricular CSF. Epithelial cells rest on a basement membrane and have tight junctions connecting apical regions that constitute the blood-CSF barrier. The underlying connective tissue stroma contains capillaries with fenestrations. (From Carpenter and Sutin, *Human Neuroanatomy*, 1983; courtesy of Williams & Wilkins.)

may be important modifiers of local CSF composition and that subarachnoid plexuses around major cerebral blood vessels may influence local vasomotor activity and thus affect cerebral blood flow. Volatile anesthetic agents and CO_2 increase CSF formation, whereas carbonic anhydrase inhibitors and norepinephrine reduce the rate of CSF formation. The choroid plexus has both adrenergic and cholinergic innervation.

BRAIN BARRIERS

The functioning of all neurons of the CNS is dependent on the maintenance of a physical and chemical milieu within certain narrow limits. The system that regulates the exchange of water and solutes between the plasma, the CSF, and the brain involves membranes with selective permeability and carrier-mediated transport. This multicompartmental "barrier" arrangement regulates the transport of chemical substances between the arterial blood, the CSF, and the brain. The "barrier" system maintains the physiochemical composition of the microenvironment of neurons, axons, and glia within the narrow limits required for neuronal survival. The blood-brain barrier separates the two major compartments of the CNS, the brain and the CSF, from the third compartment, the blood vascular system. The sites of the barrier are the interfaces between the blood vascular system and these two compartments of the CNS. Two separate barriers, a "blood-CSF barrier" and a "blood-brain barrier," have been recognized in order to explain why intravascular substances enter the CSF and the brain differently. Many substances do not cross brain capillaries (e.g., acidic dyes) or cross only at very slow rates (e.g., ions). The concept of restrictive passage of dissolved substances from the blood into the brain was based on the demonstration that intravenous trypan blue stained virtually all tissues of the body except the brain. Transport of certain ions (e.g., K^+, Na^+) from capillaries to brain is much slower than in other tissues. The rates of movement of amino acids into brain are variable, and some are virtually excluded (e.g., proline, glutamic acid, glycine, and gamma-aminobutyric acid). The concentrations of many substances in the CSF are independent of their

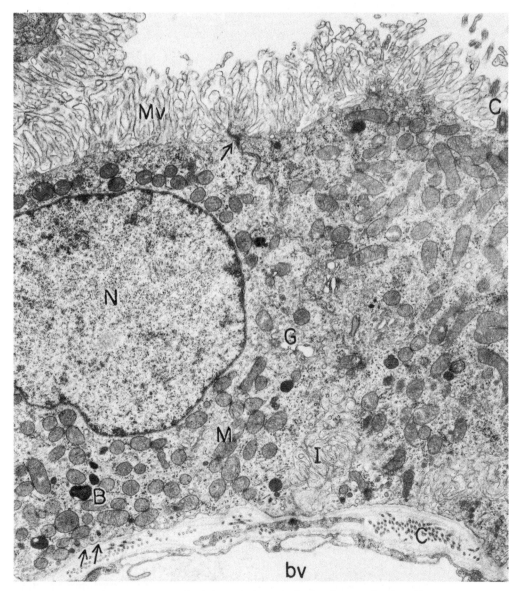

Figure 1.15.   An electron micrograph of choroid plexus in the fourth ventricle of a rabbit. Cuboidal epithelial cells have a large nucleus (N) and polypoidal microvilli (MV) and occasional cilia (C) on the ventricular surface. A tight junction (arrow) seals the adjacent cell near the apex, while elaborate infoldings (I) occur near the base. A paranuclear Golgi complex (G), numerous mitochondria (M), heterogeneous dense bodies (B), and vesicles are present in the cytoplasm. A basement membrane (double arrow) separates the choroidal epithelial cells from the connective tissue (C), which contains interstitial cells and blood vessels (bv). × 8000. (Courtesy of Virginia Tennyson, Columbia University.)

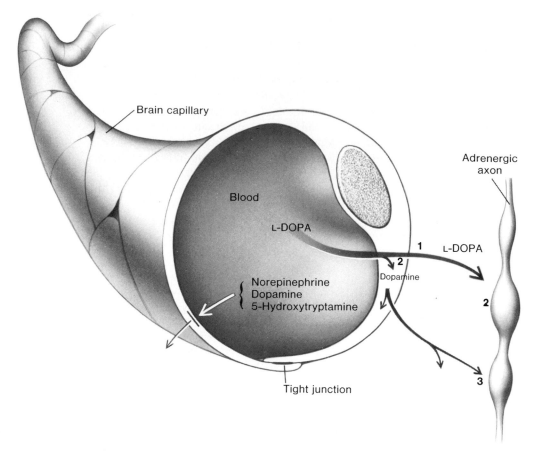

Figure 1.16. Diagrammatic drawing of a brain capillary demonstrating a tight junction between endothelial cells that constitute the blood-brain barrier. Endothelial cells of brain capillaries contain enzymes that regulate the specific transport of biogenic amines (norepinephrine, dopamine, and 5-hydroxytryptamine) and amino acids. L-DOPA passes the blood-brain barrier (1), is decarboxylated to dopamine in the capillary endothelium (2), and enters neural tissue (3), where it is degraded by monoamine oxidase. Decarboxylation of L-DOPA to dopamine (2) also takes place after its incorporation into axonal varicosities of aminergic neurons. (From Carpenter and Sutin, *Human Neuroanatomy*, 1983; courtesy of Williams & Wilkins.)

concentrations in the plasma, indicating that there also is a blood-CSF barrier with distinctive features and varying rates of transfer.

These two barriers differ greatly in surface area; the surface area of the blood-brain barrier is estimated to be 5000 times greater than that of the blood-CSF barrier. The brain barriers are considered to develop at an early stage when the blood vessels invade the brain.

The ependyma surfaces of the cerebral ventricles and the pia-glial membrane on the brain surface do not impede the exchange of substances between the CSF and the brain. Thus the brain-CSF interface does not constitute a barrier. Ependymal cells lining the ventricles are not connected by tight junctions and do not hinder macromolecular exchange between the CSF and the brain. Drugs injected into the cerebral ventricles easily cross the ependymal lining and produce prompt pharmacological and behavioral effects. A schematic diagram of relationships between the blood-brain barrier, the blood-CSF barrier, and the brain-CSF interface is shown in Figure 1.17.

Blood-Brain Barrier

The pia and the subjacent glial membrane blend with the vessel wall before it penetrates the substance of the brain or spinal cord (Fig. 1.12). Smaller arterial branches have only thin neuroglial investments that persist to the capillary level. The capillary endothelium, a continuous homogeneous basement membrane, and numerous astrocytic processes are all that separate the plasma from the extracellular space (i.e., interstitial) within the CNS. Ultrastructural studies indicate that the *blood-brain barrier* is formed by the capillary endothelium, which has tight junctions between contiguous cells (Fig. 1.16).

The wall of a brain capillary consists only of flattened endothelial cells resting on a basement membrane surrounded by a thin adventitial layer. Capillaries within the CNS contain a continuous inner layer of endothelial cells connected by tight junctions, derived totally or partially from neuroectoderm. The tight junctions between endothelial cells of brain capillaries restrict intercellular diffusion of solutes and in essence form a continuous cell layer with the permeability properties of a plasma membrane (Fig. 1.16). The basement membrane surrounding the endothelial cells has approximately 85% of its surface covered by glial cells. The tight junctions between endothelial cells prevent the transfer of microperoxidase, HRP, and ferritin from the capillary lumen to the basement membrane surrounding the capillary. One gram of brain has about 240 cm^2 of capillary surface. Cerebral blood vessels have neither a well-developed small pore system nor a vesicular transport system, and pinocytotic vesicles are rare in endothelial cells of cerebral capillaries.

Movement of molecules across the blood-brain barrier involves diffusion, carrier-mediated transport, and active transport requiring energy. Water is the most important substance entering the brain by diffusion; its rate of exchange is rapid but limited by the permeability of the capillary endothelium and the rate of cerebral blood flow. Many drugs (e.g., barbiturates, heroin, and alcohol) diffuse across the blood-brain barrier in proportion to their lipid solubility. Intrinsically lipid-soluble molecules bound to protein do not permeate the barrier. D-Glucose rapidly passes the barrier by carrier-mediated transport, but L-glucose, a stereoisomer, is excluded. 2-Deoxyglucose, an analogue of D-glucose, readily passes the barrier and competitively inhibits the transport of glucose. [^{14}C] 2-Deoxyglucose in tracer amounts is used in conjunction with autoradiography to identify pathways and neural systems by their metabolic activity. In the CNS capillary endothelial cells are metabolically active with respect to both oxidative and hydrolytic enzymes. Enzymes within these cells regulate and transport amines and amino acids (Fig. 1.16). An example of this regulation is seen in Parkinson's disease (paralysis agitans) in which there is a deficiency of dopamine in neurons of the substantia nigra, which synthesize and convey this neurotransmitter to a part of the basal ganglia known as the striatum. Although dopamine cannot cross the blood-brain barrier, L-DOPA, an amino acid precursor of dopamine and norepinephrine, readily enters brain capillaries where it is decarboxylated to dopamine. DOPA decarboxylase also decarboxylates 5-hydroxytryptophan, the precursor of serotonin (5-HT). Thus large doses of L-DOPA given to patients with Parkinson's disease can result in a therapeutically effective brain level of the biogenic amine dopamine, which ameliorates many of the disturbances of this syndrome (Fig. 1.16).

Large neutral amino acids, required for the synthesis of neurotransmitters and protein, are transported into brain by well-defined carrier

Figure 1.17. Schematic diagram of the blood-brain barrier, the blood-CSF barrier, and the brain-CSF interface that separate the brain and CSF from the cerebral vascular compartment. The blood-brain barrier is a series of interfaces between arterial blood, CSF, and neural tissue that regulates the transport of chemical substances. Tight junctions between endothelial cells (see Fig. 1.16) of cerebral capillaries (the blood-brain barrier) and a paucity of pinocytosis restrict the passage of solutes from the blood into the extracellular compartment (i.e., interstitial fluid). The blood-CSF barrier is formed by tight junctions surrounding apical regions of the cuboidal epithelium of the choroid plexus (see Fig. 1.14). The brain-CSF interface, consisting of the ependymal lining of the cerebral ventricles and the pia-glial membrane on the external surface of the brain, does not impede the exchange of solutes between the CSF and the brain. The extracellular compartment has been estimated to constitute about 18% of wet brain weight. (From Carpenter and Sutin, *Human Neuroanatomy*, 1983; courtesy of Williams & Wilkins.)

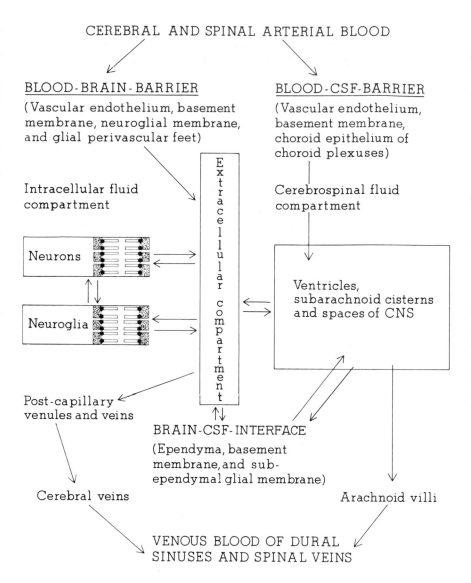

systems, although rates of movement are variable and several compete for entry into endothelial cells by the same transport mechanism. Small neutral amino acids are not transported from blood to brain, but many of these small molecules can be synthesized by neurons. Active transport mechanisms are not required to move molecules into brain, but they operate to move weak organic acids, halides, and extracellular K^+ from brain and CSF into plasma against a concentration gradient.

Capillaries in skeletal muscle, in contrast to brain capillaries, contain endothelial cells separated by 10-nm clefts, have abundant pinocytotic vesicles for transport of macromolecules, and contain contractile proteins. Although occasional tight junctions between endothelial cells are seen in muscle capillaries, they are not uniformly present as in brain capillaries. The blood-brain barrier in the CNS is not everywhere complete. In certain regions of the brain, capillary endothelia with tight junctions are replaced by capillaries with fenestrated endothelia. Regions of the brain devoid of a blood-brain barrier include the pineal body, the subfornical organ, the organum vasculosum of the lamina terminalis (or supraoptic crest), the median eminence of the hypothalamus, the neurohypophysis, and the area postrema (Fig. 1.18). These structures are known as the *circumventricular organs*, and all except the area postrema bear relationships to the diencephalon and the third ventricle. In the regions of the circumventricular organs, capillary fenestrations provide specific sites for the transfer of proteins and solutes, irrespective of molecular size and lipid solubility.

Blood-Cerebrospinal Fluid Barrier

The epithelium and adnexa of the choroid plexus in the lateral, third, and fourth ventricles actively secrete CSF, which has higher concentrations of Na^+, Cl^-, and Mg^{2+} and lower concentrations of K^+, Ca^{2+}, glucose, and protein than the plasma. The barrier to passive exchange of protein and solutes between blood and CSF is not at the choroidal capillaries that have fenestrated endothelial cells. The blood-CSF barrier is located at tight junctions, which surround and connect apical regions of cuboidal epithelial cells near the surface of the choroid plexus (Figs. 1.14 and 1.15). Protein tracers and HRP injected intravascularly stain the stroma of the choroid plexus by passing through pores in the choroidal capillaries, but they do not pass beyond the tight junctions of the epithelial cells and they do not enter the CSF.

The movement of substances from the blood into the CSF is similar to that from blood into brain, in spite of structural differences between the choroid plexus and brain capillaries. Water, gases, and lipid-soluble substances move freely from blood to CSF. Glucose, amino acids, and cations (K^+, Ca^{2+}, and Mg^{2+}) are transported by carrier-mediated processes. It seems likely that a Cl^- pump may be responsible for the higher level of this anion in the CSF. Proteins and most hexoses, other than glucose, do not enter the CSF from the blood.

A probenecid-sensitive organic acid transport system in both the choroid plexus and brain capillaries controls the movement of penicillin into the brain. Penicillin concentrations in the CSF are much lower than in the plasma, which is fortunate, because penicillin even in low concentrations may produce seizures. Alterations in the blood-brain barrier in bacterial meningitis tend to increase penicillin concentrations at inflammatory sites.

The surface area of the blood-CSF barrier is only about 0.02% of the surface area of the blood-brain barrier. In spite of great quantitative differences in surface area, some circulating substances probably enter the brain via the blood-CSF barrier. Circulating peptides (insulin) and plasma proteins may be selectively transported into the CSF via the blood-CSF barrier. The ependymal lining of the ventricles and the pia-glial membrane on the surface of the brain do not impede exchanges between the CSF and the brain.

BRAIN EXTRACELLULAR SPACE

Neurons and neuroglial comprise the *intracellular fluid compartment* of the brain (Fig. 1.17). Passage of solutes into, and out of, neurons and glial takes place from the *extracellular space* (i.e., interstitial space) through the cell membranes. Estimates of the total extracellular space vary widely as determined by different methods. Ultrastructural studies suggest that neurons, neuroglia, and their processes take up most of the available space, except for a fairly constant 20-nm cleft between adjacent cellular elements (estimate 4%). Neurochemical data, based on the assumption that the chloride ion is distributed mainly in extracellular space, suggest the extracellular space ranges from 25 to 40%. Other data indicate that the extracellular space equals approximately 18% of wet brain weight.

The water content of the rhesus monkey brain progressively diminishes during fetal development and postpartum maturation. The developing and immature brain have an expanded extracellular space, although tight junctions surrounding epithelial cells of the choroid plexus at early developmental stages do not differ qualitatively from the adult. The increased extracellular space appears to account for the observation that trypan blue given intravenously stains the brains of very immature animals. Although the dye enters the brain only at nonbarrier sites, it extends further into the extracellular space than it does in the mature brain.

CIRCUMVENTRICULAR ORGANS

Specialized tissues located at strategic positions in the midline ventricular system that lack a blood-brain barrier collectively are referred to as the circumventricular organs (Fig. 1.18). Included under this designation are (1) the pineal body, (2) the subcommissural organ, (3) the subfornical organ, (4) the organum vasculosum of the lamina terminalis (supraoptic crest), (5) the median eminence, (6) the neurohypophysis, and (7) the area postrema. With the exception of the area postrema, located bilaterally along the caudal margins of the fourth ventricle (Figs. 1.18 and 5.7), all of these structures are unpaired and occupy midline positions related to portions of the diencephalon. All of these structures, except the subcommissural organ, contain fenestrated capillaries and are excluded from the blood-brain barrier. The *neurohypophysis* receives fibers from magnocellular hypothalamic nuclei (i.e., paraventricular and supraoptic nuclei) that terminate around fenestrated capillaries. These terminal fibers contain vasopressin and oxytocin, which are stored and released into the general circulation from the neural lobe of the hypophysis. The *organum vasculosum of the lamina terminalis* (OVLT) may also serve as a neurohemal outlet for hypothalamic peptides. In addition, it may serve a neurohemal function in which certain peptides, amines, and proteins in the blood are sensed by neurons with receptor properties. The *median eminence* serves as a neuroendocrine transducer. The final common pathway for neuroendocrine control of the anterior pituitary by the hypothalamus is provided by neurosecretory neurons whose axons discharge hormone-releasing factors into the hypophysial portal system (Fig. 10.15). The *subfornical organ*, located between the interventricular foramina, has connections with the choroid plexus and may serve to regulate body fluids. The *pineal body*, containing pinealocytes, produces melatonin in animals deprived of photic stimuli and has been considered as a biological clock, which regulates circadian rhythms. The *subcommissural organ* is located beneath the posterior commissure at the junction of the third ventricle and cerebral aqueduct. The function of this structure is unknown. The *area postrema*, the only pair circumventricular organ, is located along the caudal margins of the fourth ventricle (Fig. 5.7) and has a structure similar to that of the subfornical organ. The area postrema serves as a chemoreceptor that triggers vomiting in response to circulating emetic substances, such as digitalis glycosides and apomorphine. The circumventricular organs may be sites where the brain monitors a variety of substances contained in the blood.

The widespread distribution of peptides in the CNS suggests that the CSF may be a conduit by which peptides modulate neuronal function in different regions of the brain. Neural peptides have limited access to the CNS across the blood-brain barrier but have been detected in high concentrations in the circumventricular organs. Peptides identified in the CSF include (1) thyroid-releasing hormone, (2) luteinizing hormone-

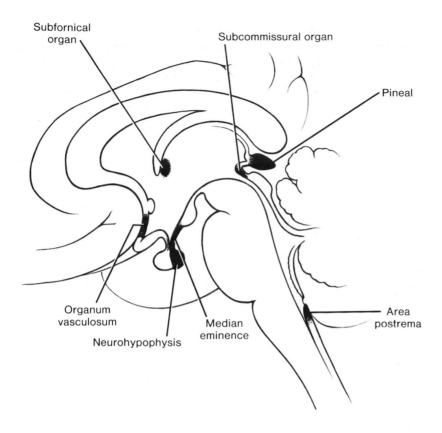

Subfornical organ

Subcommissural organ

Pineal

Organum vasculosum

Neurohypophysis

Median eminence

Area postrema

Figure 1.18. Drawing of a midsagittal section of the human brain indicating the locations of the circumventricular organs. All of these structures, except the *area postrema*, are unpaired, situated in the midline, and related to diencephalic structures. All, except the *subcommissural organ*, are highly vascularized and lack a blood-brain barrier. Neuropeptides have limited transport across the blood-brain barrier but can enter and leave the brain, via the CSF, in regions of the circumventricular organs. The *organum vasculosum of the lamina terminalis* (OVLT) resembles the median eminence, but its function has not been clarified; this structure, particularly prominent in rodents, is also designated as the supraoptic crest. The *median eminence* serves as a neuroendocrine transducer and the final common pathway by which releasing hormones are discharged into the hypophysial portal system. (From Carpenter and Sutin, *Human Neuroanatomy*, 1983; courtesy of Williams & Wilkins.)

releasing hormone, (3) somatostatin, (4) opioid peptides, (5) cholecystokinin, (6) angiotensin II, (7) substance P, (8) adenohypophysial hormones, and (9) neurohypophysial hormones.

SUGGESTED READINGS

AKERT, K., POTTER, H. D., AND ANDERSON, J. W. 1961. The subfornical organ in mammals. I. Comparative and topographical anatomy. J. Comp. Neurol., **116**: 1–14.

BÁRÁNY, E. H. 1972. Inhibition by hippurate and probenecid of *in vitro* uptake of iodipamide and o-iodohippurate: A composite uptake system for iodipamide in choroid plexus, kidney cortex and anterior uvea of several species. Acta Physiol Scand., **86**: 12–27.

BRIGHTMAN, M. W. 1965. The distribution within the brain of ferritin injected into cerebrospinal fluid compartments. I. Ependymal distribution. J. Cell Biol., **26**: 99–123.

BRIGHTMAN, M. W., AND REESE, T. S. 1969. Junctions between intimately apposed cell membranes in the vertebrate brain. J. Cell Biol., **40**: 648–677.

BRIGHTMAN, M. W., REESE, T. S., AND FEDER, N. 1970. Assessment with the electron microscope of the permeability to peroxidase of cerebral endothelium and epithelium in mice and sharks. In C. CRONE AND N. A. LASSEN (Editors), *Capillary Permeability*. Academic Press, New York, pp. 468–476.

BORISON, H. L., AND WANG, S. C. 1949. Functional localization of central coordinating mechanisms for emesis in cat. J. Neurophysiol., **12**: 305–313.

BORISON, H. L., AND WANG, S. C. 1953. Physiology and pharmacology of vomiting. Pharmacol. Rev., **5**: 193–230.

BROADWELL, R. D., AND BRIGHTMAN, M. W. 1976. Entry of peroxidase into neurons of the central and peripheral nervous systems from extracerebral and cerebral blood. J. Comp. Neurol., **166**: 257–284.

CARPENTER, M. B., AND SUTIN, J. 1983. *Human Neuroanatomy*, Ed. 8. Williams & Wilkins, Baltimore.

CHAN-PALAY, V. 1976. Serotonin axons in supraependymal and subependymal plexuses in leptomeninges: Their roles in local alterations of cerebrospinal fluid and vasomotor activity. Brain Res., **102**: 103–130.

CORNING, H. K. 1922. *Lehrbuch der topographischem Anatomie für Studierende und Ärtzte*. J. F. Bergmann, Munich, pp. 609–614.

DAVSON, H. 1967. *Physiology of the Cerebrospinal Fluid*. Little, Brown and Company, Boston.

EHRLICH, P. 1885. *Das Sauerstoff-Bedürfnis des Organismus. Eine Farbenanalytische Studie*. Herschwald, Berlin, pp. 69–72.

ELLIOTT, K. A. C., AND JASPER, H. 1949. Measurement of experimentally induced brain swelling and shrinkage. Am. J. Physiol., **157**: 122–129.

FENSTERMACHER, J. D., AND RALL, D. P. 1973. Physiology and pharmacology of cerebrospinal fluid. In *Pharmacology of the Cerebral Circulation*. Pergamon Press, Oxford, Vol. 1, pp. 35–79.

GOLDSTEIN, G. W., AND BETZ, A. L. 1986. The blood-brain barrier. Scientific American, **255**: 74–83.

GOMEZ, D. G., CHAMBERS, A. A., DIBENEDETTO, A. T., AND POTTS, D. G. 1974. The spinal cerebrospinal fluid absorptive pathways. Neuroradiology. **8**: 61–66.

GOMEZ, D. G., POTTS, D. G., AND DEONARINE, J. 1974. Arachnoid granulations of sheep: Structural and ultrastructural changes with varying pressure differences. Arch. Neurol., **30**: 169–175.

HAMILTON, W. J., AND MOSSMAN, H. W. 1972. *Human Embryology*. Williams & Wilkins, Baltimore, pp. 478–481.

JACKSON, I. M. D. 1981. Neural peptides in the cerebrospinal fluid. Adv. Biochem. Psychopharmacol., **28**: 337–356.

JAYATILAKA, A. D. P. 1965. Arachnoid granulations in sheep. J. Anatomy, **99**: 315–327.

JAYATILAKA, A. D. P. 1965. An electron microscope study of sheep arachnoid granulations. J. Anat., **99**: 635–649.

KATZMAN, R. 1981. Blood-brain-CSF barriers. In G. J. SIEGEL et al. (Editors), *Basic Neurochemistry*. Little, Brown and Company, Boston, pp. 497–510.

KENNEDY, C., DES ROSIERS, M. H., SAKURADA, O., SHINOHARA, M., REIVICH, M., JEHLE, J. W., AND SOKOLOFF, L. 1976. Metabolic mapping of the primary visual system of the monkey by means of autoradiographic [^{14}C] deoxyglucose technique. Proc. Natl. Acad. Sci. USA, **73**: 4230–4234.

KNIGGE, K. M., AND SILVERMAN, A. J. 1974. The anatomy of the endocrine hypothalamus. In R. O. GREEP AND E. B. ASTWOOD (Editors), *Handbook of Physiology*, Sect. 7, Vol. IV. American Physiological Society, Washington, D.C., Ch. 1, pp. 1–32.

METTLER, F. A. 1948. *Neuroanatomy*, Ed. 2, C. V. Mosby Company, St. Louis.

MILLEN, J. W., AND WOOLLAM, D. H. M. 1961. Observations of the nature of the pia mater. Brain, **84**: 514–520.

MINER, L. C., AND REED, D. J. 1972. Composition of fluid obtained from choroid plexus tissue isolated in a chamber in situ. J. Physiol. (Lond.), **227**: 127–139.

PARDRIDGE, W. M., FRANK, H. J. L., CORNFORD, E. M., BRAUN, L. D., CRANE, P. D., AND OLDENDORF, W. H. 1981. Neuropeptides and the blood-brain barrier. Adv. Biochem, Psycho-pharmacol., **28**: 321–328.

RAICHLE, M. E., EICHLING, J. O., AND GRUBB, R. L. 1974. Brain permeability of water. Arch. Neurol., **30**: 319–321.

RAPOPORT, S. I. 1976. *Blood-Brain Barrier in Physiology and Medicine*. Raven Press, New York.

VATES, T. S., BONTING, S. L., AND OPPELT, W. W. 1964. Na-K activated adenosine triphosphatase formation of cerebrospinal fluid in the cat. Am. J. Physiol., **206**: 1165–1172.

WELCH, K. 1963. Secretion of cerebrospinal fluid by choroid plexus of the rabbit. Am. J. Physiol., **205**: 617–624.

WELCH, K., AND FRIEDMAN, J. 1960. The cerebrospinal fluid valves. Brain, **83**: 454–469.

2

Gross Anatomy of the Brain

The nervous system is composed of two parts, the central nervous system and the peripheral nervous system. The *peripheral nervous system* consists of the spinal and cranial nerves, while the *central nervous system* is represented by the brain and spinal cord. The autonomic nervous system, often considered as a separate functional entity, is part central and part peripheral.

The human brain is a relatively small structure weighing about 1400 g and constituting about 2% of the total body weight. The brain commonly is regarded as the organ solely concerned with thought, memory, and consciousness. While these are some of its most complex functions, there are many others. All information we have concerning the world about us is conveyed centrally to the brain by an elaborate sensory system. Receptors of many kinds act as transducers that change physical and chemical stimuli in our environment into nerve impulses that the brain can read and give meaning to. The ability to discriminate between stimuli of the same and different types forms one of the bases for learning. Attention, consciousness, emotional experience, and sleep are all central neural functions. Such higher neural functions as memory, imagination, thought, and creative ability are poorly understood but must be related to complex neuronal activity. The brain also is concerned with all kinds of motor activity; with the regulation of visceral, endocrine, and somatic functions; and with the receptive and expressive use of symbols and signs that underlie communication. While the gross features of the human brain are not especially impressive, its versatility, potential capabilities, efficiency, and self-programming nature put it in a class beyond any "electronic brain."

The brain consists of three basic subdivisions: the cerebral hemispheres, the brain stem, and the cerebellum. The massive paired *cerebral hemispheres* are derived from the *telencephalon*, the most rostral cerebral vesicle. The brain stem consists of four distinct parts: (1) the *diencephalon,* (2) the *mesencephalon,* (3) the *metencephalon,* and (4) the *myelencephalon.* The diencephalon, the most rostral brain stem segment, is the part of the brain stem most intimately related to the forebrain (i.e., telencephalon). The mesencephalon, or midbrain, is the smallest and least differentiated division of the brain stem. The metencephalon (pons) and myelencephalon (medulla) together constitute the *rhombencephalon* or hindbrain. The cerebellum, a derivative of the metencephalon, develops from ectodermal thickenings about the rostral borders of the fourth ventricle, known as the rhombic lip.

CEREBRAL HEMISPHERES

The paired cerebral hemispheres are mirror image duplicates consisting of a highly convoluted gray cortex (pallium), an underlying white

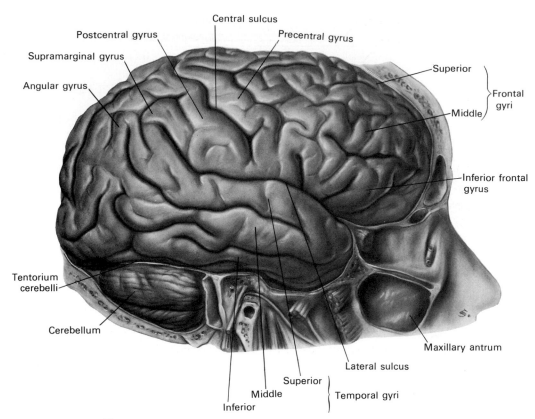

Central sulcus
Postcentral gyrus
Precentral gyrus
Supramarginal gyrus
Superior
Angular gyrus
Frontal gyri
Middle
Inferior frontal gyrus
Tentorium cerebelli
Cerebellum
Maxillary antrum
Lateral sulcus
Superior
Middle
Temporal gyri
Inferior

Figure 2.1.   Lateral view of the brain exposed in the skull to show topographical relationships. (From Mettler's *Neuroanatomy*, 1948; courtesy of The C. V. Mosby Company.)

matter, and a collection of deep neuronal masses, known as the basal ganglia. The cerebral hemispheres are partially separated from each other by the *longitudinal fissure* (Fig. 2.3). This fissure in situ contains the falx cerebri (Fig. 1.2). In frontal and occipital regions the separation of the hemispheres is complete, but in the central region the fissure extends only to fibers of the broad interhemispheric commissure, the corpus callosum (Fig. 2.6). Each cerebral hemisphere is subdivided into lobes by various sulci (Figs. 2.1 and 2.2). The major lobes of the brain are named for the overlying bones of the skull. Although the boundaries of the various lobes as seen in the gross specimen are somewhat arbitrary, cortical areas in each lobe are histologically distinctive. The gray cellular mantle of the cerebral cortex in man is highly convoluted. The crest of a single convolution is referred to as a *gyrus*; *sulci* separate the various gyri, producing a pattern with more or less constant features. On the basis of the more constant sulci and gyri, the cerebrum is divided into six so-called lobes: (1) frontal, (2) temporal, (3) parietal, (4) occipital, (5) insular, and (6) limbic. Neither the insular nor the limbic lobe is a true lobe. The insular cortex lies buried in the depths of the lateral sulcus. The limbic lobe is a synthetic lobe on the medial aspects of the hemisphere consisting of marginal portions (i.e., limbus) of the frontal, parietal, occipital, and temporal lobes, which are in continuity. This cortex, which partially encircles the rostral brain stem, is concerned particularly with visceral and behavioral functions.

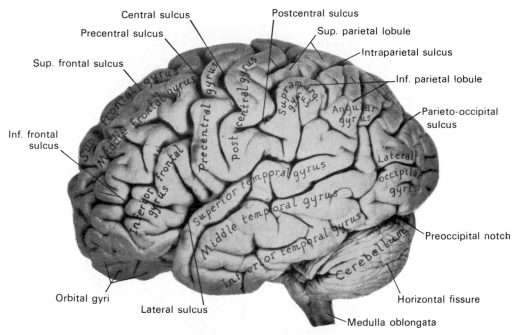

Figure 2.2.   Photograph of the lateral surface of the brain. (From Carpenter and Sutin, *Human Neuroanatomy*, 1983; courtesy of Williams & Wilkins.)

Lateral Surface

The two most important sulci for topographical orientation on the lateral convexity of the hemisphere are the lateral and central sulci (Figs. 2.1 and 2.2).

The *lateral sulcus* begins inferiorly in the Sylvian fossa and extends obliquely posterior, separating the frontal and temporal lobes. Caudally this sulcus separates portions of the parietal and temporal lobes. The terminal ascending ramus of the sulcus extends into the inferior part of the parietal lobe. Portions of the frontal, parietal, and temporal lobes, adjacent to the lateral sulcus, that overlie the insular region are referred to as the *opercular portions* of these lobes (Fig. 2.4).

The *central sulcus* is a prominent sulcus running from the superior margin of the hemisphere downward and forward toward the lateral sulcus (Figs. 2.1 and 2.2). Usually this sulcus is bowed in two locations, and superiorly it does not extend onto the medial surface of the hemisphere. The depths of the sulcus constitute the boundary between the frontal and parietal lobes.

FRONTAL LOBE

This, the largest of all the lobes of the brain, comprises about one-third of hemispheric surface. The frontal lobe extends rostrally from the central sulcus to the frontal pole (Fig. 2.3); its inferior boundary is the lateral sulcus. The convexity of the frontal lobe has four principal convolutions: a *precentral* gyrus that parallels the central sulcus and three horizontally oriented convolutions, the *superior, middle,* and *inferior frontal gyri* (Figs. 2.1 and 2.2). The anterior boundary of the precentral gyrus is the *precentral sulcus,* which, unlike the central sulcus, extends onto the medial surface of the hemisphere. The precentral gyrus and the anterior bank of the central sulcus comprise the *primary motor area* where all parts of the body are represented in a distorted but topographical

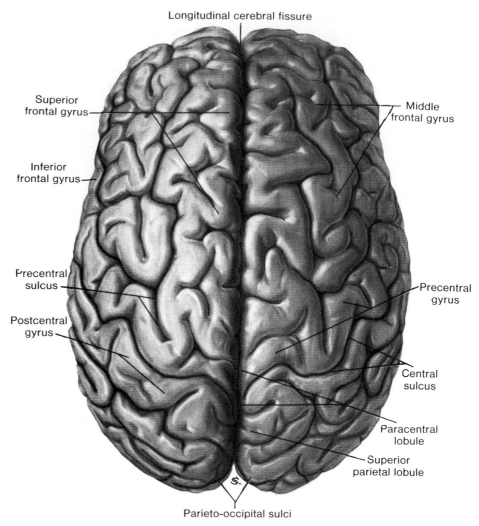

Longitudinal cerebral fissure

Superior frontal gyrus

Middle frontal gyrus

Inferior frontal gyrus

Precentral sulcus

Precentral gyrus

Postcentral gyrus

Central sulcus

Paracentral lobule

Superior parietal lobule

Parieto-occipital sulci

Figure 2.3. Superior view of the brain indicating the main sulci and gyri. (From Mettler's *Neuroanatomy*, 1948; courtesy of The C. V. Mosby Company.)

manner (Fig. 13-13). Regions of the frontal lobe rostral to the primary motor area are referred to as *premotor* and *prefrontal* areas. The broad middle frontal gyrus often is divided by a shallow horizontal sulcus into upper and lower tiers (Figs. 2.1 and 2.2). The inferior frontal gyrus is divided by anterior ascending rami of the lateral sulcus into three parts: (1) *pars orbitale*, (2) *pars triangularis*, and (3) *pars opercularis*. The pars triangularis and opercularis in the dominant hemisphere (usually the left in right-handed individuals) are referred to as *Broca's speech area*, a region concerned with the motor mechanisms of speech formulation. The inferior surface of the frontal lobe lies on the superior surface of the orbital part of the frontal bone and is slightly concave (Fig. 2.1).

PARIETAL LOBE

The boundaries of the parietal lobe are less precise, except for its anterior border on the lateral convexity formed by the central sulcus (Fig. 2.2). Its best defined posterior border lies on the medial aspect of the hemisphere (*parieto-occipital sulcus*) (Fig. 2.6). On the convexity of the hemisphere the posterior boundary is arbitrarily considered as an extrapolated line projected from the superior limit of the parieto-occipital sulcus to the small indentation on the inferior surface known as the *preoccipital notch* (Fig. 2.2). Three parts of the parietal lobe are

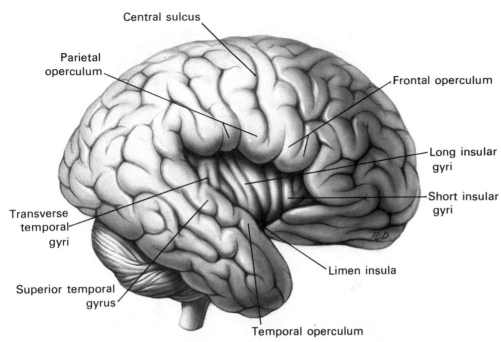

Figure 2.4. View of the right cerebral hemisphere with the banks of the lateral sulcus drawn apart to expose the insular cortex and the transverse gyrus of Heschl.

distinguished: (1) a *postcentral gyrus* running parallel and caudal to the central sulcus, (2) a *superior parietal lobule,* and (3) an *inferior parietal lobule,* the latter both located caudal to the postcentral gyrus. The postcentral gyrus, usually not continuous, but broken up into superior and inferior segments, lies between the central and postcentral sulci. The *postcentral sulcus* extends over the superior margin of the hemisphere and demarcates the caudal limit of the paracentral lobule (Fig. 2.6). The posterior bank of the central sulcus and the postcentral gyrus constitute the *primary somesthetic area,* the cortical region where tactile and kinesthetic sense from superficial and deep receptors are somatotopically represented. The majority of cortical neurons in the postcentral gyrus are concerned with fixed receptive fields on the contralateral side of the body that are place specific, modality specific, and related to discriminative aspects of sensation.

The *intraparietal sulcus,* a horizontally oriented sulcus, divides portions of the parietal lobe caudal to the postcentral gyrus into superior and inferior parietal lobules (Fig. 2.2). The *inferior parietal lobule* consists of two gyri, the *supramarginal,* about both banks of an ascending ramus of the lateral sulcus, and the *angular,* which surrounds the ascending terminal part of the superior temporal sulcus (Figs. 2.1 and 2.2). The inferior parietal lobule represents a cortical association area where multisensory signals form the adjacent parietal, temporal, and occipital regions converge. This region is especially concerned with mnemonic constellations that from the basis for understanding and interpreting sensory signals. This is one region of the cortex where strikingly different disturbances occur as a consequence of lesions in the dominant and nondominant hemispheres (see p. 429).

TEMPORAL LOBE

This large lobe lies inferior to the lateral sulcus and on its lateral surface displays three obliquely oriented convolutions, the *superior, middle,* and *inferior temporal gyri* (Figs. 2.1 and 2.2). The *superior temporal*

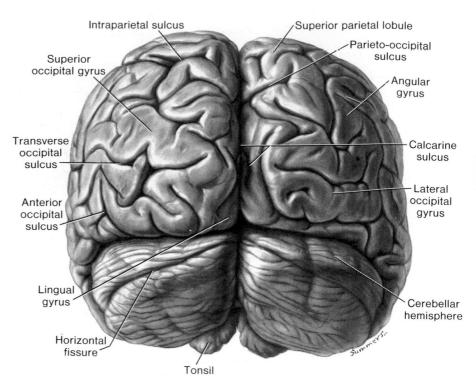

Figure 2.5.   Posterior view of the cerebral hemispheres and cerebellum. (From Mettler's *Neuroanatomy*, 1948; courtesy of The C. V. Mosby Company.)

sulcus lies parallel with the lateral sulcus, and posteriorly it has an ascending ramus that terminates in the angular gyrus. On the outer bank of the lateral sulcus several short, oblique convolutions form the transverse gyri of Heschl; these relatively short transverse gyri medial to the posterior part of the superior temporal gyri constitute the *primary auditory cortex* in man (Figs. 2.4 and 2.9). The inferior surface of the temporal lobe, which lies in the middle fossa of the skull, reveals part of the *inferior temporal gyrus*, the broad *occipitotemporal gyrus*, and the *parahippocampal gyrus* (Figs. 2.7 and 2.8). The parahippocampal gyrus and its most medial protrusion, the *uncus*, are separated from the occipitotemporal gyrus by the *collateral sulcus*. The rostral part of the parahippocampal gyrus, the uncus, and the lateral olfactory stria form the pyriform lobe, which constitutes the *primary olfactory cortex* (Figs. 2.7 and 2.8).

OCCIPITAL LOBE

The small occipital lobe rests on the tentorium cerebelli and constitutes the caudal pole of the hemisphere (Figs. 2.1 and 2.5); its rostral boundary is the parieto-occipital sulcus, present on the medial aspect of the hemisphere (Fig. 2.6). The lateral surface of the occipital lobe, poorly delimited from the parietal lobe, is composed of a number of irregular lateral *occipital gyri,* which are separated into groups by a more constant *lateral occipital sulcus* (Fig. 2.2). On the medial aspect of the hemisphere the occipital lobe is divided by the *calcarine sulcus* into the cuneus and the *lingual gyrus* (Fig. 2.6). The calcarine sulcus joins the parieto-occipital sulcus rostrally in a Y-shaped formation. The cortex on both banks of the calcarine sulcus represents the *primary visual cortex* (i.e., striate). The visual cortex in each hemisphere receives inputs from the temporal half of the ipsilateral retina and the nasal half of the contralateral retina and is concerned with perception from the contralateral half of the visual field. Binocular fusion occurs in layers of the visual cortex even though

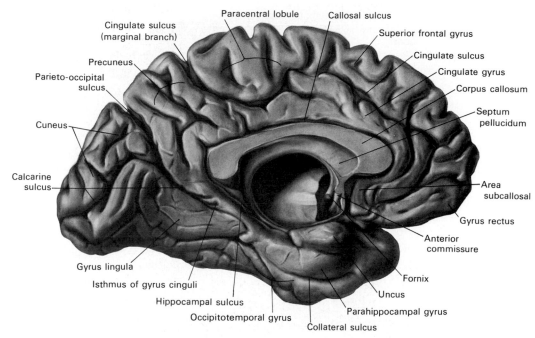

Figure 2.6.   Medial surface of the cerebral hemisphere with diencephalic structures removed. (From Mettler's *Neuroanatomy*, 1948; courtesy of The C. V. Mosby Company.)

fibers of the visual radiation conducting impulses from each eye terminate in alternate columns in the principal receptive layer of the cortex. Central (macular) vision is represented nearest the occipital pole (Figs. 2.5 and 2.6). Fibers conveying signals from the upper halves of the retinae terminate on the superior bank of the calcarine sulcus, while the inferior bank of the sulcus receives impulses from the lower halves of the retinae.

INSULA

This invaginated cortical area, buried in the depths of the lateral sulcus, can be seen only when the temporal and frontal lobes are separated. The insular lobe is a triangular cortical area, the apex of which is directed forward and downward to open into the lateral fossa (Figs. 2.4 and 2.9). The *gyri breves* and *longus*, which cover the surface, course nearly parallel to the lateral sulcus. The extent and relationships of this region can be appreciated in horizontal and transverse sections of the hemisphere (Figs. 2.11, 2.12, 2.16 and 2.17). The surface opening leading to the insular region is called the *limen insula*. The temporal, frontal, and parietal opercular regions cover the insula.

Medial Surface

In a hemisected brain, convolutions on the medial surface can be studied. The convolutions on the medial surface of the cerebral hemisphere are somewhat flatter than those on the convexity. The most prominent structure on the medial surface is the massive interhemispheric commissure, the *corpus callosum* (Fig. 2.6). This structure, composed of myelinated fibers, reciprocally interconnects nearly all cortical regions of the two hemispheres. Different parts of the corpus callosum are referred to as the *rostrum, genu, body*, and *splenium* (Figs. 2.9 and 2.15). Fibers in this structure spread out as a mass of radiations to nearly all parts of the cortex. Callosal fibers, projecting to parts of the frontal and occipital

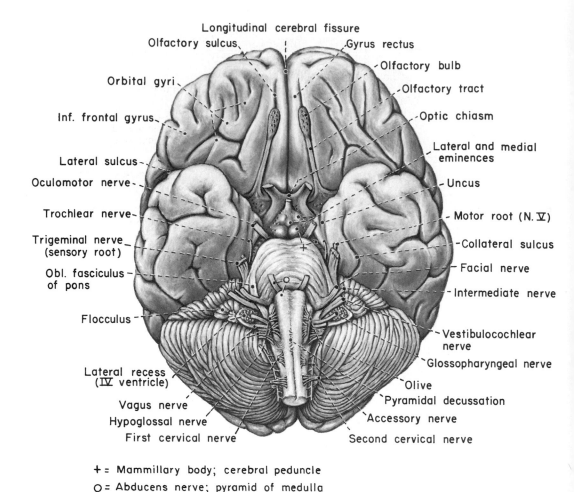

Longitudinal cerebral fissure
Olfactory sulcus
Gyrus rectus
Olfactory bulb
Orbital gyri
Olfactory tract
Inf. frontal gyrus
Optic chiasm
Lateral sulcus
Lateral and medial
eminences
Oculomotor nerve
Uncus
Trochlear nerve
Motor root (N. V)
Trigeminal nerve
(sensory root)
Collateral sulcus
Obl. fasciculus
of pons
Facial nerve
Intermediate nerve
Flocculus
Vestibulocochlear
nerve
Lateral recess
(IV ventricle)
Glossopharyngeal nerve
Olive
Vagus nerve
Pyramidal decussation
Hypoglossal nerve
Accessory nerve
First cervical nerve
Second cervical nerve

+ = Mammillary body; cerebral peduncle
O = Abducens nerve; pyramid of medulla

Figure 2.7. Inferior surface of the brain showing the cranial nerves. (From Truex and Kellner's *Detailed Atlas of the Head and Neck*, 1958; courtesy of Oxford University Press.)

lobes, form the so-called *anterior* and *posterior forceps* (Figs. 2.9 and 2.11). The corpus callosum forms the floor of the longitudinal fissure, as well as the roof of the lateral ventricle. The corpus callosum plays an important role in interhemispheric transfer of learned discriminations, sensory experience, and memory. Complete surgical section of the corpus callosum does not result in obvious neurological deficits, but these patients show a striking functional independence of the two hemispheres with respect to perceptual, cognitive, mnemonic, learned, and volitional activities. The activities of the separated hemispheres are not known to each other, and information perceived exclusively by, or generated in, the nondominant (right) hemisphere cannot be communicated in speech or writing. No impairment of linguistic expression is noted in information processed by the dominant (left) hemisphere. Linguistic expression and analytic functions are organized almost exclusively in the dominant hemisphere. The nondominant hemisphere is concerned with spatial concepts, recognition of faces, and some elements of music (see p. 428).

The *callosal sulcus* separates the corpus callosum from the cingulate gyrus; posteriorly this sulcus curves around the splenium to be continued into the temporal lobe as the *hippocampal sulcus* (Fig. 2.6). The *cingulate gyrus*, dorsal to the callosal sulcus, encircles the corpus callosum and consists of two tiers. The *cingulate sulcus*, superior to the cingulate gyrus, runs parallel to the callosal sulcus but near the splenium projects dorsally

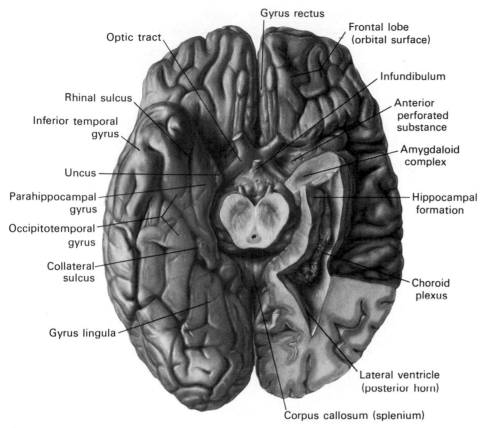

Figure 2.8. View of the inferior surface of the brain following transection of the midbrain. The inferior and posterior horns of the left lateral ventricle have been opened and portions of the temporal and occipital lobes have been removed. (From Mettler's *Neuroanatomy*, 1948; courtesy of The C. V. Mosby Company.)

as the *marginal sulcus*. In the frontal lobe the cortex superior to the cingulate gyrus is the medial surface of the superior frontal gyrus. The *paracentral lobule*, formed by the precentral and postcentral gyri which extend onto the medial surface of the hemisphere, is notched by the central sulcus (Fig. 2.6). The *paracentral sulcus*, continuous with the precentral sulcus, forms the rostral border of this lobule, while the *marginal sulcus*, continuous with the postcentral gyrus, forms the caudal border (Fig. 2.6). The portion of the parietal lobe caudal to the paracentral lobule and rostral to the parieto-occipital sulcus is known as the *precuneus* (Fig. 2.6).

LIMBIC LOBE

This is a synthetic lobe, consisting of the most medial margins (i.e., the limbus) of the frontal, parietal, and temporal lobes, which surround the interhemispheric commissure (Fig. 12.17). The limbic lobe includes the *subcallosal, cingulate,* and *parahippocampal gyri*, as well as primitive cortical derivatives, the *hippocampal formation* and the *dentate gyrus*, which in the course of development have become invaginated within the temporal lobe (Fig. 2.8). The parahippocampal gyrus is directly continuous with the cingulate gyrus by a narrow strip of cortex, posterior and inferior to the splenium of the corpus callosum, known as the *isthmus of the cingulate gyrus* (Fig. 2.6). The parahippocampal gyrus, the most medial convolution of the temporal lobe, is bounded laterally by the *rhinal* and *collateral sulci* and superiorly and medially by the *hippocampal sulcus*

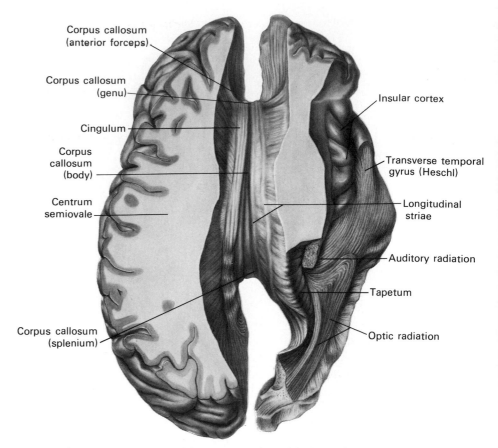

Corpus callosum
(anterior forceps)

Corpus callosum
(genu)

Cingulum

Corpus
callosum
(body)

Centrum
semiovale

Corpus callosum
(splenium)

Insular cortex

Transverse temporal
gyrus (Heschl)

Longitudinal
striae

Auditory radiation

Tapetum

Optic radiation

Figure 2.9. Dissection of the superior surface of the hemispheres exposing the corpus callosum, cingulum, longitudinal striae, and the optic and auditory radiations. (From Mettler's *Neuroanatomy*, 1948; courtesy of The C. V. Mosby Company.)

(Figs. 2.6, 2.7, and 2.8). Rostrally the parahippocampal gyrus hooks around the hippocampal sulcus to form a medially protruding convolution, the *uncus* (Figs. 2.7 and 2.8). The proximity of the uncus to the cerebral peduncle is of clinical importance because it may herniate through the tentorial notch and compress the brain stem. Structures composing the limbic lobe appear early in phylogenesis, and physiological evidence suggests functional differences between various components, although most are related to visceral and behavioral activities.

Inferior Surface

The inferior surface of the hemisphere consists of two parts: (1) a larger posterior portion, representing the inferior surfaces of the temporal and occipital lobes, and (2) the orbital surface of the frontal lobe (Figs. 2.7 and 2.8). The inferior surface of the occipital lobe and the posterior part of the temporal lobe lie on the tentorium cerebelli (Figs. 1.2, 2.1, and 2.5), while rostral parts of the temporal lobe lie in the middle cranial fossa. Gyri present in this posterior part include (1) the lingual gyrus, (2) the extensive occipitotemporal gyrus, and (3) the parahippocampal gyrus and uncus (Fig. 2.8). The inferior temporal gyrus lies lateral to the occipitotemporal gyrus. The narrow isthmus of the cingulate gyrus lies medially posterior to the splenium of the corpus callosum.

The orbital surface of the frontal lobe has a deep, straight sulcus medially, the olfactory sulcus, which contains both the olfactory bulb and tract (Figs. 2.7 and 2.8). The *gyrus rectus* lies along the ventromedial

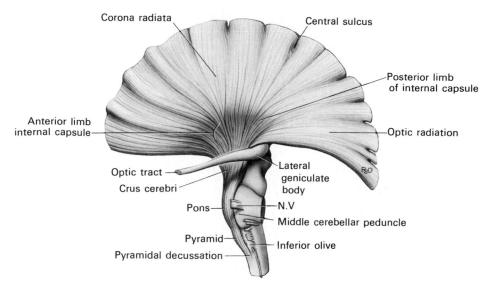

Figure 2.10. Drawing of a dissection demonstrating the continuity and relationships of the corona radiata, the internal capsule, the crus cerebri, and the medullary pyramids.

margin of the frontal lobe medial to the olfactory sulcus. The region lateral to the olfactory sulcus contains the orbital gyri whose convolutional patterns are variable. Posteriorly the olfactory tract divides into medial and *lateral olfactory striae* (Fig. 12.2). Caudal to this is the olfactory trigone and the *anterior perforated substance,* a region studded with small openings through which numerous small arteries (lateral striate) pass to subcortical structures (Figs. 2.7, 2.8, 2.20, and 14.8).

White Matter

The massive white matter beneath the cerebral cortex extends to the subcortical nuclei and the ventricular system and forms the medullary core of the hemisphere. Myelinated fibers within the white matter are of three types: (1) *projection fibers* that convey impulses either from or to the cortex, (2) *association fibers* that interconnect various cortical regions of the same hemisphere, and (3) *commissural fibers* that interconnect corresponding cortical regions of the two hemispheres (Figs. 2.9, 2.16, and 2.17). The common central mass of white matter, containing commissural, association, and projection fibers, has an oval appearance in horizontal sections of the brain and is termed the *semioval center* (Fig. 2.9).

PROJECTION FIBERS

Afferent and efferent fibers conveying impulses to and from the entire cerebral cortex enter the white matter in radially arranged bundles that converge toward the brain stem (Fig. 2.10). These radiating projection fibers form the *corona radiata*. Near the rostral part of the brain stem these fibers form a compact band of fibers known as the *internal capsule,* flanked medially and laterally by nuclear masses (Figs. 2.11 and 2.12). Two distinct parts of the internal capsule are evident in horizontal sections of the hemispheres: (1) an anterior limb and (2) a posterior limb (Fig. 2.11).

The *anterior limb of the internal capsule* partially separates two of the largest components of the corpus striatum, the caudate nucleus and the putamen. Fibers in the anterior limb of the internal capsule are di-

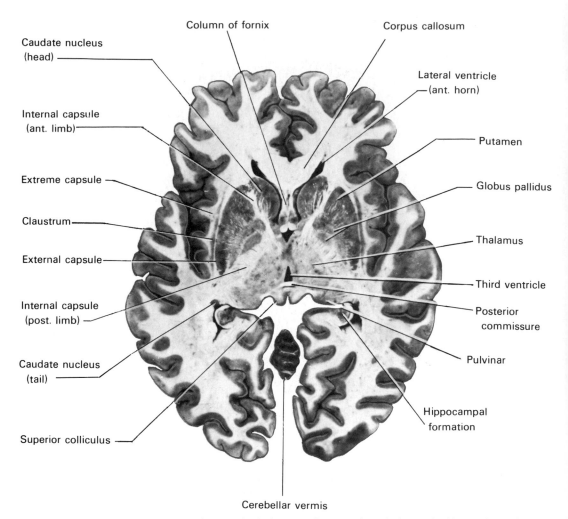

Figure 2.11. Photograph of a horizontal section through the cerebral hemispheres showing relationships of internal structures to the internal capsule. (From Carpenter and Sutin, *Human Neuroanatomy*, 1983; courtesy of Williams & Wilkins.)

rected horizontally, obliquely laterally, and upward toward the frontal lobe, and in horizontal sections of the hemisphere they appear to be cut longitudinally (Figs. 2.10, 2.11, and 2.12). In horizontal sections of the hemisphere, the anterior and posterior limbs of the internal capsule meet at an obtuse angle with the apex directed medially. The junction between the anterior and posterior limbs of the internal capsule is referred to as the *genu* (Figs. 2.11 and 9.24 and 9.25).

The *posterior limb of the internal capsule* is flanked medially by the diencephalon (thalamus) and laterally by parts of the corpus striatum known as the lentiform nucleus. Fibers in the posterior limb of the internal capsule course in nearly a vertical plane toward the brain stem, and in horizontal sections fibers are cut transversely (Fig. 2.11). The most posterior component of the posterior limb of the internal capsule contains fibers radiating toward the calcarine sulcus, known as the *optic radiation* (Figs. 2.9 and 2.14). Afferent fibers in the internal capsule arise mainly from the thalamus and project to nearly all regions of the cortex; such fibers are referred to as the *thalamocortical radiations*. Efferent fibers in the internal capsule arise from cells in deep layers of various regions of the cerebral cortex; these fibers project to nuclear masses in the brain stem and to spinal cord. Fibers projecting away from the cerebral cortex

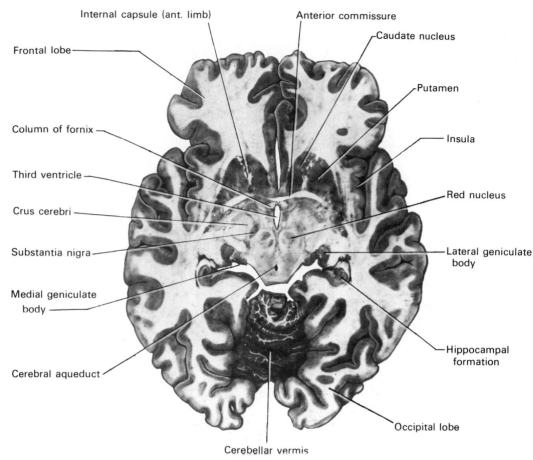

Internal capsule (ant. limb)

Anterior commissure

Caudate nucleus

Frontal lobe

Putamen

Column of fornix

Insula

Third ventricle

Crus cerebri

Red nucleus

Substantia nigra

Lateral geniculate
body

Medial geniculate
body

Hippocampal
formation

Cerebral aqueduct

Occipital lobe

Cerebellar vermis

Figure 2.12.   Photograph of a horizontal section through the cerebral hemispheres passing through the anterior commissure and the crus cerebri. (From Carpenter and Sutin, *Human Neuroanatomy*, 1983; courtesy of Williams & Wilkins.)

(i.e., corticofugal) include corticostriate, corticothalamic, corticopontine, corticobulbar, and corticospinal fibers.

ASSOCIATION FIBERS

Fibers interconnecting various cortical regions within the same hemisphere are divided into long and short groups (Fig. 2.13). *Short association fibers* arching through the floor of each sulcus connect cells in adjacent convolutions; these fibers course transversely to the long axis of the sulci. *Long association fibers,* interconnecting cortical regions in different lobes within the same hemisphere, form three main bundles: (1) the uncinate fasciculus, (2) the arcuate fasciculus, and (3) the cingulum.

The *uncinate fasciculus* is a compact bundle beneath the limen insula that connects the orbital frontal gyri with anterior portions of the temporal lobe (Fig. 2.13). A deeply placed part of this fasciculus is thought to connect the frontal and occipital lobes (i.e., inferior occipitofrontal fasciculus).

The *arcuate fasciculus* sweeps around the insular region, and its fan-shaped ends connect the superior and middle frontal gyri with parts of the temporal lobe. A group of superiorly situated fibers in this bundle extends caudally into portions of the parietal and occipital lobe and is known as the *superior longitudinal fasciculus* (Fig. 2.13).

The *cingulum*, the principal association bundle on the medial aspect of the hemisphere, lies in the white matter of the cingulate gyrus. This

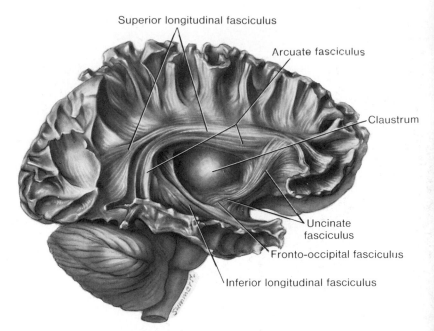

Figure 2.13. Dissection of the lateral surface of the right hemisphere revealing the long association fibers interconnecting cortical regions in different lobes. (From Mettler's *Neuroanatomy*, 1948; courtesy of The C. V. Mosby Company.)

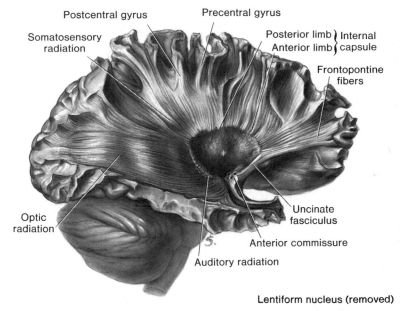

Figure 2.14. Dissection of the lateral aspect of the right cerebral hemisphere to reveal the corona radiata and the optic radiation. The lentiform nucleus (*) has been removed. (From Mettler's *Neuroanatomy*, 1948; courtesy of The C. V. Mosby Company.)

bundle contains fibers of variable length that connect medial regions of the frontal and parietal lobes with parahippocampal and adjacent temporal cortical regions (Figs. 2.9 and 2.15).

The cortical area deep to the insula contains association fibers in the *extreme* and *external capsules* (Figs. 2.11, 2.16, and 2.17). These thin capsules composed of white matter are separated by a sheet of gray matter, known as the *claustrum*. All three of these structures lie lateral to the corpus striatum.

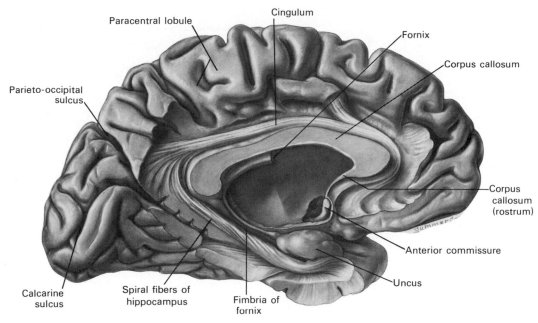

Paracentral lobule

Cingulum

Fornix

Corpus callosum

Parieto-occipital sulcus

Corpus callosum (rostrum)

Anterior commissure

Uncus

Calcarine sulcus

Spiral fibers of hippocampus

Fimbria of fornix

Figure 2.15. Dissection of the medial surface to the left cerebral hemisphere exposing the cingulum. The diencephalon has been removed. (From Mettler's *Neuroanatomy*, 1948; courtesy of The C. V. Mosby Company.)

COMMISSURAL FIBERS

Fibers interconnecting corresponding cortical regions of the two hemispheres are represented by two structures: (1) the corpus callosum and (2) the anterior commissure.

The *corpus callosum* is a broad thick plate of dense myelinated fibers that reciprocally interconnect broad regions of the cortex in all lobes with corresponding regions of the opposite hemisphere (Figs. 2.6, 2.9, and 2.15). These fibers traverse the floor of the hemispheric fissure, form most of the roof of the lateral ventricles, and fan out in a massive callosal radiation distributed to various cortical regions. The parts of the corpus callosum are designated as (1) rostrum, (2) genu, (3) body, and (4) splenium. The genu contains fibers interconnecting anterior parts of the frontal lobes; fibers from the remaining parts of the frontal lobe and the parietal lobe traverse the body of the corpus callosum. Fibers traversing the splenium relate corresponding regions of the temporal and occipital lobes. Fibers in the splenium of the corpus callosum, which sweep inferiorly along the lateral margin of the posterior horn of the lateral ventricle and separate the ventricle from the optic radiation, form the *tapetum* (Figs. 2.9 and 2.19).

The *anterior commissure* is a small compact bundle that crosses the midline rostral to the columns of the fornix (Figs. 2.6, 2.12, 2.15 and 2.16). This commissure has a general shape not unlike bicycle handlebars and consists of two parts that cannot be distinguished in the gross specimen (Figs. 2.12 and 12.9). A small anterior part of the commissure (not evident on gross inspection) interconnects the olfactory bulbs on the two sides (Fig. 12.3); the larger posterior part mainly interconnects regions of the middle and inferior temporal gyri.

BASAL GANGLIA

The basal ganglia are large subcortical nuclear masses derived mainly from the telencephalon (Figs. 2.11, 2.12, 2.16, and 2.17). Struc-

Figure 2.16. Photograph of a frontal section of the brain passing through the columns of the fornix and the anterior commissure. (From Carpenter and Sutin, *Human Neuroanatomy*, 1983; courtesy of Williams & Wilkins.)

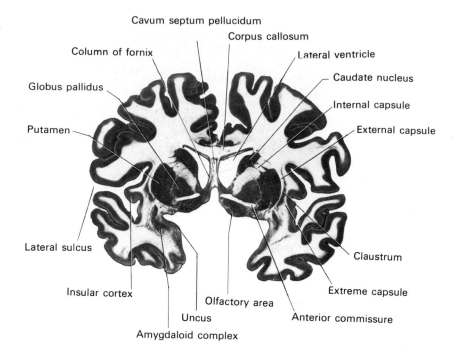

Cavum septum pellucidum
Corpus callosum
Column of fornix
Lateral ventricle
Globus pallidus
Caudate nucleus
Internal capsule
Putamen
External capsule
Lateral sulcus
Claustrum
Extreme capsule
Insular cortex
Olfactory area
Uncus
Anterior commissure
Amygdaloid complex

Figure 2.17. Photograph of a frontal section of the brain at the level of the mammillary bodies. In this section, the main nuclear groups of the thalamus are identified and portions of all components of the basal ganglia are present. The amygdaloid nuclear complex lies in the temporal lobe internal to the uncus and ventral to the lentiform nucleus (i.e., putamen and globus pallidus). (From Carpenter and Sutin, *Human Neuroanatomy*, 1983; courtesy of Williams & Wilkins.)

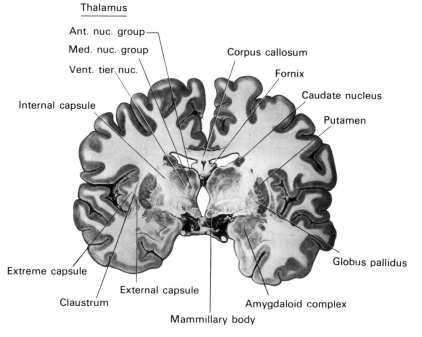

Thalamus
Ant. nuc. group
Med. nuc. group
Vent. tier nuc.
Corpus callosum
Fornix
Internal capsule
Caudate nucleus
Putamen
Extreme capsule
Globus pallidus
Claustrum
External capsule
Amygdaloid complex
Mammillary body

tures composing the basal ganglia are the *caudate nucleus*, the *putamen*, the *globus pallidus,* and the *amygdaloid nuclear complex*. The caudate nucleus, putamen, and globus pallidus constitute the *corpus striatum.*

The term *lentiform nucleus* refers to the putamen and the globus pallidus. The lentiform nucleus, with the size and shape of a Brazil nut, in transverse sections appears as a wedge with the apex directed medially. This nuclear mass lies between the internal and the external capsules. A slightly curved vertical lamina of white matter divides the lentiform nucleus into an outer portion, the putamen, and an inner portion, the globus pallidus.

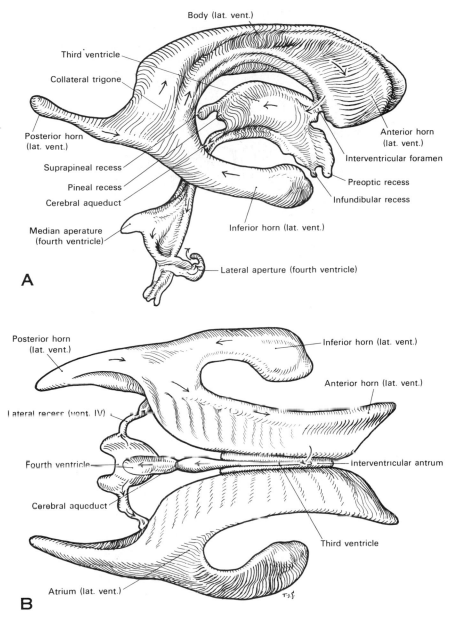

Figure 2.18. Diagrams of the ventricular system in lateral (*A*) and superior (*B*) views. (After Bailey, 1948.)

PUTAMEN

This is the largest and most lateral part of the corpus striatum; it lies between the lateral medullary lamina of the globus pallidus and the external capsule (Figs. 2.11, 2.16, and 2.17). It is traversed by fascicles of myelinated fibers directed ventromedially toward the globus pallidus, but these are seen clearly only in stained sections. The rostral part of the putamen is continuous ventromedially with the head of the caudate nucleus.

CAUDATE NUCLEUS

This nucleus is an elongated arched gray cellular mass related throughout its extent to the lateral cerebral ventricle (Figs 2.11, 2.16, and 2.17). It consists of an enlarged rostral part, called the head of the caudate

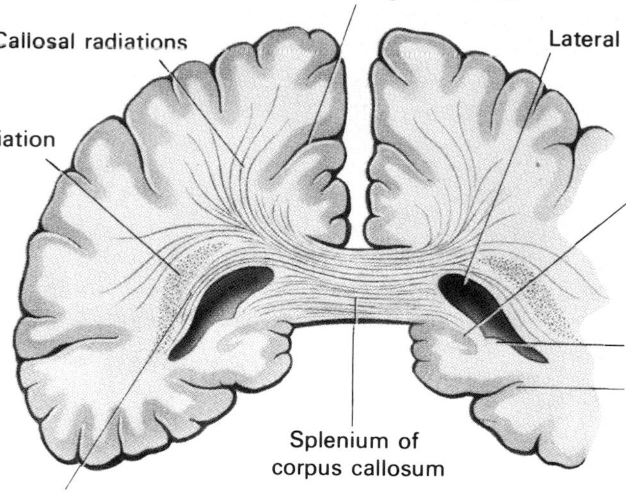

Figure 2.19. Drawing of a frontal section at the level of the splenium of the corpus callosum. Callosal fibers lateral to the ventricle are known as the tapetum. The optic radiation lies lateral to the tapetum.

nucleus, which protrudes into the anterior horn of the lateral ventricle, and a narrower body and tail (Fig. 2.26). The body of the caudate nucleus lies dorsolateral to the thalamus near the lateral wall of the lateral ventricle. The tail of the caudate nucleus follows the curvature of the inferior horn of the lateral ventricle and enters the temporal lobe. The tail of the caudate nucleus terminates in the region of the amygdaloid nuclear complex (Figs. 2.17 and 11.3).

GLOBUS PALLIDUS

The most medial part of the lentiform nucleus, the globus pallidus, is a diencephalic derivative consisting of two parallel segments (Figs. 2.11, 2.16, and 2.17). Segments of the globus pallidus are separated by a thin medullary lamina. The globus pallidus appears pale and homogeneous in freshly sectioned brains. Its medial border is formed by the fibers of the posterior limb of the internal capsule.

AMYGDALOID NUCLEAR COMPLEX

This is a gray cellular mass in the dorsomedial part of the temporal lobe that underlies the uncus (Figs. 2.8 and 2.17). This complex lies dorsal to the hippocampal formation and rostral to the tip of the inferior horn of the lateral ventricle. The amygdaloid complex arises from the same telencephalic anlage as the caudate nucleus. Cells of the amygdala give rise to fibers of the *stria terminalis*, which arch along the entire medial border of the caudate nucleus and are especially evident near the junction of the caudate nucleus and thalamus (Figs. 2.21 and 2.26). The terminal vein lies adjacent to the stria terminalis.

LATERAL VENTRICLES

The ependymal-lined cavities of the cerebral hemisphere constitute the lateral ventricles. The arch-shaped lateral ventricles contain cerebrospinal fluid and conform to the general shape of the hemispheres (Figs. 1.10, 1.11, and 2.18). The paired lateral ventricles can be divided into five parts: (1) the anterior (frontal) horn, (2) the ventricular body, (3) the collateral (atrium) trigone, (4) the inferior (temporal) horn, and (5) the posterior (occipital) horn. Each lateral ventricle communicates with the narrow, slitlike, midline third ventricle by two short channels, known as the interventricular foramina (Munro). These foramina serve as a basic reference point of great radiographic importance (Figs 1.10 and 2.18).

ANTERIOR (FRONTAL) HORN

This horn of the lateral ventricle lies rostral to the interventricular foramen; has a triangular shape in frontal section; and extends forward, laterally, and ventrally to a blunt rounded termination in the substance of the frontal lobe (Figs. 2.11 and 2.16). The roof and rostral wall of this horn are formed by the corpus callosum, while its medial boundary is the *septum pellucidum*, which rostrally separates the ventricles of the two hemispheres (Figs. 2.6, 2.23, 2.24, and 2.26). The septum pellucidi are thin paired membranes near the midline that frequently are fused. The lateral wall of the ventricle is formed by the head of the caudate nucleus whose convex surface bulges into the cavity (Figs. 2.11, 2.12, 2.16, and 2.26).

BODY OF THE LATERAL VENTRICLE

This arched part of the lateral ventricle extends caudally from the interventricular foramen to an ill-defined point near the splenium of the corpus callosum. Caudally this part of the ventricle widens into the collateral trigone (referred to by neuroradiologists as the atrium). The *collateral trigone* comprises that part of the lateral ventricle near the splenium of the corpus callosum where the body of the lateral ventricle is confluent with the temporal and occipital horns (Fig. 2.18).

INFERIOR (TEMPORAL) HORN

This horn of the ventricle curves downward and forward around the caudal aspect of the thalamus and extends rostrally into the medial part of the temporal lobe to end approximately 3 cm from the temporal pole (Fig. 2.18). The roof and lateral wall of the horn are formed by fibers of the tapetum (Figs. 2.9 and 2.19) and the optic radiation; the floor contains the *collateral eminence* caused by the deep collateral sulcus (Figs. 2.8 and 2.19). The inferior horn of the lateral ventricle contains the *hippocampal formation* in its medial wall, which extends from the region of the splenium to the rostral tip of the ventricle (Figs. 2.8, 2.11, and 2.12). The hippocampal formation, representing the phylogenetically oldest type of cortex, has become folded into the ventricle along the hippocampal sulcus. Along the superior and medial surfaces of the hippocampus is a flattened band of fibers, known as the fimbria, which extends from the region of the uncus toward the splenium of the corpus callosum (Figs. 12.8 and 12.9). The fimbria continues rostrally under the corpus callosum and becomes the fornix (Figs. 2.15, 2.26, and 2.27).

POSTERIOR (OCCIPITAL) HORN

This horn of the lateral ventricle extends from the collateral trigone into the occipital lobe. The horn varies greatly in size and often is rudimentary (Fig. 2.18). The occipital horn has the appearance of a small fingerlike projection with a rounded tip. The roof and lateral wall of this horn are formed by tapetal fibers of the corpus callosum, while its floor is the white matter of the occipital lobe. The *calcar avis*, a medial lon-

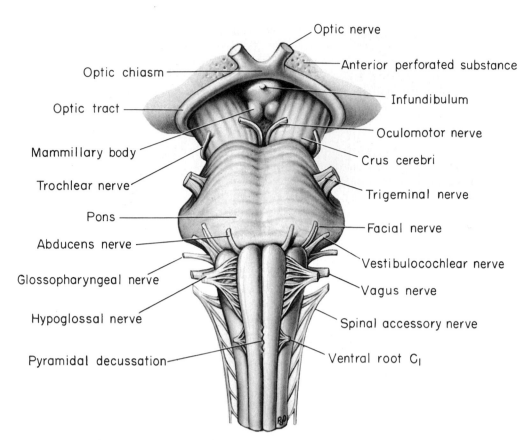

Figure 2.20. Drawing of the anterior surface of the medulla, pons, and midbrain. (From Carpenter and Sutin, *Human Neuroanatomy*, 1983; courtesy of Williams & Wilkins.)

gitudinal prominence, is produced by the deep indentation of the calcarine sulcus.

Portions of the lateral ventricles contain *choroid plexus,* which is formed by the invagination of the ependymal roof plate into the ventricular cavities. Choroid plexus develops at sites where ependyma and pia mater containing blood vessels come together. This plexus is present in the body, the collateral trigone, and in the inferior horn of the lateral ventricle and extends through the interventricular foramen to lie in the roof of the third ventricle (Figs. 1.9, 1.10, and 2.26).

BRAIN STEM

In the intact brain only the anterior, or ventral, surface of the brain stem can be seen throughout its extent, because the cerebral hemispheres and cerebellum overlap the lateral and posterior surfaces. On the anterior surface of the brain stem the medulla, pons, midbrain, and part of the hypothalamus (diencephalon) can be identified (Figs. 2.7 and 2.20). The most rostral portion of the brain stem, the diencephalon, is surrounded by hemispheric structures on all sides except for a small region between the *optic chiasm* and the *mammillary bodies.* The midbrain appears very small, but root fibers of the oculomotor nerve can be seen emerging between two massive fiber bundles, the *crura cerebri* (Figs. 2.7, 2.20, and 2.22). The ventral surface of the pons produces a convex protrusion covered by transversely oriented fiber bundles that laterally enter the substance of the cerebellum. The medulla, caudal to the pons, reveals the paired *medullary pyramids* medially and the oval *olivary eminences* dorsolaterally (Fig. 2.22). The transition from medulla to spinal cord is

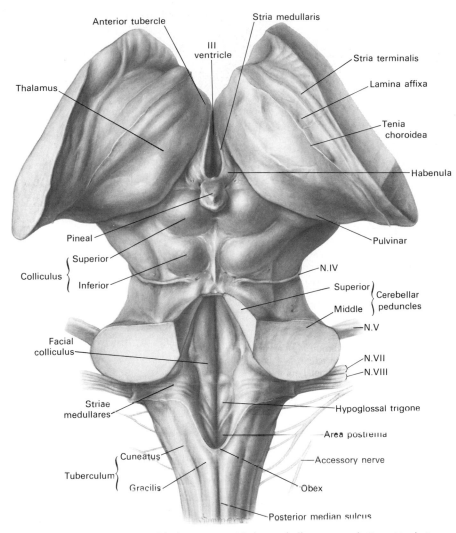

Figure 2.21. Posterior aspect of the brain stem with the cerebellum removed. (From Mettler's *Neuroanatomy*, 1948; courtesy of The C. V. Mosby Company.)

characterized by the disappearance of the medullary pyramids, the development of the anterior median fissure of the spinal cord, a conspicuous reduction in size, and the appearance of paired spinal nerves.

Removal of the cerebral hemispheres and cerebellum reveals the posterior and lateral surfaces of the brain stem (Figs. 2.21 and 2.22). The expanded diencephalon appears as two paired oval nuclear masses on each side of a vertical slitlike third ventricle (Fig. 2.21). The *thalamus* and *epithalamus*, seen in a posterior view of the brain stem, lie between the fibers of the internal capsule and are flanked dorsolaterally by the body and tail of the caudate nucleus and the *stria terminalis* (Fig. 2.21). Along the dorsomedial margin of the thalamus is the *stria medullaris*, a band of fibers coursing posteriorly toward the base of the pineal gland (Figs. 2.21, 2.23, 2.24, and 2.26). The most caudal part of the thalamus, the pulvinar, overlies lateral parts of the midbrain.

The posterior aspect of the midbrain reveals the *superior* and *inferior colliculi* and their *brachia*, which relate these structures to particular parts of the thalamus. The crossed trochlear nerves emerge dorsally, caudal to the inferior colliculus (Fig. 2.21).

The posterior aspect of the hindbrain, revealed by removing the cerebellum (Figs. 2.21 and 2.22), discloses the rhomboid fossa, an un-

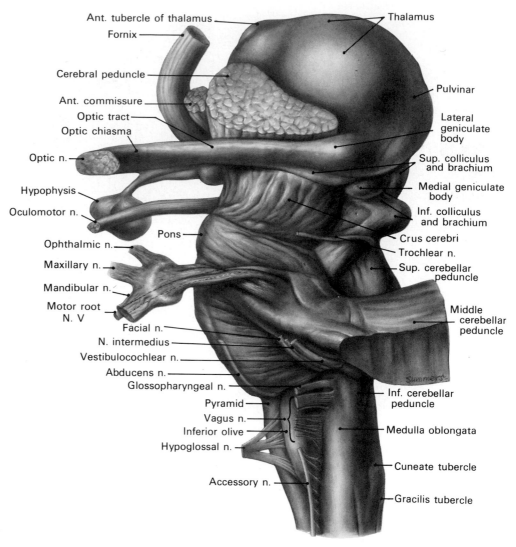

Figure 2.22. Lateral view of the brain stem with the cerebellum removed showing the sites of emergence and entrance of most of the cranial nerves. (From Mettler's *Neuroanatomy*, 1948; courtesy of The C. V. Mosby Company.)

paired symmetrical ventricle that overlies the pons and medulla. The rhomboid-shaped fourth ventricle is surrounded by three paired cerebellar peduncles, which relate the three lowest brain stem segments to the cerebellum (Fig. 2.21). The fourth ventricle contains several eminences that overlie nuclear masses in the pons and medulla, the most evident of which are the *facial colliculus* and the *hypoglossal eminence* or trigone (Fig. 2.21). Caudal to the fourth ventricle on the posterior surface of the medulla are nuclear masses related to ascending spinal systems, namely, the *cuneate* and *gracilis tubercles*.

Structurally the midbrain and hindbrain consist of three distinctive parts: (1) a roof plate superior to the ventricular system, (2) a central core of cells and fibers beneath the ventricular system known as the tegmentum, and (3) a massive collection of ventrally located fibers derived from cells of the cerebral cortex (Figs. 2.23 and 2.24). The *roof plate* of the midbrain is represented by the tectum or *quadrigeminal plate*, consisting of the superior and inferior colliculi; in the hindbrain the roof plate is represented by the *cerebellum* and the *tela choroidea*. The *tegmentum* of the midbrain, pons, and medulla represents the brain stem *reticular*

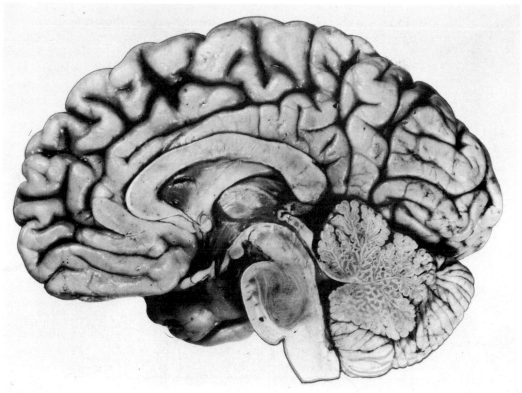

x = superior colliculi
• = inferior colliculi

Figure 2.23. Photograph of a midsagittal section of the brain. Brain stem structures are identified in Figure 2.24. (From Carpenter and Sutin, *Human Neuroanatomy*, 1983; courtesy of Williams & Wilkins.)

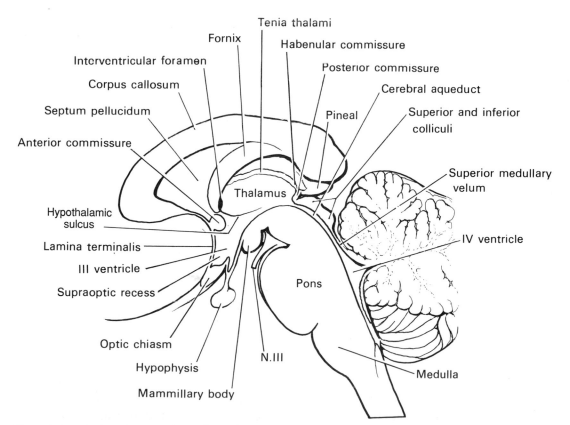

Figure 2.24. Outline drawing of a midsagittal section of the brain identifying structures shown in Figure 2.23. (From Carpenter and Sutin, *Human Neuroanatomy*, 1983; courtesy of Williams & Wilkins.)

formation, a large collection of cells and intermingled fibers that subserve multiple integrative functions. The *cortically derived ventral fiber system* forms the *crus cerebri* at midbrain levels, one of the principal constituents of the *ventral* or *basilar part of the pons*, and the *medullary pyramids* of the medulla (Figs. 2.20 and 2.22). Both the reticular formation and the cortically derived ventral fiber system are continuous within the brain stem but undergo changes at various levels (Fig. 2.10).

Medulla

The medulla (myelencephalon), the most caudal basic subdivision of the brain stem, extends from the level of the foramen magnum to the caudal border of the pons. The transition from spinal cord to medulla is gradual and characterized by (1) the obliteration of the anterior median fissure ventrally and the decussation of the medullary pyramids, (2) the appearance of the gracilis and cuneate tubercles dorsally (Fig. 2.21), (3) the disappearance of spinal nerves, (4) the appearance of cranial nerves, and (5) the development of the fourth ventricle (Figs. 2.20, 2.21, 2.23, and 2.24). The full development of the medullary pyramids, the appearance of the eminence of the inferior olivary complex, the widening of the fourth ventricle, and the gradual increase in size of the inferior cerebellar peduncle give the medulla its characteristic configuration. Cranial nerves associated with the medulla are (1) the hypoglossal (N. XII), whose fibers emerge ventrolaterally between the pyramid and the inferior olivary complex; (2) the accessory (N. XI), the vagus (N. X), and the glossopharyngeal (N. IX), whose fibers emerge from the postolivary sulcus (Fig. 2.22); and (3) the vestibulocochlear nerve (N. VIII), whose components enter the brain stem separately at the cerebellopontine angle, formed by the junction of the pons, medulla, and cerebellum (Figs. 2.20, 2.21, 2.22, and 2.25). Auditory fibers are most dorsal and caudal and partially arch over the lateral aspect of the inferior cerebellar peduncle. Vestibular fibers enter the brain stem ventral to the inferior cerebellar peduncle.

Fourth Ventricle

The fourth ventricle is a broad shallow rhomboid-shaped cavity overlying the pons and medulla that extends from the central canal of the upper cervical spinal cord to the cerebral aqueduct of the midbrain (Figs. 2.18 and 2.21). Its roof is formed by the *superior* and *inferior medullary veli*, which extend toward an apex within the cerebellum known as the *fastigium* (Figs. 2.23, 2.24, 2.30, and 2.31). The superior medullary velum forms the roof of the pontine part of the ventricle, while the inferior medullary velum and the *tela choroidea* roof over the medullary part of this ventricle. *Choroid plexus* attached to the tela choroidea caudally passes into the lateral recess of the fourth ventricle on each side (Figs. 1.10 and 2.18). The widest part of the fourth ventricle is immediately caudal to where the *middle cerebellar peduncles* enter the cerebellum (Fig. 2.21). In this region a *lateral recess* on each side extends over the surface of the inferior cerebellar peduncle to open into the *cerebello-medullary* (magna) *cistern* (Figs. 1.8 and 1.9). The lateral recesses contain choroid plexus that protrudes through the *foramina of Luschka* into the subarachnoid space (Figs. 2.7 and 2.18). A small median aperture in the caudal part of the ventricle is known as the *foramen of Magendie*. Through these three apertures cerebrospinal fluid flows from the ventricular system into the subarachnoid spaces.

The *rhomboid fossa*, which forms the floor of the fourth ventricle,

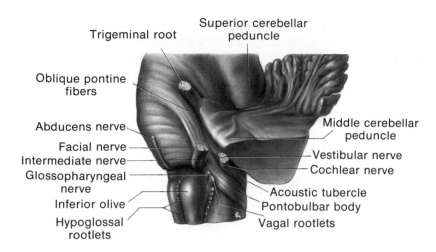

Trigeminal root

Superior cerebellar peduncle

Oblique pontine fibers

Abducens nerve

Facial nerve

Intermediate nerve

Glossopharyngeal nerve

Inferior olive

Hypoglossal rootlets

Middle cerebellar peduncle

Vestibular nerve

Cochlear nerve

Acoustic tubercle

Pontobulbar body

Vagal rootlets

Figure 2.25. Lateral view of the cerebellopontine angle from a dissection of the brain stem and cerebellum. (From Mettler's *Neuroanatomy*, 1948; courtesy of The C. V. Mosby Company.)

is divided symmetrically by the *median sulcus*. The sulcus limitans divides each half into a *medial eminence* and a lateral region known as the *vestibular area* (Fig. 5.1). The vestibular nuclei lie beneath the vestibular area. The *facial colliculus* and the *hypoglossal trigone* lie within the medial eminence, with the latter near the caudal border of the ventricle. Transversely coursing fibers of the *striae medullares* run from the region of the lateral recess toward the midline and disappear in the median sulcus (Fig. 2.21); most of these strands of myelinated fibers lie rostral to the hypoglossal trigone. The *vagal trigone* lies lateral to the hypoglossal trigone. The most caudal end of the rhomboid fossa resembles a pen and is called the *calamus scriptorius*. The point of caudal junction of the walls of the fourth ventricle is known as the *obex* (Fig. 2.21). Immediately rostral to the obex on each side of the fourth ventricle is a slightly rounded eminence, the *area postrema*, the only paired circumventricular organ (Figs. 1.18 and 5.7).

Pons

The pons (metencephalon), representing the rostral part of the hindbrain, is well delimited on the anterior surface of the brain stem (Figs. 2.20, 2.22, 2.23, and 2.24). The massive pontine protuberance is covered ventrally by broad bands of transversely oriented fibers and is separated from (1) the midbrain by the superior pontine sulcus and (2) the medulla by the inferior pontine sulcus (Fig. 2.20). Laterally the transverse fibers in the ventral part of the pons form the *middle cerebellar peduncle*. An anterior median depression, the *basilar sulcus*, indicates the position occupied by the basilar artery (Figs. 2.20 and 14.3).

Transverse sections of the pons reveal the basic organization (Fig. 6.1). The pons consists of a massive *ventral part* composed of (1) longitudinal descending fiber bundles, (2) pontine nuclei, and (3) transversely oriented fibers projecting into the cerebellum. A smaller dorsal part, known as the *tegmentum*, contains aggregations of cells and fibers that form a central core known as the reticular formation. The pontine tegmentum is continuous with the reticular formation of the medulla and midbrain. Cranial nerve nuclei, ascending sensory systems, and older descending motor pathways arising from brain stem nuclei are found within the tegmentum. Cranial nerve nuclei associated with the pons are the trigeminal (N. V), abducens (N. VI), facial (N. VII), and the two components of the vestibulocochlear nerve (N. VIII) (Fig. 2.7). The *abducens nucleus* lies in the floor of the fourth ventricle and is partially encircled by fibers of the facial nerve. Facial nerve fibers and cells of the abducens nucleus underlie the *facial colliculus* in the floor of the fourth ventricle (Fig. 2.21). Fibers of the abducens nerve emerge from the ventral surface of the brain stem at the junction of the pons and medulla. The facial and vestibulocochlear nerves emerge and enter the lateral surface of the pons at the *cerebellopontine angle*, formed by the junction of pons, medulla, and cerebellum (Fig. 2.25). The trigeminal nerve, consisting of motor and sensory fibers, traverses rostrolateral parts of the middle cerebellar peduncle to reach nuclei in the dorsolateral pontine tegmentum (Figs. 2.20 and 2.22).

The *middle cerebellar peduncle,* consisting of massive collections of crossed fibers, arising from the pontine nuclei, projects to the opposite cerebellar hemisphere. This is the largest of the three cerebellar peduncles (Figs. 2.21 and 2.22).

Midbrain

The midbrain (mesencephalon) is the smallest and least differentiated brain stem segment (Figs. 2.20, 2.21, 2.22, 2.23, and 2.24). It consists of (1) the *tectum*, represented by the superior and inferior colliculi; (2) the *tegmentum*, ventral to the cerebral aqueduct; and (3) the massive *crura cerebri* (Figs. 2.10, 2.12, 2.20, 2.21, and 2.23). The tegmentum and *crura cerebri* are separated by a large pigmented nuclear mass, the *substantia nigra* (Fig. 7.1). The cells of the substantia nigra contain melanin pigment, synthesize dopamine, and can be readily identified in fresh cut sections of the midbrain. The superior colliculus and a region immediately rostral to it, known as the *pretectum*, are important structures that receive inputs from the optic tract; these structures are involved in visual reflexes and the processing of visual information. The inferior colliculus relays auditory impulses to thalamic nuclei that in turn project to specific cortical areas.

Two cranial nerves are associated with the midbrain, the oculomotor (N. III) and the trochlear (N. IV). The oculomotor nerve emerges from the *interpeduncular fossa*, between the massive crura cerebri (Figs. 2.7, 2.20, and 2.22). The slender trochlear nerve exits from the posterior surface of the brain stem, caudal to the inferior colliculus; fibers of this nerve cross in the superior medullary velum (Fig. 2.21). The fibers of the *superior cerebellar peduncle*, seen on each side of the upper part of the fourth ventricle (Fig. 2.21), constitute the largest cerebellar efferent system. Fibers in this peduncle decussate completely in the caudal midbrain tegmentum. Crossed fibers of this peduncle traverse and surround cells in a discrete nuclear mass in the midbrain tegmentum called the *red nucleus* (Figs. 2.12 and 7.1). A large proportion of these crossed fibers ascend to terminations in diencephalic (thalamic) nuclei.

CRUS CEREBRI

On the ventral surface of the midbrain are collections of fibers originating from broad areas of the cerebral cortex that pass through the internal capsule (Figs. 2.10 and 2.20). Fibers forming the crus cerebri project to (1) spinal cord (i.e., corticospinal), (2) pontine nuclei (i.e., corticopontine), and (3) specific regions of the lower brain stem (i.e., corticobulbar). A large part of the so-called corticobulbar fibers project to portions of the reticular formation.

The pigmented *substantia nigra*, situated along the superior border of the crus cerebri, is the largest single nuclear mass in the midbrain.

Different parts of this nucleus have connections with parts of the corpus striatum and thalamus considered to subserve motor functions (Figs. 2.12 and 7.1).

Diencephalon

The diencephalon, the most rostral part of the brain stem, is a paired structure on each side of the third ventricle (Figs. 2.21, 2.22, 2.23, 2.24, and 2.26). The lateral ventricles, corpus callosum, fornix, and velum interpositum lie superior to the diencephalon. Fibers of the posterior limb of the internal capsule and the body and tail of the caudate nucleus lie along its lateral border (Fig. 2.11). Caudally the diencephalon appears continuous with the tegmentum of the midbrain; the posterior commissure demarcates the junctional zone between the diencephalon and mesencephalon (Figs. 2.11, 2.23 and 2.24). The rostral boundary of the diencephalon is near the interventricular foramen, but portions of the hypothalamus extend almost to the *lamina terminalis* (Figs. 2.23 and 2.24). The diencephalon consists of four subdivisions: (1) the epithalamus, (2) the thalamus, (3) the hypothalamus, and (4) the subthalamus (Figs. 2.21, 2.22, 2.23, 2.24, 2.26, and 2.27).

The epithalamus, evident on the superior surface of the diencephalon, consists of (1) the pineal body, (2) the habenular nuclei, (3) the striae medullares, and (4) the tenia thalami (Figs. 2.21 and 2.24).

Thalamus

The largest diencephalic subdivision is an obliquely oriented, egg-shaped nuclear mass at the rostral end of the brain stem (Figs. 2.21, 2.22, 2.23, and 2.24). This nuclear complex lies between the interventricular foramen and the posterior commissure and extends from the third ventricle to the medial border of the posterior limb of the internal capsule (Fig. 2.11). The thalamus lies dorsal to the hypothalamic sulcus, a shallow groove on the lateral wall of the third ventricle (Figs. 2.24, 2.27, and 9.5). The lateral and caudal parts of the thalamus are enlarged and overlie midbrain structures. The superior surface of the thalamus is covered by a thin layer of fibers known as the *stratum zonale* (Fig. 9.5). A narrow lateral strip on the superior surface, adjacent to the body and tail of the caudate nucleus, is covered by ependyma and forms part of the floor of the lateral ventricle. This strip is called the *lamina affixa* (Fig. 2.21). The *stria terminalis* and the terminal vein are present dorsally at the junction of thalamus and caudate nucleus. The *stria medullaris* extends along the dorsomedial margin of the thalamus near the roof of the third ventricle (Fig. 2.24). The medial surfaces of thalami on each side of the third ventricle are partially fused in about 80% of human brains. This fusion of the thalami is called the *interthalamic adhesion* or *massa intermedia*.

Although most subdivisions of the thalamus are not evident in gross specimens, the *anterior tubercle* of the thalamus is discernible rostrally as a distinct swelling (Fig. 2.22). The expanded posterior part of the thalamus that overhangs part of the midbrain is known as the *pulvinar* (Figs. 2.11 and 2.21). The *medial* and *lateral geniculate bodies,* important relay nuclei concerned with audition and vision, lie ventral to the pulvinar (Fig. 2.12). Together these structures are referred to as the *metathalamus.* The thalamus is divided into anterior, lateral, medial, and ventral nuclear groups by a thin layer of myelinated fibers known as the *internal medullary lamina* of the thalamus, which can be seen grossly in some transverse sections

Figure 2.26. Drawing of a brain dissection showing the gross relationships of the thalamus, internal capsule, corpus striatum, and the ventricular system. (From Carpenter and Sutin, *Human Neuroanatomy*, 1983; courtesy of Williams & Wilkins.)

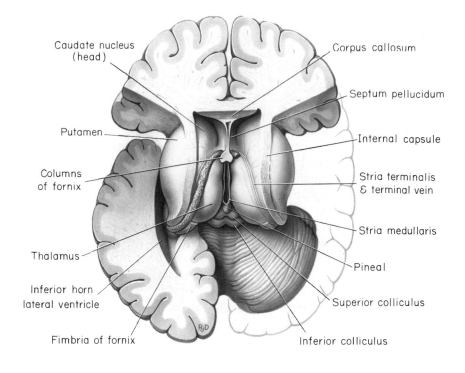

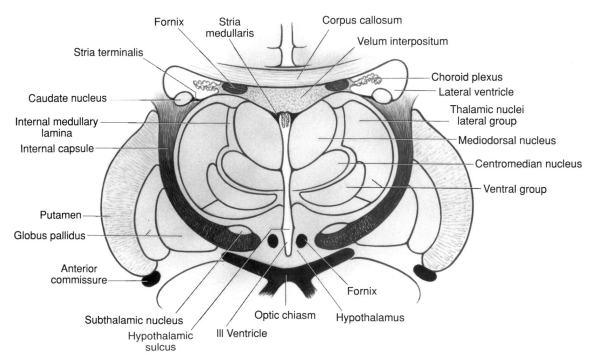

Figure 2.27. Schematic drawing of a frontal section through the diencephalon and adjacent structures indicating the major nuclear groups of the thalamus. The hypothalamus lies ventral to the thalamus, on both sides of the third ventricle, and is continuous across the floor of this ventricle. The subthalamic region lies lateral and caudal to the hypothalamus.

of the brain (Figs. 2.11 and 2.17). Nuclear groups within the internal medullary lamina are collectively referred to as the *intralaminar thalamic nuclei* (Fig. 2.27).

The thalamus is the neural structure whose relationships with other parts of the neuraxis provide the key to understanding the organization of the central nervous system. Like most keys it is small but of great importance. This small part of the diencephalon is concerned with (1) distributing most of the afferent input to the cerebral cortex, (2) controlling the electrocortical activity of the cerebral cortex, and (3) integrating motor functions by providing the relays through which impulses from the corpus striatum and cerebellum can reach the motor regions of the cerebral cortex. The functions of the thalamus are much more complex and elaborate than that of a simple relay station. The thalamus is concerned with input selection, output tuning, high fidelity impulse transmission, synchronization and desynchronization of cortical activities, parallel processing of sensory signals, and the integration of inputs that modify most activities. This structure plays a dominant role in the maintenance and regulation of states of consciousness, alertness, and attention. The thalamus may be regarded as the chief integrating and tuning mechanism of the neuraxis.

Hypothalamus

This structure lies ventral to the hypothalamic sulcus and forms the floor and lateral walls of the third ventricle (Figs. 2.23, 2.24, 2.27, 9.5, and 10.1). This subdivision of the diencephalon extends from the region of the optic chiasm to the caudal border of the mammillary bodies. The gross structures visible on the ventral surface include the *optic chiasm*, *infundibulum*, *tuber cinereum*, and *mammillary bodies* (Fig. 2.8). The hypothalamus is divided into medial and lateral nuclear groups by fibers of the fornix, most of which end in the mammillary body. Three rostrocaudal regions of the hypothalamus are recognized: (1) a supraoptic, dorsal to the optic chiasm; (2) a tuberal region centrally near the infundibulum; and (3) a mammillary region caudally (Fig. 10.1). The zone forming the floor of the third ventricle is called the *median eminence*; portions of this eminence lie both rostral and caudal to the infundibular stem. The median eminence is the anatomical interface between central neural pathways and the anterior pituitary (Fig. 10.8).

The hypothalamus has a rostrocaudal extent of about 10 mm. This subdivision of the diencephalon is concerned with visceral, endocrine, and metabolic activity, as well as with temperature regulation, sleep, and emotional behavior.

Subthalamic Region

This transitional diencephalon zone lies ventral to the thalamus and lateral to the hypothalamus. It is bounded by the thalamus above, the hypothalamus medially, and the internal capsule laterally (Figs. 2.7 and 2.27). The largest discrete nuclear mass is the *subthalamic nucleus*, a lens-shaped structure on the inner aspect of the internal capsule (Fig. 9.5). This region is traversed by important fiber systems in their projection to thalamic nuclei. A small, relatively clear area dorsal and rostral to the subthalamic nucleus, known as the *zona incerta*, serves as an important landmark in distinguishing fiber bundles with specific origins and trajectories. The subthalamic nucleus and pathways traversing this region are concerned with somatic motor function.

CEREBELLUM

The cerebellum overlies the posterior aspect of the pons and medulla and extends laterally under the tentorium to fill the greater part of the posterior fossa (Figs. 2.1 and 2.5). The superior surface is somewhat flattened, while the inferior surface is convex. A shallow *anterior cerebellar incisure* is present superiorly (Fig. 2.28). A deeper and narrower *posterior cerebellar incisure* contains a fold of dura mater, the *falx cerebelli* (Fig. 1.2).

The cerebellum consists of a midline portion, the *vermis*, and two lateral lobes or *hemispheres*. This structure is essentially wedge-shaped, having a superior surface that is covered by a tentorium, a posterior surface in the suboccipital region, and an inferior surface that overlies the fourth ventricle. On the superior surface the distinction between vermis and hemispheres is not sharp (Fig. 2.28). On the inferior surface two deep sulci clearly separate the vermis from the hemispheres. Inferiorly a deep median fossa, the *vallecula cerebelli*, is continuous with the posterior incisure. The floor of this fossa is formed by the inferior vermis (Fig. 2.29).

Structurally the cerebellum consists of a gray cortical mantle, the cerebellar cortex, a medullary core of white matter, and four pairs of intrinsic nuclei. Three paired cerebellar peduncles connect the cerebellum with the three lower segments of the brain stem (Figs. 2.21, 2.22, and 2.30).

The cerebellar cortex consists of a large number of narrow leaflike laminae known as cerebellar folia. Surface cerebellar folia are nearly parallel with each other and for the most part are transversely oriented. Each lamina contains several secondary and tertiary folia.

Five transversely oriented fissures divide the cerebellum into lobes and lobules (Fig. 8.1). These fissures and the various lobular subdivisions can be identified on the isolated cerebellum or in midsagittal section (Fig. 2.30). On the superior surface of the cerebellum two fissures can be identified: (1) the *primary* and (2) the *posterior superior* (Fig. 2.28). The primary fissure. is the deepest of all cerebellar fissures. The *horizontal fissure* roughly divides the cerebellum into superior and inferior halves (Fig. 2.28). On the inferior surface the *prepyramidal* and *posterolateral fissures* are found (Fig. 2.31). The prepyramidal fissure lies between the *tuber* and the pyramidal-shaped *pyramis* in the cerebellar vermis (Figs. 2.31 and 8.1). In the cerebellar hemisphere this fissure separates gracile and biventer lobules, which constitute parts of the *paramedian lobule*. The posterolateral fissure separates the *nodulus*, which lies in the roof of the fourth ventricle, from the rest of the cerebellar vermis.

The cerebellar vermis is the key to the gross organization of the cerebellum, but in this part there is no median raphe and the midline is difficult to establish.

The *anterior lobe of the cerebellum* lies rostral to the primary fissure (Figs. 2.28 and 8.1). In the vermis the lobules consist of the lingula, the central lobule, and the culmen (Fig. 2.31); in the hemisphere the lingula has no corresponding part, but the *alar central lobule* and the *anterior quadrangular lobule* correspond to the central lobule and the culmen. The anterior lobe of the cerebellum, known as the *paleocerebellum*, receives inputs from the spinal cord and exerts major influences on muscle tone.

The *posterior lobe* of the cerebellum lies between the primary and posterolateral fissures and represents the largest subdivision (Figs. 2.31

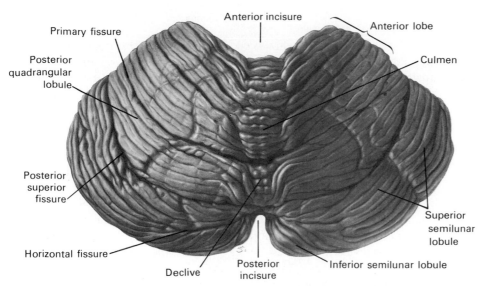

Figure 2.28.   Superior surface of cerebellum. (From Mettler's *Neuroanatomy*, 1948; courtesy of The C. V. Mosby Company.)

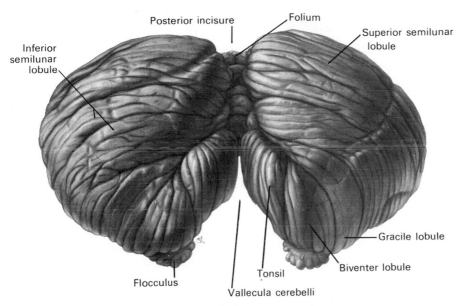

Figure 2.29.   Posteroinferior view of the cerebellum. (From Mettler's *Neuroanatomy*, 1948; courtesy of The C. V. Mosby Company.)

and 8.1). Vermal parts of the posterior lobe in sequence are the *declive*, *folium*, *tuber*, *pyramis*, and *uvula* (Fig. 2.31). The *simple lobule,* between the primary and posterior superior fissure, corresponds to the declive of the vermis (Fig. 8.1). The *ansiform lobule* is that part of the cerebellar hemisphere between the posterior superior fissure and the *gracile lobule*. The horizontal fissure divides the ansiform lobule into the *superior semilunar lobule* (crus I) and the *inferior semilunar lobule* (crus II) (Fig. 2.29). The vermal counterparts of the ansiform lobule are the folium and tuber. Between the prepyramidal and posterolateral fissures are the *pyramis* and *uvula* in the vermis and the *biventer lobule* and the *cerebellar tonsil* in the hemisphere (Figs. 2.30 and 2.31). The posterior lobe of the cerebellum, known as the *neocerebellum*, receives massive inputs from the con-

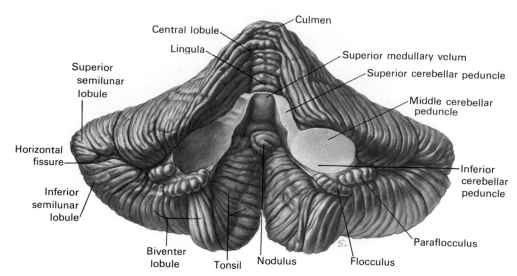

Figure 2.30. Inferior surface of cerebellum removed from brain stem by transection of cerebellar peduncles. (From Mettler's *Neuroanatomy*, 1948; courtesy of The C. V. Mosby Company.)

tralateral cerebral cortex and is concerned with coordination of motor function.

The *flocculonodular lobule* lies rostral to the posterolateral fissure and consists of the vermal nodulus and the paired flocculi (Fig. 2.30). The *nodulus* lies immediately caudal to the inferior medullary velum (Fig. 2.31). The flocculonodular lobule and portions of the uvula constitute the *archicerebellum*, the part most intimately related to the vestibular system.

In midsagittal section the relationships of the cerebellum to the brain stem are evident (Fig. 2.24). The complex branching of the medullary core and the treelike appearance of the laminae and folia in sagittal section have given rise to the descriptive term *arbor vitae* (Figs. 2.23 and 2.31). The intrinsic deep nuclei of the cerebellum can be seen only in sections. These nuclei are the dentate (most lateral), the emboliform, the globose, and the fastigial (most medial) (Fig. 6.22). The fastigial nuclei, commonly called the roof nuclei, lie in the roof of the fourth ventricle.

Although the cerebellum is derived from the metencephalon, this portion of the neuraxis functions in a suprasegmental manner. It is concerned primarily with coordination of somatic motor function, the control of muscle tone, and the maintenance of equilibrium. Sensory signals generated in nearly every kind of receptor are projected to the cerebellum, but none of these give rise to conscious sensory perceptions. The cerebellum functions as a special kind of computer that processes, organizes, and integrates sensory inputs and provides an output that contributes to the smooth and effective control of somatic motor function. Output systems of the cerebellum arise largely, but not exclusively, from the deep cerebellar nuclei and exert their major influences on brain stem nuclei at multiple levels.

IMAGING TECHNICS

Several roentgenographic technics have been used to visualize structures in and around the brain. These technics have involved introduction of air or contrast media into the ventricles or subarachnoid space (i.e., ventriculography and pneumoencephalography) or injection of a water-

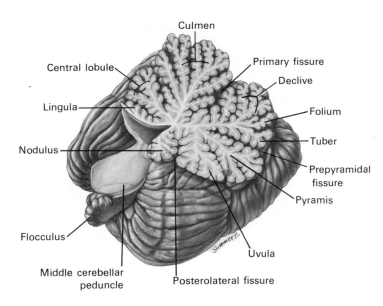

Culmen

Central lobule

Primary fissure

Declive

Lingula

Folium

Nodulus

Tuber

Prepyramidal
fissure

Pyramis

Flocculus

Uvula

Middle cerebellar
peduncle

Posterolateral fissure

Figure 2.31. Sagittal view of the sectioned cerebellum showing the lobules of the cerebellar vermis. The primary fissure is the deepest of all cerebellar fissures. (From Mettler's *Neuroanatomy*, 1948; courtesy of The C. V. Mosby Company.)

soluble contrast media into the common carotid or the vertebral arteries (cerebral angiography; see Figs. 14.7, 14.12, and 14.13). Plain films of the head do not reveal images of the brain because of its homogeneous radiodensity.

Computerized tomography, a technic capable of presenting an image of a cross section of the brain or body, uses scintillation counters rather than x-ray film and feeds data into a computer capable of direct imaging. The scanning unit and the detectors rotate so that scans are taken 1 degree apart.

Magnetic resonance imaging (MRI) has emerged as the imaging modality that can provide the most specific and the greatest range of information, particularly in soft tissue. By selecting the appropriate MRI technics, virtually all regions of the brain and spinal cord can be imaged in detail. This method also can provide information concerning a variety of space-occupying lesions (i.e., tumors), demyelinating diseases, degenerative diseases, areas of edema or hemorrhage and can be used to identify vascular structures and cranial nerves. MRI is based on the biochemistry of tissue and anatomical delineation results from the characteristic biochemical nature of individual structures and organs. MRI is noninvasive, does not use ionizing radiation, and can produce a quality image in a variety of planes.

Atomic nuclei with an odd number of protons and neutrons, such as hydrogen, have a property called spin. Since the nuclei have a charge and are in angular motion about an axis, they have a "magnetic moment," which represents a directional magnetic force. Normally the random orientations of the nuclear spins cause the magnetic moments to cancel each other, so that there is no net magnetic field. In a strong magnetic field, magnetic moments of nuclear particles tend to become aligned either parallel or antiparallel to the magnetic field. Application of an appropriate pulsed radiofrequency (RF) wave at 90° to the direction of the magnetic field causes the nuclear spins to become reoriented at 90° from their aligned prepulsed positions. When the RF pulse is complete, the nuclear spins gradually return to their prepulsed positions. The combined magnetic moments of all protons altered by the RF pulse produce RF signals that are recorded by a receiver and fed into a computer. The computer transforms the frequencies and amplitudes of the RF signals into an image.

This technic also is referred to as nuclear magnetic resonance

Figure 2.32. Magnetic resonance imaging (MRI) in the midsagittal plane of the head showing the definition of brain structures. In this image the cerebrospinal fluid in the cisterns and ventricles appears dark. (Courtesy of John Sherman, M.D., Washington, D.C.).

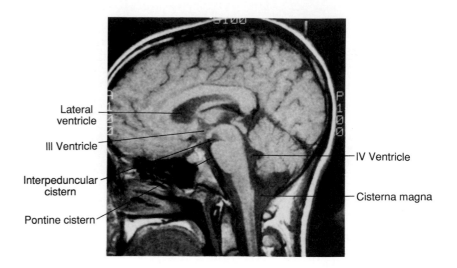

Lateral ventricle

III Ventricle

Interpeduncular cistern

Pontine cistern

IV Ventricle

Cisterna magna

(NMR): (1) *nuclear* because the magnetic moments are generated by the spinning charged nuclear particles, such as the proton in hydrogen; (2) *magnetic* because the tissue must be in a strong static magnetic field to align the spinning nuclear particles parallel and antiparallel; and (3) *resonance* because the frequencies of the pulsed RF waves and the spinning nuclear particles must be identical in order to interact and produce a magnetic resonance signal that can be transformed by a computer into a quality image. Examples of MRI taken in different planes are shown in Figures 1.11 and 2.32.

SUGGESTED READING

BAILEY, P. 1948. *Intracranial Tumors*, Ed. 2. Charles C Thomas, Publishers, Springfield, IL.

BROCA, P. 1878. Anatomie comparée circonvolutions cérébrales: Le grand lobe limbique et la scissure limbique dans la série des mammifères. Rev. Anthropol. Ser. 2, **1**: 384–498.

BRODAL, A. 1981. *Neurological Anatomy in Relation to Clinical Medicine*, Ed. 3. Oxford University Press, New York.

CARPENTER, M. B., AND SUTIN, J. 1983. *Human Neuroanatomy*, Ed. 8, Williams & Wilkins, Baltimore.

GAZZANIGA, M. S., AND SPERRY, R. W. 1967. Language after section of the cerebral commissures. Brain, **90**: 131–148.

GROSSMAN, C. B. 1990. *Magnetic Resonance Imaging and Computed Tomography of the Head and Spine*. Williams & Wilkins, Baltimore.

HANAWAY, J., SCOTT, W. R., AND STROTHER, C. M. 1980. *Atlas of the Human Brain and the Orbit for Computer Tomography*, Ed. 2. Warren H. Green, II, Inc., St. Louis.

HEIMER, L. 1983. *The Human Brain and Spinal Cord*. Springer-Verlag, New York.

JACOBS, E. R. 1987. *Medical Imaging. A Concise Textbook*. Igaku-Shoin, New York.

MADIGAN, J. C., JR., AND CARPENTER, M. B. 1971. *Cerebellum of the Rhesus Monkey: Atlas of Lobules, Laminae, and Folia, in Sections*. University Park Press, Baltimore.

METTLER, F. A. 1948. *Neuroanatomy*, Ed. 2. C. V. Mosby, St. Louis.

NIEUWENHUYS, R., VOOGD, J., AND VAN HUIZEN, C. 1981. *The Human Central Nervous System*, Ed. 2. Springer-Verlag, Berlin.

NOBACK, C. R., AND DEMAREST, R. J. 1981. *The Human Nervous System*, Ed. 3. McGraw-Hill Book Company, New York.

PURPURA, D. P. 1970. Operations and processes in thalamic and synaptically related neural subsystems. In F. O. SCHMITT (Editor), *The Neurosciences, Second Study Program*. Rockefeller University Press, New York, Ch. 42, pp. 458–470.

TRUEX, R. C., AND KELLNER, C. E. 1948. *Detailed Atlas of the Head and Neck*. Oxford University Press, New York.

YOUNG, S. W. 1988. *Magnetic Resonance Imaging: Basic Principles*. Raven Press, New York.

3

Spinal Cord: Gross Anatomy and Internal Structure

The spinal cord is the least modified and most caudal portion of the embryonic neural tube. Although the spinal cord is a continuous unsegmented structure, pairs of spinal nerves associated with local regions impose an external segmentation.

GROSS ANATOMY

The spinal cord is a long cylindrical structure, invested by meninges, that lies in the vertebral canal. It extends from the foramen magnum (Fig. 1.4), where it is continuous with the medulla, to the lower border of the first lumbar vertebra (Fig. 1.7). Two enlargements of the spinal cord are recognized, cervical and lumbar, each associated with nerve roots that innervate, respectively, the upper and lower extremities (Fig. 3.1). Caudal to the lumbar enlargement, the spinal cord has a conical termination, the *conus medullaris* (Figs. 1.7 and 3.1). A condensation of pia mater, extending caudally from the conus medullaris, forms the *filum terminale*; the latter structure penetrates the dural tube at levels of the second sacral vertebra, becomes invested by dura, and continues as the coccygeal ligament to the posterior surface of the coccyx (Fig. 1.7).

The 31 pairs of spinal nerves associated with localized regions of the spinal cord produce an external segmentation. On this basis, the spinal cord is considered to consist of 31 segments, each of which receives and furnishes paired dorsal and ventral root filaments (Fig. 3.1). The spinal cord is divided into the following segments: 8 cervical, 12 thoracic, 5 lumbar, 5 sacral, and 1 coccygeal. Up to the third month of fetal life the spinal cord occupies the entire length of the vertebral canal, but after that time the differential rate of growth of the vertebral column exceeds that of the spinal cord. At birth the conus medullaris is located near the L3 vertebra; in the adult it is between the L1 and L2 vertebrae and occupies only the upper two-thirds of the vertebral canal. The sites of emergence of the spinal nerves do not change, but there is a lengthening of root filaments between the intervertebral foramina and the spinal cord, most marked for the lumbar and sacral spinal roots (Figs. 3.1 and 3.2). These spinal roots descend for a considerable distance within the dural sac before reaching their respective intervertebral foramina. Collectively lumbosacral roots surrounding the filum terminale are known as the *cauda equina* (Fig. 1.7). Spinal nerves emerge from the vertebral canal via the intervertebral foramina. The first cervical nerve emerges between the atlas and the occiput (Fig. 1.4). The eighth cervical root emerges from the intervertebral foramen between C7 and T1; all other spinal nerves emerge from the intervertebral foramina beneath the vertebrae of their

Figure 3.1. Posterior view of spinal cord showing attached dorsal root filaments and spinal ganglia. *Letters* and *numbers* indicate corresponding spinal nerves. (From Carpenter and Sutin, *Human Neuroanatomy*, 1983; courtesy of Williams & Wilkins.)

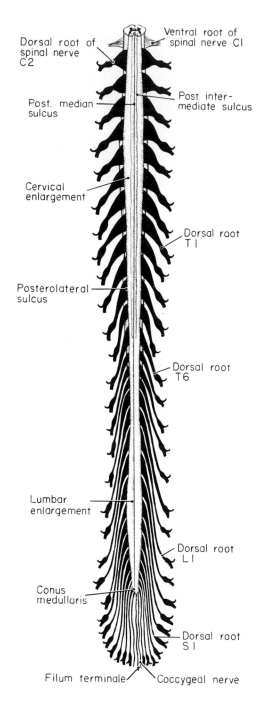

Dorsal root of spinal nerve C2

Ventral root of spinal nerve Cl

Post. median sulcus

Post. inter-mediate sulcus

Cervical enlargement

Dorsal root T I

Posterolateral sulcus

Dorsal root T 6

Lumbar enlargement

Dorsal root L I

Conus medullaris

Dorsal root S I

Filum terminale

Coccygeal nerve

same number (Fig. 3.2). Dorsal root fibers usually are absent in the first cervical and the coccygeal roots, and there are no corresponding dermatomes for these segments.

The spinal cord, like the entire central nervous system, is derived from the embryonic neural tube. The central canal, lined by ependymal cells, represents the vestigial lumen.

Topography

On the anterior surface a deep *anterior median fissure* penetrates the spinal cord almost to the gray commissure (Figs. 3.3 and 3.4). On the posterior surface of the spinal cord a small *posterior median sulcus* is

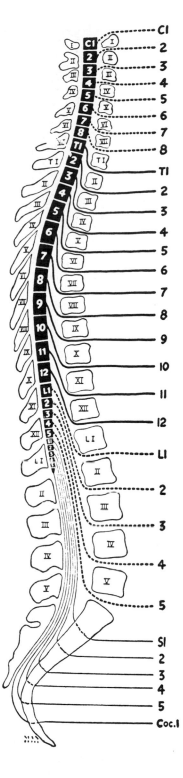

Figure 3.2. Diagram of the position of the spinal cord segments with reference to the bodies and spinous processes of the vertebrae. Locations of emergence and entrance of spinal roots are indicated. (From Carpenter and Sutin, *Human Neuroanatomy*, 1983; courtesy of Williams & Wilkins.)

continuous with a delicate glial partition, the *posterior median septum*, which extends to the spinal gray. Lateral to the midline posteriorly are two *posterolateral sulci* located near the dorsal root entry zones. Ascending and descending fibers occupying particular regions of the white matter are organized into more or less distinct bundles. Fiber bundles having the same origin, course, and termination are known as *tracts* or *fasciculi*. The white matter of the spinal cord is divided into three paired *funiculi*: posterior, lateral, and anterior. The *posterior funiculus* lies be-

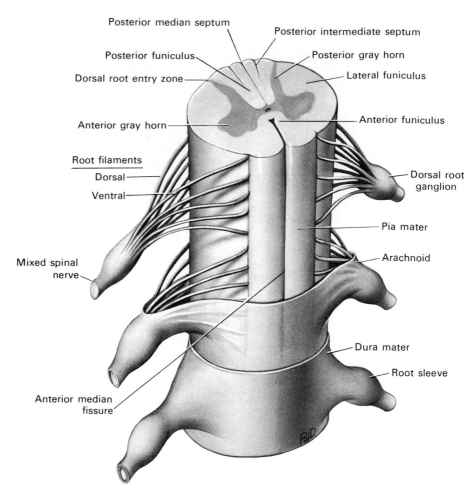

Figure 3.3. Drawing of the spinal cord, nerve roots, and meninges. The blood supply and venous drainage of the spinal cord are shown in Figures 14.1 and 14.2.

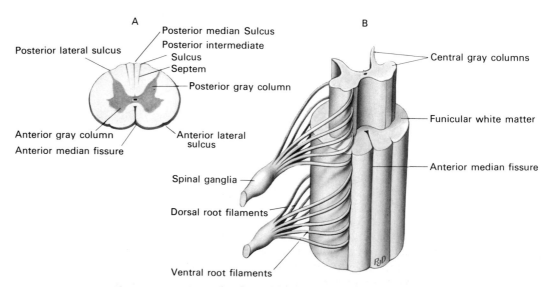

Figure 3.4. *A,* External and internal topography of cervical spinal cord. *B,* Diagram showing internal arrangement of gray and white matter of the spinal cord. (From Carpenter and Sutin, *Human Neuroanatomy,* 1983; courtesy of Williams & Wilkins.)

tween the posterior horn and the posterior median septum. In upper thoracic and cervical regions a smaller, less definite *posterior intermediate septum* divides each posterior funiculus into two white columns (Figs. 3.3, 3.4, and 3.5). The *lateral funiculus* lies between the dorsal root entry zone and the site where ventral root fibers emerge from the spinal cord. The anterior lateral sulcus marks the site at which ventral root fibers emerge (Fig. 3.4). The *anterior funiculus* lies between the anterior median fissure and the emerging ventral root filaments. The posterior funiculus is the largest and is composed almost exclusively of long ascending and short descending fibers that arise from cells in the spinal ganglia. Tracts composing the lateral and anterior funiculi are both ascending and descending. Ascending tracts in these funiculi arise from cells within the spinal gray; long descending tracts arise from nuclei in the brain stem and the cerebral cortex.

The *cervical enlargement*, consisting of the four lowest cervical segments and the first thoracic segment, gives rise to nerve roots that form the *brachial plexus* (Fig. 3.1). The *lumbar enlargement* gives rise to fibers that form the *lumbar plexus* (L1 to L4) and the *sacral plexus* (L4 to S2).

Although the spinal cord constitutes only 2% of the central nervous system, its functions are of great importance since it contains (1) afferent pathways that conduct sensory impulses from most of the body, (2) descending pathways that mediate voluntary motor function and modify muscle tone, and (3) fiber systems and neurons that mediate segmental reflexes and provide autonomic innervation.

INTERNAL STRUCTURE

In transverse section the spinal cord consists of (1) a butterfly-shaped central gray substance composed of collections of cell bodies and their processes, and (2) a surrounding mantle of white matter composed of bundles of myelinated fibers that are either ascending or descending in the three paired funiculi (Figs. 3.3 and 3.4). The symmetrical butterfly-shaped gray consists of cell columns that extend the length of the spinal cord and vary in configuration at different levels. Each half of the spinal cord has a *posterior gray column* or *posterior horn* that extends postero-laterally almost to the surface. An *anterior gray column* or *anterior horn* extends ventrally but does not reach the surface. In thoracic spinal segments a small, pointed *lateral horn* is evident near the base of the anterior horn (Figs. 1.6 and 3.5). A *gray commissure*, connecting the gray substance of the two sides, encompasses the central canal.

The gray and white matter of the spinal cord are composed of neural elements and their supporting neuroglial framework. Sections stained with hematoxylin and eosin, thionin, or cresyl violet reveal the cellular elements of the gray matter but leave the fibrous elements of the neuropil unstained. Only neuronal perikarya, glia, and endothelial nuclei are stained (Figs. 3.9 and 3.11). Myelin sheath stains such as the Weigert method, Marchi method, and Luxol fast blue reveal the bundles of myelinated fibers that compose the white matter and enter and leave the gray matter (Figs. 3.6 and 3.8). Golgi silver technics reveal cell bodies and their processes in minute detail. Information concerning the internal structure and organization of the spinal cord has been based on these classic histological technics, as well as on silver impregnation methods. Methods utilizing the physiological property of axoplasmic transport and radioactive amino acids, the enzyme horseradish peroxidase (HRP), and a variety of fluorescent dyes have further expanded knowledge of the organization of the nervous system. Immunocytochemical methods have

Figure 3.5. Diagrams of transverse sections of the spinal cord at various levels showing the variations in the size, shape, and topography of the gray and white matter. Variations in the cytoarchitectural laminations of Rexed (indicated by *Roman numerals*) are indicated at cervical, thoracic, and lumbar levels.

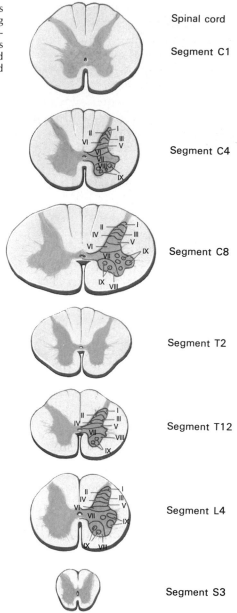

Spinal cord

Segment C1

Segment C4

Segment C8

Segment T2

Segment T12

Segment L4

Segment S3

provided information concerning neurotransmitters in cells and fiber systems that have important functional correlations.

Spinal Cord Levels

Different levels of the spinal cord vary in (1) size and shape, (2) the relative amounts of gray and white matter, and (3) the disposition and configuration of the gray matter (Fig. 3.5). Cervical spinal segments contain the largest number of fibers in the white matter because (1) descending fiber systems have not yet contributed fibers to lower segmental levels, and (2) ascending fiber systems, augmented at each successive rostral segment, reach their maximum. The gray columns are maximal in the cervical and lumbar enlargements, which are associated with larger nerves that innervate the extremities. Lumbosacral segments

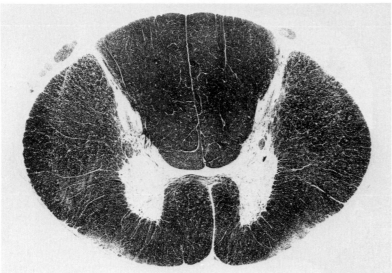

Figure 3.6. Photomicrograph of a transverse section through the second cervical segment of the adult human spinal cord. Note the narrowness of the anterior and posterior gray horns and the abundant white matter. Weigert's myelin stain. (From Carpenter and Sutin, *Human Neuroanatomy*, 1983; courtesy of Williams & Wilkins.)

contain the largest amount of gray matter, relative to both the size of the cord segments and the amount of white matter.

Cervical

These segments are characterized by their relatively large size, relatively large amounts of white matter, and an oval shape (Figs. 3.5 and 3.6). The transverse diameter exceeds the anteroposterior diameter at nearly all levels (Fig. 3.8). The posterior funiculus on each side is divided by a prominent posterior intermediate septum into a *fasciculus gracilis* (medial) and a *fasciculus cuneatus* (lateral) (Figs. 3.3, 3.4, and 3.5). In the lower cervical segments (C5 and below) the posterior horns are enlarged, and well-developed anterior horns extend into the lateral funiculi. Near the neck of the posterior horn is a serrated cellular area known as the reticular process, present throughout all cervical segments. In upper cervical segments (C1 and C2) the posterior horn is enlarged, but the anterior horn is relatively small (Fig. 3.6).

Thoracic

These segments show considerable variation in size at different levels. The small diameter of thoracic segments is due primarily to a marked reduction in gray matter (Fig. 3.5). Both the fasciculi gracilis and cuneatus are present in upper thoracic segments (T1 to T6) while only the fasciculus gracilis is seen at more caudal levels (Figs. 3.10 and 3.13). The anterior and posterior horns generally are small and somewhat tapered; the first thoracic segment is an exception in that it forms the lowest segment of the cervical enlargement. A small lateral horn, present at all thoracic levels, contains the intermediolateral cell column, which gives rise to preganglionic sympathetic efferent fibers (Figs. 3.10 and 3.11). At the base of the medial aspect of the posterior horn is a rounded collection of large cells, the *dorsal nucleus of Clarke* or *nucleus thoracicus* (Fig. 3.10). While this nucleus is present in all thoracic segments, it is particularly well developed at T10 through L2 (Fig. 3.13).

Lumbar

These segments are nearly circular in transverse section, have massive anterior and posterior horns, and contain relatively and absolutely less white matter than cervical segments (Fig. 3.5). The fasciculi gracilis

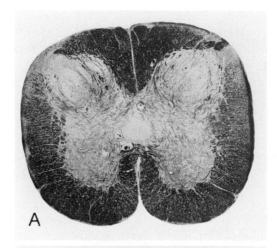

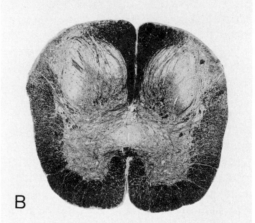

in the posterior funiculus is not as broad as at higher levels, especially near the gray commissure, and has a highly characteristic configuration (Fig. 3.14). The well-developed anterior horns have a blunt process that extends into the lateral funiculi; motor cells in this process in segments L3 through L5 innervate large muscle groups in the lower extremities. Upper lumbar levels (L1 and L2) resemble lower thoracic spinal segments in that they contain a large well-developed dorsal nucleus and an intermediolateral cell column.

Sacral

These segments are characterized by their small size; relatively large amounts of gray matter; relatively small amounts of white matter; and a short, thick gray commissure (Figs. 3.5 and 3.7). The anterior and posterior horns are large and thick, but the anterior horn is not bayed out laterally as in lumbar spinal segments. In caudal sequence sacral segments conspicuously diminish in overall diameter but retain relatively large proportions of gray matter (Figs. 3.16 and 3.17). Coccygeal segments resemble lower sacral spinal segments but are greatly reduced in size (Fig. 3.7). Fibers in the posterior columns tend to spread laterally over the enlarged posterior horns.

Nuclei and Cell Groups

The butterfly-shaped gray matter of the spinal cord contains an enormous number of neurons of varying size and shape. Basically these cells can be classified as root cells and column cells.

Root cells lie in the anterior and lateral horns and give rise to axons that exit via the ventral root to innervate somatic or visceral effectors.

Column cells are neurons whose peripheral processes are confined within the central nervous system. On the basis of the length, course, and axonal synaptic articulations, these cells can be classified as *central, internuncial, commissural,* or *association neurons.* A large number of column cells give rise to fibers that enter the white matter, bifurcate, and ascend or descend for variable distances. Some of these fibers form part of an intersegmental fiber system. Other fibers have long processes that ascend to higher levels of the neuraxis and transmit impulses related to specific sensory modalities. Nerve cells are organized in the gray matter into more or less definite groups that extend longitudinally and are referred to as cell columns or nuclei. In the neuroanatomical sense, a nucleus consists of a collection of cells with common cytological characteristics, which give rise to fibers that follow a common path, have a common termination, and subserve the same function. Most of our information concerning the structural organization of the central nervous system is centered around this concept. The spinal gray also contains Golgi type II cells whose short unmyelinated axons may be commissural, intersegmental, or terminate close to their origin.

Cytoarchitectural Lamination

A variety of inconsistent terminologies based on cytological features and topographical locations of cell groups within the spinal gray have been replaced by a terminology based on cytoarchitectural lamination of the spinal gray (Fig. 3.5). Although Rexed described this neuronal lamination in thick sections (80 to 100 μm) of the cat spinal cord, it is generally accepted that a similar lamination exists in the spinal gray in all mammals, including man. Examples of this cytoarchitectural lamination in man have been used to illustrate this chapter (Figs. 3.9, 3.11, 3.15, and 3.17).

Studies of the *cytoarchitectonic organization* of the spinal cord indicate nine distinct cellular laminae identified by Roman numerals and an area X, representing the gray surrounding the central canal (Figs. 3.5 and 3.9). There are differences in configuration of laminae at various segmental levels of the spinal cord. These laminae constitute regions with characteristic cytological features, but their boundaries are zones of transition where changes may occur either gradually or abruptly. While most laminae are present in some form at all spinal levels, lamina VI represents an exception in that it is absent between T4 and L2 (Fig. 3.11). Lamina VII occupies a large heterogeneous region extending across the central part of the spinal gray with boundaries that vary at different levels. In the spinal enlargements lamina VII extends ventrally into the anterior gray horn (Figs. 3.5 and 3.9), while in thoracic segments it occupies a zone between the anterior and posterior horns (Fig. 3.11), referred to as the *zona intermedia* (intermediate gray). Only the principal features of the individual lamina are described here. Some of the laminae, or cell aggregations within specific lamina, correspond to recognized cell columns or nuclei, while others are regional admixtures of cells.

Lamina I is a thin veil of gray substance that caps the surface of the posterior horn and bends around its margins (Figs. 3.9, 3.11, and 3.12). It contains small and medium-sized cells and scattered fairly large spindle-shaped cells oriented parallel to convex surface of the posterior horn. Arrays of nonmyelinated axons, small dendrites, and synaptic knobs lie within this lamina, which corresponds to the *posteromarginal nucleus*

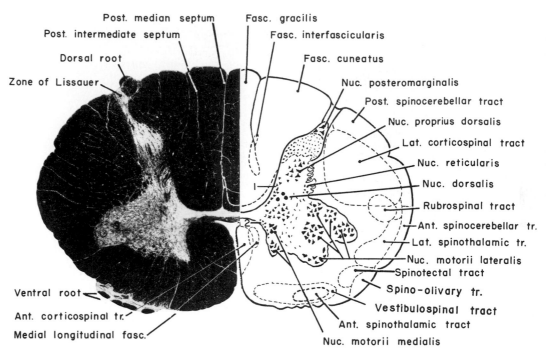

Post. median septum
Post. intermediate septum
Dorsal root
Zone of Lissauer

Fasc. gracilis
Fasc. interfascicularis
Fasc. cuneatus
Nuc. posteromarginalis
Post. spinocerebellar tract
Nuc. proprius dorsalis
Lat. corticospinal tract
Nuc. reticularis
Nuc. dorsalis
Rubrospinal tract
Ant. spinocerebellar tr.
Lat. spinothalamic tr.
Nuc. motorii lateralis
Spinotectal tract
Spino-olivary tr.
Vestibulospinal tract
Ant. spinothalamic tract
Nuc. motorii medialis

Ventral root
Ant. corticospinal tr.
Medial longitudinal fasc.

Figure 3.8. Section through eighth cervical segment of adult human spinal cord. The important cell groups and fiber tracts are identified. *1*, Nucleus cornucommissuralis posterior; *2*, nucleus cornucommissuralis anterior. Weigert's myelin stain. Photograph. (From Carpenter and Sutin, *Human Neuroanatomy*, 1983; courtesy of Williams & Wilkins.)

Figure 3.9. Cytoarchitectural lamination of the gray matter of the C6 segment indicated on a thick section of the human spinal cord. The central canal (*CC*) and intermediomedial nucleus (*IM*) are identified. Compare with Figure 3.8. Thionin stain. Photograph. ×9. (From Carpenter and Sutin, *Human Neuroanatomy*, 1983; courtesy of Williams & Wilkins.)

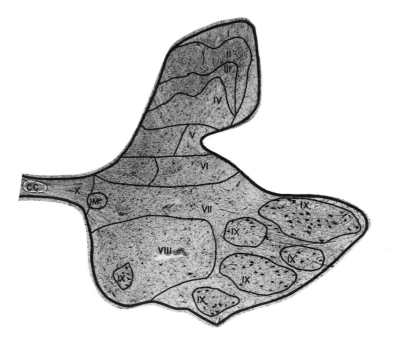

(Figs. 3.14 and 3.15). Axons from neurons in lamina II end axosomatically upon cells in lamina I, while primarily afferent fibers terminate axodendritically upon the same cell population (Fig. 3.12). A large proportion of axons from both of these sources reach lamina I via the *dorsolateral fasciculus of Lissauer* (Figs. 3.8 and 3.14). Cells in lamina I respond specifically to noxious and thermal stimuli and contribute fibers to the contralateral spinothalamic tract. Immunocytochemical studies indicate that lamina I contains cells positive for substance P (SP) and enkephalin

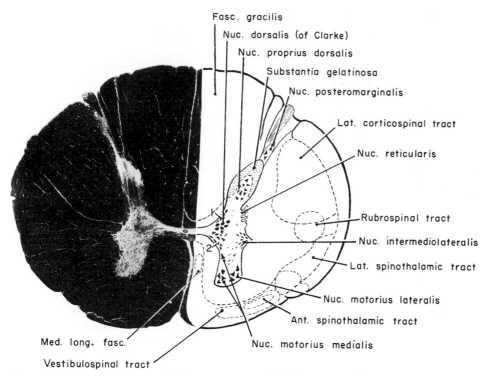

Figure 3.10.   Section through the fifth thoracic segment of adult human spinal cord. Important cell groups and fiber tracts are identified. *1*, Nucleus cornucommissuralis posterior; *2*, nucleus cornucommissuralis anterior. Weigert's myelin stain. Photograph. (From Carpenter and Sutin, *Human Neuroanatomy*, 1983; courtesy of Williams & Wilkins.)

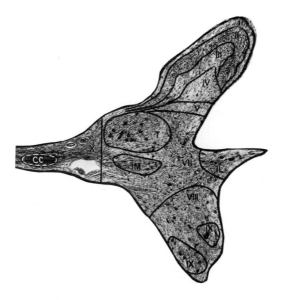

Figure 3.11.   Cytoarchitectural lamination of the gray matter of the T10 segment indicated on a thick section of the human spinal cord. The central canal (*CC*), intermediomedial nucleus (*IM*), and the dorsal nucleus of Clarke (nucleus thoracicus, *T*) are identified. Compare with Figure 3.10. Thionin stain. Photograph. ×14. (From Carpenter and Sutin, *Human Neuroanatomy*, 1983; courtesy of Williams & Wilkins.)

(ENK), as well as fibers immunoreactive for SP, ENK, somatostatin (SRIF), and serotonin (5-HT).

Lamina II forms a well-delineated, fairly broad band around the apex of the posterior horn readily identified in cell and myelin sheath stains (Figs. 3.5, 3.8, 3.10, 3.14, and 3.15). This highly cellular band is covered dorsolaterally by lamina I, but its medial border is the posterior funiculus (Fig. 3.8). Lamina II, composed of tightly packed small cells, corresponds to the *substantia gelatinosa* and is found at all spinal levels. Two zones are recognized within lamina II: (1) a narrower *outer zone* with slightly smaller cells and (2) a broader *inner zone*. In both zones

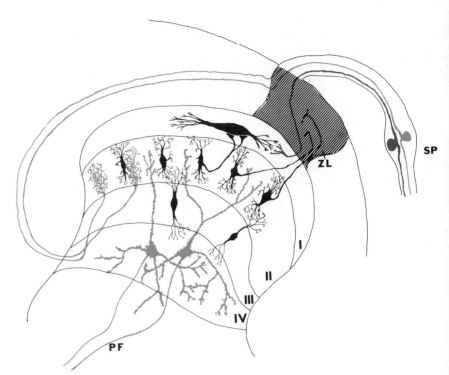

Figure 3.12. Schematic diagram of cutaneous input into the posterior gray horn. I, II, III, and IV represent laminae of Rexed; SP is the spinal ganglion, and ZL (shaded area) is the zone of Lissauer. Primary nociceptive afferents (*red*) enter lateral parts of the root entry zone, traverse the zone of Lissauer, and synapse upon distal dendrites of larger cells in the posteromarginal nucleus (lamina I). Substantia gelatinosa neurons in lamina II provide axons, or axon collaterals, that synapse on the soma of cells in lamina I and longer axons that ascend or descend in the zone of Lissauer to ultimately return to lamina II at other levels. Nonnociceptive primary afferents (*blue*) enter as part of the medial division of root fibers by passing either medial to or through the superficial gray laminae. These larger caliber fibers enter lamina II from its ventral aspect and end in terminal arbors near substantia gelatinosa neurons and in relation to dendrites of large cells of the proper sensory nucleus in lamina IV. Large cells in lamina IV give rise to projection fibers (PF), which cross in the anterior white commissure and project to the thalamus. Some cells in laminae I and V also give rise to projections that reach the thalamus. (From Carpenter and Sutin, *Human Neuroanatomy*, 1983; courtesy of Williams & Wilkins.)

round or elliptical neurons are oriented radially to the surface (Fig. 3.12). Spindle-shaped cell bodies, hardly larger than the nucleus, give rise to rich dendritic trees from one or both poles. The absence of discrete Nissl bodies in light microscopy is correlated with a paucity of granular endoplasmic reticulum at the ultrastructural level. Numerous bundles of unmyelinated axons in lamina II run parallel and perpendicular to the axis of the spinal cord, while myelinated axons pass radially through lamina II to deeper regions of the spinal gray.

As central processes of spinal ganglion cells approach the dorsal root entry zone, small, fine fibers shift to lateral portions of the rootlets while larger fibers are segregated medially. Upon entering the spinal cord, root fibers bifurcate into ascending and descending branches (Fig. 3.22). Small unmyelinated and poorly myelinated fibers in the lateral division (Fig. 3.20) contribute to the dorsolateral fasciculus of Lissauer (Fig. 3.14). Afferent fibers to lamina II are derived from (1) the dorsolateral fasciculus, (2) the posterior funiculus, and (3) adjacent parts of the lateral funiculus. Collateral fibers from these sources enter lamina II in a radial fashion forming flame-shaped terminal arborizations that make synaptic contacts with large numbers of neurons (Fig. 3.12). Terminal arborizations within lamina II have a columnar arrangement with little overlap.

The finest afferent fibers terminate in the outer zone of lamina II, while small myelinated fibers end in the inner zone. Physiological observations on morphologically identified cells indicate that cell bodies of nociceptive and thermoreceptive neurons tend to be located in lamina I and the outer zone of lamina II, while neurons responding to innocuous mechanoreceptive stimuli are located in the inner zone of lamina II.

The majority of neurons in lamina II send axons into the dorsolateral fasciculus or the fasciculus proprius (Fig. 3.12). Axons from cells in lamina II also have been traced into this same lamina at other spinal levels. None of the axons from cells in this lamina have been traced into other structures that could relay impulses into recognized ascending sensory pathways. Lamina II has been regarded as a "closed system," which can influence larger neurons in deeper layers of the spinal gray whose dendrites extend into lamina II (Fig. 3.12). Because neurons in lamina II appear organized to exert influences on larger cells in laminae III and IV, these neurons have been considered to play a modulating role in the transmission of sensory signals.

Laminae I and II contain high concentrations of substance P (Fig. 3.21), an undecapeptide synthesized in spinal ganglia and transported to terminals of dorsal root fibers. This peptide, selectively distributed in the central nervous system, has especially high concentrations in areas receiving sensory afferents. Substance P is considered to have an excitatory role in the central transmission of impulses associated with pain. Opiate receptors, which mediate all pharmacological effects of opiates, are highly concentrated in laminae I and II. Unilateral section of multiple dorsal roots has demonstrated a 50% loss of opiate receptor binding sites in spinal segments on the side of the dorsal rhizotomies. The distribution of enkephalin, an endogenous opioid peptide, appears to parallel the distribution of opiate receptor binding sites in the primate brain (Fig. 3.19A). Thus opiate receptors and their natural ligand compose an endogenous "pain suppression system."

Lamina III forms a band across the posterior horn parallel with laminae I and II in which larger cells are oriented vertically with their dendritic arborization extending dorsally into laminae I and II (Fig. 3.12). Axons of these neurons bifurcate a number of times to form a dense plexus in laminae III and IV. Thus, most cells in lamina III are anatomically organized to function as interneurons.

Lamina IV, the thickest of the first four laminae of the posterior horn, extends across the width of the posterior horn and is composed of round, triangular, or star-shaped neurons, a few of which are quite large (Figs. 3.8 and 3.12). Dendrites of neurons in lamina IV radiate upward into lamina II in a candelabra fashion parallel to primary sensory fibers and intrinsic neurons of that lamina. Cells in laminae III and IV correspond to the *proper sensory nucleus* of the older terminology (Figs. 3.8, 3.10, and 3.13). Neurons of lamina IV respond to low intensity stimuli, such as light touch. Axons of some cells in this lamina cross at spinal levels and ascend to the thalamus.

Lamina V is a broad zone extending across the neck of the posterior horn, which is divided into medial and lateral parts, except in thoracic segments (Figs. 3.9 and 3.12). Lateral parts of lamina V give rise to the reticular process, which is most prominent at cervical levels (Fig. 3.9). Neurons of lamina V are variable in size and shape, and dendrites of some cells extend upward into lamina II where they are contacted by dorsal root fibers.

Lamina VI extends across the base of the posterior horn and is

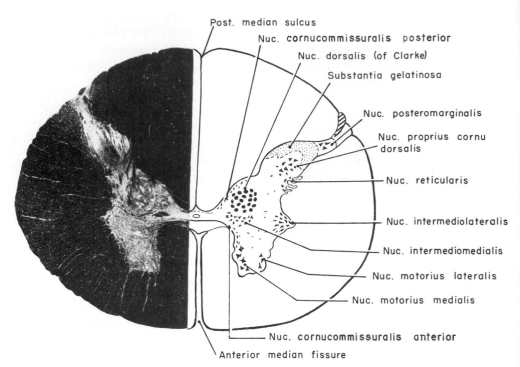

Post. median sulcus
Nuc. cornucommissuralis posterior
Nuc. dorsalis (of Clarke)
Substantia gelatinosa
Nuc. posteromarginalis
Nuc. proprius cornu dorsalis
Nuc. reticularis
Nuc. intermediolateralis
Nuc. intermediomedialis
Nuc. motorius lateralis
Nuc. motorius medialis
Nuc. cornucommissuralis anterior
Anterior median fissure

Figure 3.13. Section through the twelfth thoracic segment of the adult human spinal cord. Important cell groups are identified on the right. Weigert's myelin stain. Photograph. (From Carpenter and Sutin, *Human Neuroanatomy*, 1983; courtesy of Williams & Wilkins.)

present only in the cord enlargements. This lamina is divided into medial and lateral regions; group I muscle afferents terminate in the medial zone, while descending spinal pathways project to the lateral zone.

Lamina VII, also known as the *zona intermedia*, lies between the anterior and posterior horns. The boundaries of this lamina vary at different levels; in the spinal enlargements lamina VII extends ventrally into the anterior horn (Fig. 3.5 and 3.9), but at other levels it forms a narrower band across the spinal gray and includes the lateral horn (Fig. 3.11). Light-staining neurons, a large number of which are internuncial, are evenly distributed in this lamina. Well-defined cell columns that extend for some rostrocaudal distance within this lamina include the dorsal, the intermediolateral, and the intermediomedial nuclei.

The *dorsal nucleus of Clarke* (nucleus thoracicus) forms a prominent round or oval cell column in the medial part of lamina VII that extends from C8 to L2 (Figs. 3.11 and 3.13). Large multipolar or oval cells of this nucleus with coarse Nissl granules have characteristic eccentric nuclei. Collaterals of dorsal root afferents establish secure synapses upon cells of this nucleus at multiple levels. Cells of the dorsal nucleus give rise to uncrossed fibers of the *posterior spinocerebellar tract*. Cells in lamina VII and adjacent parts of laminae V and VI, which do not form a discrete nucleus, give rise to crossed fibers that form the *anterior spinocerebellar tract*.

The *intermediolateral nucleus* forms a cell column in the apical region of the lateral horn in thoracic and upper lumbar spinal segments (T1 through L2 or L3). Spindle-shaped cells of this nucleus give rise to preganglionic sympathetic fibers that emerge via the ventral roots and project to various sympathetic ganglia via the white rami communicants (Figs. 3.10 and 3.11).

Sacral autonomic nuclei occupy corresponding positions in lateral

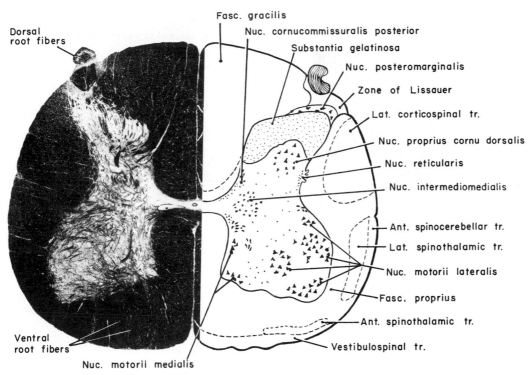

Figure 3.14. Section through the fourth lumbar segment of the adult human spinal cord. The important cell groups and fiber tracts are identified. Weigert's myelin stain. Photograph. (From Carpenter and Sutin, *Human Neuroanatomy*, 1983; courtesy of Williams & Wilkins.)

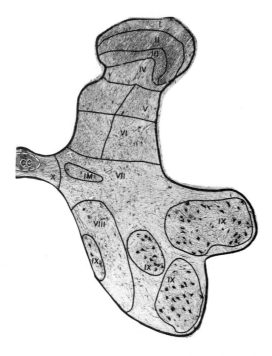

Figure 3.15. Cytoarchitectural lamination of the gray matter of the L5 segment indicated on a thick section of the human spinal cord. The central canal (*CC*) and the intermedio-medial nucleus (*IM*) are identified. Compare with Figure 3.14. Thionin stain. Photograph. ×7.5. (From Carpenter and Sutin, *Human Neuroanatomy*, 1983; courtesy of Williams & Wilkins.)

regions of lamina VII in segments S2, 3, and S4, even though no lateral horn is present. These neurons resemble those of the intermedio-lateral cell column but give rise to preganglionic parasympathetic fibers that exit via sacral ventral roots and form the "pelvic nerves." Cells of the intermediolateral cell column in thoracic and upper lumbar spinal segments and sacral visceral neurons are cholinergic and immunoreactive to choline acetyltransferase (ChAT) (Fig. 3.19*B*).

Figure 3.16. Section through third sacral segment of adult human spinal cord. The important cell groups and fiber tracts are identified. *1*, Nucleus cornucommissuralis posterior; *2*, nucleus cornucommissuralis anterior. Weigert's myelin stain. Photograph. (From Carpenter and Sutin, *Human Neuroanatomy*, 1983; courtesy of Williams & Wilkins.)

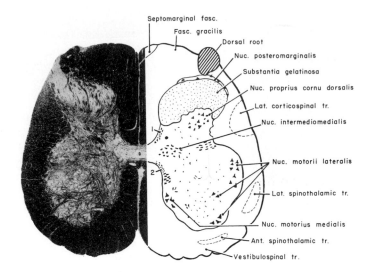

Figure 3.17. Cytoarchitectural lamination of the gray matter of the S4 segment of a thick section of the human spinal cord. Structures identified are the commissural nucleus (*C*), the central canal (*CC*), and the intermediomedial nucleus (*IM*). Compare with Figure 3.16. Thionin stain. Photograph. ×15. (From Carpenter and Sutin, *Human Neuroanatomy*, 1983; courtesy of Williams & Wilkins.)

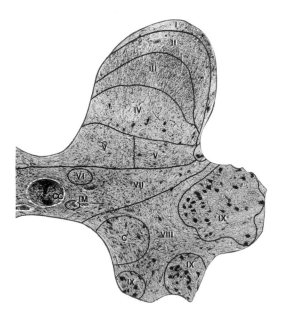

The *intermediomedial nucleus* forms a small cell column in the medial part of lamina VII, lateral to the central canal that extends the length of the spinal cord (Figs. 3.10 and 3.13). This nucleus receives visceral afferents at all spinal levels.

The *central cervical nucleus* forms an interrupted cell column in the upper four cervical spinal segments that extend into the caudal medulla. Large polygonal cells of this nucleus lie lateral to the intermediomedial nucleus. Cells of the central cervical nucleus receive dorsal root fibers and give rise to crossed projections to the cerebellum and the inferior vestibular nucleus.

Lamina VIII is a zone of heterogeneous cells at the base of the anterior horn that varies in size and configuration at different levels (Figs. 3.5, 3.9, and 3.11). In the cord enlargements, lamina VIII occupies only the medial part of the anterior horn, but at other levels it extends across the base of the anterior horn ventral to lamina VII. This lamina constitutes a discrete entity, in part, because fibers of a number of specific descending tracts terminate upon cells within its boundaries.

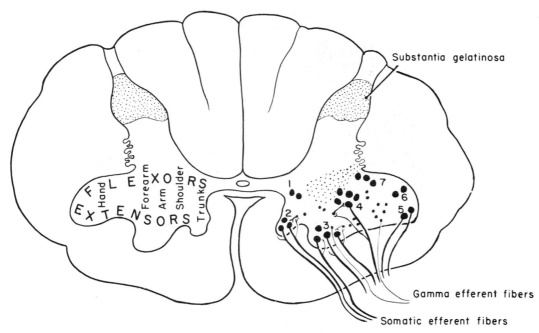

Figure 3.18. Diagram of motor nuclei in anterior gray horn of a lower cervical spinal segment. On the *left* the general location of anterior horn cells innervating the muscle groups of the upper extremity are shown. Groups of motor nuclei indicated on the *right* are *1*, posteromedial; *2*, anteromedial; *3*, anterior; *4*, central; *5*, anterolateral; *6*, posterolateral; *7*, retroposterolateral. Smaller anterior horn cells (gamma neurons) supply the intrafusal muscle fibers of neuromuscular spindle (Fig. 3.23). Note the collaterals from somatic efferent axons that return to gray matter and synapse on small medially placed "Renshaw cells." Smaller cells represented as dots in the intermediate gray (lamina VII) indicate the area of the internuncial neurons. (From Carpenter and Sutin, *Human Neuroanatomy*, 1983; courtesy of Williams & Wilkins.)

Lamina IX consists of several distinct clusters of large somatic motor neurons that occupy somewhat different positions within the anterior gray horn at various spinal levels (Figs. 3.5, 3.9, 3.11, and 3.15). In thoracic spinal segments, smaller islands of motor neurons occupy ventral parts of the anterior horn (Fig. 3.11), but in the cord enlargements, larger numbers of motor neurons form more numerous groups (Fig. 3.9). Anterior horn cells of this lamina are large multipolar neurons (30 to 70 μm) with central nuclei, coarse Nissl granules, multiple dendrites, and large axons that exit via the ventral root. Large somatic motor cells of the anterior horn that innervate striate muscle are referred to as alpha (α) motor neurons. Scattered among these large motor cells are smaller gamma (γ) neurons that give rise to efferent fibers that emerge via the ventral root and innervate the contractile elements of the muscle spindle (i.e., intrafusal muscle fibers). Gamma efferent fibers play an essential role in the maintenance of muscle tone and bring the muscle spindle under control of spinal and supraspinal influences (Figs. 3.23 and 3.24).

Anterior horn cells are organized into medial and lateral groups, each with several subdivisions. The *medial nuclear group* extends the entire length of the spinal cord and consists of posteromedial and anteromedial subdivisions (Figs. 3.8 and 3.18). The anteromedial subgroup is larger and most prominent in upper cervical, upper thoracic, and in certain lumbosacral segments (L3, S4, S2, and S3). The smaller posteromedial subgroup is most distinct in the cord enlargements. The medial motor cell column innervates axial muscle groups. Cells of the *lateral nuclear*

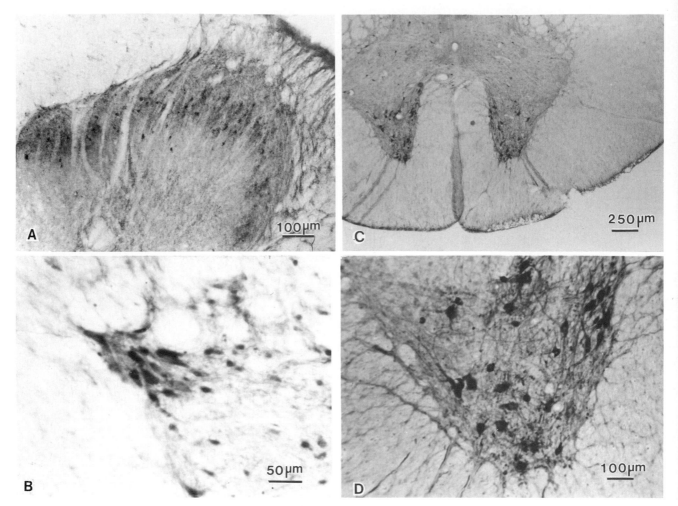

Figure 3.19. Immunocytochemical staining of spinal neurons in the monkey. *A*, Neurons in deep portions of lamina II at C1 immunoreactive to leucine enkephalin. *B*, Visceral neurons in the intermediolateral cell column at a thoracic level immunoreactive to choline acetyl-transferase (ChAT). *C and D*, Spinal motor neurons in the anterior horn immunoreactive to ChAT.

group show considerable variations in number and size and innervate the remaining body musculature (Figs. 3.9 and 3.18). In thoracic segments a relatively small number of cells innervate the intercostal and anterolateral trunk muscles (Fig. 3.10). In the cervical and lumbar enlargements the lateral nuclear groups are enlarged and several subgroups can be distinguished. Lateral cell groups innervate the appendicular musculature (Fig. 3.18). In general the more distal muscles are supplied by the more lateral cell groups. Passing in an arc from the most medial part of the anterior horn to its lateral periphery, motor neurons successively innervate muscles of the trunk, shoulder and pelvic girdle, proximal arm and leg, and distal arm and leg (Fig. 3.18). The retroposterolateral cell groups supply the small intrinsic muscles of the hand and foot.

Alpha motor neurons of the anterior horn contain and release ace-tylcholine (ACh) at their terminals; this is evidenced by immunoreactivity to choline acetyltransferase (ChAT), the synthesizing enzyme (Fig. 3.19*C*, *D*). Some of the small cells in the anterior horn are immunoreactive to gamma-aminobutyric acid (GABA), an inhibitory neurotransmitter.

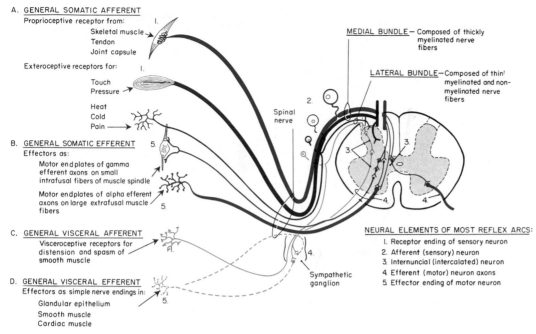

A. GENERAL SOMATIC AFFERENT
Proprioceptive receptor from:
    Skeletal muscle
    Tendon
    Joint capsule

Exteroceptive receptors for:
    Touch
    Pressure
    Heat
    Cold
    Pain

B. GENERAL SOMATIC EFFERENT
Effectors as:
    Motor endplates of gamma efferent axons on small intrafusal fibers of muscle spindle
    Motor endplates of alpha efferent axons on large extrafusal muscle fibers

C. GENERAL VISCERAL AFFERENT
    Visceroceptive receptors for distension and spasm of smooth muscle

D. GENERAL VISCERAL EFFERENT
Effectors as simple nerve endings in:
    Glandular epithelium
    Smooth muscle
    Cardiac muscle

MEDIAL BUNDLE — Composed of thickly myelinated nerve fibers

LATERAL BUNDLE — Composed of thinly myelinated and non-myelinated nerve fibers

Spinal nerve

Sympathetic ganglion

NEURAL ELEMENTS OF MOST REFLEX ARCS:
1. Receptor ending of sensory neuron
2. Afferent (sensory) neuron
3. Internuncial (intercalated) neuron
4. Efferent (motor) neuron axons
5. Effector ending of motor neuron

Figure 3.20.   Diagram of functional components of a thoracic spinal nerve and the arrangement of dorsal root fibers as they enter the spinal cord via medial and lateral bundles. Muscle afferent and efferent fibers are indicated in *red*. Visceral afferent and efferent fibers are shown in *blue*. An afferent fiber from a Pacinian corpuscle (*black*) and a thin pain fiber (*black*) also are shown. Numbers in the diagram correspond to neural elements that form reflex arcs. (From Carpenter and Sutin, *Human Neuroanatomy*, 1983; courtesy of Williams & Wilkins.)

DORSAL ROOT AFFERENTS

Sensory neurons within dorsal root ganglia have been divided into two classes on the basis of perikaryal size. While there is little direct evidence for relationships between perikaryal size and axon diameters, there are histochemical differences in dorsal root ganglion cells. Small cell populations of the dorsal root ganglia contain substance P (SP), somatostatin (SRIF), and cholecystokinin (CCK). Considerable evidence suggests that glutamate (GLU) may be the principal neurotransmitter of cells in spinal and sensory cranial nerve ganglia. Nearly half of the spinal ganglion cells appear to contain GLU. Many small dorsal root ganglion cells (35–65%) exhibit colocalization of SP and GLU. These two neurotransmitters may be coreleased from the same afferent terminals in portions of Rexed's lamina II.

Central processes of cells in the spinal ganglia enter the dorsolateral aspect of the spinal cord in small fascicles over a considerable distance (Fig. 3.3). Peripheral processes of these cells convey impulses centrally from various somatic and visceral receptors (Fig. 3.20). As the central processes of spinal ganglion cells approach the dorsal root entry zone, small fine fibers become segregated in lateral portions of the rootlet. Larger fibers shift medially in the rootlets and enter the posterior columns or traverse medial parts of the posterior horn (Fig. 3.20). Thus root fibers of spinal ganglia become segregated into a medial bundle of thick myelinated fibers and a lateral bundle of thinly myelinated and nonmyelinated fibers. The *medial bundle* of thickly myelinated fibers represents central

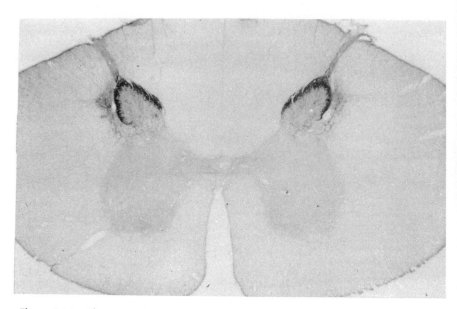

Figure 3.21. Photomicrograph of the monkey spinal cord immunoreacted with antiserum to substance P (SP). Substance P immunoreactive fibers and terminals are present in the root entry zone and in the most superficial laminae (I and outer II) of the dorsal horn. SP is considered to be associated with fibers that transmit impulses related to pain and noxious stimuli. Enkephalinergic neurons present in deep parts of lamina II (Fig. 3.19A) may modulate the release of SP at terminals. (Courtesy of Professor Stephen Hunt, University of Cambridge.)

processes of spinal ganglion cells conveying impulses from encapsulated somatic receptors, such as neuromuscular spindles, Golgi tendon organs, Pacinian corpuscles, and Meissner's corpuscles (Fig. 3.20). The *lateral bundle* represents the central processes of smaller ganglion cells related to free nerve endings, tactile, thermal, and other somatic and visceral receptors. Upon entering the spinal cord, the central processes of each dorsal root ganglion cell divide into ascending and descending branches that give rise to collateral branches (Fig. 3.22). Most of the collateral branches are given off in the segment of entry; these collaterals either participate in intrasegmental reflexes or relay impulses to other neurons. The long ascending primary branches of the medial bundle enter the ipsilateral posterior funiculus, and many, but not all, fibers ascend without synapse as far as the medulla (Figs. 3.20 and 3.22). Most of the primary afferent fibers entering laminae III and IV are intermediate to thick fibers that pass through or around lamina II and after a recurving course in the gray matter approach cells in the proper sensory nucleus from a ventral direction (Fig. 3.12). Primary afferent fibers largely terminate upon dendrites of these neurons. Most neurons in lamina IV respond to low intensity stimuli, such as light touch.

One of the principal sites of termination of large myelinated dorsal root fibers is the dorsal nucleus of Clarke (Fig. 3.13). This nucleus receives fibers at different levels from all ipsilateral dorsal roots, except upper cervical roots. There is considerable overlap of afferent fibers from different dorsal roots, which reach the nucleus via both ascending and descending collaterals. The greatest number of afferents are related to the hindlimb. Synapses of dorsal root afferents upon the cells of Clarke's nucleus appear uniquely secure. Collaterals of dorsal root fibers traverse central parts of lamina VII to enter laminae VIII and IX. Dorsal root collaterals from muscle spindle afferents (i.e., group Ia), projecting to lamina IX and synapsing upon α-motor neurons or their dendrites, participate in the monosynaptic myotatic reflex (Figs. 3.22 and 3.23).

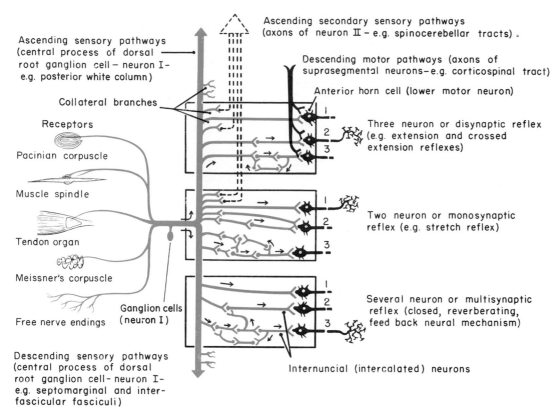

Figure 3.22.   Diagram of major branches and collaterals of spinal ganglion cells within three spinal cord segments. On the left are various receptors that generate impulses in response to different kinds of stimuli. Impulses from muscle spindles initiate the myotatic or stretch reflex involving two neurons (monosynaptic reflex). Impulses from tendon organ initiate disynaptic reflex circuits involving inhibitory mechanisms. Other reflex circuits may involve many neurons (multisynaptic). Also indicated are ascending and descending branches of dorsal root fibers in the posterior white column (see Fig. 4.1) and collateral pathways that project fibers to the cerebellum (Fig. 4.4). (From Carpenter and Sutin, *Human Neuroanatomy*, 1983; courtesy of Williams & Wilkins.)

The *zone of Lissauer* (dorsolateral fasciculus) lies dorsolateral to lamina I in the root entry zone and is composed of (1) fine myelinated and unmyelinated dorsal root fibers and (2) large numbers of endogenous propriospinal fibers that interconnect different levels of the substantia gelatinosa. Fine thinly myelinated and unmyelinated fibers in the lateral bundle of the dorsal root, conveying impulses associated with pain, thermal sense, and light tactile sense, enter the medial part of the zone of Lissauer and/or terminate directly in portions of laminae I and II (Figs. 3.12, 3.14, and 3.20). Cells in lamina I and the outer zone of lamina II receive projections from cutaneous nociceptors. Primary afferent fibers terminating in the inner zone of lamina II are related to innocuous mechanoreceptors.

PAIN MECHANISMS

Pain of varying character and intensity constitutes one of the most common complaints in medicine, yet its nature is unresolved. Pain is a sensory experience evoked by stimuli that injure or threaten to destroy tissue that is defined introspectively by every man. There are two principal theories concerning pain: (1) the theory that considers pain a specific sensory modality and (2) the pattern theory that maintains that the im-

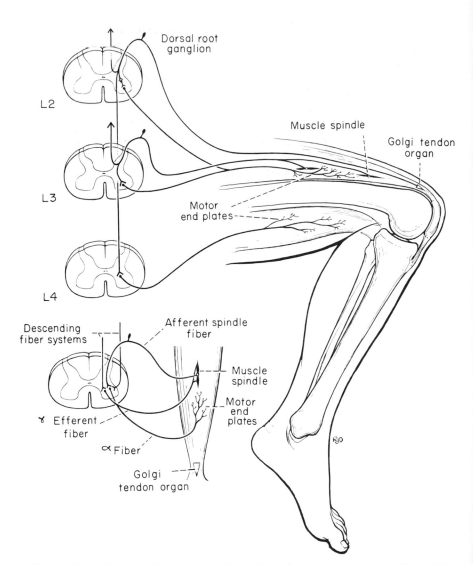

Figure 3.23. Schematic diagram of patellar tendon reflex. Motor and sensory fibers of the femoral nerve associated with spinal segments L2, L3, and L4 mediate this myotatic reflex. The principle receptors are the muscle spindles, which respond to a brisk stretching of the muscle effected usually by tapping the patellar tendon. Afferent fibers from muscle spindles are shown entering only the L3 spinal segment, while afferent fibers from the Golgi tendon organ are shown entering only the L2 spinal segment. In this monosynaptic reflex, afferent fibers entering spinal segments L2, L3, and L4 and efferent fibers issuing from the anterior horn cells of these levels complete the reflex arc. Motor fibers shown leaving the L4 spinal segment and passing to the hamstring muscles demonstrate the pathway by which inhibitory influences are exerted on an antagonistic muscle group during the reflex. The *small diagram below* illustrates the gamma (γ) loop. Gamma efferent fibers pass to the polar portions of the muscle spindle. Contractions of the intrafusal fibers in the polar parts of the spindle stretch the nuclear bag region and thus cause an afferent impulse to be conducted centrally. The afferent fibers from the spindle synapse upon an alpha (α) motor neuron, whose peripheral processes pass to extrafusal muscle fibers, thus completing the loop. Both α and γ motor neurons can be influenced by descending fiber systems from supraspinal levels. These are indicated separately. (From Carpenter and Sutin, *Human Neuroanatomy*, 1983; courtesy of Williams & Wilkins.)

pulse pattern for pain is produced by intense stimulation of nonspecific receptors. The *gate control theory*, proposed to explain neural mechanisms associated with pain, is based on three points: (1) while small diameter fibers respond only to noxious stimuli, other larger fibers also may respond to the same stimulus; (2) spinal neurons excited by noxious stimuli may be influenced by afferents signaling innocuous stimuli; and (3) descending systems may modulate the excitability of neurons responding to noxious stimuli.

The most important advance in the understanding of pain mechanisms has been the identification of opiate receptor binding sites upon synaptic membranes. These binding sites mediate all pharmacological effects of opiates, the most powerful agents in alleviating pain. In the spinal gray, opiate receptor binding sites are especially concentrated in Rexed's laminae I and II. The central nervous system contains endogenous opioids: enkephalin, whose distribution appears to parallel opiate receptor binding sites, and β-endorphin, identified from pituitary extracts (Fig. 3.19*A*). Thus opiate receptors and endogenous opiates compose an intrinsic "pain suppression system." Opiate receptor binding sites concentrated in laminae I and II probably represent the first level at which this intrinsic mechanism could modulate pain. Enkephalin may in some fashion inhibit the release of substance P (Figs. 3.19*A* and 3.21), which is associated with the transmission of impulses related to noxious stimuli. Descending spinal projections originating from various brain stem nuclei also contain a variety of neurotransmitters. Large numbers of raphe neurons projecting to spinal cord contain both enkephalin (ENK) and serotonin (5-HT). These neurotransmitters also exert modulating influences on pain mechanisms.

SPINAL REFLEXES

Most spinal reflexes require (1) peripheral receptors, (2) sensory neurons, (3) internuncial neurons, (4) motor neurons, and (5) terminal effectors.

The *myotatic* or *stretch reflex* is a monosynaptic reflex dependent on two neurons, one in the spinal ganglion and one α motor neuron in the anterior horn. Receptor endings in the muscle spindle responding to a brisk stretch of the muscle initiate impulses transmitted centrally to α motor neurons (one synapse involved) that cause these neurons to fire (Fig. 3.23). The result is a reflex contraction of the muscle stretched. In the illustrated example in Figure 3.23, striking the patellar tendon produces a forceful reflex contraction of the quadriceps femoris muscle and brisk extension of the leg at the knee. Afferent volleys in the femoral nerve, transmitted centrally to spinal segments L2, L3, and L4, cause α motor neurons in the same segments to discharge and produce contraction in the muscle stretched. The myotatic reflex is useful in determining the levels of motor integrity of the nervous system but may also reveal evidence of release of higher control.

The *muscle spindle* consists of several bundles of intrafusal muscle fibers surrounded by a connective tissue capsule. The central part of this specialized structure is a noncontractile nuclear bag region. Stretching the noncontractile nuclear bag region by contraction of the polar intrafusal fibers, or stretching the extrafusal muscle fibers to which spindle fibers are attached, constitutes the mechanical stimulus required to fire the annulospiral or primary afferent fiber (group Ia) of this receptor (Fig. 3.24). Group Ia afferents from the muscle spindle make synaptic contact with the cells of the dorsal nucleus and with α motor neurons. (Fig. 3.20). Gamma efferent fibers (originating from γ-motor neurons in the anterior horn) terminating in the polar (contractile) portions of the muscle spindle bring this receptor under the control of spinal and supraspinal influences. (Fig. 3.18 and 3.23).

Figure 3.24. Diagram showing the anatomical and functional relationships of the muscle spindle and the Golgi tendon organ to extrafusal muscle fibers. The muscle spindles are arranged in "parallel" with the extrafusal muscle fibers, so that stretching the muscle causes the spindles to discharge. Contraction of the muscle tends to "unload" or "silence" the muscle spindles. The Golgi tendon organs are arranged in "series" with respect to the extrafusal muscle fibers. Thus, the Golgi tendon organs can be discharged by either a stretch of the tendon or a contraction of the muscle. The threshold of the Golgi tendon organ is relatively higher than that of the muscle spindle. The *lower diagram* summarizes the functional characteristics of the muscle spindle and Golgi tendon in relation to changes in muscle length. At *A*, the muscle is shown at its resting length, and the slow spontaneous discharge of the tendon organ and muscle spindle is indicated. At *B*, the muscle is stretched and both receptors discharge, though the adaptation of the muscle spindle is more rapid. At A^1, the muscle resumes its original length and tension, and there is a temporary reduction in the frequency of spontaneous firing of the muscle spindle. At *C*, where the muscle is contracted and shortened, the muscle spindle is silenced, but the rate of discharge of the tendon organ is increased. At A^2, the muscle is stretched out to its resting length, and the muscle spindles are therefore discharged, while the tendon organs are silenced by the drop in tension. (From Carpenter and Sutin, *Human Neuroanatomy*, 1983; courtesy of Williams & Wilkins.)

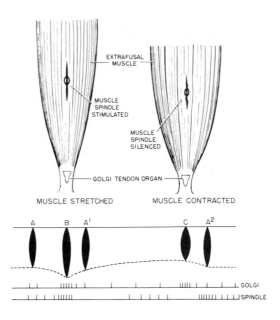

The *Golgi tendon organs* are located in tendons close to their muscular attachments. This relatively high threshold stretch-receptor is considered to be in "series" with the extrafusal muscle fibers, in that it can be caused to discharge by either a powerful stretch or a contraction of the muscle (Fig. 3.24). Afferent fibers from the Golgi tendon organ (group Ib) have a disynaptic inhibitory influence on α motor neurons. In contrast, the muscle spindle is considered to be arranged in "parallel" with extrafusal muscle fibers, in that stretching of extrafusal muscles causes the spindle to discharge while contraction of the muscle "unloads" or "silences" the spindle (Figs. 3.23 and 3.24). An anterior horn cell (lower motor neuron) may be facilitated, or inhibited, by the sum total of all impulses that impinge upon it via thousands of synaptic terminals. Such synaptic endings may be terminals of incoming sensory fibers, internuncial neurons, or fibers of several different descending pathways arising from higher levels of the neuraxis.

SUGGESTED READINGS

Barber, R. P., Phelps, P. E., Houser, C. R., Crawford, G. D., Salvaterra, P. M., and Vaughn, J. E. 1984. The morphology and distribution of neurons containing choline acetyltransferase in the adult rat spinal cord: An immunocytochemical study. J. Comp. Neurol., **229**: 329–346.

Barber, R. P., Vaughn, J. E., and Roberts, E. 1982. The cytoarchitecture of GABAergic neurons in rat spinal cord. Brain Res., **238**: 305–328.

BASBAUM, A. I., RALSTON, D. D., AND RALSTON, H. J. 1986. Bulbospinal projections in the primate: A light and electron microscopic study of a pain modulating system. J. Comp. Neurol., **250**: 311–323.

BATTAGLIA, G., AND RUSTIONI, A. 1988. Coexistence of glutamate and substance P in dorsal root ganglion neurons of the rat and monkey. J. Comp. Neurol., **277**: 302–312.

BENTIVOGLIO, M., KUYPERS, H. G. J. M., CATSMAN-BERREVOETS, C. E., AND DANN, O. 1979. Fluorescent retrograde neuronal labeling in rat by means of substances binding specifically to adenine-thymine rich DNA. Neurosci. Lett., **12**: 235–240.

CARLETON, S. C., AND CARPENTER, M. B. 1983. Afferent and efferent connections of the medial, inferior and lateral vestibular nuclei in the cat and monkey. Brain Res., **278**: 29–51.

CARPENTER, M. B., STEIN, B. M., AND SHRIVER, J. E. 1968. Central projections of spinal dorsal roots in the monkey. II. Lower thoracic lumbosacral and coccygeal dorsal roots. Am. J. Anat., **123**: 75–118.

CARPENTER, M. B., AND SUTIN, J. 1983. *Human Neuroanatomy*, Ed. 8. Williams & Wilkins, Baltimore.

COWAN, W. M., AND CUÉNOD, M. 1975. The use of axonal transport for study of neuronal connections: A retrospective survey. In *The Use of Axonal Transport for Studies of Neuronal Connectivity*. Elsevier, Amsterdam, pp. 2–23.

CUMMINGS, J. F., AND PETRAS, J. M. 1977. The origin of spinocerebellar pathways. I. The nucelus cervicalis centralis of the cranial cervical spinal cord. J. Comp. Neurol., **173**: 655–692.

DeBIASI, S., AND RUSTIONI, A. 1988. Glutamate and substance P coexist in primary afferent terminals in the superficial laminae of spinal cord. Proc. Natl. Acad. Sci. USA, **85**: 7820–7824.

DEMÊMES, D., RAYMOND, J., AND SANS, A. 1984. Selective retrograde labeling of neurons of the cat vestibular ganglion with [^{3}H]D-aspartate. Brain Res., **304**: 188–191.

FINK, R. P., AND HEIMER, L. 1967. Two methods for selective silver impregnation of degenerating axons and their synaptic endings in the central nervous system. Brain Res., **4**: 369–374.

GERFEN, C. R., AND SAWCHENKO, P. E. 1984. An anterograde neuroanatomical tracing method that shows detailed morphology on neurons, their axons and terminals: Immunohistochemical localization of an axonally transported plant lectin, *Phaseolus vulgaris* leucoagglutinin (PhAL-L). Brain Res., **290**: 219–238.

GRANIT, R. 1955. *Receptors and Sensory Perception*. Yale University Press, New Haven, CT.

HAYMAKER, W., AND WOODHALL, B. 1945. *Peripheral Nerve Injuries: Principles of Diagnosis*. W. B. Saunders, Philadelphia.

HEIMER, L., AND ROBARDS, M. J. (Editors) 1981. *Neuroanatomical Tract-Tracing Methods*. Plenum Press, New York.

HÖKFELT, T., TERENIUS, L., KUYPERS, H. G. J. M., AND DANN, O. 1979. Evidence for enkephalin immunoreactive neurons in the medulla oblongata projecting to the spinal cord. Neurosci. Lett., **14**: 55–60.

HUNT, S. P. 1983. Cytochemistry of the spinal cord. In P. C. EMSON (Editor), *Chemical Neuroanatomy*. Raven Press, New York, pp. 53–84.

INAGAKI, N., KAMISAKI, Y., KIYAMA, H., HORIO, Y., TOHYAMA, M., AND WADA, H. 1987. Immunocytochemical localization of cytosolic and mitochondrial glutamine oxaloacetic transaminase isozymes in rat primary sensory neurons as a marker for the glutamate neuronal system. Brain Res., **402**: 197–200.

JESSELL, T. M., AND IVERSEN, L. L. 1977. Opiate analgesics inhibit substance P release from rat trigeminal nucleus. Nature, **268**: 549–551.

KIMURA, H., McGEER, P. L., PENG, J. H., AND McGEER, E. G. 1981. The central cholinergic system studies by choline acetyltransferase immunohistochemistry in the cat. J. Comp. Neurol., **200**: 151–201.

LaMOTTE, C. C., PERT, C. B., AND SNYDER, S. H. 1976. Opiate receptor binding in primate spinal cord: Distribution and changes after dorsal root section. Brain Res., **155**: 374–379.

LIGHT, A. R., AND PERL, E. R. 1979. Reexamination of the dorsal root projection to the spinal dorsal horn including observations on the differential termination of coarse and fine fibers. J. Comp. Neurol., **186**: 117–132.

LIGHT, A. R., AND PERL, E. R. 1979. Spinal terminations of functionally identified primary afferent neurons with slowly conducting myelinated fibers. J. Comp. Neurol., **186** 133–150.

LIGHT, A. R., TREVINO, D. L., AND PERL, E. R. 1979. Morphological features of functionally defined neurons in the marginal zone and substantia gelatinosa of the spinal dorsal horn. J. Comp. Neurol., **186**: 151–172.

MOUNTCASTLE, V. B. 1974. Sensory receptors and neural encoding: Introduction to sensory processes. In V. B. MOUNTCASTLE (Editor), *Medical Physiology*, Vol. 1. C. V. Mosby, St. Louis, pp. 285–306 and 348–381.

NAUTA, W. J. H., AND GYGAX, P. A. 1954. Silver impregnation of degenerating axons in the central nervous system: A modified technic. Stain Technol., **29**: 91–93.

OLIVER, D. L., POTASHER, S. J., JONES, D. R., AND MOREST, D. K. 1983. Selective labeling of spinal ganglion and granule cells with D-aspartate in the auditory system of cat and guinea pig. J. Neuroscience, **3**: 455–472.

PERT, C. B. 1978. Opiate receptors and pain pathways. Neurosci. Res. Program Bull., **16**: 133–141.

PETRAS, J. M., AND CUMMINGS, J. F. 1971. Autonomic neurons in the spinal cord of the Rhesus monkey: A correlation of the findings of cytoarchitectonics and sympathectomy with fiber degeneration following dorsal rhizotomy. J. Comp. Neurol., **146**: 189–218.

PRICE, D. D., AND MAYER, D. J. 1974. Physiological laminar organization of dorsal horn of *M. mulatta*. Brain Res., **79**: 321–325.

REXED, B. 1952. The cytoarchitectonic organization of the spinal cord in the cat. J. Comp. Neurol., **96**: 415–496.

REXED, B. 1954. A cytoarchitectonic atlas of the spinal cord in the cat. J. Comp. Neurol., **100**: 297–400.

SHRIVER, J. E., STEIN, B. M., AND CARPENTER, M. B. 1968. Central projections of spinal dorsal roots in the monkey I. Cervical and upper thoracic dorsal roots. Amer. J. Anat., **123**: 27–74.

SIMANTOV, R., KUHAR, M. J., PASTERNAK, G. W., AND SNYDER, S. H. 1976. The regional distribution of a morphine-like factor enkephalin in monkey brain. Brain Res., **106**: 189–197.

STEWARD, O. 1981. Horseradish peroxidase and fluorescent substance and their combination with other techniques. In L. H. HEIMER AND M. J. ROBARDS (Editors), *Neuroanatomical Tract-Tracing Methods*. Plenum Press, New York, pp. 279–310.

SZENTÁGOTHAI, J. 1964. Neuronal and synaptic arrangement in the substantia gelatinosa Rolandi. J. Comp. Neurol., **122**: 219–239.

TREVINO, D. L., AND CARSTENS, E. 1975. Confirmation of the location of spinothalamic neurons in the cat and monkey by the retrograde transport of horseradish peroxidase. Brain Res., **98**: 177–182.

TREVINO, D. L., COULTER, J. D., AND WILLIS, W. D. 1973. Location of cells of origin of spinothalamic tract in lumbar enlargement of the monkey. J. Neurophysiol., **36**: 750–761.

WALL, P. D. 1978. The gate control theory of pain mechanism: A reexamination and restatement. Brain, **101**: 1–18.

4

Tracts of the Spinal Cord

Ascending and descending fibers in the spinal cord are organized into more or less distinct bundles that occupy particular regions in the white matter. Bundles of fibers having the same origin, course, and terminations are known as tracts or fasciculi. Since the white matter of the spinal cord is divided into three funiculi, all ascending and descending tracts lie in one or more funiculi (Figs. 3.3 and 3.4). A funiculus may contain several different tracts conducting impulses in different directions. Because certain spinal tracts are partially intermingled, or overlap fibers in other tracts, special technics must be used to demonstrate these tracts. In general, long tracts tend to be located peripherally in the white matter, while shorter tracts are found near the gray matter.

ASCENDING SPINAL TRACTS

Although dorsal root afferent fibers entering the spinal cord convey impulses from all general types of somatic and visceral receptors, the signals transmitted rostrally in the spinal cord are segregated so that impulses concerned with pain, thermal sense, touch, and kinesthesis (sense of movement and joint position) from various body segments ascend together in more or less specific tracts, sometimes widely separated from each other (Fig. 3.22). Ascending tracts not only transmit impulses concerned with specific sensory modalities that reach consciousness, but they also transmit impulses from stretch receptors and tactile receptors that project directly, or via relay nuclei, to the cerebellum. The cerebellum receives sensory inputs from all types of receptors but is not concerned with conscious sensory perception. Impulses projected to the cerebellum play an important role in the regulation of muscle tone and the coordination of motor function.

Posterior White Columns

A large proportion of the heavily myelinated fibers of the dorsal root curve medially around the posterior horn and enter the posterior funiculus (Fig. 3.20). These fibers, arising from cells of spinal ganglia at all levels, bifurcate into long ascending and short descending branches. Ascending fibers from caudal segmental levels shift medially and dorsally as they ascend in the posterior funiculus (Fig. 4.1). Branches of fibers from cervical dorsal roots ascend lateral to those of thoracic roots. This patterned arrangement of ascending fibers produces an overlapping laminar arrangement in which longer sacral fibers are most medial and posterior, shorter cervical fibers are most lateral, and lumbar and thoracic fibers occupy intermediate positions. The number of ascending fibers derived from a particular root bears a relationship to the size of the root;

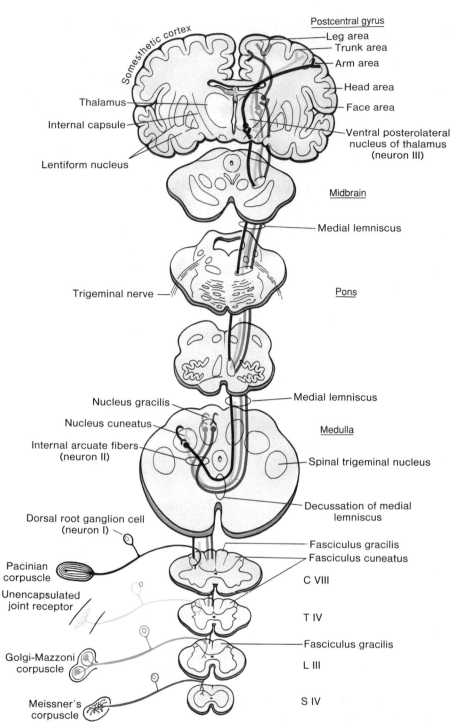

Figure 4.1. Schematic diagram of the formation and course of the posterior white columns in the spinal cord and the medial lemniscus in the brain stem. The posterior white columns are formed from uncrossed ascending and descending branches of spinal ganglion cells. Ascending fibers in the fasciculi gracilis and cuneatus synapse upon cells of the nuclei gracilis and cuneatus. Fibers forming the medial lemniscus arise from cells of the nuclei gracilis and cuneatus, cross in the lower medulla, and ascend to the thalamus. Impulses mediated by this pathway largely concern discriminating tactile sense (touch and pressure) and kinesthetic sense (position and movement). Different receptors shown at various spinal levels on the left generate impulses conveyed centrally by this system. Spinal ganglia and afferent fibers entering the spinal cord at different levels (*red*, sacral; *blue*, lumbar; *yellow*, thoracic; *black*, cervical) are color-coded. *Letters* and *numbers* indicate segmental levels of the spinal cord. (From Carpenter and Sutin, *Human Neuroanatomy*, 1983; courtesy of Williams & Wilkins.)

dorsal roots of the cervical and lumbar enlargements contribute the greatest number of fibers.

The posterior funiculus on each side is divided by a posterior intermediate septum in the upper thoracic and cervical regions (Figs. 3.3 and 3.4). This septum, which becomes discernible at about T6, separates the *fasciculus gracilis* (medial) from the *fasciculus cuneatus* (lateral). The fasciculus gracilis, present at all spinal levels, contains the long ascending branches of fibers from sacral, lumbar, and the lower six thoracic dorsal roots (Figs. 3.13, 3.14, and 3.16). The fasciculus cuneatus first appears at about T6 and contains long ascending branches of the upper six thoracic and all cervical dorsal roots (Fig. 3.8). Fibers in the fasciculus gracilis and cuneatus ascend ipsilaterally and terminate upon the posterior column medullary relay nuclei, namely, the nucleus gracilis and the nucleus cuneatus. Dorsal root fibers projecting to the nuclei gracilis and cuneatus terminate somatotopically; the degree of overlap in the nucleus cuneatus is moderate, but that in the nucleus gracilis is more extensive.

The nuclei gracilis and cuneatus give rise to second-order fibers, which sweep ventromedially, as *internal arcuate fibers*, decussate, and form a single compact fiber bundle, the *medial lemniscus* (Fig. 4.1). The medial lemniscus ascends through the contralateral half of the brain stem and its fibers terminate in the ventral posterolateral nucleus, pars caudalis (VPL$_c$), of the thalamus. The central processes of spinal ganglion cells that enter the spinal cord and ascend ipsilaterally in either the fasciculus gracilis or fasciculus cuneatus, depending on the level of ganglion, constitute the first-order neuron (neuron I). Fibers of the first-order terminate upon cells in posterior column nuclei (i.e., nuclei gracilis or cuneatus) in the caudal medulla (Fig. 4.1). The posterior column nuclei give rise to fibers that decussate in the medulla, form the medial lemniscus, and ascend to the contralateral thalamus. Neurons in the nuclei gracilis and cuneatus (Fig. 4.1) are of the second order (neuron II).

Ascending fibers in the posterior columns and medial lemniscus convey impulses concerned with touch-pressure and kinesthesis. These fibers constitute parts of a large, highly specific sensory pathway in which single elements are responsive to one or the other of these forms of physiological stimuli but not to both. Fibers of this system are highly specific with respect to place and endowed with an exquisite capacity for temporal and spatial discrimination. These fibers convey tactile impulses for precise localization and for two-point discrimination. Ascending impulses from receptors on joint surfaces and in joint capsules, which are excited by movement, convey information concerning the position of different parts of the body. Rapid successive stimuli perceived on bone or skin by Pacinian corpuscles result in a sense of vibration. "Vibratory sense" is not a specific sensory modality but a temporal modulation of tactile sense; impulses concerned with this form of temporally modulated tactile sense are considered to ascend in both the posterior and lateral funiculi.

The posterior columns also contain group Ia muscle spindle afferents and group Ib Golgi tendon organ afferents. Most of the lower limb group I afferents ascending in the funiculus gracilis project to the dorsal nucleus of Clarke at levels of L2 and above (Fig. 3.13) and do not reach the nucleus gracilis. Muscle spindle afferents (Ia) and Golgi tendon afferents (Ib) from the upper extremity enter the spinal cord rostral to the dorsal nucleus of Clarke. These afferents ascend in the fasciculus cuneatus and terminate somatotopically upon portions of the accessory cuneate nucleus. Cells of the accessory cuneate nucleus resemble those of Clarke's nucleus and, like that nucleus, project fibers to the cerebellum (Fig. 5.6).

The descending branches of dorsal root fibers in the posterior columns project for variable distances. These fibers terminate upon parts of the dorsal nucleus and cells in medial parts of lamina VI. Bundles of descending fibers in cervical and upper thoracic spinal segments are known as the *fasciculus interfascicularis* and in the lumbar region as the *septomarginal fasciculus* (Fig. 4.17). Cells in the posterior column nuclei also give rise to descending axons in the ipsilateral posterior columns, which terminate in parts of laminae IV, V, and possibly I. These descending projections may regulate ascending transmission of sensory information.

Lesions involving the posterior columns diminish or abolish discriminating tactile and kinesthetic sense. These disturbances are most evident in the distal parts of the extremities (i.e., in the digits of the hands and feet). Loss of position sense in the lower extremities, as in tabes dorsalis, greatly impairs equilibrium, stance, and gait (posterior column ataxia). Since a nerve fiber severed from its cell of origin degenerates, injury to fibers of the posterior columns (Fig. 4.5), or to dorsal root fibers proximal to the spinal ganglia (Fig. 4.18), will cause degeneration in the posterior white columns in a specific location depending on the level of the lesion.

Anterior Spinothalamic Tract

The spinothalamic tracts, unlike the fibers in the posterior white columns, arise from neurons within the spinal cord (Figs. 4.2 and 4.3). Cells within the spinal gray give rise to fibers that cross and ascend to the thalamus. Although it has long been known that fibers in these tracts cross within the spinal cord and ascend to the thalamus, the cells of origin of these tracts have only recently been established. The cells of origin of the spinothalamic tracts have been identified: (1) physiologically by antidromic stimulation of the specific sensory relay nucleus of the thalamus and (2) anatomically by tracing the retrograde transport of the enzyme horseradish peroxidase (HRP). These data agree that fibers of the spinothalamic tracts arise contralaterally in the spinal cord from cells mainly in laminae I, IV, and V, although some fibers arise from cells in laminae VI and VII (Fig. 3.10). After large HRP injections in the primate thalamus, the largest number of spinothalamic neurons is found in contralateral lower lumbar segments. For each region of the spinal cord, ipsilateral labeled spinothalamic neurons constitute about 10% of the total. Neurons that form the spinothalamic tract constitute a heterogeneous cell population that varies in size, shape, and number among the different segments and spinal laminae. Details concerning the terminations of primary sensory fibers in the posterior gray horn and subsequent synaptic articulations are unclear, but it is presumed that afferent fibers (Fig. 3.12) contact dendrites of cells in laminae IV and V. Spinothalamic fibers cross in the anterior white commissure in a decussation that involves several spinal segments and ascend contralaterally (Fig. 4.2). Fibers forming the anterior spinothalamic tract ascend in the anterior and anterolateral funiculi and are somatotopically arranged, so that those arising from sacral and lumbar segments are most lateral and those from thoracic and cervical segments are most medial (Fig. 4.2). A small number of uncrossed fibers in this tract are not indicated in Figure 4.2.

The anterior spinothalamic tract is reduced in size at medullary

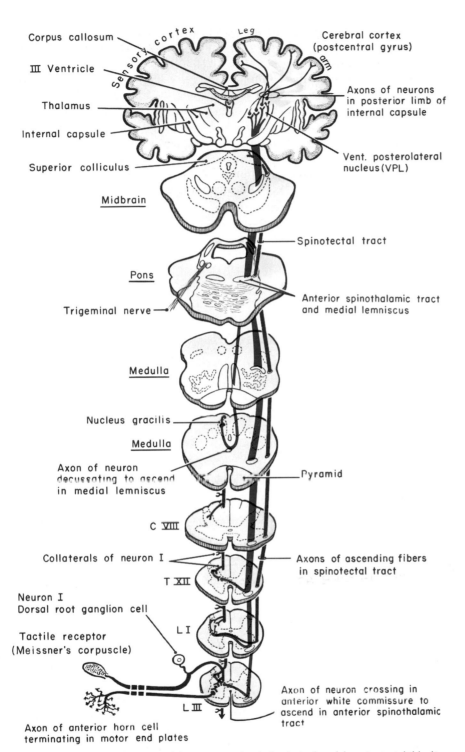

Corpus callosum
III Ventricle
Thalamus
Internal capsule
Superior colliculus
Sensory cortex
Leg
arm
Cerebral cortex
(postcentral gyrus)
Axons of neurons
in posterior limb of
internal capsule
Vent. posterolateral
nucleus (VPL)

Midbrain

Spinotectal tract

Pons

Trigeminal nerve

Anterior spinothalamic tract
and medial lemniscus

Medulla

Nucleus gracilis
Medulla

Axon of neuron
decussating to ascend
in medial lemniscus

Pyramid

C VIII

Collaterals of neuron I

Axons of ascending fibers
in spinotectal tract

T XII

Neuron I
Dorsal root ganglion cell

Tactile receptor
(Meissner's corpuscle)

L I

L III

Axon of anterior horn cell
terminating in motor end plates

Axon of neuron crossing in
anterior white commissure to
ascend in anterior spinothalamic
tract

Figure 4.2. Schematic diagram of the anterior spinothalamic (*red*) and the spinotectal (*black*) tracts. These tracts arise from cells in multiple laminae of the spinal gray at all levels. The largest number of spinothalamic fibers arise from cells in laminae I, IV, and V contralaterally. The anterior spinothalamic tract conveys impulses associated with "light touch," the sensation produced by stroking glabrous skin with a wisp of cotton. The spinotectal tract ascends in association with the anterior spinothalamic tract but terminates in deep layers of the contra-lateral superior colliculus and in parts of the periaquedectal gray; this tract conveys noci-ceptive impulses. *Letters* and *numbers* indicate segmental spinal levels. (From Carpenter and Sutin, *Human Neuroanatomy*, 1983; courtesy of Williams & Wilkins.)

levels because some fibers, or collaterals, project to nuclei in the reticular formation. The spinothalamic component of this tract becomes closely associated with the medial lemniscus in the pons and midbrain. At midbrain levels the anterior spinothalamic tract consists of two components. Fibers of the larger lateral component terminate in caudal parts of the ventral posterolateral, pars caudalis (VPL$_c$), thalamic nucleus (Fig. 4.2). Fibers of the medial component of the tract project into the periaqueductal gray and bilaterally into the intralaminar thalamic nuclei.

Fibers of the anterior spinothalamic tract convey impulses associated with what is called "light touch"; this sensation is provoked by stroking skin, devoid of hair, with a feather or wisp of cotton. Injury to the anterior spinothalamic tract produces little, if any, disturbance because tactile sense also is conveyed by the posterior white columns.

Lateral Spinothalamic Tract

This tract is closely related to the anterior spinothalamic tract but is of greater clinical importance because it transmits impulses concerned with pain and thermal sense. Fibers of this tract are more concentrated and contain more long fibers that project directly to the thalamus. Statements made concerning the cells of origin of the anterior spinothalamic tract apply also to the lateral spinothalamic tract. Cells largely in laminae I, IV, and V give rise to most of the axons that cross in the anterior white commissure and ascend in the contralateral lateral funiculus as the lateral spinothalamic tract (Fig. 4.3). Fibers of this tract cross obliquely to the opposite side, usually within one spinal segment. This tract is somatotopically organized in a manner similar to that of the anterior spinothalamic tract; the tract lies medial to the anterior spinocerebellar tract. There is an incomplete segregation of fibers concerned with pain and thermal sense; fibers related to thermal sense tend to be posterior to those related to pain. In the brain stem this tract sends branches into the reticular formation while the main fibers terminate in the VPL$_c$ nucleus of the thalamus.

Anterolateral cordotomy in the monkey indicates that the thalamic projections of the spinothalamic system are far more complex than classic descriptions suggest. Unilateral anterolateral cordotomy produces (1) ipsilateral degeneration in the VPL$_c$ nucleus, (2) bilateral degeneration in certain intralaminar thalamic nuclei, and (3) bilateral degeneration in a posterior thalamic nucleus. In the VPL$_c$ nucleus of the thalamus (1) the body surface is represented in an orderly, distorted topographic manner, and (2) cells of this nucleus are related to small contralateral receptive fields (Fig. 9.15). In the posterior thalamic nucleus cells are activated from large receptive fields, both ipsilaterally and contralaterally.

Unilateral section of the lateral spinothalamic tract produces loss of pain and thermal sense on the opposite side of the body beginning about one segment below the level of the lesion. Even though such lesions concomitantly interrupt fibers of the anterior spinothalamic tract, tactile sense remains intact because it is also transmitted centrally by uncrossed fibers in the posterior funiculus. The position of degenerated fibers in the lateral spinothalamic tracts after a crush of the lumbosacral region of the spinal cord is demonstrated in Figure 4.5.

Spinotectal Tract

Cells of origin of the tectospinal tract lie in laminae I and V of the posterior horn. Fibers of this crossed tract ascend in the anterolateral

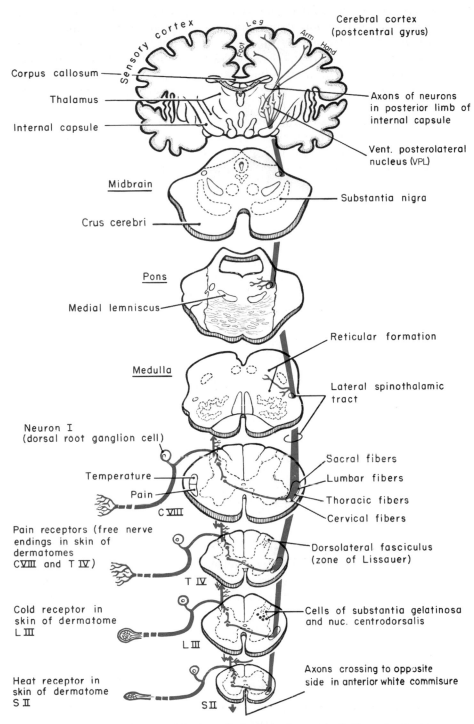

Figure 4.3. Schematic diagram of the lateral spinothalamic tract (*red*). The cells of origin of the lateral spinothalamic tract appear to be largely in laminae I, IV, and V of Rexed. Fibers of this tract cross to the opposite side within one segment in the anterior white commissure. The lateral spinothalamic tract has a more complex termination in the thalamus than indicated here, conveys impulses associated with pain and thermal sense, and has a somatotopic lamination. *Letters* and *numbers* indicate segmental spinal levels. (From Carpenter and Sutin, *Human Neuroanatomy*, 1983; courtesy of Williams & Wilkins.)

part of the spinal cord in association with the spinothalamic system but at midbrain levels project into the intermediate and deep layers of the superior colliculus and lateral regions of the periaqueductal gray (Fig. 4.2). The functional significance of this tract is unknown, but evidence suggests it may be part of a multisynaptic pathway transmitting nociceptive impulses. The intermediate and deep layers of the superior colliculus receive multiple sensory inputs while projections to the superficial layer are all related to the visual system.

Posterior Spinocerebellar Tract

This uncrossed tract, which ascends along the posterolateral periphery of the spinal cord, arises from the large cells of the dorsal nucleus of Clarke (Figs. 3.11 and 3.13). Dorsal root afferents reach the dorsal nuclei directly and after ascending and descending in the posterior columns (Fig. 3.22). The cells of Clarke's nucleus give rise to large fibers that ascend in the posterolateral part of the lateral funiculus (i.e., lateral to the corticospinal tract) (Fig. 4.4). In the medulla the fibers of this tract become incorporated in the inferior cerebellar peduncle, enter the cerebellum, and terminate ipsilaterally in rostral and caudal portions of the vermis. In the anterior vermis fibers end in lobules I to IV; posteriorly fibers terminate mainly in parts of the pyramis and paramedian lobule.

Since the dorsal nucleus is not present caudal to L3, some dorsal root fibers from more caudal segments ascend first in the posterior columns to upper lumbar segments and then terminate upon cells of the dorsal nucleus. Impulses relayed to the cerebellum via the posterior spinocerebellar tract arise from muscle spindles, Golgi tendon organs, and from touch and pressure receptors. Neurons of Clarke's nucleus receive monosynaptic excitation mainly via group Ia, Ib, and group II afferent fibers. The synaptic linkage between group I afferents and the dorsal nucleus allows transmission of impulses at high frequencies. Exteroceptive impulses, also transmitted via the posterior spinocerebellar tract, are related to touch and pressure receptors in skin and slowly adapting pressure receptors. The posterior spinocerebellar tract is somatotopically organized at spinal levels and in its cerebellar terminations. None of the impulses conveyed by this tract reaches conscious levels. Impulses transmitted by these tracts are utilized in the fine coordination of posture and movement of individual limb muscles.

Anterior Spinocerebellar Tract

This tract ascends along the lateral periphery of the spinal cord anterior to the posterior spinocerebellar tract (Fig. 4.4). The tract makes its first appearance at lower lumbar levels, but its cells of origin do not constitute a discrete entity such as the dorsal nucleus of Clarke. Fibers of the anterior spinocerebellar tract arise from cells in parts of laminae V, VI, and VII. Cells giving rise to this tract extend from coccygeal and sacral spinal segments as far rostrally as the L1 segment. Fibers of the anterior spinocerebellar tract are less numerous than those of the posterior spinocerebellar tract, are uniformly large, and are virtually all crossed. Like the posterior spinocerebellar tract, it is concerned with the transmission of impulses mainly from the lower extremity. Cells that give rise to the anterior spinocerebellar tract receive monosynaptic excitation from group Ib afferents from Golgi tendon organs whose receptive fields often include one synergic muscle group at each joint of the lower limb.

This pathway to the cerebellum is composed of two neurons:

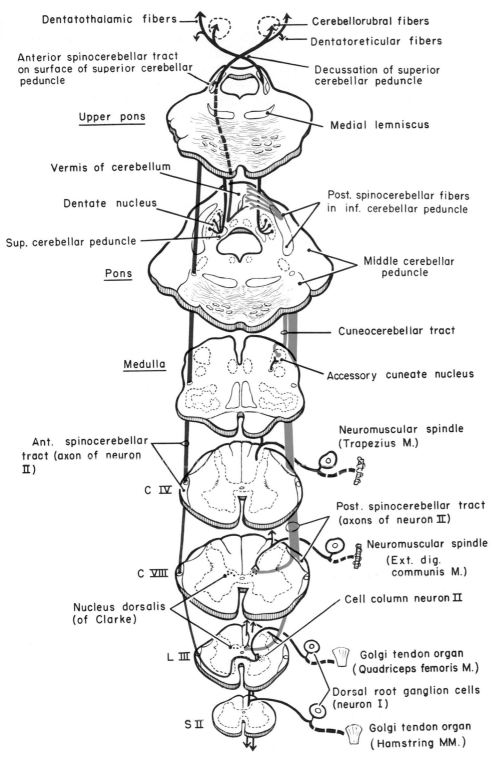

Figure 4.4. Schematic diagram of the anterior (*red*) and posterior (*blue*) spinocerebellar tracts and the cuneocerebellar tract (*blue*). The posterior spinocerebellar tract arises from cells of the dorsal nucleus of Clarke (nucleus thoracicus) and is uncrossed; it conveys impulses arising from muscle spindles and Golgi tendon organs. Fibers of the anterior spinocerebellar tract are crossed and arise from cells in parts of laminae V, VI, and VIII; fibers of this tract are activated by impulses from Golgi tendon organs. The cuneocerebellar tract, arising from cells of the accessory cuneate nucleus in the medulla, is considered the upper limb equivalent of the posterior spinocerebellar tract; this tract is uncrossed. *Letters* and *numbers* indicate spinal levels. (From Carpenter and Sutin, *Human Neuroanatomy*, 1983; courtesy of Williams & Wilkins.)

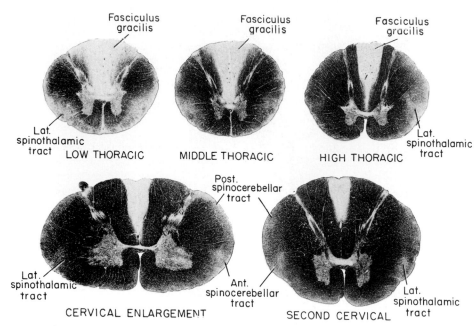

Figure 4.5. Transverse sections of human spinal cord crushed some time previously in the lumbosacral region. In the posterior white columns the progressive diminution of the degenerated area is due to passage into the gray matter of short and medium length ascending branches of lumbosacral dorsal root fibers. The progressive increase in normal fibers adjacent to the posterior horns is due to the addition of ascending branches of dorsal root fibers entering above the level of the injury. Degeneration is seen also in the spinothalamic tracts and both the anterior and posterior spinocerebellar tracts. Weigert's myelin stain. (From Carpenter and Sutin, *Human Neuroanatomy*, 1983; courtesy of Williams & Wilkins.)

(1) neuron I in the spinal ganglia and (2) neuron II in scattered cell groups at the base of the anterior and posterior horns in lumbar, sacral, and coccygeal spinal segments (Fig. 4.4). Fibers of neuron II cross in the spinal cord and ascend peripheral to fibers of the lateral spinothalamic tract. At upper pontine levels the tract enters the cerebellum by coursing along the dorsal surface of the superior cerebellar peduncle. The majority of the fibers of this tract terminate contralaterally in the anterior cerebellar vermis in lobules I to IV. Fibers of this tract convey impulses concerned with the coordinated movement and posture of the entire lower limb.

Clinically it is virtually impossible to determine the effects of injury to the spinocerebellar tracts, because other spinal tracts usually are involved. No loss of tactile or kinesthetic sense results from such lesions, since impulses projected to the cerebellum do not enter the conscious sphere.

Cuneocerebellar Tract

Some uncrossed dorsal root fibers that ascend in the fasciculus cuneatus convey impulses from muscle afferents (group Ia) and Golgi tendon organ afferents (group Ib); these fibers terminate somatotopically upon cells of the accessory cuneate nucleus in the medulla (Fig. 5.6). These fibers follow this course because the dorsal nucleus of Clarke is not present above C8. The accessory cuneate nucleus in the dorsolateral part of the medulla is considered to be homologous to the dorsal nucleus. Cells of the accessory cuneate nucleus give rise to *cuneocerebellar fibers*, which enter the cerebellum via the inferior cerebellar peduncle (Fig. 4.4). These fibers terminate ipsilaterally in lobule V of the cerebellar cortex. The

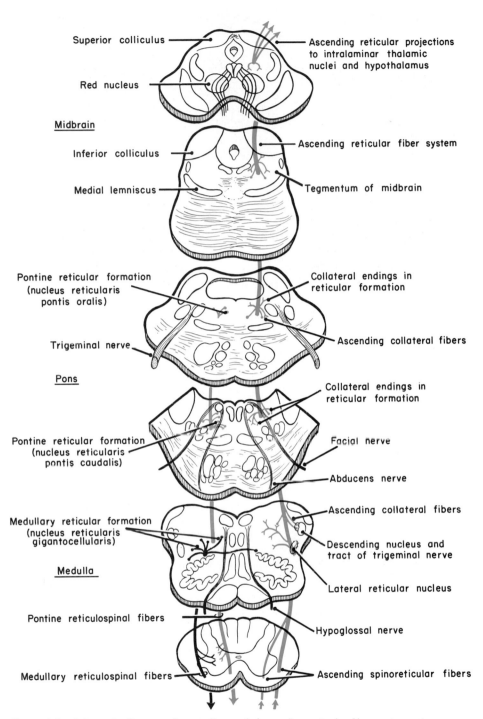

Superior colliculus

Ascending reticular projections
to intralaminar thalamic
nuclei and hypothalamus

Red nucleus

Midbrain

Inferior colliculus

Ascending reticular fiber system

Medial lemniscus

Tegmentum of midbrain

Pontine reticular formation
(nucleus reticularis
pontis oralis)

Collateral endings in
reticular formation

Trigeminal nerve

Ascending collateral fibers

Pons

Collateral endings in
reticular formation

Pontine reticular formation
(nucleus reticularis
pontis caudalis)

Facial nerve

Abducens nerve

Ascending collateral fibers

Medullary reticular formation
(nucleus reticularis
gigantocellularis)

Descending nucleus and
tract of trigeminal nerve

Medulla

Lateral reticular nucleus

Pontine reticulospinal fibers

Hypoglossal nerve

Medullary reticulospinal fibers

Ascending spinoreticular fibers

Figure 4.6. Schematic diagram of ascending and descending reticular fiber systems. Ascending spinoreticular projections and collaterals are shown on the *right* (*blue*). In this system collaterals are given off at various brain stem levels and the pathway is augmented by rostrally projecting reticular fibers. Pontine reticulospinal fibers (*red*) are uncrossed and originate largely from the nucleus reticularis pontis caudalis. Medullary reticulospinal fibers (*black*) arise from the nucleus reticularis gigantocellularis and project bilaterally to spinal levels in the anterior part of the lateral funiculi. Descending fibers from these sources are not topographically organized or sharply segregated in the spinal cord. (From Carpenter and Sutin, *Human Neuroanatomy*, 1983; courtesy of Williams & Wilkins.)

cuneocerebellar tract is considered to be the upper limb equivalent of the posterior spinocerebellar tract.

Spino-olivary Pathways

Spino-olivary pathways constitute another component of spinocerebellar circuitry in which impulses from the spinal cord are relayed to the cerebellum via parts of the inferior olive. The two best defined tracts are the posterior and anterior spino-olivary tracts. Fibers of the posterior spino-olivary tract ascend in the posterior white columns and synapse upon cells of the nuclei cuneatus and gracilis that relay impulses to the accessory olivary nuclei. Multiple anterior spinocerebellar fibers ascending contralaterally in the anterior funiculus terminate upon portions of the dorsal and medial accessory olivary nuclei. Fibers contributing to spino-olivary tracts arise at all levels of the spinal cord and are activated by stimulation of cutaneous and group Ib receptors. The accessory olivary nuclei give rise to crossed olivocerebellar fibers, which project mainly to the anterior lobe of the cerebellum.

Spinoreticular Fibers

A considerable number of spinoreticular fibers, arising from cells of the posterior horn, ascend in the anterolateral part of the spinal cord and are distributed to widespread regions of the brain stem reticular formation. Predominantly uncrossed fibers terminate chiefly upon cells of the nucleus reticularis gigantocellularis of the medulla (Fig. 4.6). Spinoreticular fibers passing to pontine reticular nuclei are distributed bilaterally. A smaller number of spinoreticular fibers reach the midbrain reticular formation. Functionally, spinoreticular fibers represent a component of a phylogenetically older, polysynaptic system, which plays a significant role in behavioral awareness, modification of motor and sensory activities, and in the modulation of electrocortical activity.

DESCENDING SPINAL TRACTS

The descending spinal tracts are concerned with somatic motor function, visceral innervation, the modification of muscle tone, segmental reflexes, and central transmission of sensory impulses. The largest and most important of these tracts arises from the cerebral cortex; all other descending spinal tracts arise from localized cell groups within the three lowest segments of the brain stem.

Corticospinal System

These tracts consist of all fibers that (1) arise from cells in the cerebral cortex, (2) pass through the medullary pyramid, and (3) descend into the spinal cord (Figs. 4.7, 4.8, and 4.9). At the medullary level each pyramid consists of about one million fibers; about two-thirds of these fibers have appreciable myelin sheaths. Nearly 90% of these fibers are between 1 and 4 μm in diameter; remaining fibers range from 5 to 22 μm, but only about 3.5% of these are above 20 μm. Fibers of the corticospinal tract arise from cells in the deeper part of lamina V in the precentral motor area (area 4), the premotor area (area 6), and the postcentral gyrus (areas 3a, 3b, 1, 2) and adjacent parietal cortex (area 5). Cells of origin are arranged in strips or clusters and vary in size in different cortical areas (Fig. 4.7). The largest fibers arise from the giant pyramidal cells of Betz in the precentral gyrus (Fig. 13.2). These fibers converge in the corona radiata, enter the internal capsule, and descend to form the crus cerebri at midbrain levels (Fig. 2.10). As this tract descends in the ventral part of the infratentorial brain stem, its fibers pass close to the emerging root fibers of the cranial nerves III, VI, and XII. In the medulla the fibers form the massive pyramids (Figs. 5.2 and 5.5). At the junction of medulla and spinal cord, the corticospinal tract undergoes an incomplete decussation (Figs. 4.8 and 5.4) and divides into three separate tracts: (1) the large lateral corticospinal tract (crossed), (2) the small anterior corticospinal tract (uncrossed), and (3) the relatively minute uncrossed anterolateral corticospinal tract. Between 75 and 90% of the fibers in the corticospinal tract decussate at caudal medullary levels and enter the posterior part of the lateral funiculus where they form the lateral corticospinal tract (Fig. 4.8). Fibers of this tract lie medial to the posterior spinocerebellar tract and lateral to the fasciculus proprius (Fig. 4.10).

The *lateral corticospinal tract* descends the length of the spinal cord, gives off fibers to the spinal gray at all levels, and progressively diminishes in size at more caudal levels. In lower lumbar and sacral spinal segments, caudal to the posterior spinocerebellar tract, fibers of the lateral corticospinal tract reach the dorsolateral surface of the spinal cord (Fig. 4.19). Fibers of the crossed lateral corticospinal tract enter the spinal gray in the intermediate zone and are distributed to parts of laminae IV, V, VI, and VII. In the monkey a small number of fibers end directly upon anterior horn cells or their processes in lamina IX.

The *anterior corticospinal tract*, formed from a smaller portion of pyramidal fibers, descends uncrossed into the spinal cord and occupies an oval area adjacent to the anterior median fissure. This tract is distinguishable mainly in cervical segments (Figs. 4.7, 4.8, and 4.9). Most fibers of this tract cross at upper cervical spinal levels in the anterior white commissure and terminate in lamina VII.

Fibers of the *anterolateral corticospinal tract* are uncrossed, of fine caliber, and descend in a more ventral position in the lateral funiculus than those of the crossed lateral corticospinal tract (Fig. 4.8). These fibers remain uncrossed and terminate in the base of the posterior horn and the intermediate gray. Demyelination in the lateral and anterior corticospinal tract can be detected readily in Weigert-stained preparations, but this stain is not sensitive enough to reveal the small number of fibers in the anterolateral corticospinal tract (Fig. 4.10).

Autoradiographic studies indicate that fibers from the precentral motor cortex terminate extensively in lamina VII and in dorsolateral parts of lamina IX, while fibers from somatosensory cortex (areas 3, 1, 2, and 5) terminate in overlapping zones in parts of the posterior horn. Although some corticospinal fibers establish synaptic contact with anterior horn cells, the majority terminate on internuncial neurons in lamina VII.

Corticospinal neurons in the motor cortex have multiple axonal branches that project to different spinal segments. Corticospinal neurons with axonal collaterals terminating at different spinal levels are distributed over a wide area of the motor cortex. Multiple collateral branches of corticospinal axons explain (1) why a small horseradish peroxidase (HRP) injection in the spinal gray retrogradely labels widely scattered projection neurons in the motor cortex, and (2) why a small lesion in the motor cortex produces corticospinal degeneration distributed over many segments. Collaterals of individual corticospinal axons project to multiple motor neuronal pools in the cervical and lumbar enlargements innervating different muscles. Thus corticospinal axons exert multiple influences upon

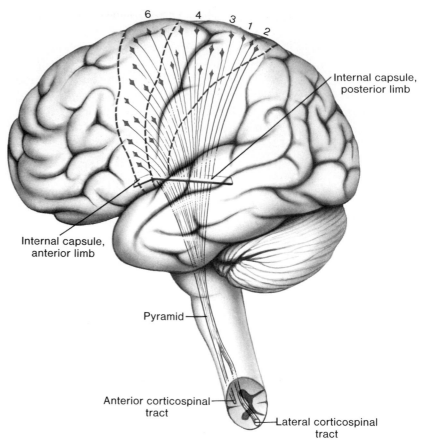

different groups of spinal neurons in widely separated spinal segments via their collateral branches. These data indicate that the corticospinal tract is not somatotopically organized.

Immunocytochemical studies in the rat combined with retrograde tracing methods suggest that glutamate and/or aspartate may be the excitatory neurotransmitters of corticospinal neurons. Approximately 30% of identified corticospinal neurons in layer V were positive for either glutamate or aspartate, and 50% of these neurons were positive for both substances (Fig. 13.6). The corticospinal tract is phylogenetically new, is present only in mammals, and becomes myelinated in the human during the first two years of life.

The corticospinal tract is universally regarded as the descending pathway most concerned with voluntary, discrete, skilled movements. Lesions destroying portions of this tract at any level result in variable degrees of paresis (i.e., paralysis). Such lesions usually are associated with (1) initial loss of muscle tone, succeeded by gradually increased muscle tone in antigravity muscles; (2) hyperactive deep tendon (myotatic) reflexes; (3) loss of superficial abdominal and cremasteric reflexes; and (4) the appearance of an extensor toe response (Babinski sign) on stroking the sole of the foot. The Babinski sign is interpreted to mean injury to the corticospinal system, but it is not an infallible sign, for it can be elicited in the newborn, the sleeping or intoxicated adult, or following a generalized seizure.

Paralysis of both arm and leg on the same side is termed *hemiplegia*. The term *paraplegia* denotes paralysis of both legs, while *quadraplegia* refers to paralysis of all four extremities.

All major descending spinal tracts, other than the corticospinal tract, arise from the brain stem. Three descending spinal tracts arise from the

Corticospinal tract

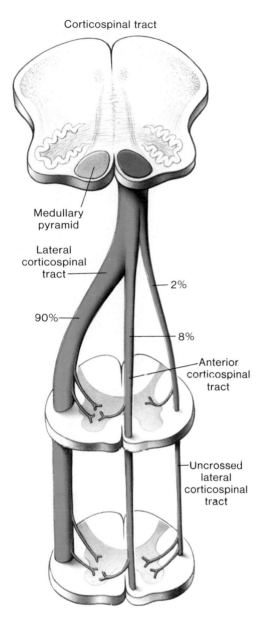

Medullary
pyramid

Lateral
corticospinal
tract

2%

90%

8%

Anterior
corticospinal
tract

Uncrossed
lateral
corticospinal
tract

Figure 4.8. Schematic diagram of the decussation of the human corticospinal tract (*red*). Approximately 90% of the corticospinal tract crosses in the lower medulla to form the *lateral corticospinal tract*. Of the fibers that do not decussate in the medulla approximately 8% form the *anterior corticospinal tract*, which descends in the anterior funiculus; most of these fibers cross in cervical spinal segments. The small number of fibers in the *uncrossed lateral corticospinal tract* (Barnes) remain uncrossed. (From Carpenter and Sutin, *Human Neuroanatomy*, 1983; courtesy of Williams & Wilkins.)

midbrain. These are the tectospinal, rubrospinal, and interstitiospinal tracts.

Tectospinal Tract

Fibers of this tract arise from cells in the deeper layers of the superior colliculus, sweep anteromedially around the periaqueductal gray, cross in the *dorsal tegmental decussation*, and descend near the median raphe anterior to the medial longitudinal fasciculus (Fig. 4.11). At medullary levels tectospinal fibers become incorporated in the medial longitudinal fasciculus (abbreviated MLF). In the spinal cord tectospinal fibers, located in the anterior funiculus near the anterior median fissure, descend only through cervical levels (Fig. 4.11). The majority of the fibers terminate in the upper four cervical segments in laminae VIII, VII, and parts of VI. None of these fibers end directly upon alpha motor neurons. The tectospinal tract mediates reflex postural movements in response to visual and, perhaps, auditory stimuli.

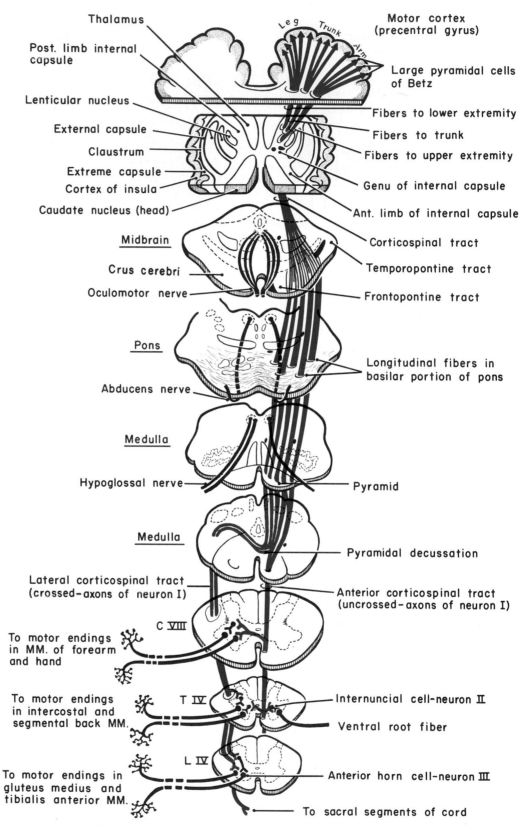

Figure 4.9.   Schematic diagram of lateral and anterior corticospinal tracts—the principal descending pathway concerned with skilled, voluntary motor activity. The locations of the corticobulbar tracts at each level of the brain stem are indicated by *black areas* (*right side*). *Letters* and *numbers* indicate corresponding segments of the spinal cord. (From Carpenter and Sutin, *Human Neuroanatomy*, 1983; courtesy of Williams & Wilkins.)

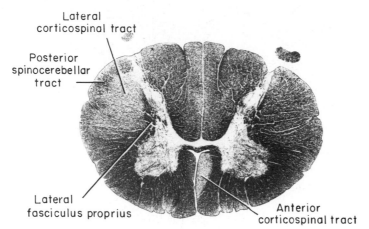

Lateral
corticospinal tract

Posterior
spinocerebellar
tract

Lateral
fasciculus proprius

Anterior
corticospinal tract

Figure 4.10. Transverse section through the cervical enlargement of the spinal cord of an individual sustaining a vascular lesion of one medullary pyramid. The lateral corticospinal tract on the left and the anterior corticospinal tract on the side of the lesion are degenerated and demyelinated. Weigert's myelin stain. Photograph. (From Carpenter and Sutin, *Human Neuroanatomy*, 1983; courtesy of Williams & Wilkins.)

Rubrospinal Tract

Fibers of this tract arise from the red nucleus, an oval cell mass in the central part of the midbrain tegmentum (Fig. 4.11). The red nucleus consists of a rostral parvicellular part and a caudal magnocellular part, which vary in size in different animals. The rubrospinal tract arises from the magnocellular region of the red nucleus. Rubrospinal fibers cross completely in the *ventral tegmental decussation* and descend to spinal levels where they lie anterior to, and partially intermingled with, fibers of the corticospinal tract in the lateral funiculus (Fig. 4.11). Fibers of the rubrospinal tract are somatotopically organized, meaning that cells in particular parts of the nucleus project selectively to defined spinal levels. Fibers projecting to cervical spinal segments arise from dorsal and dorsomedial parts of the red nucleus, while fibers projecting to lumbosacral spinal segments arise from ventral and ventrolateral parts of the nucleus. Thoracic spinal segments receive fibers that arise from an intermediate region of the nucleus. Rubrospinal fibers (1) descend the length of the spinal cord and (2) terminate in the lateral half of lamina V, lamina VI, and dorsal and central parts of lamina VII.

The red nucleus receives fibers from the cerebral cortex and the cerebellum. Corticorubral fibers from the "motor" cortex project bilaterally to the parvicellular part of the red nucleus and ipsilaterally to the magnocellular division. These projections are somatotopically organized with respect to origin and termination. The synaptic linkage of corticorubral and rubrospinal fibers together constitute a somatotopically organized nonpyramidal pathway between the motor cortex and particular spinal levels. All parts of the red nucleus receive crossed cerebellar efferent fibers via the superior cerebellar peduncle. Fibers from the interposed nuclei (equivalent to globose and emboliform nuclei) relate portions of the cerebellar cortex somatotopically with the magnocellular part of the red nucleus (Fig. 8.16). Stimulation of cells in the red nucleus produces excitatory postsynaptic potentials in contralateral flexor alpha (α) motor neurons and inhibitory postsynaptic potentials in extensor alpha motor neurons. The most important function of the rubrospinal tract concerns control of tone in flexor muscle groups.

The *interstitiospinal tract* is a small uncrossed tract forming a component of the descending MLF; it will be discussed with that composite bundle.

Two major descending spinal tracts arise from the pons. These are the vestibulospinal and pontine reticulospinal tracts. The pontine and medullary reticulospinal tracts will be discussed together.

Figure 4.11. Schematic diagram of the rubrospinal (*red*) and the tectospinal (*blue*) tracts. The rubrospinal tract arises somatotopically from the magnocellular part of the red nucleus, crosses in the ventral tegmental decussation, and descends to spinal levels where fibers terminate in parts of laminae V, VI, and VII. Tectospinal fibers arise from cells in deep layers of the superior colliculus, cross in the dorsal tegmental decussation, and descend in association with the medial longitudinal fasciculus. Fibers of the tectospinal tract are distributed to parts of laminae VIII, VII, and VI only in cervical spinal segments.

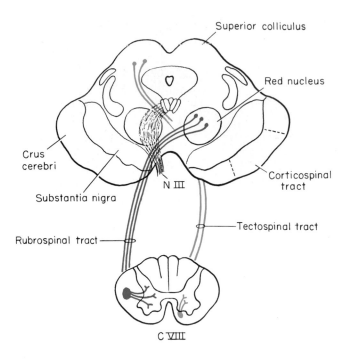

Vestibulospinal Tract

The vestibular nuclei constitute a cytological complex in the floor of the fourth ventricle in both the pons and medulla. The four major nuclei of this complex receive afferents from the vestibular nerve and parts of the cerebellum that are distributed differentially (Fig. 6.14). The vestibulospinal tract, the principal descending spinal pathway from this complex, arises mainly from the lateral vestibular nucleus. The lateral vestibular nucleus consists of a collection of giant cells in the lateral part of the complex near the entry of the vestibular nerve root. Practically all cells of the lateral vestibular nucleus contribute fibers to the formation of this ipsilateral tract, which descends the length of the spinal cord in the anterior part of the lateral funiculus (Figs. 4.12 and 4.13).

The vestibulospinal tract is considered to be somatotopically organized because cells in dorsocaudal parts of the lateral vestibular nucleus project to lumbosacral spinal segments and cells in rostroventral regions project mainly to cervical spinal segments. Somatotopic features are somewhat blurred by the observation that fibers of the tract give off collaterals that innervate several spinal segments, particularly in the enlargements. The vestibulospinal tract has a three- to four-fold stronger influence on cervical and lower lumbar spinal regions than on thoracic spinal segments. Fibers of the vestibulospinal tract in cervical segments give off collaterals that enter laminae IX and adjacent parts of VII and VIII. Synaptic contacts are made with interneurons and with proximal dendrites and somata of large motor neurons. Physiological evidence indicates monosynaptic excitation of motor neurons in the lumbosacral region and direct connections with gamma-motor neurons.

Vestibular influences, and certain cerebellar influences, upon spinal cord activities are mediated by the vestibulospinal tract. This tract is considered to exert a facilitatory influence on somatic spinal reflex activity and spinal mechanisms that control extensor muscle tone. Stimulation of the lateral vestibular nucleus in the cat produces excitatory postsynaptic potentials in extensor motor neurons. A large part of these facilitatory effects on extensor α motor neurons are considered to be mediated both

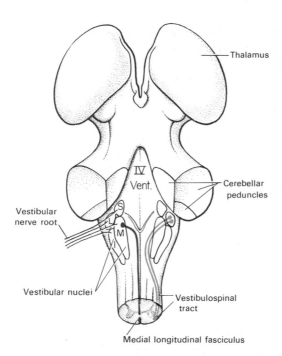

Figure 4.12. Schematic diagram of the spinal projections from the vestibular nuclei. The vestibulospinal tract (*blue*) arises from cells of the lateral vestibular nucleus. This tract is uncrossed, somatotopically organized, extends the length of the spinal cord, and is concerned with the facilitation of extensor muscle tone. Vestibular fibers descending in the medial longitudinal fasciculus (*red*) arise largely from the medial vestibular nucleus and are mainly uncrossed. *S* indicates superior vestibular nucleus, *L* indicates the lateral vestibular nucleus, and *I* and *M* indicate the inferior and medial vestibular nuclei.

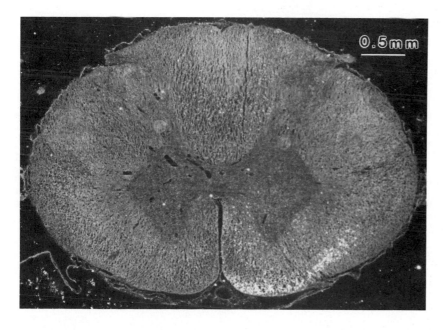

Figure 4.13. Autoradiograph of an upper cervical spinal segment in a monkey demonstrating labeling of fibers in the vestibulospinal tract (VST).

monosynaptically and disynaptically via interneurons in laminae VII and VIII.

Reticulospinal Tracts

Two relatively large regions of the brain stem reticular formation give rise to fibers that descend to spinal levels. One of these regions is in the pontine tegmentum while the other lies in the medulla, hence it is proper to refer to these as the pontine and medullary reticulospinal tracts (Fig. 4.6 and 4.14).

The *pontine reticulospinal tract* arises from aggregation of cells in the medial pontine tegmentum (Fig. 4.6) referred to as the *nuclei reticularis pontis caudalis* and *oralis*. The caudal pontine reticular nucleus begins in the caudal pontine tegmentum and extends rostrally to the level of the motor trigeminal nucleus. This nucleus contains a number of giant cells in addition to various types of smaller cells. The pontine reticulospinal tract is almost entirely ipsilateral and descends chiefly in the medial part of the anterior funiculus (i.e., sulcomarginal area). In the brain stem and spinal cord these fibers descend in association with the MLF. Pontine reticulospinal fibers are more numerous than those arising in the medulla, descend the entire length of the spinal cord, and terminate in lamina VIII and adjacent parts of lamina VII. A large proportion of these reticulospinal fibers give off collateral branches to more than one level of the spinal cord, suggesting they may be involved in activities at multiple spinal levels. Stimulation of the pontine reticulospinal pathway evokes both monosynaptic and polysynaptic excitation of motor neurons supplying

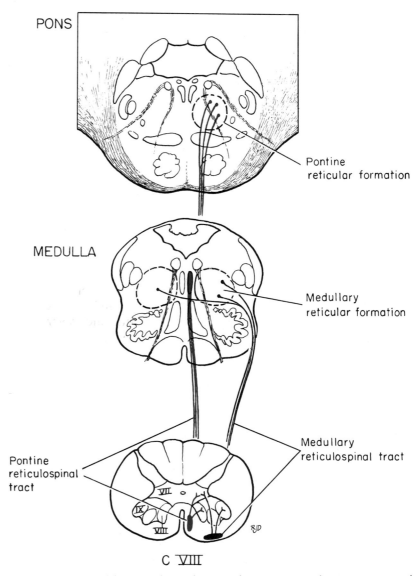

Figure 4.14.   Diagram of the recticulospinal tracts indicating regions of origin, course, and terminations. Pontine reticulospinal fibers (*red*) descend in the sulcomarginal region of the anterior funiculus, are uncrossed, descend the length of the spinal cord, and give off collaterals and terminals at nearly all levels that end in lamina VIII and parts of lamina VII. Medullary reticulospinal fibers (*black*) arise bilaterally, descend in the anterior part of the lateral funiculus, and terminate in laminae VII and IX. Neither of these tracts is somatotopically organized.

axial and limb muscles; direct effects are strongest upon axial muscles particularly in the neck.

The *medullary reticulospinal tract* arises from the medial two-thirds of the medullary reticular formation. The largest number of fibers arise from the *nucleus reticularis gigantocellularis*, lying dorsal to the inferior olivary complex and lateral to the paramedian region (Figs. 4.6 and 4.14). As the name of this nucleus implies, it is composed of some characteristic large cells, but in addition it contains many medium-sized and small cells. Fibers of the medullary reticulospinal tract project bilateral to spinal levels (crossed and uncrossed) and mainly descend in the anterior part of the lateral funiculi. Fibers crossing to the opposite side do so in the medulla and are less numerous than uncrossed fibers. Some fibers of the medullary reticulospinal tract descend the length of the spinal cord. Reticulospinal fibers from the pons and medulla are not segregated sharply in the spinal cord. Medullary reticulospinal fibers terminate chiefly in lamina VII, but some fibers terminate in lamina IX. Several components of the medullary reticulospinal tract have been identified physiologically: (1) long projections that provide collaterals to multiple spinal levels and (2) short projections to cervical segments arising mainly from dorsorostral regions of the nucleus reticularis gigantocellularis.

Reticulospinal fibers, arising in both the pons and medulla, largely terminate upon the somata and dendrites of internuncial neurons, although some medullary projections end directly upon motor neurons. Most impulses from the reticular formation that influence gamma (γ) motor neurons probably are mediated at segmental levels by internuncial neurons in laminae VII and VIII. Anatomically neither the pontine nor the medullary reticulospinal tract is somatotopically organized, although physiological data suggest that localized regions of the pontine and rostrodorsal portion of the medullary reticular formation may exert their major influences at particular spinal levels. Regions in which pontine reticulospinal fibers terminate are similar to those in which vestibulospinal fibers end; both of these systems are considered to convey facilitatory impulses. Medullary reticulospinal fibers terminate in portions of the gray laminae that also receive fibers from corticospinal and rubrospinal tracts.

Autonomic fibers from higher levels descend and traverse portions of the reticular formation that give rise to the reticulospinal tracts. Ventrolateral regions of the medulla and pons contain several groups of noradrenergic neurons that receive inputs from rostral autonomic structures and project fibers into parts of the reticular formation. One large group in the ventrolateral pons project fibers directly to spinal cord (Fig. 4.16). Stimulation of this ventrolateral region, known as the *lateral tegmental system*, produces a variety of sympathetic responses, including increases in arterial blood pressure.

Experimental studies indicate that stimulation of the brain stem reticular formation can (1) facilitate and inhibit voluntary movement, cortically induced movement, and reflex activity; (2) influence muscle tone, probably via the gamma system; (3) affect phasic activities associated with respiration; (4) exert pressor and depressor effects on the circulatory system; and (5) exert facilitating and inhibiting influences on the central transmission of sensory impulses. Areas of the medullary reticular formation from which the medullary reticulospinal tract arises correspond to regions from which inhibitory effects are elicited. Facilitatory effects are obtained from far larger rostral regions of the reticular formation.

The brain stem reticular formation receives input from many sources, but direct corticoreticular projections are particularly abundant.

Corticoreticular fibers arise from widespread areas of the cortex, although the greatest number originate from the "motor area." These fibers terminate in two fairly restricted regions of the reticular formation, one in the pons and one in the medulla. Corticoreticular fibers are distributed bilaterally with some crossed preponderance. The terminations within the reticular formation correspond to those regions that give rise to the reticulospinal tracts. Thus, the synaptic linkage of corticoreticular and reticulospinal fibers forms a pathway from the cortex to spinal levels. There is no evidence of a somatotopic linkage within this system.

The nuclei of the raphe that have serotonin (5-hydroxytryptamine, 5-HT) as their neurotransmitter give rise to projections distributed extensively in the reticular formation. Only the nucleus raphe magnus (medulla) and perhaps nucleus raphe pontis appear to project to spinal levels. Cells of the nucleus raphe magnus give rise to bilateral spinal projections that descend in the dorsolateral funiculus (Fig. 5.14). These fibers terminate most profusely in laminae I, II, and V in the cervical enlargement. Stimulation of the nucleus raphe magnus produces an analgesic effect by inhibitory actions of 5-HT and other neurotransmitters upon sensory neurons.

Medial Longitudinal Fasciculus (MLF)

The posterior part of the anterior funiculus contains a composite bundle of descending fibers that originate from different nuclei at various brain stem levels. This composite bundle is known as the MLF. Spinal portions of this bundle represent only a part of the brain stem tract designated by the same name. Descending fibers in the spinal MLF arise from the medial and inferior vestibular nuclei, the pontine reticular formation, the superior colliculus (tectospinal), and the interstitial nucleus of Cajal (interstitiospinal) (Figs. 4.11, 4.12, and 4.14). This bundle forms a well-defined tract only in cervical spinal segments, but component fiber systems descend to sacral levels. Fibers of this bundle arising from the medial vestibular nucleus are predominantly ipsilateral in the spinal cord and terminate in portions of laminae VIII and VII (Fig. 4.12). The largest component of the spinal MLF, the pontine reticulospinal tract, has been described previously. The interstitiospinal tract arises from a small mesencephalic nucleus lateral to the MLF and oculomotor complex. Fibers of this tract are uncrossed and terminate in parts of laminae VIII and VII at all spinal levels.

Descending Autonomic Pathways

The spinal cord contains descending autonomic fibers that terminate upon visceral cell groups (i.e., intermediolateral cell column and sacral preganglionic cell groups) that innervate smooth muscle, heart muscle, glands, and body viscera. The principal nuclei giving rise to descending autonomic fibers are (1) in several regions of the hypothalamus, (2) visceral nuclei of the oculomotor complex, (3) the locus ceruleus, and (4) portions of the nucleus of the solitary tract (Fig. 4.15). In addition some neurons in the reticular formation are concerned with visceral activities. Hypothalamic neurons projecting to spinal levels include cells in the (1) paraventricular nucleus and (2) lateral and posterior regions of the hypothalamus. Fibers from these hypothalamic nuclei project to visceral nuclei in the medulla as well as to spinal levels (Fig. 4.15). Direct hypothalamic-spinal fibers descend in the lateral funiculus and terminate

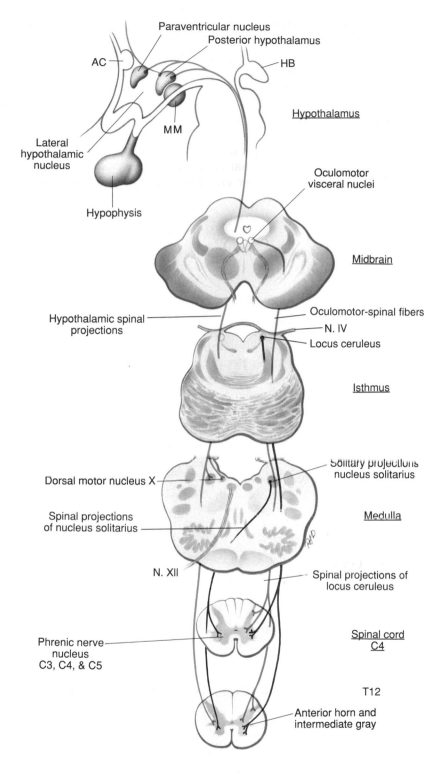

Paraventricular nucleus
Posterior hypothalamus
AC
HB
Lateral
hypothalamic
nucleus
MM
Hypothalamus
Hypophysis
Oculomotor
visceral nuclei
Midbrain
Hypothalamic spinal
projections
Oculomotor-spinal fibers
N. IV
Locus ceruleus
Isthmus
Dorsal motor nucleus X
Solitary projections
nucleus solitarius
Spinal projections
of nucleus solitarius
Medulla
N. XII
Spinal projections of
locus ceruleus
Phrenic nerve
nucleus
C3, C4, & C5
Spinal cord
C4
T12
Anterior horn and
intermediate gray

Figure 4.15. Schematic diagram of descending autonomic projections to the spinal cord. Projections from hypothalamic nuclei (parvicellular paraventricular nucleus, lateral hypothalamic nucleus, and the posterior hypothalamus) descend to terminate upon cells of the ipsilateral intermediolateral column in thoracic and upper lumbar spinal segments (*blue*). Hypothalamic nuclei are shown in a sagittal plane. Parasympathetic visceral neurons in the oculomotor nuclear complex supply intrinsic ocular structures and project fibers to the spinal cord that terminate in parts of laminae I and V (*green*). At isthmus levels cells of the pigmented locus ceruleus, containing noradrenergic fibers, project descending fibers to spinal levels that end in parts of the anterior horn and the intermediate gray (*red*). Cells in the ventrolateral part of the nucleus solitarius project crossed fibers to the phrenic nerve nucleus (C3, C4, and C5) and to parts of the anterior horn in thoracic spinal segments (*black*). Noradrenergic projections to the spinal cord from the ventrolateral pontine tegmentum (cell group A5) are shown in Figure 4.16.

upon cells of the intermediolateral cell column in thoracic, lumbar, and sacral segments. These uncrossed fibers appear to directly influence preganglionic sympathetic and parasympathetic neurons.

Although the visceral nuclei of the oculomotor nuclear complex (Fig. 7.10) project large numbers preganglionic parasympathetic fibers into third nerve, these neurons also project fibers directly to spinal levels. Descending fibers from the Edinger-Westphal nucleus contribute fibers to the posterior column nuclei and spinal projections that descend to lumbar levels (Fig. 4.15). In the spinal cord most of these fibers end in lamina I and parts of lamina V.

A small pigmented nucleus in the rostral pons, known as the locus ceruleus (Figs. 4.15, 6.28, and 6.29), has been demonstrated to synthesize, store, and release the neurotransmitter norepinephrine. Immunocytochemically noradrenergic neurons can be identified by using antiserum to dopamine-β-hydroxylase. The locus ceruleus distributes fibers widely in the neuraxis and is regarded as the principal source of norepinephrine in the central nervous system. Spinal projections from this nucleus descend in the anterior and lateral funiculi; are mainly uncrossed; and terminate in the anterior horn, intermediate gray, and dorsal regions of the posterior horn.

Cells in ventrolateral parts of the nucleus of the solitary tract (Figs. 4.15 and 5.22) project to cervical and thoracic spinal segments. The solitariospinal tract is predominantly crossed and terminates in the region of phrenic motor neurons at C3–C5 levels and the anterior horn and intermediolateral cell column at thoracic levels. Fibers of this tract provide excitatory inputs to phrenic and inspiratory motor neurons.

Major noradrenergic projections to spinal cord originate from cells lateral to the facial nucleus in the pons (i.e., group A5). These fibers descend ipsilaterally through the ventrolateral medulla; provide collaterals to the reticular formation, nucleus solitarius, and the dorsal motor nucleus of the vagus; and enter the ipsilateral ventral funiculus of the spinal cord (Fig. 4.16). This bilateral, but predominantly uncrossed, noradrenergic spinal system terminates upon cells of the intermediolateral cell column in thoracic and upper lumbar segments. No medullary noradrenergic neurons in the lateral tegmental system project to spinal cord.

With the exception of some descending autonomic pathways and the corticospinal tract, the neurotransmitters of the long ascending and descending tracts of the spinal cord have not been identified. While it seems likely that glutamate and/or aspartate are the principal neurotransmitters of cortical projections, highly specific antisera may recognize other substances. The ubiquitous nature of glutamate in the CNS and its involvement in the basic metabolic activities of neurons make it difficult to determine if immunocytochemical glutamate is in the "transmitter pool" or the "metabolic pool."

Fasciculi Proprii

Short ascending and descending fiber systems, both crossed and uncrossed, which begin and end within the spinal cord, constitute the fasciculi proprii or spinospinal fasciculi (Fig. 4.17). This intrinsic spinal pathway interconnects cell groups at various levels and within the same level. Descending collaterals of dorsal root fibers in the posterior columns frequently are regarded as part of this system. Fibers of this system participate in intersegmental spinal reflexes. The fasciculi proprii, adjacent to the spinal gray in all funiculi, are most numerous in anterolateral regions. These tracts and the major ascending and descending spinal tracts are shown schematically in Figure 4.17.

UPPER AND LOWER MOTOR NEURONS

Lower Motor Neuron

The anterior horn cells and their axons, projecting via the ventral root to striated muscle, constitute an anatomical and physiological unit

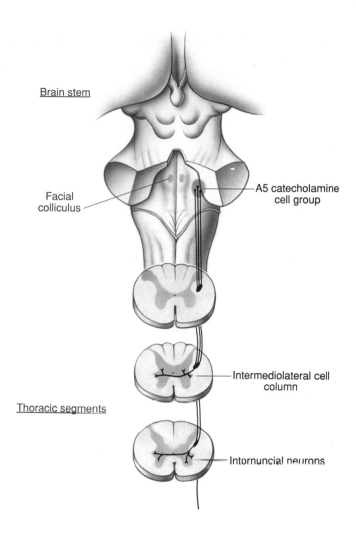

Figure 4.16. Schematic diagram of the spinal projections from the pontine catecholamine cell group (A5). Noradrenergic fibers from this cell group descend ipsilaterally but are distributed bilaterally to the intermediolateral cell column and internuncial neurons in thoracic spinal segments. Preganglionic and postganglionic sympathetic fibers project to the cardiovascular system.

Brain stem

Facial
colliculus

A5 catecholamine
cell group

Intermediolateral cell
column

Thoracic segments

Intornuncial neurons

referred to as the final common pathway or the lower motor neuron. Injury or disease of the anterior horn cells or their projecting axons results in paralysis of the muscles innervated by these fibers, loss of muscle tone, and prompt atrophy of the denervated muscle. Myotatic reflexes in the denervated muscle will be abolished because the reflex is broken. This sequence of events is seen in poliomyelitis, other diseases involving the anterior horn cells, and following severance of the ventral roots.

Upper Motor Neuron

The anterior horn cells can be directly and indirectly activated by impulses transmitted by descending fiber systems. Although virtually all of the descending spinal systems influence the activity of the lower motor neuron to some degree, the overwhelming clinical importance of the corticospinal tract has caused it to be equated with the *upper motor neuron*. Lesions of the upper motor neuron are characterized by paresis (i.e., incomplete loss of muscle power) or paralysis and initial loss of muscle tone, followed in time by increased tone in antigravity muscles (i.e., spasticity), hyperactive myotatic reflexes, the Babinski sign, and loss of the superficial abdominal and cremasteric reflexes. Muscle atrophy is not seen in the early stages, because segmental innervation of striated muscles remains intact; however, with long standing upper motor neuron paralysis, atrophy of disuse becomes evident. The concepts of the upper and lower motor neuron constitute one of the basic corner stones of

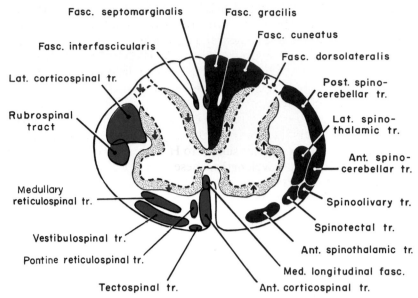

Figure 4.17.   Diagram of ascending (*black*) and descending (*red*) pathways of the spinal cord. The fasciculus proprius system (*stippled*) and dorsolateral fasciculus contain both ascending and descending nerve fibers. (From Carpenter and Sutin, *Human Neuroanatomy*, 1983; courtesy of Williams & Wilkins.)

clinical neurology and the simple distinctions outlined previously must be considered in the neurological examination of every patient.

SPINAL CORD LESIONS

Determination of the origin, course, and termination of most spinal cord pathways from the study of normal Weigert- and Nissl-stained sections is virtually impossible, but such sections provide valuable information concerning spinal cord organization and cytoarchitecture. The most precise data concerning spinal pathways has been derived from anatomical and physiological studies in animals. Secondary degeneration in nerve fibers (severed from cell bodies), studied in sections stained by the Marchi, Nauta, or other silver impregnation technics, provided valuable information concerning the course and termination of fiber bundles. Lesions in nerve fibers also produce alterations of the cell bodies, giving rise to these fibers, which can be detected in Nissl-stained sections within a few days. These cell changes, referred to as *retrograde cell changes*, are characterized by swelling and distortion of the perikaryon, eccentric nuclei, and dissolution of Nissl substance. Retrograde cellular provides precise data concerning the cells of origin of particular fiber bundles.

More precise information concerning fiber connections in the central nervous system can be obtained using tritiated amino acids and autoradiographic technics. This method is based on the physiological principle of axoplasmic flow. Since the neuronal soma is the principal site of synthesis of protein and other materials, injection of neurons with radioactive precursors (^{3}H amino acids) labels substances synthesized in the soma and transported via the axon to the terminals. (Figs. 6.13, 6.20, 7.19, 8.17, and 11.19). The enzyme horseradish peroxidase (HRP) and certain lectins (wheat germ agglutinin) are transported by axons in both anterograde and retrograde fashion. HRP taken up at axonal terminals and neuromuscular junctions is transported retrogradely to the cell somata where it is sequestered in lysosomes or in multivesicular bodies. The demonstration of HRP granules in neurons and their processes depends on the ability of the enzyme to oxidize a chromagen (diaminobenzidine, benzidine dihydrochloride, or tetramethylbenzidine) in the presence of hydrogen peroxide to form a dense, dark precipitate. Tissue reacted with these chromagens and hydrogen peroxide reveals fine, dark granules within retrogradely labeled neurons. HRP taken up by neurons or injured axons is transported distally (anterograde) to terminals where it appears as very fine grains in reacted tissue. Reaction product in cells, fibers, and terminals can be identified microscopically under bright or dark-field illumination. Certain fluorescent compounds also are transported intraaxonally in a retrograde manner similar to HRP. Because these compounds fluoresce at different wavelengths, these substances lend themselves to double-labeling studies. Fluorescent dyes injected into two separate fields of terminals will retrogradely double-label neurons projecting collaterals to both fields.

Root Lesions

Section of the dorsal roots (dorsal rhizotomy) abolishes all input supplied by these roots and interrupts segmental reflex arcs. Because of extensive overlap, section of one dorsal root does not result in detectable sensory loss. If multiple dorsal roots are sectioned, for example C5 through T1, cutaneous sensibility will be lost or greatly impaired, in the C6, C7, and C8 dermatomes, but input from stretch receptors entering all five dorsal roots will be abolished. As a consequence muscle tone and myotatic reflexes will be absent in most of the muscles of the upper extremity. Although the muscles can be contracted because the ventral roots remain intact, the deafferented extremity is virtually useless due to loss of cutaneous and kinesthetic sense. Monkeys with such rhizotomies do not use the deafferented limb for walking, climbing, or grasping.

Spinal cord degeneration resulting from multiple dorsal rhizotomies (C5 through T1) is distributed most profusely at the level of the sectioned roots to portions of the posterior horn, to selected cell groups within lamina VII, and to parts of lamina IX (Fig. 3.9). Particularly profuse ascending and descending degeneration is present in the ipsilateral fasciculus cuneatus. No ascending degeneration is present in other ascending spinal tracts, because these tracts arise from cell groups within the spinal cord. In other words, degeneration is limited to the primary afferent fibers and does not involve intrinsic spinal neurons or their processes. A diagrammatic representation of degeneration resulting from section of a single lumbar dorsal root is shown at *1* in Figure 4.18.

Injury or section of the ventral root produces a lower motor neuron paralysis of the muscle units innervated by the particular root (*4*, in Fig. 4.18). If the lesion involves thoracic or upper lumbar ventral roots, preganglionic sympathetic fibers also will be interrupted (*3*, in Fig. 4.18). Secondary (Wallerian) degeneration will result in somatic and visceral efferent fibers; postganglionic neurons and their processes will remain intact. Section of a mixed nerve distal to the sympathetic ganglion in the lower thoracic region (*2* in Fig. 4.18) results in degeneration in motor, sensory, and postganglionic sympathetic nerve fibers distal to the lesion.

Spinal Cord Transection

Complete spinal cord transection results in the immediate loss of all neural function below the level of the lesion. There is a complete loss below the level of the lesion of (1) all somatic sensation, (2) all motor function, (3) all visceral sensation, (4) all reflex activity, (5) all muscle tone, and (6) thermoregulatory control. This complete cessation of all neural function in the isolated spinal cord caudal to the lesion is called *spinal shock* and persists for 1 to 6 weeks (averages 3 weeks) in humans. The termination of the period of spinal shock is heralded by the appear-

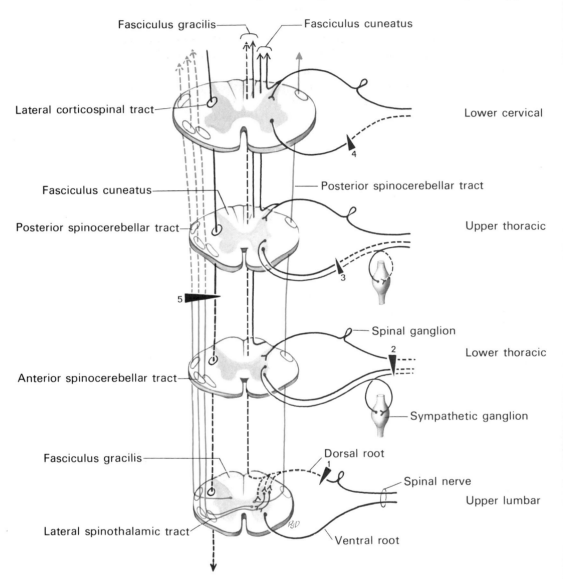

Figure 4.18. Simplified schematic diagram of degeneration resulting from certain lesions of the spinal nerves, spinal roots, and spinal cord. Sites of lesions are indicated by black wedges. Dorsal and ventral root fibers, peripheral nerve fibers, fibers in the posterior white columns, and short relays are in *black*; ascending spinal tracts are *blue*, and the corticospinal tract is *red*. A lesion of the dorsal root, *1*, at upper lumbar levels produces degeneration (dashed lines) in the posterior and anterior gray horns (not shown) and in parts of the fasciculus gracilis. No degeneration is present in other ascending spinal tracts because degeneration does not pass beyond the synapse. A lesion of spinal nerve as at *2* produces peripheral degeneration (dashed lines) in somatic motor, sensory, and postganglionic sympathetic fibers. A lesion of the ventral root at site *3* produces degeneration in somatic motor and preganglionic sympathetic fibers. A lesion at *4* produces degeneration only in somatic motor fibers distal to the lesion. The lesion at *5* destroys the lateral funiculus and produces ascending degeneration (dashed lines) in the posterior and anterior spinocerebellar tracts (*blue*) and in the spinothalamic tracts [only the lateral spinothalamic tract (*blue*) shown here] above the level of the lesion. This lesion also produces descending degeneration (dashed lines) in the corticospinal tract (*red*) below the level of the lesion. Although other spinal tracts that would degenerate are not indicated, the same principle applies. (From Carpenter and Sutin, *Human Neuroanatomy*, 1983; courtesy of Williams & Wilkins.)

ance of the Babinski sign (i.e., an extensor toe response to stroking the sole of the foot) and evidence of *minimal reflex responses* to painful stimuli. In time recovery of flexor reflex activity leads to a phase characterized by *flexor muscle spasms*. These spasms, which are bilateral, may in time result in the *triple flexion response* of Sherrington, characterized by flexion of the lower extremity at the hip and knee and dorsoflexion of the foot. The most extreme form of the triple flexion response is the *mass reflex*, in which repeated discharge in flexor motor units occurs spontaneously or in response to minimal and nonspecific stimuli. Beginning about 4 months after injury there is a slow, gradual, and progressive increase in extensor muscle tone. During this period there may be episodes of alternate flexor and extensor muscle spasm. Extensor muscle tone ultimately becomes predominant. Examination of the patient at this time reveals (1) marked extensor muscle tone, (2) spasticity, (3) hyperactive myotatic reflexes, (4) sustained clonus (a self-perpetuating myotatic reflex activity), (5) bilateral Babinski signs, (6) loss of the superficial abdominal and cremastoric (male) reflexor and (7) loss of all sensation and voluntary motor function below the level of the lesion. Spasticity is characterized by increased tone in the antigravity muscles (extensors in the lower extremity and flexors in the upper extremity), increased resistance to passive movement, and a sudden reduction in tone as the limb is flexed or extended passively. The abrupt melting away of muscle tone, referred to as the *knife-clasp phenomenon*, is due to disynaptic inhibition of extensor or flexor motor neurons caused by stimulating Gogli tendon organs in passively stretching the involved muscles (Fig. 3.23).

Disturbances of bowel and bladder function produce distressing problems in the management of paraplegic patients. Initially there is urinary retention; this is followed by overflow incontinence. This problem usually is handled by a system of tidal drainage, which automatically fills and empties the bladder at regular intervals.

Degeneration resulting from complete transection of the spinal cord follows a well-established pattern. Above the level of the lesion, ascending tracts will be degenerated, while below the lesion level, they will appear intact. The reverse is seen in the descending tracts. Thus by studying spinal cord sections above and below the level of the lesion, it is possible to predict fairly closely the level of the lesion (Figs. 4.5 and 4.19).

Spinal Cord Hemisection

While spinal cord hemisection is less common than complete cord transection, it presents a highly characteristic syndrome (Brown-Séquard) and is instructive for teaching purposes. This type of lesion is not associated with a period of spinal shock and the neurological disturbances on the two sides are different. On the side of the lesion the following are found below the level of the lesion: (1) an upper motor neuron syndrome, (2) greatly impaired discriminatory tactile sense, (3) loss of kinesthetic sense, and (4) reduced muscle tone. At the level of the lesion, there usually is bilateral impairment of pain and thermal sense and variable degrees of lower motor neuron involvement dependent on the size of the lesion side. Contralateral to the lesion there is (1) loss of pain sensibility from one segment below the level of the lesion and (2) loss of thermal sense from about two segments below the level of the lesion. Sensory disturbances contralateral to the lesion are due to interruption of crossed ascending fibers in the spinothalamic tracts. The spinal degeneration seen in the Brown-Séguard syndrome is almost entirely on the side of the

Figure 4.19. Section through fourth lumbar segment of a human spinal cord that had been crushed in the lower cervical region. The degenerated long descending tracts are unstained. Note that the lateral corticospinal tract reaches the lateral periphery of the spinal cord at this level and the vestibulospinal tract lies on the anterior surface of the cord. Weigert's myelin stain. Photograph. (From Carpenter and Sutin, *Human Neuroanatomy*, 1983; courtesy of Williams & Wilkins.)

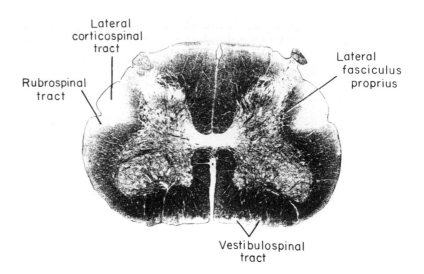

lesion and conforms to the same principle as described for complete spinal cord transection (5, in Fig. 4.18).

Spinal Cord Syndromes

There are many varieties of spinal cord lesions and syndromes. *Amyotrophic lateral sclerosis* is a progressive degenerative disease involving both upper and lower motor neurons bilaterally. There is degeneration and demyelinization of the corticospinal tracts and degeneration of anterior horn cells bilaterally at some segmental levels. Involvement of the anterior horn cells results in marked weakness, fasciculation (twitching of groups of muscle fibers), and progressive atrophy. *Combined system disease*, representing the neurological manifestations of pernicious anemia, is associated with degenerative changes in peripheral nerves and in the central nervous system. Degeneration in the spinal cord is evident bilaterally in the posterior white columns (fasciculi gracilis) and in the corticospinal tracts but is not confined to these systems. *Syringomyelia* is a chronic disease characterized by cavities that develop in relationship to the central canal of the spinal cord. The hallmark of the disease is an early impairment, or loss, of pain and thermal sense with preservation of tactile sense. This differential loss of pain and thermal sense is called "sensory dissociation." The central cavities that develop in this disease interrupt the decussating fibers of the spinothalamic tracts in the ventral white commissure in several consecutive segments. *Tabes dorsalis* is a central nervous system form of syphilis that produces degeneration in the central processes of spinal ganglion cells. Sensory loss, impairment of position and vibratory sense, radicular (i.e., root) pains, and paresthesias all are related to dorsal root pathology. Ataxia and difficulty in walking are related to loss of position and kinesthetic sense. Muscle tone and myotatic reflexes are greatly reduced in the lower extremities. Vascular lesions of the spinal cord are not common but sometimes occur in relationship to surgical procedures. The blood supply of the spinal cord is discussed in Chapter 14 (Figs. 14.1 and 14.2).

SUGGESTED READINGS

ALBE-FESSARD, D., LEVANTE, A., AND LAMOUR, Y. 1974. Origin of spinothalamic tract in monkeys. Brain Res., **65**: 503–509.

AKAIKE, T. 1983. Neuronal organization of the vestibulospinal system in the cat. Brain Res., **259**: 217–227.

APKARIAN, A. V., AND HODGE, C. J. 1989. Primate spinothalamic pathways: I. A quantitative study of the cells of origin of the spinothalamic pathway. J. Comp. Neurol., **288**: 447–473.

ASANUMA, H., ZARZECKI, P., JANKOWSKA, E., HONGO, T., AND MARCUS, S. 1979. Projection of individual pyramidal tract neurons to lumbar motoneuron pool of the monkey. Exp. Brain Res., **34**: 73–89.

BARNES, S. 1901. Degeneration in hemiplegia: With special reference to a ventrolateral pyramidal tract, the accessory fillet and Pick's bundle. Brain, **24**: 463–501.

BASBAUM, A. I., CLANTON, C. H., AND FIELDS, H. L. 1976. Opiate and stimulus-produced analgesia: Functional anatomy of medullospinal pathways. Proc. Natl. Acad. Sci., USA, **73**: 4685–4688.

BASBAUM, A. I., CLANTON, C. H., AND FIELDS, H. L. 1978. Three bulbospinal pathways from the rostral medulla of the cat: An autoradiographic study of pain modulating systems. J. Comp. Neurol., **178**: 209–224.

BASBAUM, A. I., RALSTON, D. D., AND RALSTON, H. J. 1986. Bulbospinal projections in the primate: A light and electron microscopic study of a pain modulating system. J. Comp. Neurol., **250**: 311–323.

BRODAL, A. 1957. *The Reticular Formation of the Brain Stem. Anatomical Aspects and Functional Correlations.* Charles C Thomas, Springfield, IL.

CARPENTER, M. B., STEIN, B. M., AND SHRIVER, J. E. 1968. Central projections of spinal dorsal roots in the monkey. II. Lower thoracic, lumbosacral and coccygeal dorsal roots. Am. J. Anat., **123**: 75–118.

CAVERSON, M. M., CIRIELLO, J., AND CALARESU, F. R. 1983. Direct pathway from cardiovascular neurons in the ventrolateral medulla to the region of the intermediolateral nucleus of upper thoracic cord: An anatomical and electrophysiological investigation in the cat. J. Aut. Nerv. System, **9**: 451–475.

COULTER, J. D., EWING, L., AND CARTER, C. 1976. Origin of primary sensorimotor cortical projections to lumbar spinal cord of cat and monkey. Brain Res., **103**: 366–372.

COULTER, J. D., AND JONES, E. G. 1977. Differential distribution of corticospinal projections from individual cytoarchitectonic fields in the monkey. Brain Res., **129**: 335–340.

COWAN, W. M., AND CUÉNOD, M. 1975. The use of axonal transport for study of neuronal connections: A retrospective survey. In *The Use of Axonal Transport for Studies of Neuronal Connectivity.* Elsevier, Amsterdam, pp. 2–23.

DAMPNEY, R. A. L., CZACHURSKI, J., DEMBOWSKY, K., GOODCHILD, A. K., AND SELLER, H. 1987. Afferent connections and spinal projections of the pressor region in the rostral ventrolateral medulla of the cat. J. Aut. Nerv. System, **20**: 73–86.

GIUFFRIDA, R., AND RUSTIONI, A. 1989. Glutamate and aspartate immunoreactivity in corticospinal neurons of rats. J. Comp. Neurol., **288**: 154–164.

GRANT, G. 1962. Spinal course and somatotopically localized termination of the spinocerebellar tracts: An experimental study in the cat. Acta Physiol. Scand., **56** (suppl. 193): 1–45.

GRILLNER, S., HONGO, T., AND LUND, S. 1969. Descending monosynaptic and reflex control of γ motoneurones. Acta Physiol. Scand., **75**: 592–614.

GRILLNER, S., HONGO, T., AND LUND, S. 1970. The vestibulospinal tract. Effects on alpha-motoneurons in the lumbosacral spinal cord in the cat. Exp. Brain Res., **10**: 94–120.

GROOS, W., EWING, L. K., CARTER, C. M., AND COULTER, J. D. 1978. Organization of corticospinal neurons in the cat. Brain Res., **143**: 393–419.

HA, H., AND LIU, C. N. 1968. Cell origin of the ventral spinocerebellar tract. J. Comp. Neurol., **133**: 185–205.

HARTMANN-VON MONAKOW, K., AKERT, K., AND KÜNZLE, H. 1979. Projections of the precentral and premotor cortex to the red nucleus and other midbrain areas in *Macaca fascicularis.* Exp. Brain Res., **34**: 91–105.

HUBBARD, J. I., AND OSCARSSON, O. 1962. Localization of the cell bodies of the ventral spinocerebellar tract in lumbar segments of the cat. J. Comp. Neurol., **118**: 199–204.

JONES, E. G., AND WISE, S. P. 1977. Size, laminar and columnar distribution of efferent cells in the sensory-motor cortex of monkeys. J. Comp. Neurol., **175**: 391–438.

LOEWY, A. D., AND BURTON, H. 1978. Nuclei of the solitary tract: Efferent projections to the lower brain stem and spinal cord of the cat. J. Comp. Neurol., **181**: 421–450.

LOEWY, A. D., SAPER, C. B., AND YAMODIS, N. D. 1978. Reevaluation of the efferent projections of the Edinger-Westphal nucleus. Brain Res., **141**: 153–159.

LOEWY, A. D., McKELLAR, S., AND SAPER, C. D. 1979. Direct projections of the A5 catecholamine cell group to the intermediolateral cell column. Brain Res., **174**: 309–314.

MATSUSHITA, M. 1988. Spinocerebellar projections from the lowest lumbar and sacral-caudal segments in the cat, as studied by anterograde transport of wheat germ agglutinin-horseradish peroxidase. J. Comp. Neurol., **274**: 23–254.

MEHLER, W. R., FEFERMAN, M. E., AND NAUTA, W. J. H. 1960. Ascending axon degeneration following anterolateral cordotomy: An experimental study in the monkey. Brain, **83**: 718–750.

MESULAM, M. M. 1978. Tetramethylbenzidine for horseradish peroxidase neurohistochemistry: A non-carcinogenic blue reaction-product with superior sensitivity for visualizing neural afferents and efferents. J. Histochem. Cytochem., **26**: 106–117.

NYBERG-HANSEN, R. 1966. Functional organization of descending supraspinal fibre system to the spinal cord: Anatomical observations and physiological correlations. Ergeb. Anat. Entwicklungsgesch., **39**: 1–48.

OSCARSSON, O. 1965. Functional organization of the spino- and cuneocerebellar tracts. Physiol. Rev., **45**: 495–522.

OSCARSSON, O., AND SJÖLUND, B. 1977. The ventral spino-olivocerebellar system in the cat. I. Identification of five paths and their terminations in the cerebellar anterior lobe. Exp. Brain Res., **28**: 469–486.

OLSZEWSKI, J., AND BAXTER, D. 1954. *Cytoarchitecture of the Human Brain Stem.* J. B. Lippincott, Philadelphia.

OTTERSEN, O. P., AND STORM-MATHISEN, J. 1984. Glutamate and GABA-containing neurons in the mouse and rat brain, as demonstrated with a new immunocytochemical technique. J. Comp. Neurol., **239**: 374–392.

PETERSON, B. 1979. Reticulo-motor pathways: Their connections and possible roles in motor behavior. In H. ASANUMA and V. J. WILSON (Editors), *Integration in the Nervous System*, Igaku Shoin, Tokyo, pp. 185–201.

PETERSON, B. 1980. Participation of pontomedullary reticular neurons in specific motor activity. In J. A. HOBSON and M. A. B. BRAZIER (Editors), *The Reticular Formation Revisited.* Raven Press, New York, pp. 171–192.

PETERSON, B. W., MAUNZ, R. A., PITTS, N. G., AND MACKEL, R. G. 1975. Patterns of projection and branching of reticulospinal neurons. Exp. Brain Res., **23**: 333–351.

POGGIO, G. F., AND MOUNTCASTLE, V. B. 1960. A study of the functional contributions of the lemniscal and spinothalamic systems to somatic sensibility. Bull. Johns Hopkins Hosp., **106**: 266–316.

POMPEIANO, O., AND BRODAL, A. 1957. Experimental demonstration of a somatotopical origin of rubrospinal fibers in the cat. J. Comp. Neurol., **108**: 225–251.

POMPEIANO, O., AND BRODAL, A. 1957. The origin of the vestibulospinal fibres in the cat: An experimental-anatomical study, with comments on the descending and medial longitudinal fasciculus. Arch. Ital. Biol., **95**: 166–195.

ROSSI, G. F., AND BRODAL, A. 1956. Corticofugal fibers to the brain stem reticular formation: An experimental study in the cat. J. Anat., **90**: 42–62.

SAPER, C. B., LOEWY, A. D., SWANSON, L. W., AND COWAN, W. M. 1976. Direct hypothalamo-automatic connections. Brain Res., **117**: 305–312.

SCHWINDT, P. C. 1981. Control of motoneuron output by pathways descending from the brain stem. In A. L. TOWE AND E. S. LUSCHEI (Editors), *Handbook of Behavioral Neurobiology, Motor Coordination.* Plenum Press, New York, Vol. 5, pp. 139–230.

SHINODA, Y., ARNOLD, A., AND ASANUMA, H. 1976. Spinal branching of corticospinal axons in the cat. Exp. Brain Res., **26**: 215–234.

SHINODA, Y., GHAZ, C., AND ARNOLD, A. 1977. Spinal branching of rubrospinal axons in the cat. Exp. Brain Res., **30**: 203–218.

SHINODA, Y., OHGAKI, T., AND FUTAMI, T. 1986. The morphology of single lateral vestibulospinal tract axons in the lower cervical spinal cord of the cat. J. Comp. Neurol., **249**: 226–241.

SHINODA, Y., YAMAGUCHI, T., AND FUTAMI, T. 1986. Multiple axon collaterals of single corticospinal axons in the cat spinal cord. J. Neurophysiol., **55**: 425–448.

SHINODA, Y., ZARZECKI, P., AND ASANUMA, H. 1979. Spinal branching of pyramidal tract neurons in the monkey. Exp. Brain Res., **34**: 59–72.

SHRIVER, J. E., STEIN, B. M., AND CARPENTER, M. B. 1968. Central projections of spinal dorsal roots in the monkey. I. Cervical and upper thoracic dorsal roots. Am. J. Anat., **123**: 27–74.

TREVINO, D. L., AND CARSTENS, E. 1975. Confirmation of the location of spinothalamic neurons in the cat and monkey by retrograde transport of horseradish peroxidase. Brain Res., **98**: 177–182.

TREVINO, D. L., COULTER, J. D., AND WILLIS, W. D. 1973. Location of cells of origin in spinothalamic tract in lumbar enlargement of the monkey. J. Neurophysiol., **36**: 750–761.

TYNER, C. F. 1974. Anatomical specificity in the feline corticospinal system. Brain Res., **69**: 336–340.

WESTLUND, K. N., BOWKER, R. M., ZIEGLER, M. G., AND COULTER, J. D. 1984. Origins and terminations of descending noradrenergic projections to spinal cord of monkey. Brain Res., **292**: 1–16.

WESTLUND, K. N., AND COULTER, J. D. 1980. Descending projections of the locus coeruleus and subcoeruleus/medial parabrachial nuclei in monkey: Axonal transport studies and dopamine-β-hydroxylase immunocytochemistry. Brain Res. Rev., **2**: 235–264.

5

The Medulla

The medulla (myelencephalon), the most caudal brain stem segment, begins rostral to the highest rootlets of the first cervical spinal nerve. The external transition from upper cervical spinal cord to medulla is gradual and appears as a cylindrical expansion. Above the level of transition, the medulla increases in size and develops distinctive external features (Figs. 5.1 and 5.2). The development of the fourth ventricle causes structures located posteriorly to shift posterolaterally. The medullary pyramids rostral to the corticospinal decussation obliterate the anterior median fissure, and the development of the inferior olivary complex above the transitional zone produces an oval eminence posterolateral to the pyramids. Internal changes in the transition from spinal cord to medulla are (1) the decussation of the medullary pyramids (Figs. 4.7, 4.8, 4.9, 5.3, and 5.4); (2) the termination of the fasciculi gracilis and cuneatus upon their respective nuclei and the decussation of internal arcuate fibers to form the medial lemniscus (Figs. 4.1 and 5.5); (3) the replacement of fibers in the zone of Lissauer by descending fibers of the spinal trigeminal tract (Fig. 5.5); (4) replacement of the spinal gray by the reticular formation; and (5) the development of cranial nerve nuclei (Figs. 5.7 and 5.8).

SPINOMEDULLARY TRANSITION

Transverse sections at the junction of spinal cord and medulla resemble those of upper cervical spinal segments (Fig. 5.3). The substantia gelatinosa has increased in size, and coarse descending fibers of the spinal trigeminal tract are found posterolateral to it. These fibers arise from cells of the trigeminal ganglion, enter the brain stem at pontine levels, and descend caudally as far as the second cervical segment (Fig. 5.8). The substantia gelatinosa gradually becomes the spinal trigeminal nucleus at high cervical levels, and this nucleus retains its position and size throughout the medulla. The lateral corticospinal tract, caudal to the pyramidal decussation, presents a reticulated appearance as its fibers project dorsally, laterally, and caudally into the lateral funiculus of the spinal cord. The anterior horn appears small and is covered anteromedially by fibers of the medial longitudinal fasciculus (MLF) and anterolaterally by fibers of the vestibulospinal tract. A few fibers of the spinal part of the spinal accessory nerve arch posterolaterally to emerge from the lateral aspect of the spinal cord (Fig. 5.3). Anterior horn cells that extend into the lower medulla constitute the *supraspinal nucleus*.

Corticospinal Decussation

The most conspicuous feature of the spinomedullary transition is the corticospinal decussation (Figs. 4.8 and 5.4). Fibers in the medullary pyramid cross the midline in large fascicles anterior to the central gray

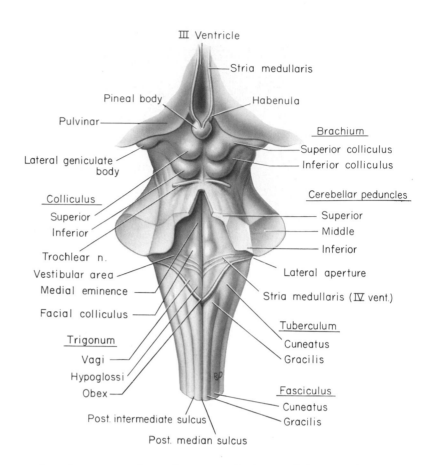

and project posterolaterally across the base of the anterior horn. Interdigitating fiber bundles, often of unequal size, project downward and posteriorly so that in transverse sections most of the bundles are cut obliquely. The crossed fibers of the lateral corticospinal tract descend in the dorsal part of the lateral funiculus, while uncrossed fibers of the anterior corticospinal tract descend in the anterior funiculus (Figs. 4.8, 4.9, and 4.10). In a graded series of ascending sections the corticospinal decussation is seen in reverse sequence. The corticospinal decussation forms the anatomical basis for voluntary motor control of one half of the body by signals from the contralateral cerebral cortex.

Decussation of the Medial Lemniscus

At levels through the corticospinal decussation, relatively large nuclear masses begin to appear in the posterior white columns. These are the nuclei gracilis and cuneatus (Figs. 5.4 and 5.5). The long ascending branches of cells in the spinal ganglia, contained in the fasciculi gracilis and cuneatus, terminate respectively upon these nuclei (Figs. 4.1 and 5.5). The nuclei gracilis appear first as slender collections of cells posterior to the central gray and anterior to the fibers of the fasciculi gracilis (Fig. 5.4). The nuclei cuneatus develop at more rostral levels as triangular-shaped cell aggregations in the most anterior part of the fasciculi cuneatus. At higher levels the posterior column nuclei progressively enlarge and fibers of the posterior white columns show a corresponding reduction (Fig. 5.5). Fibers in the posterior white column terminate somatotopically throughout most of the rostrocaudal extent of the nuclei gracilis and cuneatus.

Three cytological regions of the nucleus gracilis have been recog-

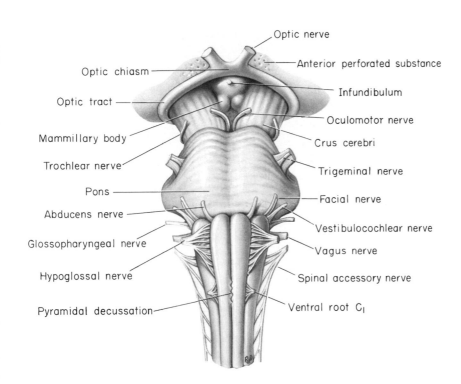

Optic nerve

Optic chiasm

Optic tract

Mammillary body

Trochlear nerve

Pons

Abducens nerve

Glossopharyngeal nerve

Hypoglossal nerve

Pyramidal decussation

Anterior perforated substance

Infundibulum

Oculomotor nerve

Crus cerebri

Trigeminal nerve

Facial nerve

Vestibulocochlear nerve

Vagus nerve

Spinal accessory nerve

Ventral root C$_I$

Figure 5.2. Drawing of the anterior aspect of the medulla, pons, and midbrain. (From Carpenter and Sutin, *Human Neuroanatomy,* 1983; courtesy of Williams & Wilkins.)

nized: (1) a rostral reticular region characterized by a loose cellular organization, (2) a central "cell nest" region made up of cell clusters, and (3) a caudal region of scattered cells. Ascending branches of dorsal root fibers projecting upon the nucleus gracilis exhibit a crude somatotopic lamination in the "cell nest" region; terminals in the reticular region are diffuse. The nucleus cuneatus also exhibits regional differences in cytoarchitecture. Dorsal regions of the cuneate nucleus contain clusters of round cells with bushy dendrites, while basal areas contain triangular, multipolar, and fusiform cells. Clusters of round cells, considered to receive the principal ascending afferents from distal parts of the upper extremity, are related to small cutaneous receptive fields, while triangular cells receive afferents from proximal parts of limb related to larger cutaneous receptive fields. The somatotopic organization of the posterior columns and the medial lemniscus is maintained at the level of the posterior column nuclei, and neural elements related to kinesthesis and tactile sense are intermingled in a single and mutual somatotopic pattern.

Myelinated fibers arising from the nuclei gracilis and cuneatus sweep anteromedially around the central gray, as *internal arcuate fibers* (Figs. 4.1 and 5.5). These fibers decussate completely and form a well-defined ascending bundle, the *medial lemniscus*. Fibers of the medial lemniscus form a compact L-shaped bundle adjacent to the median raphe and medial to the inferior olivary complex at higher medullary levels (Figs. 5.7 and 5.9). Projections originating from the nucleus gracilis are located ventrally in the medial lemniscus, and those from the nucleus cuneatus are dorsal. Unlike most other ascending systems from the spinal cord, fibers of the medial lemniscus do not give off collaterals as they course through the brain stem to the ventral posterolateral (VPLc) nucleus of the thalamus. The decussation of the medial lemniscus provides part of the anatomical basis for the sensory representation of half of the body in the contralateral cerebral cortex.

Cells in rostral parts of the nuclei gracilis and cuneatus give rise to fibers that cross the midline with the internal arcuate fibers but terminate

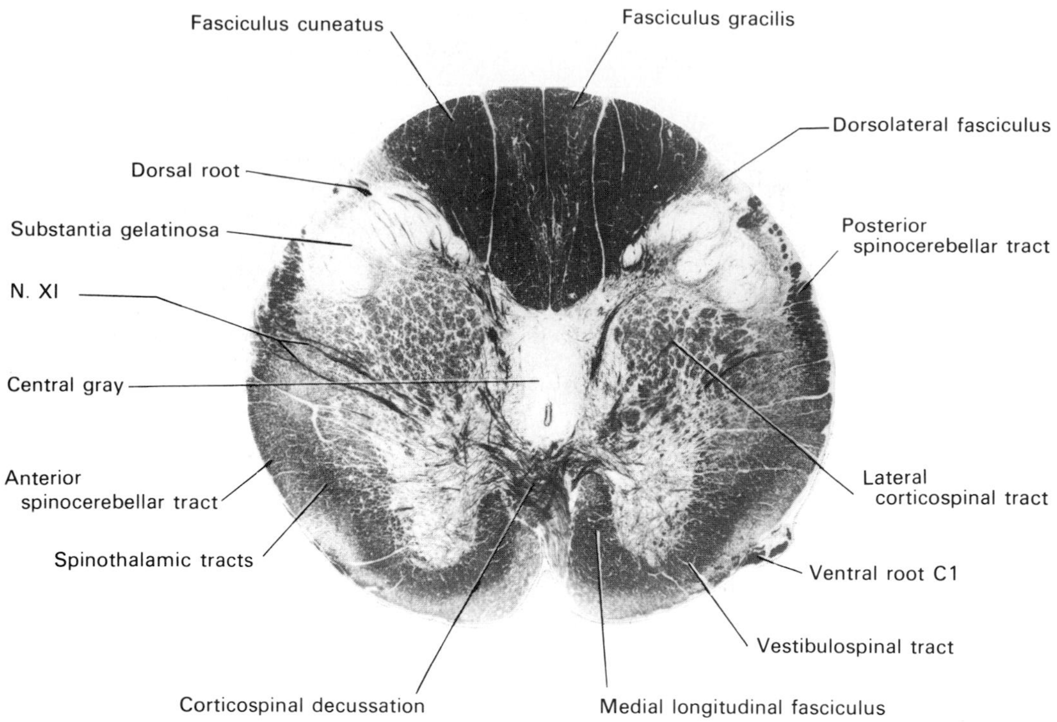

Fasciculus cuneatus

Fasciculus gracilis

Dorsolateral fasciculus

Dorsal root

Substantia gelatinosa

Posterior spinocerebellar tract

N. XI

Central gray

Anterior spinocerebellar tract

Lateral corticospinal tract

Spinothalamic tracts

Ventral root C1

Vestibulospinal tract

Corticospinal decussation

Medial longitudinal fasciculus

Figure 5.3. Transverse section through the junction of spinal cord and medulla. The most caudally decussating fibers of the corticospinal tract can be seen passing into the posterior part of the lateral funiculus. The substantia gelatinosa at this level contains cell groups of the spinal trigeminal nucleus. Fibers of the spinal part of the accessory nerve can be seen emerging laterally on the left. Weigert's myelin stain.

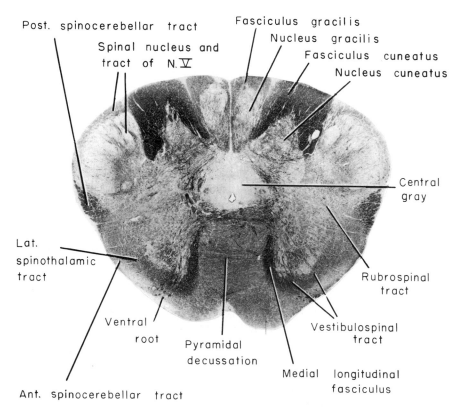

Post. spinocerebellar tract

Spinal nucleus and tract of N. V

Fasciculus gracilis

Nucleus gracilis

Fasciculus cuneatus

Nucleus cuneatus

Central gray

Lat. spinothalamic tract

Rubrospinal tract

Ventral root

Pyramidal decussation

Vestibulospinal tract

Medial longitudinal fasciculus

Ant. spinocerebellar tract

Figure 5.4. Transverse section of the medulla through the upper part of the corticospinal decussation. Weigert's myelin stain. Photograph. (From Carpenter and Sutin, *Human Neuroanatomy*, 1983; courtesy of Williams & Wilkins.)

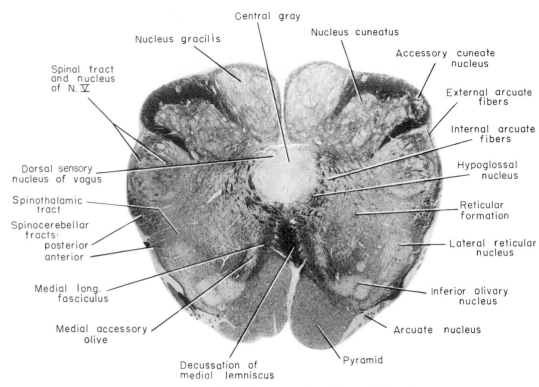

Central gray

Nucleus gracilis

Nucleus cuneatus

Accessory cuneate
nucleus

Spinal tract
and nucleus
of N. Ⅴ

External arcuate
fibers

Internal arcuate
fibers

Hypoglossal
nucleus

Dorsal sensory
nucleus of vagus

Spinothalamic
tract

Reticular
formation

Spinocerebellar
tracts:
posterior
anterior

Lateral reticular
nucleus

Medial long.
fasciculus

Inferior olivary
nucleus

Medial accessory
olive

Arcuate nucleus

Decussation of
medial lemniscus

Pyramid

Figure 5.5. Transverse section of medulla through the decussation of the medial lemniscus. Weigert's myelin stain. Photograph. (From Carpenter and Sutin, *Human Neuroanatomy*, 1983; courtesy of Williams & Wilkins.)

in the dorsal accessory olivary nucleus. These fibers from the posterior column nuclei form a link in the dorsal spino-olivocerebellar pathway. This pathway to the cerebellar vermis is activated exclusively by flexor reflex afferents (i.e., myelinated afferents that evoke a flexor reflex).

The *accessory cuneate nucleus*, located lateral to the cuneate nucleus at slightly more rostral levels, is composed of large cells that resemble those of the dorsal nucleus of Clarke (nucleus thoracicus) (Figs. 5.5, 5.6, and 5.7). Cells of the accessory cuneate nucleus and the dorsal nucleus of Clarke are morphologically similar (i.e., large cells with eccentric nuclei); receive afferents from spinal ganglia; give rise to uncrossed cerebellar projections; and relay information from muscle spindles, Golgi tendon organs, and cutaneous afferents. Fibers terminating in the accessory cuneate nucleus are derived from the same spinal ganglia as those projecting to the cuneate nucleus, namely cervical and upper thoracic. Ascending fibers in the fasciculus cuneatus terminate somatotopically in the accessory cuneate nucleus. Cells of the accessory cuneate nucleus give rise to uncrossed *cuneocerebellar fibers*, which enter the cerebellum via the inferior cerebellar peduncle (Fig. 4.4). The main cerebellar projection of the accessory cuneate nucleus is ipsilateral to paramedian parts in the anterior lobe (Fig. 8.1). The cuneocerebellar tract is regarded as the upper limb equivalent of the posterior spinocerebellar tract.

Spinal Trigeminal Tract

Afferent trigeminal root fibers, which enter at upper pons levels, descend in the dorsolateral part of the brain stem, and project as far caudally as the C2 spinal level, constitute the spinal trigeminal tract (Figs. 5.4, 5.5, 5.7, and 5.8). These descending fibers, originating from cells of

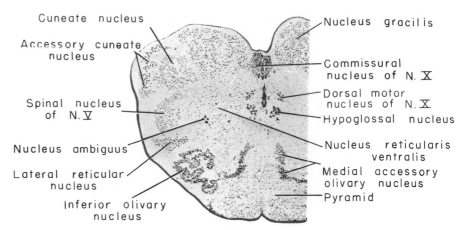

Figure 5.6. Section through medulla of 1-month-old infant about the same level as in Figure 5.5. Cresyl violet. Photograph, with cell groups blocked in schematically. (From Carpenter and Sutin, *Human Neuroanatomy*, 1983; courtesy of Williams & Wilkins.)

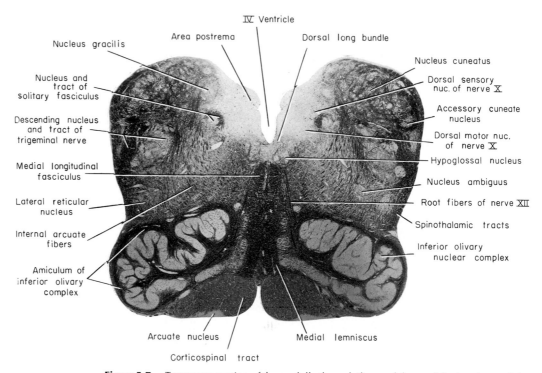

Figure 5.7. Transverse section of the medulla through the caudal part of the fourth ventricle, the area postrema, and the caudal part of the inferior olivary nucleus. Weigert's myelin stain. Photograph. (From Carpenter and Sutin, *Human Neuroanatomy*, 1983; courtesy of Williams & Wilkins.)

the trigeminal ganglion, have a definite topographic organization, so that: (1) fibers of the mandibular division are most dorsal, (2) fibers of the ophthalmic division are most ventral, and (3) fibers of the maxillary division are intermediate (Fig. 5.8). Some trigeminal root fibers from all divisions extend into upper cervical spinal segments. As this tract descends, it becomes progressively smaller as fibers of the tract terminate upon cells of the adjacent spinal trigeminal nucleus (Fig. 5.6). The tract contains general somatic afferent fibers from the trigeminal nerve, as well as fibers of the same functional category from the vagus, glossopharyngeal, and facial nerves that descend. A few visceral afferent fibers descending in the dorsal part of the spinal trigeminal tract project medially and terminate in ventrolateral parts of the nucleus solitarius.

Spinal Trigeminal Nucleus

This nucleus lies along the medial border of the tract from the level of the trigeminal root in the pons to the second cervical spinal segment (Figs. 5.5, 5.6, 5.7, and 5.8). Fibers of the spinal trigeminal tract terminate upon cells of the nucleus throughout its extent. Cytoarchitecturally, the spinal trigeminal nucleus is subdivided into three parts: (1) *pars oralis*, which extends caudally to the rostral pole of the hypoglossal nucleus; (2) *pars interpolaris*, which extends caudally to the level of the obex; and (3) *pars caudalis*, which begins near the level of the obex and extends into the upper cervical spinal cord. The caudal part of the spinal trigeminal nucleus has a cytological lamination similar to that of the dorsal horn of the spinal gray (Fig. 5.9). Four laminae are recognized: (1) lamina I (corresponding to the posteromarginal zone); (2) lamina II (corresponding to the substantia gelatinosa); and (3) laminae III and IV, which form the magnocellular layers. Laminae I and II in the caudal part of the spinal trigeminal nucleus contain afferent fibers positive for substance P; cells in lamina II are immunoreactive for enkephalin (Fig. 5.10). Cells in laminae III and IV are referred to as the magnocellular subnucleus. Lamina I and parts of lamina II in the caudal spinal trigeminal nucleus are uniquely concerned with pain and nociceptive stimuli. Substance P fibers and cells positive for enkephalin are not found in rostral portions of the spinal trigeminal nucleus.

Fibers in different parts of the spinal trigeminal tract terminate in corresponding circumscribed parts of the spinal trigeminal nucleus (e.g., mandibular fibers terminate in dorsal parts of the nucleus). Some neurons in the spinal trigeminal nucleus emit collaterals that link together different levels of the spinal trigeminal nucleus.

Fibers in the spinal trigeminal tract convey impulses concerned with pain, thermal, and tactile sense from the face, forehead, and mucous membranes of the nose and mouth. The spinal trigeminal tract and nucleus appear to be the only part of the trigeminal complex uniquely concerned with the perception of pain and thermal sense. Medullary trigeminal tractotomy (i.e., section of the spinal trigeminal tract) markedly reduces pain and thermal sense ipsilaterally without impairing tactile sense. Lesions in the dorsolateral region of the medulla involving the spinal trigeminal tract and the adjacent spinothalamic tracts produce a curious alternating hemianalgesia and hemithermo-anesthesia of the face and body (Figs. 4.3 and 5.8). This condition, known as the lateral medullary syndrome, is characterized by diminished pain and thermal sense in the face ipsilaterally (spinal trigeminal tract) and over the opposite side of the body (spinothalamic tracts).

Secondary trigeminal fibers arise from cells of the spinal trigeminal tract at multiple levels, cross through the reticular formation to the opposite side, and ascend to thalamic levels in association with the contralateral medial lemniscus (Fig. 6.24). These trigeminothalamic fibers constitute the second neuron in a sensory pathway from the face to the cortex. Other trigeminal fibers (1) terminate upon reticular neurons, (2) project to the cerebellum via the inferior cerebellar peduncle, or (3) establish reflex connections with multiple motor cranial nerve nuclei.

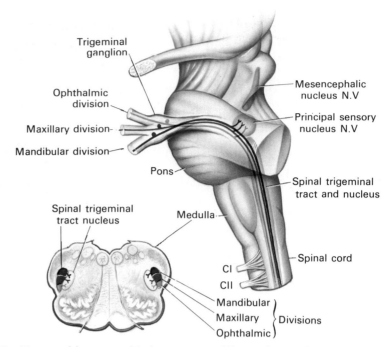

Figure 5.8. Diagram of the topographical arrangement of fibers in the spinal trigeminal tract. Fibers with cell bodies in the trigeminal ganglion enter in the upper pons and descend caudally as far as C2. Throughout the length of the tract, mandibular fibers are most dorsal and those of the ophthalmic division are most ventral. Fibers leave the spinal trigeminal tract to synapse upon cells of the spinal trigeminal nucleus.

Reticular Formation

The reticular formation represents large collections of neurons of various sizes and shapes enmeshed in a matrix of fibers that form the core of the brain stem. At the level of the decussation of the medial lemniscus the reticular formation occupies a region anterior to the posterior column nuclei, medial to the spinal trigeminal complex, and posterolateral to the pyramid (Figs. 5.5 and 5.6). Cells of various sizes arranged in more or less definite groups are traversed by both longitudinal and transverse fiber bundles. The internal arcuate fibers and many smaller bundles, including secondary trigeminal fibers, course through the reticular formation. Cells in the previously described region constitute the *ventral reticular nucleus* (Fig. 5.6).

One of the more discrete and distinct nuclei at this level is the *lateral reticular nucleus of the medulla*, located anterolaterally (Figs. 5.5, 5.6, and 5.7). This nucleus begins caudal to the inferior olivary complex and extends to midolivary regions. Three cytoarchitectonic regions of the nucleus are recognized: magnocellular, parvicellular, and subtrigeminal. Large cells are located dorsal to the inferior olive, while small cell groups are situated dorsolaterally within the nucleus. The lateral reticular nucleus of the medulla is a cerebellar relay nucleus. It receives afferent fibers from the spinal cord (i.e., spinoreticular and collaterals from the spinothalamic tracts) and descending fibers from the red nucleus (rubrobulbar). Spinal afferents to the lateral reticular nucleus are topographically organized. Fibers from all subdivisions of the lateral reticular nucleus enter the cerebellum via the inferior cerebellar peduncle and terminate as mossy fibers in the anterior lobe and in the paramedian lobule (Fig. 8.1).

On the anterior aspect of the pyramid is a small collection of cells that varies in size, position, and level. These cells, constituting the *arcuate nucleus* (Figs. 5.5 and 5.7), frequently become continuous with the pon-

Area postrema

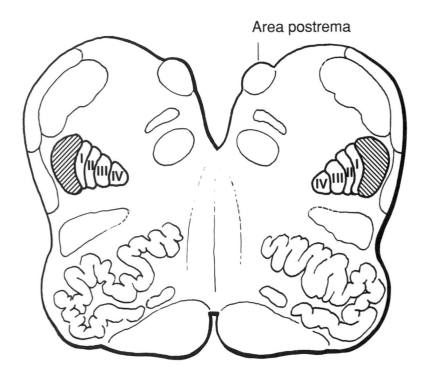

Figure 5.9. Schematic diagram of the laminar organization of the spinal trigeminal nucleus. Cells in lamina I resemble those of the posteromarginal nucleus at spinal levels. Lamina II corresponds to the substantia gelatinosa, and laminae III and IV form the magnocellular subdivision. Caudally, lamina I and the outer part of lamina II contain substance P fibers and terminals. Cells positive for enkephalin are found in deep parts of lamina II caudally.

tine nuclei at higher levels. Afferent fibers are derived from the cerebral cortex and efferents project to the cerebellum as *external arcuate fibers* (Fig. 5.5).

Area Postrema

Immediately rostral to the obex on each side of the fourth ventricle is a small rounded eminence, the *area postrema* (Figs. 5.7 and 5.9), containing astroblast-like cells, arterioles, sinusoids, and some apolar or unipolar neurons. The area postrema is one of several specialized ependymal regions that lie outside the blood-brain barrier, collectively referred to as circumventricular organs (Fig. 1.18). All of the circumventricular organs, except the area postrema, are unpaired and related to portions of the diencephalon. Fibers from the solitary nucleus and spinal cord project to the area postrema. Fields of terminals surrounding this area contain neurophysin, oxytocin, and vasopressin, although these peptides cannot be demonstrated within the area postrema. The area postrema is an emetic chemoreceptor, sensitive to apomorphine and intravenous digitalis glycosides.

Cranial Nerve Nuclei

At these levels, the cranial nerve nuclei, other than the spinal trigeminal nucleus, include the hypoglossal (N.XII) and those of the vagus (N.X) nerve (Figs. 5.6 and 5.7). Components of the vagal nuclei are in the gray surrounding the central canal. Anterolateral to the central canal are small collections of typical large motor neurons that constitute caudal portions of the hypoglossal nucleus; root fibers of N.XII project ventrally and emerge between the inferior olive and the medullary pyramid. Lateral to the central canal, collections of smaller spindle-shaped cells form the dorsal motor nucleus of the vagus nerve. These cells give rise to preganglionic parasympathetic fibers. Dorsal to the central canal on each side of the median raphe is the commissural nucleus of the vagus nerve (Fig.

Figure 5.10. Immunocytochemical features of the caudal spinal trigeminal tract and nucleus in the monkey. *A*, Fibers immunoreactive for substance P in the spinal trigeminal tract and in laminae I and II of the spinal trigeminal nucleus. *B*, Fibers and cells in the spinal trigeminal nucleus immunoreactive for leucine-enkephalin. Sections were taken from the same animal.

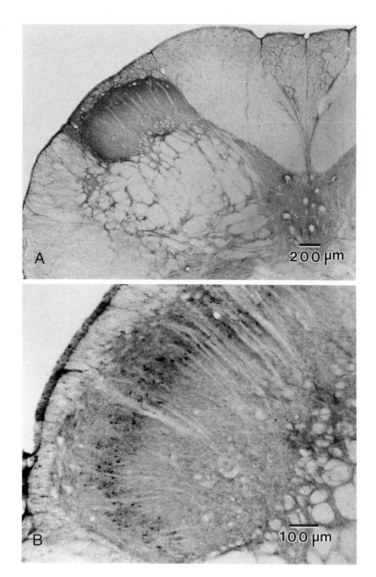

5.6). These cells, the most caudal extension of the medial portion of the nucleus solitarius, receive general visceral afferent fibers. The nucleus ambiguus lies in the reticular formation dorsal to the inferior olivary complex and medial to the lateral reticular nucleus (Figs. 5.6 and 5.7). Cells of the nucleus ambiguus, which project fibers forming components of the spinal accessory (N.XI), the vagus (N.X), and the glossopharyngeal (N.IX) nerves, are difficult to positively identify in Nissl preparations. Because these cells are cholinergic, they are easily visualized in immunocytochemical preparations using choline acetyltransferase (ChAT) (Fig. 5.16). Cells of the hypoglossal nucleus and the dorsal motor nucleus of the vagus also are immunoreactive to ChAT.

OLIVARY LEVELS OF THE MEDULLA

The most characteristic features of the medulla are present in transverse sections through the inferior olivary complex (Figs. 5.11 and 5.12). The central canal has opened into the fourth ventricle, and the roof of this ventricle is formed by the tela choroidea and the choroid plexus in the inferior medullary velum. The floor of the fourth ventricle contains three eminences, which overlie cranial nerve nuclei. The most medial is the *hypoglossal eminence* overlying the nucleus of N.XII (Figs. 5.1 and 5.18); an *intermediate eminence* overlies the vagal nuclei. The most medial of the vagal nuclei is the dorsal motor nucleus; the lateral part of the intermediate eminence overlies the nuclei of the solitary fasciculus. The sulcus limitans, often an indistinct sulcus, passes through the intermediate or vagal eminence; cranial nerve cell columns medial to the sulcus are efferent, while those lateral to it are afferent (Fig. 5.18). The most *lateral eminence* overlies the vestibular nuclei and is referred to as the *area vestibularis* (Fig. 5.12). Internal arcuate fibers sweep ventromedially through portions of the reticular formation, decussate, and enter the contralateral medial lemniscus (Fig. 5.7). The medial lemnisci occupy triangular-shaped areas on each side of the raphe, bounded ventrally by the pyramids and laterally by the inferior olivary nuclei. The accessory cuneate nucleus lies dorsolaterally, posterior to the spinal trigeminal tract and nucleus.

Inferior Olivary Nuclear Complex

The most characteristic and striking nuclear structure in the medulla is the inferior olivary complex (Figs. 5.6, 5.7, 5.11, and 5.12). This complex consists of three parts: (1) the *principal inferior olivary nucleus* appearing as a folded bag with the opening or hilus directed medially, (2) a *medial accessory olivary nucleus* located along the lateral border of the medial lemniscus, and (3) a *dorsal accessory olivary nucleus* located dorsal to the principal nucleus. These nuclei are composed of small round cells with numerous short dendrites and appear to have glutamate as their excitatory neurotransmitter. Axons of cells of the inferior olivary complex cross the median raphe, sweep posterolaterally, and enter the cerebellum via the contralateral inferior cerebellar peduncle. Crossed *olivocerebellar fibers*, constituting the largest single component of the inferior cerebellar peduncle (Figs. 5.11 and 5.17), project to all parts of the cerebellar cortex and to the deep cerebellar nuclei. Fibers of this massive projection end as climbing fibers in the cerebellar cortex that have a powerful excitatory action upon individual Purkinje cells.

The accessory olivary nuclei and the most medial part of the principal olivary nucleus project fibers to the cerebellar vermis. The larger lateral part of the principal olivary nucleus projects fibers to the contralateral cerebellar hemisphere. The principal olivary nucleus is surrounded by a band of myelinated fibers, which form the *amiculum olivae* (Fig. 5.7).

Descending fibers terminating upon cells of the inferior olivary complex arise from the cerebral cortex, the red nucleus, the periaqueductal gray of the midbrain, the inferior vestibular nucleus, parts of the spinal trigeminal nucleus, and the contralateral deep cerebellar nuclei. Spinal projections to the inferior olivary complex terminate mainly in the accessory olivary nuclei. Fibers ascending in the anterior spino-olivary tract (anterior funiculus) synapse in the accessory olivary nuclei; olivary efferents largely cross in the caudal medulla. Spino-olivary fibers, ascending in the posterior white columns, synapse upon cells in rostral parts of the nuclei gracilis and cuneatus, which in turn project fibers to the contralateral accessory olivary nuclei. Spinal afferents to parts of the inferior olivary complex constitute a link in spinocerebellar circuitry that resembles that of other spinocerebellar tracts.

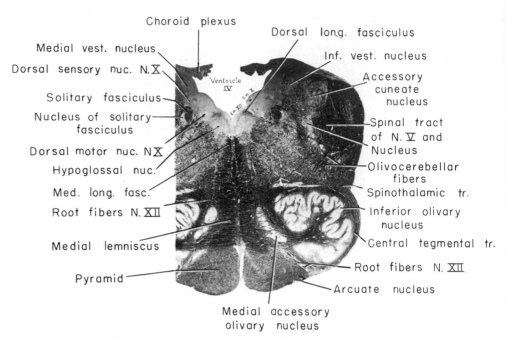

Figure 5.11. Transverse section of the medulla through the inferior olive complex rostral to that shown in Figure 5.7. *Em. X*, eminentia vagi; *Em. XII*, eminentia hypoglossi. Weigert's myelin stain. Photograph. (From Carpenter and Sutin, *Human Neuroanatomy*, 1983; courtesy of Williams & Wilkins.)

Medullary Reticular Formation

Phylogenetically, this constitutes the oldest part of the brain stem and is the matrix that forms its core. It is composed of diverse types of cells, organized in both compact and diffuse aggregations, and enmeshed in a complex fiber network (Figs. 5.5, 5.6, 5.7, 5.11, and 5.12). Anatomical studies indicate that the brain stem reticular formation can be subdivided into regions having distinctive cytoarchitecture, fiber connections, and intrinsic organization. In spite of these features, various subdivisions cannot be regarded as entirely independent entities, because fiber connections provide innumerable possibilities for interaction between subdivisions. Neurons in the reticular core project axons in both rostral and caudal directions. Primary bifurcating axons are oriented longitudinally, but collaterals pass in all directions and terminate in a variety of different endings. Many collaterals arborize about cells in both motor and sensory cranial nerve nuclei. Golgi type II cells (i.e., cells with short axons) have not been found in the reticular formation, a finding that suggests that polysynaptic transmission of impulses probably is due to dispersion of impulses along collateral fibers. The organization of the reticular formation suggests that a single reticular neuron can convey impulses both rostrally and caudally, may exert its influences both locally and at a distance, and impulses can be conducted both rapidly (primary axon) and slowly (via synapsing collateral axons).

The brain stem reticular formation begins in the caudal medulla rostral to the corticospinal decussation. Reticular nuclei present at this level are the *lateral reticular nucleus* of the medulla and the *ventral reticular nucleus* (Fig. 5.6). At midolivary levels the *gigantocellular reticular nucleus* occupies the area dorsal and medial to the inferior olivary complex (Figs. 4.6, 4.14, and 5.12). As its name implies, it has characteristic large cells, but it also contains many medium-sized and small cells. This nucleus

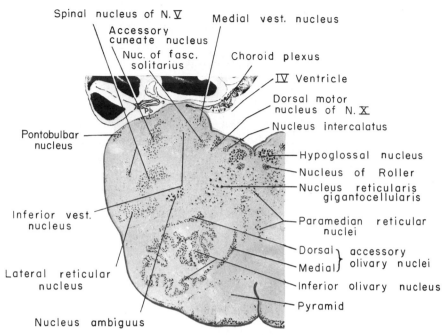

Figure 5.12. Section through midolivary region of the medulla. Cresyl violet. Photograph, with schematic representation of main cell groups. (From Carpenter and Sutin, *Human Neuroanatomy*, 1983; courtesy of Williams & Wilkins.)

occupies the medial two-thirds of the reticular formation and extends to the medullary-pontine junction.

The *parvicellular reticular nucleus* is a collection of small cells located posterolaterally, medial to the spinal trigeminal nucleus, and anterior to the vestibular nuclei. This nucleus, occupying roughly the lateral third of the medullary reticular formation, has been referred to as the "sensory" part because it receives collaterals from secondary sensory pathways.

The *paramedian reticular nuclei* consist of several small nuclear groups that lie close to, and sometimes among, fibers of the medial longitudinal fasciculus and the medial lemniscus (Fig. 5.12). These reticular neurons project most of their fibers to the cerebellar vermis.

In essence, the medullary reticular formation consists of three principal nuclear masses: (1) a *paramedian reticular nuclear group*, (2) a *central group* (i.e., the ventral reticular and gigantocellular reticular nuclei), and (3) a *lateral nuclear group* consisting of the lateral reticular and parvicellular reticular nuclei. The raphe nuclei, consisting of several distinct groups of neurons, probably also belong to the reticular formation but will be described separately.

Afferent fibers projecting into the medullary reticular formation arise in the spinal cord from secondary sensory cranial nerve nuclei and from the cerebral cortex and the deep cerebellar nuclei. *Spinoreticular fibers* ascend in the anterolateral funiculus and terminate in the caudal and lateral portions of the medullary reticular formation. A considerable number of these fibers end in the gigantocellular reticular nucleus, though some project to more rostral parts of the reticular formation. Collaterals of spinothalamic fibers terminate somatotopically upon cells of the lateral reticular nucleus, a cerebellar relay nucleus. *Collateral fibers* from second-order sensory neurons in cranial nerve nuclei [i.e., auditory, vestibular, trigeminal, and visceral (solitary fasciculus)], project to the parvicellular reticular nucleus. No collaterals of the medial lemniscus terminate in any part of the brain stem reticular formation.

Cerebelloreticular fibers terminate mainly in the paramedian reticular nuclei. These reticular projections originate from the fastigial and dentate nuclei. The paramedian reticular nuclei are involved in a feedback system in that they project and receive fibers from the cerebellum.

Corticoreticular fibers arise from widespread areas of cortex, but the largest number of these fibers are derived from sensorimotor areas. Most of these fibers terminate in portions of the reticular formation in the pons and medulla. These fibers are both crossed and uncrossed. Regions of the brain stem reticular formation receiving corticoreticular fibers give rise to reticulospinal fibers. Impulses from a wide variety of sources converge upon the reticular nuclei. The maximal overlap of afferent fibers from different sources occurs in the medullary reticular formation, which gives rise to a large number of long ascending and descending axons.

Efferent fibers arise from the medial two-thirds of the medullary reticular formation, which corresponds to the gigantocellular reticular nucleus; this nuclear mass gives rise to both long ascending and descending fibers. Ascending fibers from this nuclear mass ascend in the *central tegmental tract*, are uncrossed, and terminate mainly upon portions of the intralaminar thalamic nuclei (Figs. 2.27 and 4.6). This system plays an important role in the mechanism of arousal from sleep. Descending fibers from this medial region of the reticular formation give rise to the medullary reticulospinal tracts that are bilateral but predominantly uncrossed (Fig. 4.14). Axons of medullary reticular neurons form long descending reticulospinal projections that provide collaterals to all spinal levels and shorter projections only to cervical spinal segments. Stimulation of the rostral and dorsal part of the nucleus reticularis gigantocellularis and regions of the caudal pontine reticular formation produce monosynaptic excitatory postsynaptic potentials in motor neurons supplying the axial muscles of the neck and back. Stimulation of the caudal and medial medullary reticular formation produces disynaptic and multisynaptic inhibitory postsynaptic potentials in motor neurons at all levels. Thus the medullary reticular formation can be divided into a dorsorostral facilitatory region and a caudal inhibitory zone. Neurons in this "effector" area of the medullary reticular formation receive projections from cells in the parvicellular reticular nucleus. The latter reticular region is considered to serve "receptive" or "associative" functions, while the larger, more medial reticular region is organized to exert "effector" influences at both spinal and higher brain stem levels.

Raphe Nuclei

Cell groups lying in the midline of the medulla, pons, and midbrain collectively are called the raphe nuclei. The major raphe nuclei of the brain stem are shown in a schematized midsagittal section in Figure 5.13. Many, but not all, of the raphe nuclei have neurons that synthesize serotonin (5-hydroxytryptamine, 5-HT). A large number of raphe neurons also contain cholecystokinin (CCK). Fibers originating from cells in the raphe nuclei are distributed widely in the neuraxis and release serotonin at their terminals. In the medulla, serotonergic neurons lie in the nuclei raphe magnus, raphe obscurus, and raphe pallidus (*red* in Fig. 5.13), which give rise to descending spinal projections. Cells in the nucleus raphe magnus (Fig. 5.14) give rise to bilateral spinal projections that descend in the dorsolateral funiculus and terminate mostly in laminae I and II. Stimulation of the nucleus raphe magnus produces an analgesic effect by

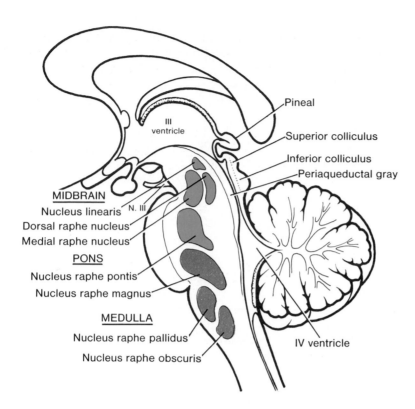

III
ventricle

Pineal

Superior colliculus

Inferior colliculus

Periaqueductal gray

MIDBRAIN
N. III
Nucleus linearis
Dorsal raphe nucleus
Medial raphe nucleus

PONS
Nucleus raphe pontis
Nucleus raphe magnus

MEDULLA
Nucleus raphe pallidus
Nucleus raphe obscuris

IV ventricle

Figure 5.13. Schematic drawing of a mid-sagittal section of the brain stem indicating the positions of the raphe nuclei. Nuclei in *red* project to spinal levels, while nuclei in *blue* have projections to brain stem nuclei and to parts of the telencephalon. Projections to diencephalic structures are most numerous from the dorsal and medial raphe nuclei and from the nucleus raphe pontis. The dorsal and medial raphe nuclei also project widely to telencephalic structures. (From Carpenter and Sutin, *Human Neuroanatomy*, 1983; courtesy of Williams & Wilkins.)

an inhibitory action upon nociceptive neurons in laminae I and II in caudal parts of the spinal trigeminal nucleus and in the spinal dorsal horn. Neurotransmitters involved in the modulation of pain probably are multiple and appear to act upon nociceptive interneurons, as well as neurons that give rise to pain pathways (i.e., spinothalamic tract neurons). While serotonin (5-HT) may be the dominant neurotransmitter of neurons in the raphe, enkephalin and other peptides have been shown to coexist within these cells. The analgesic effects of electrical stimulation of the midbrain periaqueductal gray appear to be mediated by connections with raphe nuclei in the lower brain stem.

Ascending and Descending Tracts

Ascending fibers of the medial lemniscus occupy an L-shaped area on each side of the median raphe posterior to the pyramid and medial to the inferior olivary complex (Figs. 4.1, 5.11, and 5.17). The spinothalamic tracts, which can no longer be designated as anterior and lateral, have merged and form essentially a single entity in the retro-olivary area. These tracts appear smaller than at spinal levels, because an appreciable number of fibers terminate in the lateral reticular nucleus and others have passed medially into the gigantocellular reticular nucleus. The posterior spinocerebellar tract has moved posteriorly at medullary levels and has become incorporated in the inferior cerebellar peduncle (Fig. 5.17). The anterior spinocerebellar tract maintains a retro-olivary position in the medulla and ultimately enters the cerebellum by coursing along the superior surface of the superior cerebellar peduncle (Fig. 4.4).

The medial longitudinal fasciculus (MLF) lies anterior to the hypoglossal nucleus adjacent to the median raphe (Figs. 5.7, 5.11, and 5.17). Descending fibers in this complex bundle are derived from various brain stem nuclei. Vestibular fibers in this bundle arise from the medial and inferior vestibular nuclei. The pontine reticular formation contributes the

Figure 5.14. Schematic diagram of spinal serotonergic projections from the nucleus raphe magnus (Fig. 5.23). These projections are bilateral, descend in the dorsal part of the lateral funiculus and terminate upon cells in laminae I, II, and V, considered to receive nociceptive inputs. Adjacent large reticular neurons have similar spinal projections but are not serotonergic. Both of these pathways are considered links in an endogenous analgesia-producing system. Fibers from the nuclei raphe pallidus and obscurus (not shown) descend in the ventral quadrant of the spinal cord. (From Carpenter and Sutin, *Human Neuroanatomy*, 1983; courtesy of Williams & Wilkins.)

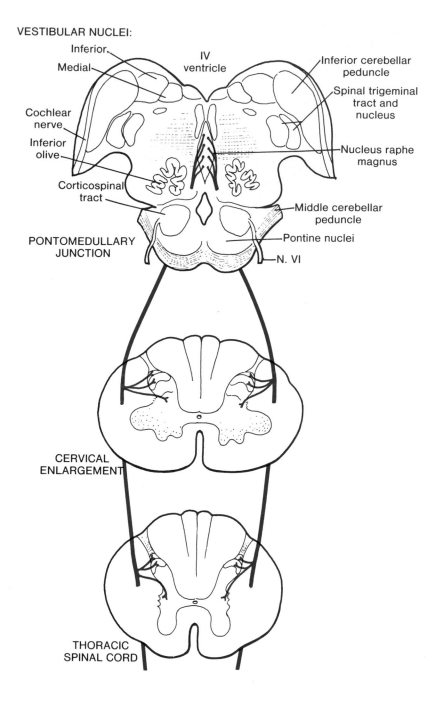

largest number of descending fibers in the MLF; smaller groups of fibers arise from the interstitial nucleus of Cajal (interstitiospinal tract) and the superior colliculus (tectospinal tract).

Rubrospinal fibers, descending in retro-olivary position, project collaterals to the lateral reticular nucleus, a cerebellar relay nucleus. Uncrossed *rubrobulbar fibers*, arising from rostral parts of the red nucleus, descend in the central tegmental tract and end upon cells in the dorsal lamella of the principal inferior olivary nucleus. At medullary levels fibers of the vestibulospinal tract are scattered in an area posterior to the inferior olivary complex (Fig. 4.12). The medullary reticulospinal tract is not evident at these levels, but its cells of origin, the gigantocellular reticular nucleus, are present posteromedial to the inferior olivary complex (Figs.

4.6, 4.14, and 5.12). The spinal trigeminal tract and nucleus occupy the same location as at more caudal levels.

Inferior Cerebellar Peduncle

This peduncle is a composite bundle that contains fibers arising from cell groups in the spinal cord and medulla that project to the cerebellum. Fibers entering this peduncle assemble along the posterolateral margin of the medulla dorsal to the spinal trigeminal tract and lateral to the accessory cuneate nucleus (Fig. 5.17). This bundle rapidly increases in size in the upper medulla by the addition of more fibers and enters the cerebellum (Figs. 5.17 and 5.27). Crossed olivocerebellar fibers constitute the largest component of the inferior cerebellar peduncle. Other medullary nuclei projecting to the cerebellum via this peduncle are (1) the lateral reticular nucleus of the medulla, (2) the accessory cuneate nucleus, (3) the paramedian reticular nuclei, (4) the arcuate nucleus, and (5) the perihypoglossal nuclei (see p. 136). Projections of the lateral reticular and accessory cuneate nuclei are uncrossed; those from other medullary relay nuclei are both crossed and uncrossed. The uncrossed posterior spinocerebellar tract also projects to the cerebellum via this peduncle.

CHEMICALLY IDENTIFIED NEURONS AND CIRCUITS

The functional organization of the central nervous system is dependent on neurotransmitters to carry impulses across synapses. Chemical coding of neurons and neural circuits are considered as essential to understanding of neuroanatomy as the cell groups and their connections. There are a large number of neurotransmitters recognized as having unique properties in certain neural circuits and probably a great many more that remain to be identified. Neurotransmitters not only turn the signals on or off as impulses arrive at the synapses, but different neurotransmitters can modify signals, act over a different time course, influence neuronal metabolism, or prepare cells for later neural events. Knowledge of neurotransmitters is essential to understanding the organization of the central nervous system, a variety of neurological diseases, and the nature of many drug actions. Immunohistochemical methods have revealed information concerning the sites of synthesis and storage of known or suspected neurotransmitters and neuromodulators. Autoradiographic technics have provided information concerning the distribution of transmitter binding sites. Retrograde labeling technics combined with immunocytochemistry or immunofluorescence make it possible to co-define neural projections and their neurotransmitters.

Acetylcholine (ACh), the first neurotransmitter identified, is the major transmitter of the peripheral nervous system but is less prominent in the central nervous system. Neurons containing ACh can be identified immunocytochemically by using antiserum to choline acetyltransferase (ChAT), the enzyme that synthesizes ACh, or histochemically by visualizing the hydrolytic enzyme acetylcholinesterase (AChE). While there is a general correspondence between ChAT immunoreactivity and the presence of AChE, AChE also is present in non-cholinergic neurons, nerve fibers, and terminals and is not considered a definitive marker. ACh is the neurotransmitter involved in producing contractions in striated muscle, and it is released at the terminals of all preganglionic neurons. All motor cranial nerve nuclei, all somatic spinal motor neurons, and all preganglionic autonomic neurons react positively to ChAT and are considered cholinergic neurons (Fig. 3.19). Postganglionic sympathetic neurons innervating the sweat glands also are cholinergic. In the medulla, cells of the hypoglossal nucleus, the dorsal motor nucleus of the vagus, and the nucleus ambiguus are all immunoreactive to ChAT (Fig. 5.16).

Biogenic amines present in the medulla are norepinephrine, epinephrine, and serotonin. The *locus ceruleus*, a blue-black pigmented nucleus located at isthmus levels, is the largest concentration of norepinephrine-containing neurons in the brain (Figs. 6.28 and 6.29). Projections of cells in the locus ceruleus distribute noradrenergic fibers throughout the central nervous system (Fig. 4.15). Although caudal parts of the locus ceruleus project via the ventral and lateral funiculi to nearly all levels of the spinal cord, these fibers do not terminate upon cells of the intermediolateral cell column in thoracolumbar spinal segments. A group of noradrenergic neurons lateral to the facial and superior olivary nuclei (A5 group) is considered to provide most of the input to the intermediolateral cell column, which gives rise to preganglionic sympathetic nerve fibers (Figs. 4.16 and 5.15). This nuclear group provides collaterals to the dorsal motor nucleus of the vagus, the nucleus solitarius, and the nucleus ambiguus (Fig. 5.15). Other noradrenergric neurons in the lower pons and medulla are scattered in lateral regions of the reticular formation. None of the noradrenergic neurons in the medulla appear to project to spinal cord. Scattered noradrenergic neurons in lateral parts of the medulla are collectively referred to as the *lateral tegmental system*. Noradrenergic neurons in the brain stem have been identified immunocytochemically using antiserum to dopamine-β-hydroxylase.

The indoleamine serotonin (5-HT) occurs largely in neurons of the raphe nuclei, although some serotonergic cells are in the reticular formation (Figs. 5.13 and 5.14). The serotonin system resembles the norepinephrine system in that both are components of the brain stem reticular formation and have widespread and partially overlapping projections. The ascending projections of the serotonin-containing neurons in the midbrain are more selective in their targets than the noradrenergic fibers (Fig. 5.14).

Two pentapeptides, methionine-enkephalin (met-enkephalin) and leucine-enkephalin (leu-enkephalin), isolated from both central and peripheral nervous tissue, appear to be endogenous ligands for opiate receptors. Both enkephalins are widely distributed in the central nervous system where their ratios differ; leu-enkephalin generally is present in higher concentrations. The distribution of opiate receptor binding sites parallels that of the opiate peptides. Enkephalin immunoreactive cell bodies in the medulla occur in laminae I and II in caudal portions of the spinal trigeminal nucleus (Fig. 5.10), in the solitary nucleus (Fig. 5.22), and in parts of reticular formation, including the raphe nuclei. These opiate-like peptides act as neurotransmitters and/or neuromodulators to suppress pain.

Substance P (SP) is a peptide of 10 amino acids found in several neural systems. About 20% of the cell bodies in spinal ganglia contain SP; fibers of these cells project via dorsal root filaments to terminations in laminae I and II of the dorsal horn (Figs. 3.21 and 5.10). Similar numbers of SP-containing cell bodies are found in the trigeminal ganglion. SP-containing cell bodies are small and associated with small, poorly myelinated fibers that encode nociceptive information. Substance P produces a prolonged excitation of central neurons. In the medulla, SP terminals are found in the superficial laminae of the caudal spinal trigeminal nucleus (Fig. 5.10), in the nucleus solitarius, and in some cells of the raphe nuclei; SP may coexist with other neurotransmitters in some cells.

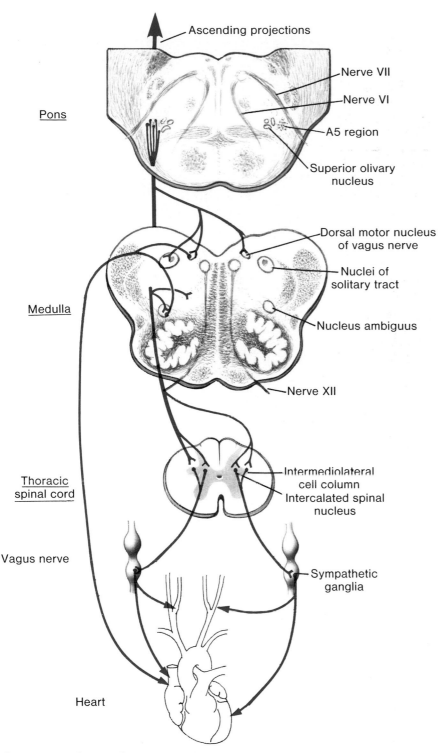

Figure 5.15. Schematic diagram of the descending projections from the pontine catechol-amine cell group (A5). This cell group, which lies lateral to the superior olivary nuclear complex, projects fibers to medullary vasomotor centers, to the intermediolateral cell column at thoracic levels, and to intercalated spinal neurons at the same levels. Medullary nuclei receiving fibers from the A5 cell group include (1) the dorsal motor nucleus of the vagus, (2) the nucleus ambiguus, (3) the nuclei of the solitary tract, and (4) portions of the medial medullary reticular formation. Descending projections to spinal cord are relayed via pre-ganglionic and postganglionic sympathetic neurons to the cardiovascular system. Stimulation of the A5 cell group produces increases in system blood and pulse pressure. Ascending projections of this cell group have not been fully characterized.

Figure 5.16. Sections of the medulla of the monkey immunoreacted with antiserum to choline acetyltransferase (ChAT), which demonstrates cholinergic neurons. *A,* Cholinergic neurons in the hypoglossal nucleus (XII), the dorsal motor nucleus of the vagus (DMN X), and the nucleus ambiguus (AMB). *B,* Cholinergic neurons in the nucleus ambiguus.

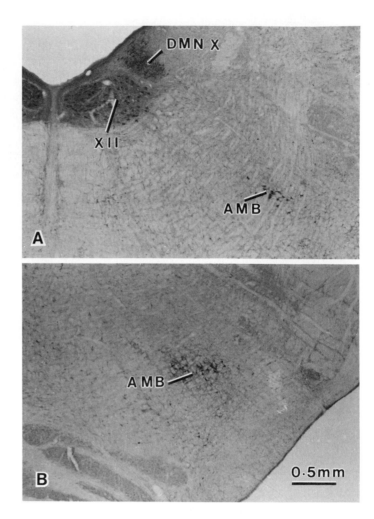

Dale's principle, which states that one neuron produces and releases only one neurotransmitter, is no longer considered a valid concept.

The nucleus of the solitary fasciculus, concerned with visceral sensation, taste sensation, and a variety of visceral reflexes, is a complex nucleus whose cell bodies have been shown to be immunoreactive to multiple neuropeptides and transmitters. Afferents to this nucleus are conveyed by the vagus, glossopharyngeal, and facial nerves, as well as neurons within the brain stem concerned with visceral functions. Neuropeptides identified within subdivisions of the nucleus solitarius include enkephalin, somatostatin, substance P, cholecystokinin, and neuropeptide Y. Cells of the nucleus solitarius contain receptors for many of these same neuropeptides. Many of these same neuropeptides have been identified in relay nuclei of ascending visceral and gustatory pathways at all levels of the neuraxis. The most numerous neuropeptides and catecholamine-containing cell bodies are located in caudal regions of the nucleus solitarius, which corresponds to the region most concerned with visceral activities.

CRANIAL NERVES OF THE MEDULLA

The schematic arrangement of the functional components of the cranial nerves of the medulla and the cell columns to which they are related are shown in Figure 5.18. The functional components of a typical spinal nerve are four: (1) *general somatic afferent* (GSA), (2) *general*

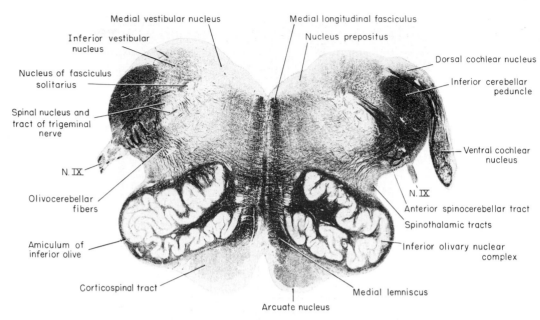

Figure 5.17.   Transverse section of medulla of 1-month-old infant through the cochlear nuclei and ninth nerve. Weigert's myelin stain. Photograph. (From Carpenter and Sutin, *Human Neuroanatomy*, 1983; courtesy of Williams & Wilkins.)

visceral afferent (GVA), (3) *general somatic efferent* (GSE), and (4) *general visceral efferent* (GVE). Functional components of the cranial nerves include the four types found in spinal nerves, plus three additional special categories: (1) *special somatic afferent* (SSA), (2) *special visceral afferent* (SVA), and (3) *special visceral efferent* (SVE). Somatic efferent fibers in both spinal and cranial nerves are regarded as a general component.

In the medulla, as in the spinal cord, the sulcus limitans divides afferent and efferent cell columns. Within the medulla special somatic afferent (SSA) cranial nerves are represented by the auditory and vestibular components of the vestibulocochlear nerve (N. VIII). General somatic afferent (GSA) fiber components of cranial nerves V, VII, IX, and X enter the brain stem at different levels and descend in the spinal trigeminal tract. Fibers conveying taste (special visceral afferent, SVA) and general visceral afferent (GVA) impulses from components of cranial nerves VII, IX, and X form a well-defined tract, the solitary fasciculus, which is embedded in the solitary nucleus (Figs. 5.7, 5.11, 5.12, and 5.23). All of the above cell columns lie posterolateral to a hypothetical extension of the sulcus limitans (Fig. 5.18). Ventromedial to this hypothetically projected line are the efferent cell columns. The dorsal motor nucleus of the vagus nerve and the inferior salivatory nucleus of the glossopharyngeal nerve give rise to general visceral efferent (GVE) fibers. Cells of the nucleus ambiguus located in the ventrolateral reticular formation posterior to the inferior olivary nuclear complex give rise to special visceral efferent (SVE) fibers that pass peripherally as components of the XI, X, and IX cranial nerves (Figs. 5.12 and 5.16). These fibers innervate muscles of the pharynx and larynx derived from the third and fourth branchial arches (i.e., branchiomeric muscles). The hypoglossal nucleus located in the floor of the fourth ventricle near the median raphe gives rise to general somatic efferent (GSE) fibers that innervate the muscles of the tongue (Fig. 5.12). The general somatic efferent cranial nerve nuclei all lie near the median raphe and in the floor of the fourth ventricle or cerebral aqueduct. Other nuclei, at more rostral levels, belonging to this group are the abducens, trochlear, and oculomotor. Schematic color-coded diagrams showing these nuclei and the intramedullary course of their fibers (Figs. 5.19 and 5.20) help to understand the organization of the cranial nerves and their various components.

Hypoglossal Nerve

This is a *general somatic efferent* (GSE) cranial nerve that supplies the somatic skeletal muscles of the tongue. The hypoglossal nucleus forms a column of typical motor cells about 18 mm long (Figs. 5.19 and 5.20). Root fibers of this nerve emerge ventrally, passing along the lateral margin of the MLF and the medial lemniscus, traversing medial parts of the inferior olivary complex, and exiting from the medulla between the pyramid and the inferior olive (Figs. 5.2, 5.7, and 5.11). In the gray matter surrounding the hypoglossal nuclei are several discrete nuclear groups, collectively known as the *perihypoglossal nuclei*. These are the *nucleus intercalatus*, the *nucleus prepositus*, and the *nucleus of Roller* (Figs. 5.12 and 5.17). The nucleus intercalatus lies between the hypoglossal and dorsal motor vagal nuclei. The nucleus prepositus extends from the rostral pole of the hypoglossal nucleus almost to the level of the abducens nucleus (Figs. 5.17 and 5.27). The nucleus of Roller lies ventrally adjacent to N.XII rootlets (Fig. 5.12). Immediately posterior to the hypoglossal nucleus is a small bundle of descending fibers in the periventricular gray known as the *dorsal longitudinal fasciculus* (Schütz). This bundle, consisting of both ascending and descending components, is considered visceral in nature (Fig. 5.11).

Lesions of the hypoglossal nerve produce a lower motor neuron paralysis of the ipsilateral tongue muscles with loss of muscle tone and, ultimately, atrophy of the muscles. Due to paralysis of the genioglossus muscle, a muscle that effects protrusion of the tongue, the tongue will deviate to the side of the lesion when protruded. The intrinsic muscles alter the shape of the tongue, while the extrinsic muscles alter its shape and position. Intramedullary lesions involving the medullary pyramid and the hypoglossal nerve (due to vascular lesions of the anterior spinal artery) produce a combined upper and lower motor neuron syndrome referred to as *inferior alternating hemiplegia*. This syndrome is characterized by (1) a contralateral hemiplegia (upper motor neuron) and (2) an ipsilateral paralysis of the tongue (lower motor neuron).

Spinal Accessory Nerve

This nerve consists of two distinct parts referred to as the cranial and spinal portions (Figs. 1.4 and 5.21). The *cranial part* of the nerve arises from cells in the most caudal part of the nucleus ambiguus. Axons of these cells emerge from the lateral surface of the medulla caudal to the filaments of the vagus nerve. Fibers of the cranial part of the accessory nerve join the vagus nerve to form the inferior (recurrent) laryngeal nerve, which innervates the intrinsic muscles of the larynx (Figs. 5.19 and 5.20). This component of the accessory nerve innervates branchiomeric musculature and is regarded as a *special visceral efferent* (SVE) component.

The *spinal portion* of the accessory nerve originates from a column of cells in the anterior horn of the upper five (or six) cervical segments (Figs. 1.4, 5.3, and 5.21). Root fibers from these cells arch posterolaterally and emerge from the lateral aspect of the spinal cord between the dorsal and ventral roots. Rootlets of the spinal portions of the nerve from upper

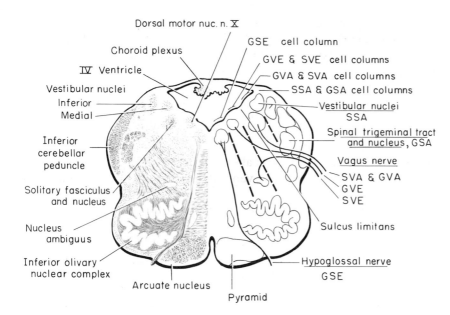

Dorsal motor nuc. n. X
GSE cell column
GVE & SVE cell columns
GVA & SVA cell columns
SSA & GSA cell columns
Choroid plexus
IV Ventricle
Vestibular nuclei
Inferior
Medial
Vestibular nuclei
SSA
Spinal trigeminal tract
and nucleus, GSA
Inferior
cerebellar
peduncle
Vagus nerve
SVA & GVA
GVE
SVE
Solitary fasciculus
and nucleus
Nucleus
ambiguus
Sulcus limitans
Inferior olivary
nuclear complex
Hypoglossal nerve
GSE
Arcuate nucleus
Pyramid

Figure 5.18. Schematic transverse section of the medulla showing relationships of cell columns to the sulcus limitans. Cell columns related to functional components of the cranial nerve are indicated on the *right*. Functional components of cranial nerves are both general and special. The vestibular nuclei shown at this level (and auditory nuclei at higher levels) form the special somatic afferent (*SSA*) cell columns. The spinal trigeminal nucleus forms the general somatic afferent (*GSA*) cell column and receives fibers from cranial nerves with this functional component (i.e., N. V, N. VII, N. IX, N. X). Functional components of the vagus nerve (except *GSA*) are shown in relation to particular nuclei. The hypoglossal nucleus (and the nuclei of N. VI, N. IV, and N. III at higher brain stem levels) gives rise to general somatic efferent (*GSE*) fibers. Heavy dashes separate the nuclei of the various cell columns on the right side. (From Carpenter and Sutin, *Human Neuroanatomy*, 1983; courtesy of Williams & Wilkins.)

cervical segments unite to form a common trunk that ascends posterior to the denticulate ligaments, enters the skull through the foramen magnum, and ultimately makes its exit from the skull via the jugular foramen in association with the vagus and glossopharyngeal nerves (Fig. 1.4). The spinal part of the accessory nerve innervates the ipsilateral sternocleidomastoid and the upper parts of the trapezius muscles. Although contraction of one sternocleidomastoid muscle turns the head to the opposite side, a unilateral lesion of the spinal accessory nerve usually does not produce any abnormality in the position of the head. Weakness in turning the head to the opposite side against resistance, however, is obvious. Paralysis of the upper part of the trapezius muscle is evidenced by (1) downward and outward rotation of the scapula, and (2) moderate sagging of the shoulder on the affected side.

Vagus Nerve

This complex mixed branchioomeric nerve contains (1) *general somatic afferent* (GSA) fibers distributed to cutaneous areas back of the ear and in the external auditory meatus; (2) *general visceral afferent* (GVA) fibers from the pharnyx, larynx, trachea, esophagus, and thoracic and abdominal viscera; (3) *special visceral afferent* (SVA) fibers from taste buds in the region of the epiglottis; (4) *general visceral efferent* (GVE) fibers distributed to parasympathetic ganglia located near to thoracic and abdominal viscera; and (5) *special visceral efferent* (SVE) fibers that innervate the striated (branchiomeric) muscles of the larynx and pharynx (Figs. 5.18 and 5.19).

General somatic afferent fibers of the vagus nerve arise from cells of the superior ganglion of the vagus nerve, located in, or immediately beneath, the jugular foramen (Fig. 5.21). Both general and special visceral afferent fibers of the vagus nerve arise from the larger inferior vagal ganglion (nodosal ganglion). Afferent vagal fibers enter the lateral surface of the medulla ventral to the inferior cerebellar peduncle by traversing parts of the spinal trigeminal tract and nucleus (Fig. 5.18). Cutaneous afferent fibers enter the dorsal part of the spinal trigeminal tract along with similar general somatic afferents from other branchiomeric cranial

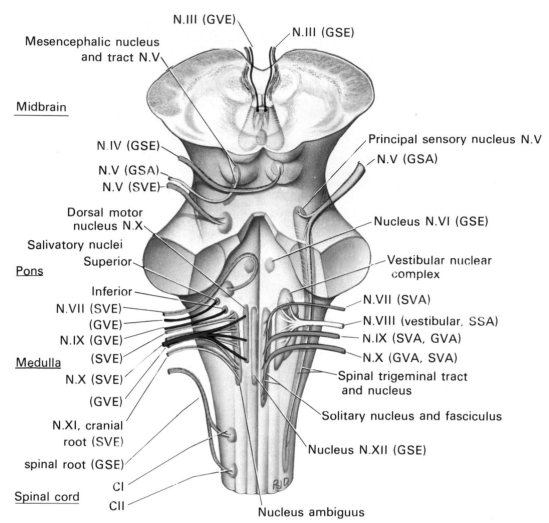

N.III (GVE)

N.III (GSE)

Mesencephalic nucleus
and tract N.V

Midbrain

N.IV (GSE)

N.V (GSA)

N.V (SVE)

Dorsal motor
nucleus N.X

Salivatory nuclei

Superior

Pons

Inferior

N.VII (SVE)

(GVE)

N.IX (GVE)

(SVE)

Medulla

N.X (SVE)

(GVE)

N.XI, cranial
root (SVE)

spinal root (GSE)

CI

Spinal cord

CII

Principal sensory nucleus N.V

N.V (GSA)

Nucleus N.VI (GSE)

Vestibular nuclear
complex

N.VII (SVA)

N.VIII (vestibular, SSA)

N.IX (SVA, GVA)

N.X (GVA, SVA)

Spinal trigeminal tract
and nucleus

Solitary nucleus and fasciculus

Nucleus N.XII (GSE)

Nucleus ambiguus

Figure 5.19. Schematic representation of the infratentorial cranial nerves showing their nuclei of origin and termination, their intramedullary course, and their functional components. The cochlear nerve and nuclei are not shown (see Fig. 6.9). General somatic afferent (*GSA*) components of the trigeminal nerve (N. V) are shown in *light blue*. General and special visceral afferent (*GVA, SVA*) components of the facial (N. VII), glossopharyngeal (N. IX), and vagus (N. X) nerves are shown in *dark blue*. The vestibular nerve, which distributes special somatic afferent (*SSA*) fibers to the vestibular nuclear complex, is *white*. Similarities in the intramedullary course of fibers in the spinal trigeminal tract, the vestibular nerve root, and the solitary fasciculus are evident on the *right*. General somatic efferent (*GSE*) fibers from the oculomotor (N. III) and trochlear (N. IV) nuclei and those of the spinal root of the accessory nerve (N. XI) are *light red*. Only contributions from the first and second cervical segments to the spinal root of the accessory nerve are shown. Root fibers of the abducens (N. VI) and hypoglossal (N. XII) nuclei, which exit ventrally and contain *GSE* fibers, are not shown. Special visceral efferent (*SVE*) fibers from the branchiomeric cranial nerves (N. V, N. VII, N. IX, N. X, and N. XI) are shown in *light red*. General visceral efferent (*GVE*) fibers, representing preganglionic parasympathetic components of the oculomotor (N. III), facial (N. VII), glossopharyngeal (N. IX), and vagus (N. X) nerves, are in *dark red*. (From Carpenter and Sutin, *Human Neuroanatomy*, 1983; courtesy of Williams & Wilkins.)

nerves. More numerous visceral afferent fibers of the vagus nerve pass dorsomedially into the nucleus and tractus solitarius (Figs. 5.19, 5.22, and 5.23). Fibers entering the solitary fasciculus bifurcate into short ascending and longer descending components. Descending vagal components in the solitary fasciculus gradually diminish in number as collaterals and terminals are given off to the solitary nucleus. Some vagal visceral fibers descend caudal to the obex, where the solitary nuclei of the two sides merge to form the *commissural nucleus* of the vagus nerve (Fig. 5.6).

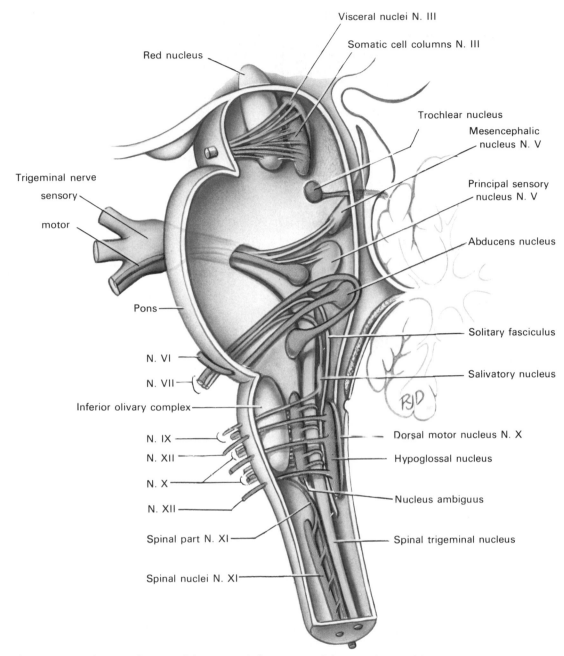

Figure 5.20. Schematic diagram of the intramedullary course of the cranial nerves in a midsagittal view. The brain stem is represented as a hollow shell except for cranial nerve components. General somatic (*GSE*) and special visceral (*SVE*) efferent components of cranial nerves innervating striated muscles are shown in *red*. General visceral efferent (*GVE*) components of cranial nerves III, VII, IX, and X, representing preganglionic parasympathetic fibers, are shown in *yellow*. General somatic (*GSA*), general visceral (*GVA*), and special visceral (*SVA*) afferent components of the cranial nerves are in *blue*. (From Carpenter and Sutin, *Human Neuroanatomy*, 1983; courtesy of Williams & Wilkins.)

The *fasciculus solitarius* is formed by visceral afferent fibers contributed by the vagus, glossopharyngeal, and facial (intermediate) nerves (Figs. 5.19 and 5.20). Fibers conveying taste from the anterior two-thirds of the tongue (chorda tympani) and from the posterior third of the tongue (glossopharyngeal nerve) mainly terminate in rostral parts of the solitary nucleus. Portions of the solitary fasciculus at the level of entry of the

Figure 5.21. Semidiagrammatic sketch of brain stem and cranial nerves showing the peripheral ganglia. (From Carpenter and Sutin, *Human Neuroanatomy*, 1983; courtesy of Williams & Wilkins.)

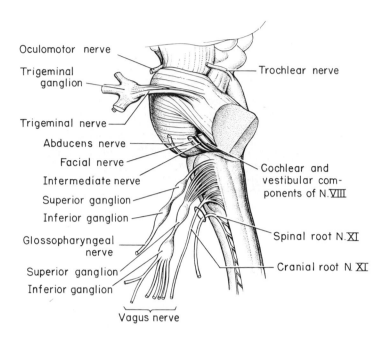

Oculomotor nerve
Trigeminal ganglion
Trigeminal nerve
Abducens nerve
Facial nerve
Intermediate nerve
Superior ganglion
Inferior ganglion
Glossopharyngeal nerve
Superior ganglion
Inferior ganglion
Vagus nerve
Trochlear nerve
Cochlear and vestibular components of N. VIII
Spinal root N. XI
Cranial root N. XI

vagus nerve, and caudal to it, contain mainly general visceral afferent fibers, largely from the vagus nerve.

The *nucleus solitarius* can be divided into several parts: (1) a medial part, dorsolateral to the dorsal motor nucleus of the vagus; (2) dorsomedial, dorsolateral, and ventrolateral subnuclei, which surround the *tractus solitarius*; and (3) a parvicellular subnucleus beneath the area postrema (Fig. 5.22). Cells of the medial part extend rostrally slightly beyond the dorsal motor nucleus of the vagus; this part of the nucleus also extends caudal to the fourth ventricle and merges with the corresponding cell column on the opposite side to form the commissural nucleus of the vagus nerve (Fig. 5.6).

The lateral nuclei form columns of larger cells that partially or completely surround the solitary fasciculus (Figs. 5.7, 5.11, and 5.22). This part of the nucleus parallels the fasciculus throughout most of its length; rostrally it extends into the lower part of the pons, while caudally its cells diminish in number and are difficult to distinguish from reticular neurons. The enlarged rostral part of the solitary nucleus (i.e., the lateral part) receives mainly special visceral afferent (taste) fibers from the facial (intermediate) and glossopharyngeal nerves and is referred to as the gustatory nucleus. The caudal and medial solitary nuclei receive most of the general visceral afferent fibers from the vagus nerve, along with some facial and glossopharyngeal fibers. As previously mentioned, cells in the medial portion of the nucleus solitarius contain a number of neuropeptides, chief among which are enkephalin, somatostatin, substance P, and cholecystokinin. Fibers containing substance P are abundant in the same area.

Secondary fiber systems arising from the solitary nucleus project ipsilaterally to (1) the nucleus ambiguus and the surrounding reticular formation; (2) the parabrachial nuclei in the rostral pons (Figs. 5.24 and 6.27); and (3) the thalamic nucleus concerned with gustatory sensation, namely the ventral posteromedial nucleus (pars parvicellularis) (Fig. 9.17). Other secondary fibers from the solitary nucleus projecting to the hypoglossal and salivatory nuclei mediate lingual and secretory reflexes. Projections from this nucleus to the dorsal motor nucleus of N. X, the phrenic nerve nucleus (at C3, C4 and C5) and anterior horn cells of

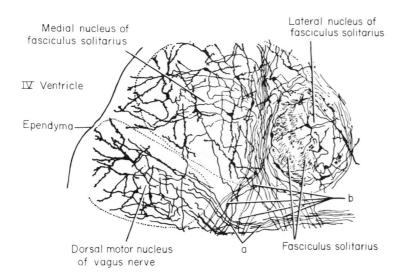

Medial nucleus of
fasciculus solitarius

Lateral nucleus of
fasciculus solitarius

IV Ventricle

Ependyma

b

Dorsal motor nucleus
of vagus nerve

a

Fasciculus solitarius

Figure 5.22. The vagal nuclei in the floor of the fourth ventricle based on a drawing of a Golgi preparation of newborn cat. Efferent (preganglionic) fibers from the dorsal motor nucleus of the vagus nerve are indicated by *a*, while *b* indicates fibers from the medial and lateral (sensory) nuclei of the fasciculus solitarius forming secondary vagoglossopharyngeal pathways. The medial nucleus of the fasciculus solitarius extends caudally to the fourth ventricle and merges with the corresponding cell group on the opposite side, forming the commissural nucleus of the vagus nerve (Fig. 5.6). The lateral nucleus of the fasciculus solitarius extends rostrally, increases in size, and parallels the fasciculus solitarius throughout most of its length. (From Carpenter and Sutin, *Human Neuroanatomy*, 1983; courtesy of Williams & Wilkins.)

thoracic spinal segments are involved in coughing and vomiting reflexes (Fig. 4.15). The nucleus of the solitary tract is coextensive with the physiologically defined medullary respiratory "center," which includes the nucleus ambiguus and surrounding portions of the reticular formation. Cells of the medullary "respiratory center" are activated by vagal impulses and directly by changes in their chemical environment (CO_2 accumulation). A medullary vasomotor "center" consisting of separate pressor and depressor zones has been poorly defined. Recent emphasis has been on neural networks concerned with cardiovascular control. A group of noradrenergic neurons (designated as group A5) (Figs. 4.16 and 5.15), located in the caudal pons between the superior olive and root fibers of the facial nerve and projecting axons to the nucleus solitarius, the nucleus ambiguus, the dorsal motor nucleus of N. X, and preganglionic sympathetic neurons in the thoracic spinal cord, appears to be part of this neural network.

The *dorsal motor nucleus* of the vagus nerve is situated in the floor of the fourth ventricle posterolateral to the hypoglossal nucleus (Figs. 5.11, 5.12, 5.16, 5.19, and 5.20). This column of small spindle-shaped cells extends both rostrally and caudally beyond the hypoglossal nucleus. Some larger cells in the nucleus contain coarse chromophilic bodies and scattered melanin pigment. Cells of this nucleus give rise to preganglionic parasympathetic fibers (GVE). Axons of these cells emerge from the lateral surface of the medulla by traversing the spinal trigeminal tract and nucleus (Fig. 5.18). The dorsal motor nucleus of the vagus is the vagal secretomotor center. Cells of the dorsal motor nucleus are strongly immunoreactive to choline acetyltransferase (ChAT) (Fig. 5.16A). Destruction of this nucleus greatly reduces insulin-induced secretion of gastric acid.

The *nucleus ambiguus* is a column of cells in the reticular formation about halfway between the spinal trigeminal nucleus and the inferior olivary complex (Figs. 5.6 and 5.12). This nucleus, extending from the level of the decussation of the medial lemniscus to levels through the rostral third of the inferior olivary complex, is composed of multipolar, cholinergic lower motor neurons (Fig. 5.16). Fibers from the nucleus arch dorsally, join efferent fibers from the dorsal motor nucleus of the vagus nerve, and emerge from the lateral surface of the medulla dorsal to the inferior olivary complex (Fig. 5.18). Caudal parts of the nucleus ambiguus give rise to the cranial part of the spinal accessory nerve, while rostral

Figure 5.23. Dark-field photomicrograph of labeled cells in the dorsal motor nucleus of the vagus (dmn X) and fibers of the tractus solitarius (TS) in a horizontal section. Section was taken from a cat in which horseradish peroxidase (HRP) was injected into the inferior vagal ganglion. Cells in the dmn X are retrogradely labeled, while fibers in the tractus solitarius are anterogradely labeled. Fine-labeled terminals occupy the region between the dmn X and the TS. (Calibration bar equals 500 μm.)

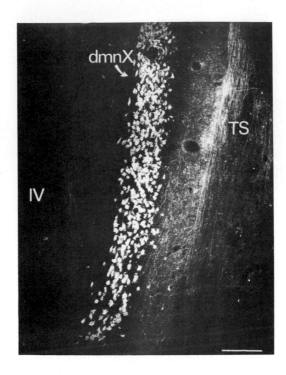

parts of this cell column give rise to glossopharyngeal special visceral efferent fibers (which innervate the stylopharyngeus muscle). Special visceral efferent fibers of the vagus nerve (and those from the cranial part of the accessory nerve that rejoin the vagus nerve) innervate the muscles of the pharynx and larynx (Figs. 5.19 and 5.20).

A unilateral lesion of the vagus nerve produces ipsilateral paralysis of the soft palate, pharynx, and larynx, which results in hoarseness of the voice, dyspnea, and dysphagia. During phonation the soft palate is elevated on the normal side and the uvula deviates to the normal side. The palatal reflex is lost on the side of the lesion. Anesthesia of the pharynx and larynx results in an ipsilateral loss of the cough reflex, while destruction of visceral motor fibers of the vagus nerve abolishes the carotid sinus reflex ipsilaterally.

Bilateral lesions of the vagus nerve cause complete paralysis of the pharynx and larynx and will result in death due to asphyxia unless a tracheostomy is performed immediately. With complete paralysis of the larynx, the vocal cords lie close to the midline and cannot be abducted on attempted inspiration. Paralysis and atonia of the esophagus and stomach produce pain and vomiting. The heart rate becomes rapid and irregular due to removal of vagal inhibition. This condition is associated with marked dysphagia and dysarthria.

Glossopharyngeal Nerve

This nerve is closely related to the vagus nerve, sharing common medullary nuclei and having similar functional components. Fibers of this nerve enter and emerge at levels rostral to the rootlets of the vagus nerve, but like the vagus nerve, they traverse the spinal trigeminal tract and nucleus (Figs. 5.17, 5.19, 5.20, and 5.21). The glossopharyngeal nerve is easier to identify than the vagus nerve, because its fibers form a single compact nerve root. Fibers of the vagus nerve enter and emerge from the brain stem by a number of small rootlets. The glossopharyngeal is a mixed branchiomeric cranial nerve with the following functional com-

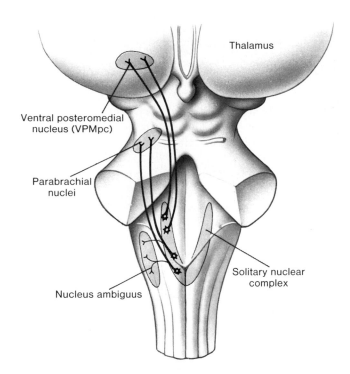

Thalamus

Ventral posteromedial
nucleus (VPMpc)

Parabrachial
nuclei

Nucleus ambiguus

Solitary nuclear
complex

Figure 5.24. Schematic diagram of ascending projections of the solitary nuclear complex. Special visceral afferent (*SVA*) neurons in the geniculate ganglion (intermediate nerve) and both special (*SVA*) and general (*GVA*) visceral neurons in the inferior ganglia of the glossopharyngeal and vagus nerves project to portions of the solitary nuclear complex (*blue*). Cells in rostral portions of the nucleus solitarius project ipsilaterally via the central tegmental tract to the small-celled part of the ventral posteromedial (VPMpc) nucleus of the thalamus (Fig. 9.17). Cells of VPMpc project thalamocortical fibers to the cortex of the parietal operculum. Caudal parts of the solitary nucleus that receive afferents from the vagus and glossopharyngeal nerves project rostrally to the ipsilateral medial and lateral parabrachial nuclei (Fig. 6.27). Caudal parts of solitary nucleus also project fibers to the ipsilateral nucleus ambiguus. The solitary nuclear complex, the nucleus ambiguus, the parabrachial nuclei, and VPMpc are shown in *blue*. (From Carpenter and Sutin, *Human Neuroanatomy*, 1983; courtesy of Williams & Wilkins.)

ponents: (1) *general visceral afferent* (GVA) fibers, (2) *special visceral afferent* (SVA) fibers (taste), (3) a few *general somatic afferent* (GSA) fibers, (4) *general visceral efferent* (GVE) fibers, and (5) a small number of *special visceral efferent* (SVE) fibers. Like the vagus nerve it has two peripheral ganglia, a small *superior ganglion* in the jugular foramen, and a larger extracranial *inferior* (*petrosal*) *ganglion* (Fig. 5.21).

Primary sensory neurons mediating general somatic sense (GSA) from cutaneous areas back of the ear lie in the superior ganglion; central processes of these cells enter the spinal trigeminal tract and nucleus. Cell bodies of visceral afferent fibers lie in the inferior ganglion. General visceral afferent fibers convey tactile sense, thermal sense, and pain from the mucous membranes of the posterior third of the tongue, the tonsil, the posterior wall of the upper pharynx, and the eustachian tube. Special visceral afferent fibers convey taste sensation from the posterior third of the tongue. Visceral afferent fibers entering the posterolateral part of the medulla are distributed to rostral portions of the solitary fasciculus and its nucleus (Figs. 5.19 and 5.20). Rostral and lateral parts of the nucleus solitarius that receive fibers from the facial (intermediate) and glossopharyngeal nerves constitute the "gustatory nucleus." The carotid sinus nerve conveys impulses from the carotid sinus, a baroreceptor, located at the bifurcation of the common carotid. Increases in carotid arterial pressure excite carotid sinus baroreceptors and impulses are conveyed centrally by the glossopharyngeal nerve to the nucleus of the solitary tract. Second-order neurons in the solitary nucleus project to the dorsal motor nucleus of the vagus nerve, which brings about reductions in heart rate and arterial blood pressure via pre- and post-ganglionic vagal fibers projecting to the sinoatrial and atrioventricular nodes, as well as to atrial heart muscle. The *carotid sinus reflex* involving glossopharyngeal visceral afferents and vagal general visceral efferents constitutes a mechanism for the regulation of arterial blood pressure.

General visceral efferent fibers, arising from the *inferior salivatory nucleus*, pass via the lesser petrosal nerve to the otic ganglion, situated below the foramen ovale and medial to the mandibular division of the trigeminal nerve. Postganglionic fibers originating from cells of the otic ganglion convey parasympathetic secretory impulses to the parotid gland. Cells of the inferior salivatory nucleus are scattered in lateral parts of the reticular formation and can be positively identified immunocytochemically by antiserum to choline acetyltransferase (ChAT). This loosely organized cluster of cholinergic neurons is considered equivalent to the dorsal motor nucleus of the vagus.

Special visceral efferent fibers, as already described, arise from rostral portions of the nucleus ambiguus (Figs. 5.12 and 5.19). These fibers, small in number, innervate the stylopharyngeus muscle and perhaps portions of the superior pharyngeal constrictor muscle.

As the previous description indicates, the glossopharyngeal nerve is predominately a sensory nerve and a nerve contributing preganglionic parasympathetic fibers to the otic ganglion. Isolated lesions of the glossopharyngeal nerve are rare. Disturbances associated with lesions of the nerve include (1) loss of the pharyngeal (gag) reflex, (2) loss of the carotid sinus reflex, and (3) loss of taste and general sensation in the posterior third of the tongue. *Glossopharyngeal neuralgia* resembles trigeminal neuralgia in that the excruciating paroxysmal pain may be triggered by seemingly trivial stimuli, such as coughing or swallowing. The pain associated with this syndrome radiates from the neck into regions behind the ear.

CORTICOBULBAR FIBERS

Corticofugal fibers projecting to, and terminating in, portions of the lower brain stem are referred to as *corticobulbar fibers*. These fibers arise from cortex on both sides of the central sulcus and project to (1) sensory relay nuclei, (2) parts of the reticular formation, and (3) directly to certain motor cranial nerve nuclei (Fig. 5.25).

Sensory relay nuclei receiving corticobulbar fibers include (1) the nuclei gracilis and cuneatus, (2) sensory trigeminal nuclei, and (3) the nucleus of the solitary fasciculus. Corticobulbar fibers to the posterior column nuclei leave the pyramid and enter these nuclei by traversing either the medial lemniscus or the reticular formation. There are suggestions of somatotopic relationships between cortical areas and the nuclei gracilis and cuneatus. Corticofugal fibers do not terminate upon the same cells of the nuclei gracilis and cuneatus that receive projections via the posterior columns.

Corticobulbar fibers projecting to all trigeminal sensory nuclei and the nucleus solitarius are derived predominantly, but not exclusively, from frontoparietal cortical areas. Fibers passing to the solitary nucleus terminate chiefly in its rostral part.

Corticobulbar fibers, projecting to the above sensory relay nuclei, underlie the physiological mechanism by which descending cortical impulses can influence the transmission of sensory impulses at the second neuronal level. Both excitatory and inhibitory influences may be exerted upon these relay nuclei.

Corticoreticular fibers projecting to the lower brain stem arise predominantly from the motor, premotor, and somesthetic cortex. Fibers descend in association with the corticospinal tract, leave the tract at various levels, and enter the reticular formation. The bulk of these fibers terminate in two fairly circumscribed areas, one in the medulla and one in the pons. In the medulla these fibers terminate in the area of the gigantocellular reticular nucleus; in the pons most of the fibers end in the

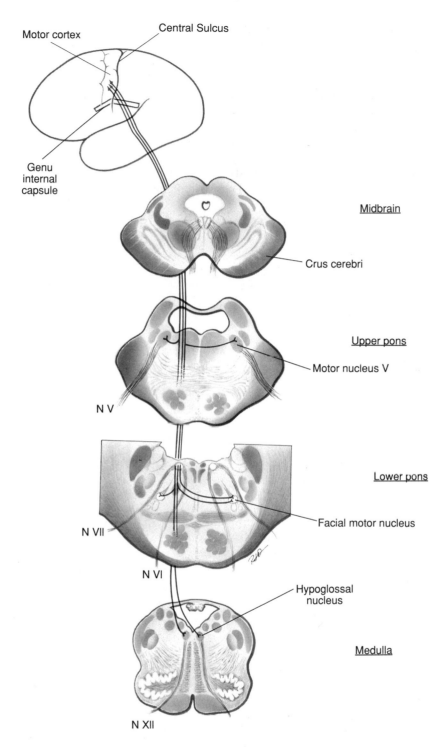

Motor cortex

Central Sulcus

Genu internal capsule

Midbrain

Crus cerebri

Upper pons

Motor nucleus V

N V

Lower pons

Facial motor nucleus

N VII

N VI

Hypoglossal nucleus

Medulla

N XII

Figure 5.25. Schematic diagram of cortico-bulbar fibers in the brain stem projecting directly to motor nuclei of the trigeminal, facial, and hypoglossal nerves. Corticobulbar fibers arise from cells in lower parts of the precentral motor cortex, pass through the region of the genu in the internal capsule, and descend in medial parts of the crus cerebri lateral to fronto-pontine fibers. Fibers projecting to the motor trigeminal nuclei, the upper part of the facial motor nuclei, and the hypoglossal nuclei are bilateral and nearly equal on the two sides. The inferior part of the facial nucleus, innervating lower facial muscles, receives only crossed corticobulbar projections. Corticoreticular projections (not shown) and synaptic articulations with reticular neurons provide supranuclear innervation for all motor cranial nerves, including those that receive direct fibers.

oral pontine reticular formation (Figs. 4.6 and 4.14). Corticoreticular fibers are distributed bilaterally but with slight contralateral preponderance. Regions of the reticular formation, receiving corticofugal fibers, give rise to (1) long ascending and descending projections, (2) projections to the cerebellum, and (3) projections to cranial nerve nuclei.

The *motor cranial nerve nuclei* innervating striated muscle receive impulses via corticobulbar pathways. These fibers arise mainly from portions of the precentral gyrus and constitute the upper motor neurons for motor cranial nerve nuclei. Most of the so-called corticobulbar fibers conveying impulses to motor cranial nerve nuclei are actually corticoreticular fibers; neurons in the reticular formation serve to relay impulses to the motor cranial nerve nuclei (Fig. 5.25). In forms below primates, it has not been possible to trace corticobulbar fibers to direct terminations in motor cranial nerve nuclei. In these animals, cortical influences upon motor cranial nerve nuclei are mediated by corticoreticular fibers and synaptically related reticular neurons projecting to the motor nuclei. This indirect system is supplemented in humans and primates by direct corticobulbar projections to particular motor cranial nerve nuclei. Nuclei receiving these direct cortical projections are the trigeminal, facial, hypoglossal, and supraspinal (Fig. 5.25). These fibers are bilateral and nearly equal in number, except for those passing to parts of the facial nucleus. The more numerous corticoreticular fibers represent a phylogenetically older indirect corticobulbar pathway in which neurons in the reticular core serve as internuncials. Direct corticobulbar fibers found in man and primates represent a more recently developed parallel system.

The *supranuclear innervation of motor cranial nerve nuclei* is largely bilateral and more complex than that present at spinal levels. Corticobulbar projections are bilateral to those cranial nerve nuclei that innervate muscle groups that, as a rule, cannot be contracted voluntarily on one side. These include laryngeal, pharyngeal, palatal, and upper facial muscles. The same principle applies to the muscles of mastication and the extraocular muscles. Because unilateral stimulation of the motor cortex produces isolated contraction of the contralateral lower facial muscles, and unilateral lesions involving corticobulbar fibers produce paralysis only of contralateral lower facial muscles, cell groups of the facial nucleus innervating lower facial musculature are regarded as receiving only crossed corticobulbar fibers.

Because the supranuclear innervation of the motor cranial nerve nuclei is bilateral, unilateral lesions interrupting corticobulbar fibers produce comparatively mild forms of paresis. Only slight weakness of tongue and jaw movements contralateral to the lesions can be detected and is expressed by modest deviation of the tongue or jaw to the side opposite the lesion. However, marked weakness in the contralateral lower facial muscles is evident with such lesions.

Pseudobulbar palsy results from bilateral lesions involving corticobulbar fibers. This syndrome is characterized by weakness or paralysis of the muscles involved in swallowing, chewing, breathing, and speaking and may occur with relatively little paralysis in the extremities. Loss of emotional control, characterized by inappropriate laughing and crying, forms an important part of this syndrome.

MEDULLARY-PONTINE JUNCTION

The fourth ventricle reaches its greatest width at the level of the lateral recess (Figs. 2.18 and 2.21). At this level the *nodulus* of the cerebellum lies in the roof of the fourth ventricle (Fig. 2.31) and the *peduncle of the flocculus* forms the dorsal surface of the lateral recess (Fig. 5.26). The cochlear nerve and the *dorsal* and *ventral cochlear nuclei* lie on the medial and ventral surfaces of the lateral recess. The *inferior cerebellar peduncle* has achieved its maximum size, and fibers of the cochlear nerve curve around its lateral and superior surfaces. At slightly more rostral levels, above the lateral recess, the inferior cerebellar peduncle enters the cerebellum by passing posterolaterally. The fibers of this peduncle lie medial to the middle cerebellar peduncle (Fig. 5.27).

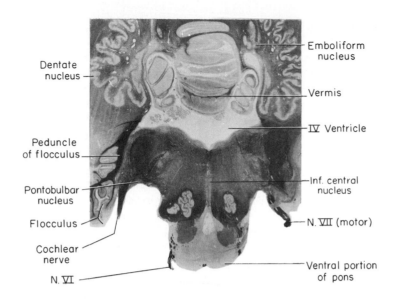

Dentate nucleus —

Peduncle of flocculus —

Pontobulbar nucleus —

Flocculus —

Cochlear nerve —

N. VI —

— Emboliform nucleus

— Vermis

— IV Ventricle

— Inf. central nucleus

— N. VII (motor)

— Ventral portion of pons

Figure 5.26. Asymmetrical transverse section through the junction of the medulla and pons in a 1-month-old infant. Attached portions of the cerebellum contain large portions of the deep cerebellar nuclei, and the peduncle of the flocculus is seen on the left near the lateral recess of the fourth ventricle. The inferior central nucleus is also known as the nucleus raphe magnus (Fig. 5.14). Other structures in the tegmentum are identified in Figure 5.27. Weigert's myelin stain. Photograph. (From Carpenter and Sutin, *Human Neuroanatomy*, 1983; courtesy of Williams & Wilkins.)

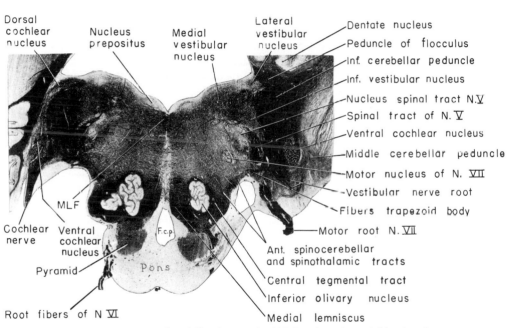

Dorsal cochlear nucleus

Nucleus prepositus

Medial vestibular nucleus

Lateral vestibular nucleus

Dentate nucleus

Peduncle of flocculus

Inf. cerebellar peduncle

Inf. vestibular nucleus

Nucleus spinal tract N.V

Spinal tract of N. V

Ventral cochlear nucleus

Middle cerebellar peduncle

Motor nucleus of N. VII

Vestibular nerve root

Fibers trapezoid body

Motor root N. VII

MLF

Cochlear nerve

Ventral cochlear nucleus

Pyramid

F.c.p.

Pons

Ant. spinocerebellar and spinothalamic tracts

Central tegmental tract

Inferior olivary nucleus

Medial lemniscus

Root fibers of N VI

Figure 5.27. Transverse section of medulla of 1-month-old infant through caudal border of pons. Fibers of the inferior cerebellar peduncle are seen entering the cerebellum on the right. *F.c.p.*, Foramen cecum posterior; *MLF*, medial longitudinal fasciculus. Weigert's myelin stain. Photograph. (From Carpenter and Sutin, *Human Neuroanatomy*, 1983; courtesy of Williams & Wilkins.)

In the floor of the fourth ventricle the nucleus prepositus lies medially in the position previously occupied by the hypoglossal nucleus. Lateral to this nucleus are the vestibular nuclei (Fig. 5.27). At this level portions of the *medial* and *inferior vestibular nuclei* are seen. The inferior vestibular nucleus, adjacent to the medial surface of the inferior cerebellar peduncle, is characterized by numerous coarse myelinated fiber bundles that course through it (Fig. 5.27). These fibers coursing longitudinally in the axis of the nucleus are descending primary vestibular fibers and cerebellar efferent fibers. The medial vestibular nucleus is highly cellular and contains finer fibers, most of which are not myelinated. In some preparations myelinated fibers of the *striae medullares* of the medulla can be seen in the floor of the fourth ventricle dorsal to the nucleus prepositus and the vestibular nuclei (Fig. 5.1). These fibers arise from the arcuate nucleus, pass dorsally in the raphe, and then project laterally in the floor of the fourth ventricle to the cerebellum.

The inferior olivary complex is reduced in size, and the accessory olivary nuclei have disappeared. Anterior to the olivary complex, the fibers of the pyramid are surrounded by pontine nuclei and some transverse fibers. The medial lemniscus and medial longitudinal fasciculus occupy the same positions as at more caudal levels, although they are separated from the corresponding tract on the opposite side by more fully developed nuclei in the median raphe (i.e., nucleus raphe magnus or inferior central nucleus). Other ascending and descending tracts maintain the same relative positions as at lower medullary levels.

The junction of medulla and pons (Fig. 5.27) is characterized by (1) passage of the inferior cerebellar peduncle into the cerebellum; (2) reduction in size and, ultimately, disappearance of the inferior olivary complex; (3) gradual incorporation of the corticospinal tracts within the ventral part of the pons; (4) enlargement of the reticular formation; and (5) appearance of cranial nerve nuclei and root fibers typical of this higher level.

Cranial nerve present at the junction of medulla and pons are the abducens, cochlear, vestibular, and facial (Fig. 5.27). The abducens nerve emerges at the lower border of the pons lateral to the pyramids. All other cranial nerves at this level are grouped together at the *cerebellopontine angle*, formed by the junction of medulla, pons, and cerebellum (Fig. 2.25). All of these nerves emerge from, or enter, the internal auditory meatus. The cochlear nerve is the most caudal and lateral, while the facial nerve is the most rostral and medial. The vestibular nerve lies between the cochlear and facial nerves (Fig. 6.2). These cranial nerves will be described and discussed in the next chapter.

Lesions of the medulla or structures within it can be produced by a variety of causes, but those due to demyelinating diseases, neoplasms, and vascular pathology are the most common. Demyelinating diseases usually are disseminated and involve multiple systems at different sites. Neoplasms tend to extend in the axis of the brain stem. Vascular lesions show great variation but often give rise to characteristic syndromes. The vascular syndrome most commonly seen in the medulla is attributed to occlusion of the posterior inferior cerebellar artery, a vessel that supplies structures in the posterolateral region (Fig. 14.14). While it seems likely that this syndrome may more frequently result from involvement of the vertebral artery and its smaller branches, the symptoms and signs are similar and unmistakable. The *lateral medullary syndrome* is characterized by (1) loss of pain and thermal sense over the ipsilateral half of the face and the contralateral half of the body, (2) nausea, (3) vertigo, (4) disturbances of equilibrium, (5) persistent hiccup, and (6) dysphonia (hoarse voice). Disturbances forming parts of this syndrome frequently can be correlated with the extent and precise location of the medullary lesion. Structures commonly involved by a single lesion in the dorsolateral part of the medulla in the lateral medullary syndrome include (1) the spinal trigeminal tract and nucleus; (2) the spinothalamic tract; (3) efferent fibers originating from the dorsal motor nucleus of the vagus and the nucleus ambiguus; (4) vagal afferent fibers projecting to the nucleus solitarius; (5) parts of the inferior cerebellar peduncle, as well as fiber systems projecting toward this peduncle; and (6) variable portion of the inferior cerebellar cortex. The blood supply of the medulla is discussed and illustrated in Chapter 14.

SUGGESTED READINGS

ANGEVINE, J. B., JR., AND COTMAN, C. W. 1981. *Principles of Neuroanatomy.* Oxford University Press, New York.

BASBAUM, A. I., RALSTON, D. D., AND RALSTON, H. J. 1986. Bulbospinal projections in the primate: A light and electron microscopic study of a pain modulating system. J. Comp. Neurol., **250**: 311–323.

BECKSTEAD, R. M., MORSE, J. R., AND NORGREN, R. 1980. The nucleus of the solitary tract in the monkey: Projections to the thalamus and brain stem nuclei. J. Comp. Neurol., **190**: 259–282.

BRODAL, A. 1940. Experimentelle Untersuchungen über die olivocerebellare Lokalisation. Z. Gesamte Neurol. Psychiat., **169**: 1–153.

BRODAL, A. 1957. *The Reticular Formation of the Brain Stem. Anatomical Aspects and Functional Correlations.* Charles C Thomas, Springfield, IL.

CUELLO, A. C., AND KANAZAWA, I. 1978. The distribution of substance P immunoreactive fibers in the rat central nervous system. J. Comp. Neurol., **178**: 129–156.

ELZE, C. 1932. Centrales Nervensystem. In H. BRAUS (Editor), *Anatomie des Menschen. Ein Lehrbuch für Studierende und Ärzte,* Vol. III. J. Springer, Berlin, p. 234.

GOBEL, S. 1978. Golgi studies of the neurons in layer I of the dorsal horn of the medulla (trigeminal nucleus caudalis). J. Comp. Neurol., **180**: 375–394.

GOBEL, S. 1978. Golgi studies of the neurons in layer II of the dorsal horn of the medulla (trigeminal nucleus caudalis). J. Comp. Neurol., **180**: 395–414.

HUNT, S. P. 1983. Cytochemistry of the spinal cord. In P. C. EMSON (Editor), *Chemical Neuroanatomy.* Raven Press, New York, pp. 53–84.

KALIA, M., AND MESULAM, M. M. 1980. Brain stem projections of sensory and motor components of the vagus complex in the cat. II. Laryngeal tracheobronchial, pulmonary, cardiac, and gastrointestinal branches. J. Comp. Neurol., **193**: 467–508.

KIMURA, H., MCGEER, P. L., PENG, J. H., AND MCGEER, E. G. 1981. The central cholinergic system studies by choline acetyltransferase immunohistochemistry in the cat. J. Comp. Neurol., **200**: 151–201.

KUYPERS, H. G. J. M. 1958. Corticobulbar connexions to the pons and lower brainstem in man An anatomical study. Brain, **81**: 364–388.

KUYPERS, H. G. J. M. 1960. Central cortical projections to motor and somatosensory cell groups. Brain, **83**: 161–184.

KUYPERS, H. G. J. M., AND TUERK, J. D. 1964. The distribution of cortical fibres within the nuclei cuneatus and gracilis in the cat. J. Anat., **98**: 143–162.

LOEWY, A. D., MCKELLAR, S., AND SAPER, C. D. 1979. Direct projections of the A5 catecholamine cell group to the intermediolateral cell column. Brain Res., **174**: 309–314.

MANTYH, P. W., AND HUNT, S. P. 1984. Neuropeptides are present in projection neurones at all levels in visceral and taste pathways: from periphery to sensory cortex. Brain Res., **299**: 297–311.

MARTIN, G. F., CULBERSEN, J., LAXSON, C., LINAUTA, M., PANNETON, M., AND TSCHISMADA, I. 1980. Afferent connections of the inferior olivary development: Studies using the North American opossum. In J. COURVILLE, C. de MONTIGNY, AND Y. LAMARRE (Editors), *The Inferior Olivary Nucleus.* Raven Press, New York, pp. 35–72.

MCGEER, P. L., ECCLES, J. C., AND MCGEER, E. G. 1987. *Molecular Neurobiology of the Mammalian Brain,* Ed. 2. Plenum Press, New York.

MCKELLAR, S., AND LOEWY, A. D. 1982. Efferent projections of the A1 catecholamine cell group in the rat: An autoradiographic study. Brain Res., **241**: 11–29.

NEWMAN, D. B. 1985. Distinguishing rat brainstem reticulospinal nuclei by their neuronal morphology. I. Medullary nuclei. J. Hirnforsch., **26**: 187–226.

OLSZEWSKI, J., AND BAXTER, D. 1954. *Cytoarchitecture of the Human Brain Stem.* J. B. Lippincott, Philadelphia.

OSCARSSON, O. 1973. Functional organization of spinocerebellar paths. In *Handbook of Sensory Physiology,* Vol. 2, Springer-Verlag, Berlin, pp. 339–380.

PANNETON, W. M., AND LOEWY, A. D. 1980. Projections of the carotid sinus nerve to the nucleus of the solitary tract in the cat. Brain Res., **191**: 239–244.

PETERSON, B. 1979. Reticulo-motor pathways: Their connections and possible roles in motor behavior. In H. ASANUMA AND V. J. WILSON (Editors), *Integration in the Nervous System,* Igaku Shoin, Tokyo, pp. 185–201.

PETERSON, B. 1980. Participation of pontomedullary reticular neurons in specific motor activity. In J. A. HOBSON AND M. A. B. BRAZIER (Editors), *The Reticular Formation Revisited.* Raven Press, New York, pp. 171–192.

POGGIO, G. F., AND MOUNTCASTLE, V. B. 1960. A study of the functional contributions of the lemniscal and spinothalamic systems to somatic sensibility. Bull. Johns Hopkins Hosp., **106**: 266–316.

SCHEIBEL, M. E., AND SCHEIBEL, A. B. 1958. Structural substrates for integrative patterns in the brain stem reticular core. In H. H. JASPERS et al. (Editors), *Reticular Formation of the Brain.* Little, Brown, Boston, Ch. 2, pp. 31–55.

SHRIVER, J. E., STEIN, B. M., AND CARPENTER, M. B. 1968. Central projections of spinal dorsal roots in the monkey. I. Cervical and upper thoracic dorsal roots. Am. J. Anat., **123**: 27–74.

STEINBUSCH, H. W. M., AND NIEUWENHUYS, R. 1983. The raphe nuclei of the rat brain stem: A cytoarchitectonic and immunohistochemical study. In P. C. EMSON (Editor), *Chemical Neuroanatomy*. Raven Press, New York, pp. 131–207.

THOR, K. B., AND HELKE, C. J. 1987. Serotonin- and substance P-containing projections to the nucleus tractus solitarii of the rat. J. Comp. Neurol., **265**: 275–293.

WALBERG, F. 1980. Olivocerebellocortical projection in the cat as determined with the method of retrograde axonal transport of horseradish peroxidase. I. Topographical pattern. In J. COURVILLE, C. de MONTIGNY, AND Y. LAMARRE (Editors), *The Inferior Olivary Nucleus*. Raven Press, New York, pp. 169–187.

WESTLUND, K. N., BOWKER, R. M., ZIEGLER, M. G., AND COULTER, J. D. 1984. Origins and terminations of descending noradrenergic projections to spinal cord of monkey. Brain Res., **292**: 1–16.

6

The Pons

The pons (metencephalon) represents the rostral part of the hindbrain. It consists of two distinctive parts: (1) an older *dorsal portion*, the pontine tegmentum, and (2) a newer *ventral portion*, referred to as the pons proper (Fig. 6.1).

CAUDAL PONS

Dorsal Portion of the Pons

The pontine tegmentum is the rostral continuation of the medullary reticular formation. It contains cranial nerve nuclei, ascending and descending tracts, and reticular nuclei (Fig. 6.1). Cranial nerve nuclei found in the pons are those of nerves V, VI, VII, and VIII (Figs. 6.2, 6.3, 6.4, 6.5, 6.6, and 6.22). The ascending tracts in the pons occupy positions similar to those in the medulla, except for the medial lemniscus. The medial lemniscus, which in the medulla was oriented vertically on each side of the median raphe, now assumes a nearly horizontal position dorsal to the ventral part of the pons (Figs. 6.1 and 6.2). Crossing fibers of the trapezoid body traverse ventral parts of the bundle on each side. The medial longitudinal fasciculi (MLF) are in the floor of the fourth ventricle on each side of the median raphe. The spinothalamic and anterior spinocerebellar tracts are difficult to distinguish but occupy positions in the anterolateral tegmentum. The spinal trigeminal tract and nucleus lie medial and ventral to the inferior cerebellar peduncle. The vestibular nuclei (i.e., medial and lateral) are present in the floor of the fourth ventricle (Fig. 6.2).

The pontine reticular formation, more extensive than the medullary reticular formation, occupies a similar region. The major part of the pontine reticular formation is represented by the *pontine reticular nuclei* (pars caudalis and pars oralis; Figs. 6.1 and 6.23). The *pars caudalis* replaces the gigantocellular reticular nucleus of the medulla and extends rostrally to the level of the trigeminal motor nucleus (Fig. 6.23). The *pars oralis*, present in more rostral pontine levels, extends into the caudal mesencephalon. The pontine reticular nuclei give rise to the pontine reticulospinal tract (Figs. 4.6 and 4.14). Lateral to the pars caudalis is a small-celled reticular nucleus (parvicellularis) similar to that described in the medulla. The median raphe contains the inferior central nucleus, also known as the nucleus raphe magnus (Figs. 5.13 and 5.26).

The reticular formation posterolateral to the medial lemniscus contains a relatively large discrete bundle not present in the medulla, known as the *central tegmental tract* (Figs. 6.1 and 6.4). This is a composite tract consisting of descending fibers from midbrain nuclei that project to the inferior olivary complex and ascending fibers from the reticular formation that project to thalamic nuclei.

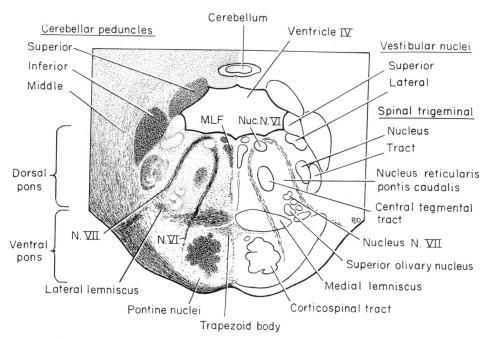

Figure 6.1. Semidiagrammatic drawing of a transverse section of the pons at the level of the abducens nucleus. The dorsal portion of the pons, constituting the tegmentum, contains the reticular formation, cranial nerve nuclei, and ascending and descending tracts. The ventral portion of the pons contains the pontine nuclei, massive bundles of corticofugal fibers, and the transverse fibers of the pons, which form the middle cerebellar peduncle. (From Carpenter and Sutin, *Human Neuroanatomy*, 1983; courtesy of Williams & Wilkins.)

Ventral Portion of the Pons

The massive ventral part of the pons consists of orderly arranged transverse and longitudinal fiber bundles, and large collections of pontine nuclei (Figs. 6.1, 6.3, and 6.5). Longitudinal fiber bundles coursing through central regions of the ventral pons are (1) corticospinal, (2) corticobulbar, and (3) corticopontine. Corticospinal fibers traverse the ventral part of the pons and in sagittal sections can be traced into the medullary pyramid (Fig. 10.9). Corticopontine fibers, arising from the frontal, parietal, temporal, and occipital cortex, descend without crossing and terminate upon the pontine nuclei. The pontine nuclei surround the fibers of the corticospinal and corticopontine tracts. These nuclei give rise to the transverse fiber bundles of the pons, which cross the midline and enter the cerebellum as the middle cerebellar peduncle (Figs. 6.1 and 6.3). Transverse pontocerebellar fibers cross above and below the fascicles of descending fibers. The ventral portion of the pons may be considered as a massive relay station in a two-neuronal pathway by which impulses from the cerebral cortex are transmitted to the contralateral cerebellar hemisphere. Corticobulbar fibers descending in the ventral part of the pons project into the pontine tegmentum (Fig. 5.25).

VESTIBULOCOCHLEAR NERVE

The eighth cranial nerve (N. VIII) consists of two distinctive parts: (1) the cochlear part concerned with audition and (2) the vestibular part conveying impulses concerned with equilibrium and orientation in three-dimensional space. These two components of the vestibulocochlear nerve run together from the internal auditory meatus to the cerebellopontine angle, where they enter the brain stem (Figs. 1.4, 2.21, 2.22, 2.25, 5.1,

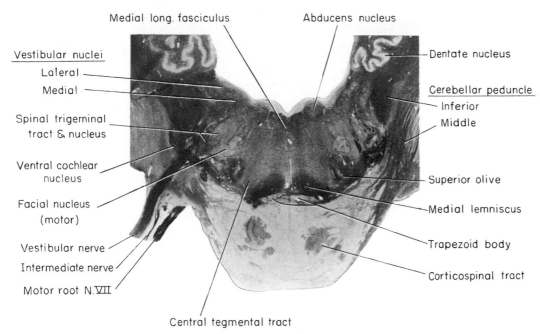

Medial long. fasciculus

Abducens nucleus

Vestibular nuclei

Lateral

Medial

Dentate nucleus

Cerebellar peduncle

Inferior

Middle

Spinal trigeminal
tract & nucleus

Ventral cochlear
nucleus

Facial nucleus
(motor)

Vestibular nerve

Intermediate nerve

Motor root N.VII

Superior olive

Medial lemniscus

Trapezoid body

Corticospinal tract

Central tegmental tract

Figure 6.2. Slightly asymmetrical section of the pons of a 1-month-old infant. Root fibers of the vestibular, intermediate, and facial nerves are present on the left at the cerebellopontine angle. Weigert's myelin stain. Photograph. (From Carpenter and Sutin, *Human Neuroanatomy*, 1983; courtesy of Williams & Wilkins.)

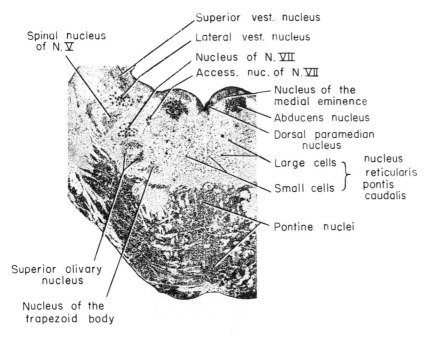

Spinal nucleus
of N. V

Superior vest. nucleus

Lateral vest. nucleus

Nucleus of N. VII

Access. nuc. of N. VII

Nucleus of the
medial eminence

Abducens nucleus

Dorsal paramedian
nucleus

Large cells ⎫
　　　　　　⎬ nucleus
Small cells ⎭ reticularis
pontis
caudalis

Pontine nuclei

Superior olivary
nucleus

Nucleus of the
trapezoid body

Figure 6.3. Section through pons and pontine tegmentum of a 3-month-old infant near same level as Figure 6.2. Cresyl violet. Photograph, with schematic representation of cell groups. (From Carpenter and Sutin, *Human Neuroanatomy*, 1983; courtesy of Williams & Wilkins.)

and 6.2). Each of these nerves arise from separate ganglia and project to distinctive central nuclei.

Cochlea

The cochlea consists of a fluid-filled coil tube of two and a half turns (Fig. 6.6) that contains the auditory transducer (Fig. 6.7). The basilar and vestibular (Reissner's) membranes partition the cochlea to form the scala vestibuli, the scala tympani, and cochlear duct (scala media). Energy

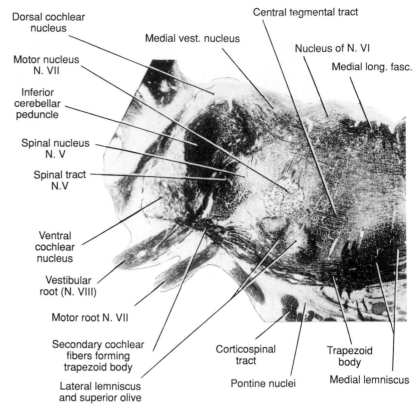

Dorsal cochlear nucleus

Motor nucleus N. VII

Inferior cerebellar peduncle

Spinal nucleus N. V

Spinal tract N.V

Ventral cochlear nucleus

Vestibular root (N. VIII)

Motor root N. VII

Secondary cochlear fibers forming trapezoid body

Lateral lemniscus and superior olive

Medial vest. nucleus

Central tegmental tract

Nucleus of N. VI

Medial long. fasc.

Corticospinal tract

Pontine nuclei

Trapezoid body

Medial lemniscus

Figure 6.4. Section of left half of the pontine tegmentum of a 3-year-old child whose brain showed a complete absence of the left cerebellar hemisphere and middle cerebellar peduncle. Fibers of the trapezoid body arising from the ventral cochlear nucleus are clearly shown. Smaller numbers of fibers in the dorsal acoustic stria are seen passing into the tegmentum from the dorsal cochlear nucleus. Weigert's myelin stain. Photograph. (From Carpenter and Sutin, *Human Neuroanatomy*, 1983; courtesy of Williams & Wilkins.)

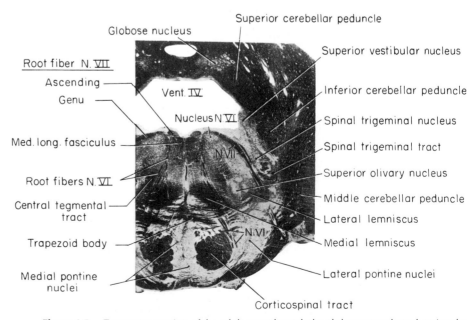

Globose nucleus

Superior cerebellar peduncle

Root fiber N. VII

Ascending

Genu

Med. long. fasciculus

Root fibers N. VI

Central tegmental tract

Trapezoid body

Medial pontine nuclei

Vent. IV

Nucleus N VI

N VII

N.VI

Superior vestibular nucleus

Inferior cerebellar peduncle

Spinal trigeminal nucleus

Spinal trigeminal tract

Superior olivary nucleus

Middle cerebellar peduncle

Lateral lemniscus

Medial lemniscus

Lateral pontine nuclei

Corticospinal tract

Figure 6.5. Transverse section of the adult pons through the abducens nucleus showing the root fibers of the abducens and facial nerves. Weigert's myelin stain. Photograph. (From Carpenter and Sutin, *Human Neuroanatomy*, 1983; courtesy of Williams & Wilkins.)

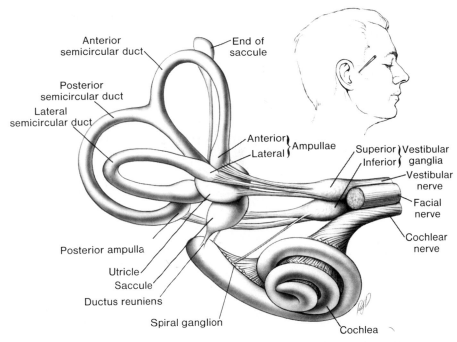

Figure 6.6.   Drawing of the labyrinthine and cochlear apparatus, their ganglia, and nerves with anatomical orientation. The cochlea has been rotated downward and laterally to expose the vestibular ganglia. (From Carpenter and Sutin, *Human Neuroanatomy*, 1983; courtesy of Williams & Wilkins.)

from sound waves reaching the tympanic membrane is transmitted via the ear ossicles to the scala vestibuli (ovale window) by the foot plate of the stapes. The membrane covering the round window at the base of the scala tympani accommodates to hydrostatic pressure changes. The *organ of Corti*, the auditory transductor, lies in the cochlear duct and consists of one row of inner hair cells and three rows of outer hair cells (Figs. 6.7 and 6.8). The tectorial membrane, attached to the spiral limbus, overlies the hair cells. The pistonlike action of the stapes transmits the energy of sound waves to the perilymph in the scala vestibuli. Energy transmitted to the perilymph produces traveling waves in the basilar membrane that move from the base of the cochlea to its apex. Displacement of the basilar membrane in response to acoustic stimuli causes bending of hair cells in contact with the tectorial membrane. Maximum displacement of the basal membrane at different distances from the stapes can be correlated with specific sound frequencies. High frequencies are perceived at the base of the cochlea and low frequencies at its apex.

Cochlear Nerve and Nuclei

The cochlear nerve originates from cells of the *spiral ganglion* situated about the modiolus of the cochlea that have glutamate as their principal neurotransmitter (Figs. 6.7 and 6.8). Peripheral processes of the bipolar cells of the spiral ganglion end in relation to the hair cells of the organ of Corti. The central processes of ganglion cells form the cochlear nerve, which enters the brain stem lateral, dorsal, and slightly caudal to the vestibular nerve. Fibers of the cochlear nerve terminate in two cell masses on the lateral surface of the inferior cerebellar peduncle, the ventral and dorsal cochlear nuclei (Figs. 5.27 and 6.9). These nuclei represent a more or less continuous cell mass, but they have distinctive cells and cytoarchitecture. The *dorsal cochlear nucleus* forms an eminence

Figure 6.7. Drawing of a radial section through the cochlea showing the cochlear duct, the basilar membrane, the organ of Corti, and the tectorial membrane. The small *diagram in the upper left* is an axial section of the cochlea. The *area enclosed in the rectangle* is reproduced in detail in the large drawing. (From Carpenter and Sutin, *Human Neuroanatomy*, 1983; courtesy of Williams & Wilkins.)

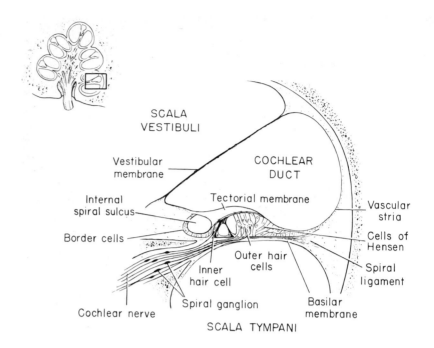

on the most lateral part of the floor of the fourth ventricle, known as the *acoustic tubercle* (Fig. 6.4). Cells of this nucleus, in most mammals, are distinctly laminated; three layers are recognized: (1) molecular, (2) fusiform, and (3) polymorphic. In humans these layers are indistinct.

The *ventral cochlear nucleus* is subdivided into anteroventral and posteroventral nuclei on a topographical and cytological basis. Cells of the *anteroventral cochlear nucleus* in the rostral region contain densely packed ovoid cells. The *posteroventral cochlear nucleus*, near the cochlear nerve root, contains several types of neurons with a predominance of multipolar cells. Each of the subdivisions of the cochlear nuclei is tonotopically organized and has a sequential representation of the auditory spectrum.

On entering the brain stem, fibers of the cochlear nerve bifurcate in orderly sequence and are distributed to both dorsal and ventral cochlear nuclei in a tonotopic fashion (Fig. 6.9). The multiple tonotopic representation in all divisions of the cochlear nuclear complex is due to the orderly bifurcation and distribution of fibers throughout the complex. In all divisions of the cochlear nuclear complex, neurons responding to higher frequencies are located dorsally. The tonotopic localization in the cochlear nuclei is the reverse of that in the cochlea with high frequencies perceived in dorsal regions and low frequencies in ventral regions.

Auditory Pathways

Secondary auditory pathways in the brain stem are complex, and many details concerning their composition are uncertain (Fig. 6.9). Fibers arising from the three subdivisions of the cochlear nuclei are grouped into three acoustic striae: (1) a *ventral acoustic stria*, which arises from the ventral cochlear nucleus and courses medially along the ventral border of the pontine tegmentum (Fig. 6.5), (2) a *dorsal acoustic stria*, which arises from the dorsal cochlear nucleus, and (3) a small *intermediate acoustic stria*, which arises from parts of both dorsal and ventral cochlear nuclei. Fibers of the dorsal and intermediate acoustic striae pass medially dorsal to the inferior cerebellar peduncle (Fig. 6.9). The dorsal acoustic

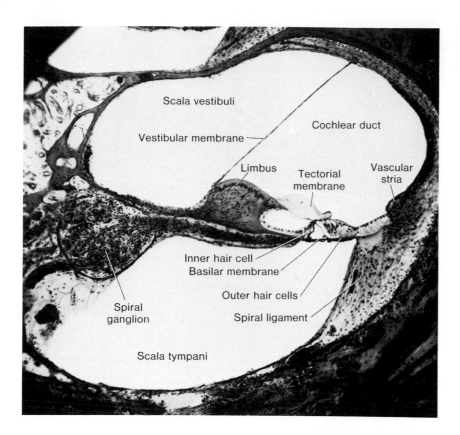

Scala vestibuli

Cochlear duct

Vestibular membrane

Limbus

Tectorial
membrane

Vascular
stria

Inner hair cell
Basilar membrane

Outer hair cells

Spiral
ganglion

Spiral ligament

Scala tympani

Figure 6.8. Photomicrograph of a radial section through the cochlea in the human similar to the schematic drawing in Figure 6.7. (From Carpenter and Sutin, *Human Neuroanatomy*, 1983; courtesy of Williams & Wilkins.)

stria crosses the median raphe ventral to the MLF, and its fibers join the lateral lemniscus of the opposite side. The intermediate stria courses through the reticular formation in a more ventral position, crosses the midline, and also enters the contralateral lateral lemniscus. The ventral acoustic stria is larger than the combined dorsal and intermediate striae and arises largely from the anteroventral cochlear nucleus. In their passage through the tegmentum, fibers of the ventral acoustic stria terminate in the reticular formation, the superior olivary nuclei, and the nuclei of the trapezoid body (Figs. 6.3 and 6.4). The superior olivary and trapezoid nuclei give rise to tertiary auditory fibers that ascend mainly in the contralateral lateral lemniscus (Fig. 6.9). No fibers from the cochlear nuclei ascend directly in the ipsilateral lateral lemniscus. Many fibers of the ventral acoustic stria pass through ventral parts of the medial lemniscus to reach the superior olivary nucleus of the opposite side. These ventrally crossing fibers form part of the trapezoid body. Intercalated cell aggregations among these fibers constitute the *nuclei of the trapezoid body* (Figs. 6.3, 6.4, and 6.9). Laterally most of the fibers of the trapezoid body enter the lateral lemniscus. Close to the place where fibers enter the lateral lemniscus there is a large collection of cells called the superior olivary nuclear complex. This complex consists of an S-shaped principal nucleus and a medial wedge-shaped accessory nucleus (Figs. 6.3, 6.4, and 6.9). The superior olivary nuclei receive secondary auditory fibers and project fibers into the lateral lemniscus. The lateral lemniscus, the principal ascending auditory pathway in the brain stem, ascends in the lateral part of the tegmentum (Fig. 6.9).

The *lateral lemniscus* ascends to midbrain levels, where most of the fibers terminate in the inferior colliculus (Figs. 6.9, 7.2, and 7.3). Interposed in the lateral lemniscus at isthmus levels are the *nuclei of the lateral lemniscus*, which receive and contribute fibers to the main bundle (Figs.

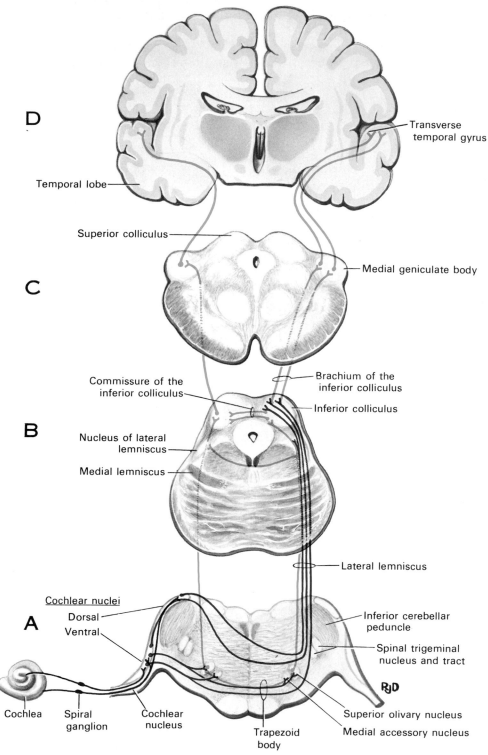

D

Transverse
temporal gyrus

Temporal lobe

Superior colliculus

C

Medial geniculate body

Commissure of the
inferior colliculus

Brachium of the
inferior colliculus

Inferior colliculus

B

Nucleus of lateral
lemniscus

Medial lemniscus

Lateral lemniscus

Cochlear nuclei

Dorsal

Ventral

A

Inferior cerebellar
peduncle

Spinal trigeminal
nucleus and tract

Cochlea

Spiral
ganglion

Cochlear
nucleus

Trapezoid
body

Superior olivary nucleus

Medial accessory nucleus

Figure 6.9.   Schematic diagram of the auditory pathways. Primary auditory fibers arising
from the spiral ganglion are in *black*. Secondary auditory fibers arising from the cochlear
nuclei and forming the acoustic striae are in *red*. Auditory fibers arising from relay nuclei
are in *blue*. *A*, Medulla; *B*, level of inferior colliculus; *C*, level of superior colliculus;
D, transverse section through the cerebral hemisphere.

6.26 and 6.27). The inferior colliculus gives rise to fibers that project to the medial geniculate body via the brachium of the inferior colliculus (Fig. 5.1).

Destruction of the cochlea, the cochlear nerve, or the cochlear nuclei (both dorsal and ventral) results in complete ipsilateral deafness. Lesions of the lateral lemniscus cause bilateral partial deafness, greatest in the contralateral ear, because fibers in this pathway are both crossed and uncrossed.

Efferent Cochlear Bundle

Crossed and uncrossed components of the *olivocochlear bundle* or the *efferent cochlear bundle* project peripherally from the brain stem to the cochlea and form a pathway by which the central nervous system may influence its own sensory input (Fig. 6.10). Electrical stimulation of the crossed fibers of this bundle in the cat inhibits auditory nerve responses to acoustic stimuli. Fibers of the olivocochlear bundle originate from cholinergic neurons surrounding the principal and accessory superior olivary nuclei (Fig. 6.11). Cochlear efferent fibers are best defined on the basis of their cells of origin into medial and lateral systems. The medial olivocochlear system originates from cells medial, ventral, and rostral to the medial superior olive; is composed of myelinated fibers; and projects bilaterally (with contralateral dominance) to the outer hair cell region of the cochlea. The lateral olivocochlear system arises from cells lateral to the medial superior olive, contains unmyelinated fibers, and projects bilaterally (with ipsilateral dominance) to the inner hair cell region of the cochlea. Crossed fibers of the olivocochlear bundle project dorsomedially toward the facial genu, cross the midline, and are joined by uncrossed fibers. Both crossed and uncrossed components of this efferent bundle emerge from the brain stem via the vestibular nerve root. In the inner ear these efferent fibers enter the cochlear nerve via the vestibulocochlear anastomosis, pass to the organ of Corti, and make synaptic contact with hair cells. The efferent cochlear bundle suppresses auditory nerve activity by inhibiting the receptivity of the end organ.

Other feedback mechanisms in the auditory system involve relay nuclei in the auditory pathway. Fibers from the inferior colliculus, the nuclei of the lateral lemniscus, and the superior olivary nuclei descend, or pass distally, to relay nuclei. These pathways differentially inhibit impulses concerned with certain frequencies of the auditory spectrum and in this way enhance frequencies not subject to central inhibition. This phenomenon is known as auditory sharpening.

Acoustic reflex mechanisms involve middle ear muscles such as the stapedius and tensor tympani. The stapedius muscle, which serves to dampen the oscillations of the ear ossicles in response to high levels of acoustic stimuli, is innervated by fibers of the facial nerve. Auditory fibers from the superior olivary complex project bilaterally to stapedius motor neurons. Contractions of the stapedius muscle, in response to loud sounds, serve to diminish amplitude. Contractions of the tensor tympani muscle, innervated by trigeminal nerve fibers, also are initiated by inputs from the superior olivary complex. The tensor tympani muscles diminish the sensitivity of the tympanic membrane to sound by tensing the membrane.

Labyrinth

The vestibular part of the inner ear consists of the *semicircular* ducts, the *utricle*, and the *saccule* (Fig. 6.6). These parts of the labyrinth are

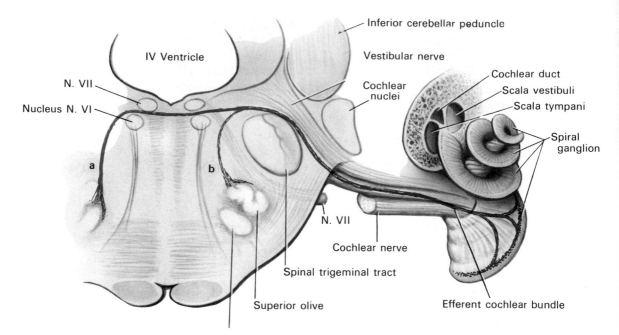

Figure 6.10. Schematic drawing of efferent cochlear fibers in the cat. Cochlear efferent fibers are defined on the basis of cells of origin into medial and lateral systems, which contain both crossed and uncrossed fibers. The *medial olivocochlear bundle* originates from cells medial and rostral to the medial superior olive (a) and is composed predominantly of crossed myelinated fibers, which terminate in outer hair cell region of the cochlea. The *lateral olivocochlear bundle* arises from cells lateral to the medial superior olive (b), contains mainly unmyelinated fibers, and projects bilaterally (with ipsilateral dominance) to the inner hair cell region of the cochlea. Crossed fibers of the olivocochlear bundle project dorsomedially toward the facial genu, cross the midline, and are joined by uncrossed fibers. Crossed and uncrossed components of this bundle emerge from the brain stem via the vestibular nerve.

concerned with orientation in three-dimensional space, maintenance of equilibrium, and modification of muscle tone. The semicircular ducts, concerned with kinetic equilibrium, are arranged at right angles to each other and represent the three planes of space. One end of each duct has a dilatation, the ampulla, containing a transversely oriented ridge, known as the *crista ampullaris*. Columnar epithelium of the crista ampullaris is composed of neuroepithelial hair cells that constitute the vestibular receptor (Fig. 6.15). Each crista has opposite it a gelatinous *cupula* that moves across the hair cells in response to movement of the endolymphatic fluid. Angular acceleration causes displacement of endolymphatic fluid and movement of the cupula, which stimulates the hair cells. Endolymphatic flow is greatest in the pair of semicircular ducts most nearly perpendicular to the axis of rotation.

The utricle and saccule (the otolithic organs) each have a similar patch of sensory epithelium known as the macula (Fig. 6.12). The maculae contain hair cells in contact with a gelatinous mass containing small calcareous particles, the otoliths. The utricular macula responds to changes in gravitational forces and to linear acceleration in the long axis of the body and conveys impulses concerning the position of the head in space (i.e., static equilibrium). The macula of the saccule is less sensitive but responds to linear acceleration in the ventrodorsal axis of the body.

Vestibular Ganglion and Nerve

The maculae and cristae are innervated by cells in the vestibular ganglion (Fig. 6.12). Most cells of the vestibular ganglion have glutamate

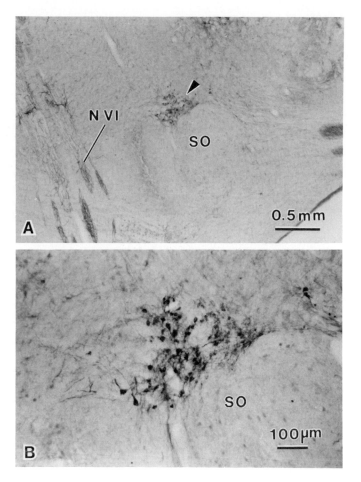

Figure 6.11. Cochlear efferent neurons identified by immunoreactivity to choline acetyltransferase (ChAT) in the monkey. In *A*, a collection of ChAT-positive neurons lies dorsal to the superior olivary nucleus (SO), identified by the arrowhead. The same group of cochlear efferent neurons is seen at a higher magnification in *B*. N. VI, abducens nerve. (From Carpenter et al., 1987. Brain Res., **408**: 275–280.)

as their neurotransmitter, but over 20% of the cells contain substance P. This ganglion can be divided into superior and inferior vestibular ganglia, which are connected by a narrow isthmus. Peripheral processes of bipolar cells located in the ganglia pass to the maculae and cristae, while the central processes form the vestibular nerve. Vestibular root fibers enter the brain stem at the cerebellopontine angle where fibers pass between the inferior cerebellar peduncle and the spinal trigeminal tract (Figs. 2.25 and 6.2). On entering the vestibular nuclear complex, the fibers bifurcate into short ascending and long descending fibers that terminate in vestibular nuclei; a small number of fibers pass directly to parts of the cerebellum.

Vestibular Nuclei

The vestibular nuclei lie in the floor of the fourth ventricle and extend from levels rostral to the hypoglossal nucleus to slightly beyond the level of the abducens nucleus. Nuclei of this complex are arranged in two longitudinal columns (Figs. 6.13 and 6.14). The lateral column consists of three distinctive nuclei, the inferior, lateral, and superior vestibular nuclei. The medial vestibular nucleus constitutes the medial cell column.

The *inferior vestibular nucleus* begins in the medulla, medial to the accessory cuneate nucleus, and extends rostrally to the level of entrance of the vestibular nerve (Figs. 5.17, 5.27, and 6.4). This nucleus is composed mostly of small and medium-sized cells, except in its most rostral

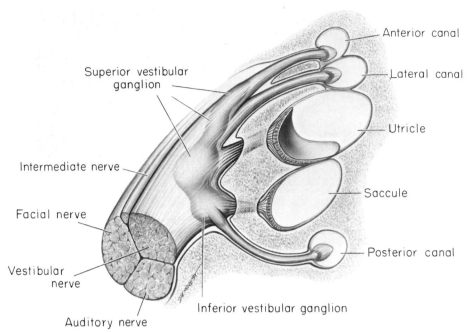

Figure 6.12. Semischematic drawing of the vestibular ganglia and peripheral branches innervating distinctive portions of the labyrinth. Cells in the superior vestibular ganglion are arranged in a spiral, and cells in the distal portion of the ganglion innervate the cristae of the anterior and lateral semicircular ducts. Cells in the broader proximal part of the superior vestibular ganglion innervate the macula of the utricle. Cells of the inferior vestibular ganglion innervate the macula of the saccule and the crista of the posterior semicircular duct. The superior and inferior vestibular ganglia are joined by an isthmus of cells. Relationships with the facial, intermediate, vestibular, and auditory nerves are shown.

part where large cells resemble those of the lateral vestibular nucleus. In fiber-stained sections, the nucleus is characterized by bundles of longitudinally oriented fibers.

The *lateral vestibular nucleus*, located at the level of entrance of the vestibular nerve, is composed of giant cells, with some regional differences in the number and size of cells (Fig. 6.3). Fibers of the vestibular root traverse ventral parts of the nucleus.

The *superior vestibular nucleus* lies dorsal and rostral to the lateral vestibular nucleus and is capped by fibers of the superior cerebellar peduncle (Fig. 6.5). Large cells in central parts of the nucleus are surrounded by smaller cells.

The *medial vestibular nucleus*, the largest of all the vestibular nuclei, is composed of small and medium-sized cells and contains relatively few fibers (Figs. 6.2, 6.3, and 6.4). This vestibular nucleus extends from the oral pole of the hypoglossal nucleus to the abducens nucleus and rostrally fuses with the superior vestibular nucleus (Fig. 6.14).

Primary Vestibular Fibers

These fibers project to all four vestibular nuclei and to the interstitial nucleus of the vestibular nerve, a collection of cells between entering vestibular root fibers (Figs. 6.13 and 6.14). Upon entering the vestibular complex, virtually all fibers bifurcate into ascending and descending branches. Ascending branches project mainly to the superior, lateral, and rostral parts of the medial vestibular nuclei. Descending branches provide fibers to the inferior vestibular nucleus and collaterals to caudal parts of the medial vestibular nucleus. Primary vestibular fibers are distributed within all vestibular nuclei, but some regions of each nucleus contain

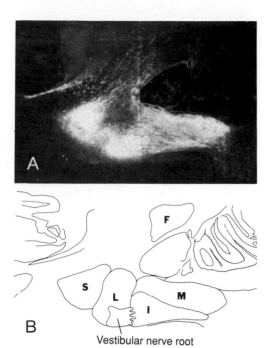

B

Vestibular nerve root

Figure 6.13. *A,* Sagittal section through the brain stem in a rhesus monkey demonstrating the transport of [³H] amino acids from the labyrinth to the vestibular nuclei in an autoradiograph. Cresyl violet, dark-field, × 20. *B,* Outline drawings of the fastigial (F) and vestibular nuclei: S, superior vestibular nucleus; L, lateral vestibular nucleus; I, inferior vestibular nucleus; M, medial vestibular nucleus. Although primary vestibular afferents project to all ipsilateral vestibular nuclei, only the ventral half of the lateral vestibular receives terminals from this source. (From Carpenter and Sutin, *Human Neuroanatomy,* 1983; courtesy of Williams & Wilkins.)

fewer endings. In the superior vestibular nucleus, primary fibers terminate most profusely about large central cells but extend into all peripheral regions. In the lateral vestibular nucleus, primary fibers terminate only in ventral regions (Fig. 6.13); the dorsal part of the lateral vestibular nucleus is the largest regional area devoid of terminal vestibular fibers. The medial vestibular nucleus receives vestibular fibers throughout its extent. Primary vestibular fibers in the inferior vestibular nucleus end most profusely in dorsal regions. The cristae of the semicircular ducts give rise to fibers that project primarily to the superior vestibular nucleus and to rostral parts of the medial vestibular nucleus. Cells of the superior vestibular ganglion, which innervate the macula of the utricle, project almost exclusively to the ventral part of the lateral vestibular nucleus (Fig. 6.13). Cells of the inferior vestibular ganglion, which innervate the macula of the saccule, give rise to central fibers that descend and terminate mainly in dorsolateral portions of the inferior vestibular nucleus and in an accessory nucleus known as cell group "y."

A small number of primary vestibular fibers enter the cerebellum via the juxtarestiform body (Fig. 6.22). In the monkey, cells in all parts of the vestibular ganglion project to the ipsilateral nodulus, uvula, and flocculus where these projections end as mossy fibers in the granular layer of the cerebellar cortex.

Afferent Projections to the Vestibular Nuclei

The vestibular nuclei, which function in conjunction with the cerebellum to maintain equilibrium, orientation in three-dimensional space, and modify muscle tone, receive important afferent projections from specific parts of the cerebellum. Afferents from the cerebellum include projections from (1) the vestibulocerebellum (i.e., the flocculus, nodulus, and uvula) to the superior and medial vestibular nuclei; (2) the anterior lobe vermis to the dorsal half of the lateral vestibular nucleus (Fig. 8.19); and (3) the fastigial nucleus bilaterally to symmetrical ventral portions of the inferior and lateral vestibular nuclei (Fig. 8.18). Projections from the

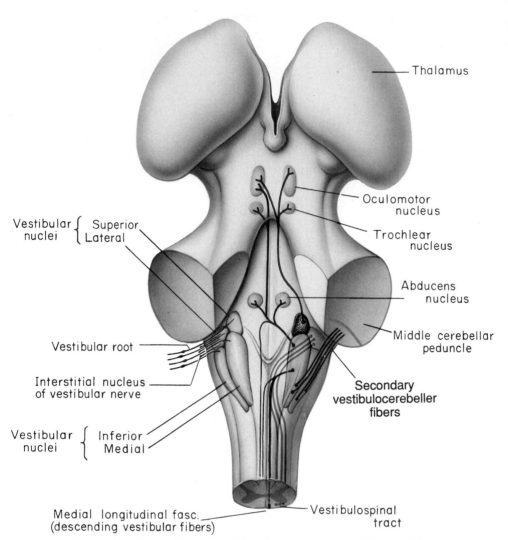

Thalamus

Oculomotor
nucleus

Trochlear
nucleus

Vestibular { Superior
nuclei { Lateral

Abducens
nucleus

Middle cerebellar
peduncle

Vestibular root

**Secondary
vestibulocerebeller
fibers**

Interstitial nucleus
of vestibular nerve

Vestibular { Inferior
nuclei { Medial

Medial longitudinal fasc.
(descending vestibular fibers)

Vestibulospinal
tract

Figure 6.14.   Schematic diagram of the principal connections of the vestibular system in the brain stem. Relationships and spatial disposition of the four main vestibular nuclei are indicated on the *left*. *Primary vestibular afferents* enter at the cerebellopontine angle and are distributed to all vestibular nuclei. The dorsal half of the lateral vestibular nucleus does not receive primary afferents. Cells of the interstitial nucleus of the vestibular nerve lie among fibers of the vestibular root. *Secondary vestibular projections* originating from the vestibular nuclei are shown on the *right*. Fibers from the superior vestibular nucleus (*red*) ascend in the ipsilateral MLF to the trochlear and oculomotor nuclei; in the caudal midbrain some fibers cross and project to parts of the oculomotor complex contralaterally. Ascending fibers from the medial vestibular nucleus (*black*) project bilaterally to the nuclei of the extraocular muscles, with contralateral dominance. Collaterals of some cells in the medial vestibular nucleus project both ascending and descending fibers in the MLF. Major descending projections from the medial vestibular nucleus are uncrossed. Cells of the lateral vestibular nucleus form the vestibulospinal tract (*blue*). Secondary vestibulocerebellar projections (*black*) arise from caudal parts of the medial and inferior vestibular nuclei.

cerebellar cortex, representing Purkinje cell axons, have inhibitory influences upon vestibular neurons mediated by γ-aminobutyric acid (GABA). Fastigial efferent projections have excitatory influences, probably mediated by the neurotransmitter glutamate.

Commissural projections from the contralateral vestibular nuclei, principally the superior and medial vestibular nuclei, have major influences on vestibular function. Vestibular neurons receiving inputs from ganglion cells innervating the cristae of the semicircular ducts have inhibitory influences on contralateral vestibular neurons via commissural projections. Vestibular neurons with inputs from ganglion cells inner-

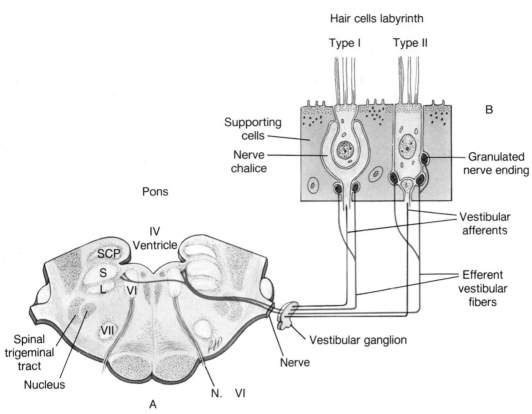

Figure 6.15.   Schematic diagram of efferent vestibular fibers (*red*) and their relationship to hair cells of the labyrinth. Efferent cholinergic vestibular fibers arise bilaterally from small groups of neurons along the lateral border of the abducens nucleus (VI) (Fig. 6.16), emerge via the vestibular nerve, and terminate in granulated nerve endings at the base of type I and type II hair cells. *A*, Schematic transverse drawing of the pons at level of abducens nuclei, and *B*, hair cells of the labyrinth. Efferent vestibular fibers exert excitatory influences upon the hair cells, which may modulate their dynamic range. Abbreviations used: L, lateral vestibular nucleus; S, superior vestibular nucleus; SCP, superior cerebellar peduncle.

vating the maculae of the otoliths exert contralateral excitatory influences via commissural projections.

Secondary Vestibular Fibers

The vestibular nuclei give rise to secondary fibers that project to specific portions of the cerebellum, to certain motor cranial nerve nuclei, and to all spinal levels. These fibers are more widely dispersed within the neuraxis than those of any special sensory system, probably because the vestibular system is concerned with the maintenance of equilibrium and orientation in three-dimensional space.

Secondary vestibulocerebellar fibers arise mainly from caudal portions of the medial and inferior vestibular nuclei and project ipsilaterally to the cortex of the nodulus, uvula, and flocculus. Vestibulocerebellar fibers, both primary and secondary, enter the cerebellum via the juxtarestiform body (Fig. 6.22). None of these fibers ends in the fastigial nucleus.

Cells of the lateral vestibular nucleus give rise to the somatotopically organized, uncrossed vestibulospinal tract (Figs. 4.12 and 4.13). In the medulla the vestibulospinal tract is a loosely organized bundle extending obliquely from the region of the medial longitudinal fasciculus (MLF) to the retroolivary area. The dorsal half of the lateral vestibular nucleus receives inhibitory influences from Purkinje cells in the anterior lobe

Figure 6.16. Vestibular efferent neurons identified by their immunoreactivity to choline acetyltransferase (ChAI) in a monkey. Vestibular efferent neurons lying lateral to cells of the abducens nucleus (VI) are indicated by an arrowhead in A. In the higher magnification of the same section, vestibular efferent neurons and one population of cells in the abducens nucleus are cholinergic (B). (From Carpenter et al., 1987. Brain Res., **408:** 275–280.)

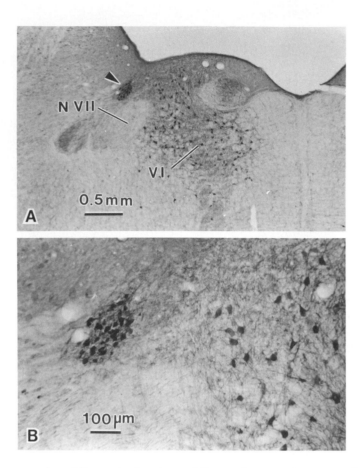

vermis, while ventral regions of the nucleus receive crossed and uncrossed excitatory inputs from the fastigial nuclei. Impulses relayed to spinal levels via the vestibulospinal tract have facilitating influences upon extensor muscle tone.

Fibers of the MLF arise from parts of the medial and inferior vestibular nuclei, and many of these fibers bifurcate into ascending and descending branches (Fig. 6.14). Although descending fibers in the MLF from these nuclei are bilateral in the medulla, at spinal levels most fibers are ipsilateral and extend only to cervical spinal segments. Some vestibular fibers in the MLF terminating monosynaptically upon anterior horn cells exert inhibitory and excitatory influences.

Medial Longitudinal Fasciculus (MLF)

Ascending fibers of the MLF arise mainly from parts of the medial and superior vestibular nuclei, are crossed and uncrossed, and project primarily to the nuclei of the extraocular muscles (i.e., the abducens, trochlear, and oculomotor). Ascending fibers from the medial vestibular nucleus are predominantly crossed and project bilaterally upon the abducens nuclei and asymmetrically upon portions of the oculomotor nuclei; projections to the trochlear nucleus are largely crossed (Fig. 6.14). Large cells in central parts of the superior vestibular nucleus give rise to uncrossed ascending fibers in the MLF distributed to the trochlear and oculomotor nuclei. Smaller cells in peripheral parts of the superior vestibular nucleus project fibers to the oculomotor nucleus via a crossed ventral tegmental pathway (outside of the MLF), which has major influences on cells innervating the opposite superior rectus muscle. Physiologically crossed ascending vestibular projections to the nuclei of the

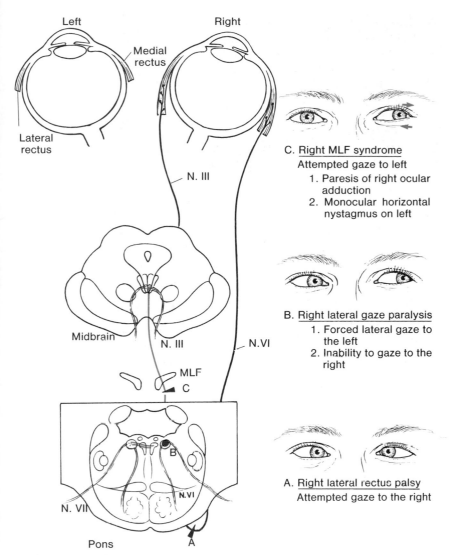

Figure 6.17. Diagrammatic drawing of lesions affecting conjugate horizontal gaze. The lesion (*red*) at *A*, involving the right abducens nerve as it leaves the brain stem, produces a paralysis of the right lateral rectus muscle. In sketch of the eyes at *A* the patient is attempting to gaze to the right; the right eye is somewhat adducted and the left eye is fully adducted. This patient would experience diplopia on attempted right lateral gaze. The lesion (*red*) in the abducens nucleus (*B*) would destroy lower motor neurons and abducens internuclear neurons whose axons enter the opposite MLF and ascend to the medial rectus subdivision of the oculomotor complex. A patient with such a lesion would have a right lateral gaze paralysis, and both eyes would be forcefully directed to the left field of gaze. A unilateral lesion (*red*) in the MLF (*blue*) at *C* would interrupt axons of abducens internuclear neurons arising from the left abducens nucleus. This lesion would produce dissociated horizontal eye movements. On attempted gaze to the left, there would be a paresis of right ocular adduction (*C*) and monocular horizontal nystagmus in the left abducting eye, indicated by arrows. (From Carpenter and Sutin, *Human Neuroanatomy*, 1983; courtesy of Williams & Wilkins.)

extraocular muscles have excitatory effects, while uncrossed fibers exert inhibition (Fig. 6.14).

In addition, the MLF contains an impressive crossed ascending projection originating from abducens internuclear neurons that terminates upon cells of the medial rectus subdivision of the oculomotor nuclear complex (Figs. 6.17 and 6.20). This projection interrelates activities of the abducens nucleus of one side with neurons of the oculomotor nucleus, which innervates the medial rectus muscle on the opposite side. This pathway provides a neural mechanism for simultaneous contractions of the lateral rectus muscle on one side and the medial rectus muscle on the opposite side, required for conjugate lateral gaze (Fig. 6.17).

A small number of ascending vestibular fibers in the MLF bypass the oculomotor nucleus and terminate in the interstitial nucleus of Cajal, a small group of neurons embedded in the MLF (Figs. 7.11 and 7.14). The medial vestibular nucleus projects to the opposite interstitial nucleus, while the superior vestibular nucleus provides terminals to the ipsilateral interstitial nucleus.

Secondary vestibular projections to thalamic relay nuclei are bilateral, modest in number, and end about cell clusters in the ventral posterolateral (VPL_c) thalamic nucleus. Vestibular projections to the thalamus only partly ascend in the MLF. Thalamic nuclei receiving vestibular inputs also respond to somatosensory signals, suggesting there is no exclusive representation of vestibular sense at thalamic levels.

Efferent Vestibular Projections

Like the cochlea, the vestibular end organ receives an efferent innervation that arises bilaterally from brain stem neurons. These cholinergic efferent neurons lie along the lateral border of the abducens nucleus and give rise to fibers that pass peripherally with the vestibular nerve on each side to innervate hair cells in the cristae of the semicircular ducts and the maculae of the utricle and saccule (Figs. 6.15 and 6.16). Efferent vestibular fibers have bilateral excitatory effects on each of the five end organs of the labyrinth. It has been postulated that the efferent vestibular projection may modulate the dynamic range of afferents to match expected accelerations. It is of interest that the efferent cochlear and vestibular neurons are both cholinergic, but efferent cochlear fibers are inhibitory and efferent vestibular fibers are excitatory (Figs. 6.11 and 6.16).

FUNCTIONAL CONSIDERATIONS

Secondary vestibular fibers contained in the MLF play an important role in conjugate eye movements. Selective stimulation of the nerve from the ampulla of individual semicircular ducts produces specific deviations of both eyes that are regarded as primary responses.

Stimulation of the ampullary nerve from the horizontal duct produces conjugate deviation of the eyes to the opposite side. Bilateral stimulation of the ampullary nerves of the anterior ducts produces upward movement of both eyes; similar bilateral stimulation of the ampullary nerves of the posterior ducts causes downward movements of the eyes. Section of the MLF rostral to the abducens nuclei abolishes these primary oculomotor responses, but nystagmus still results from labyrinthine stimulation, suggesting that pathways essential for nystagmus probably pass via the reticular formation.

Labyrinthine stimulation, irritation, or disease causes vertigo, postural deviations, unsteadiness in standing and walking, deviations of the eyes, and nystagmus. *Vertigo* implies a subjective sense of rotation, either of the individual or of the environment. The most prominent objective sign of vestibular involvement is *nystagmus*, a rhythmic, involuntary oscillation of the eyes characterized by alternate slow and rapid ocular excursions. Slow movement of the eyes in one direction is abruptly followed by rapid eye movements in the opposite direction. By convention the direction of the nystagmus is named for the rapid phase, even though the slow ocular excursion is the primary movement (the rapid phase is the automatic reflex correction). Tests of vestibular function are based on stimulation of the semicircular canals or vestibular nerve endings by (1) the rotating-chair test (Bárány chair) or (2) the caloric test (irrigation of the external auditory canal with water of temperatures appropriate to induce convection currents in the endolymphatic fluid). Following a period of rotation in the Bárány chair, the chair is abruptly stopped, but the endolymphatic fluid continues to circulate for a time. In this postrotational phase, the slow phase of the nystagmus, the deviations of the eyes, postural deviation (standing), and past-pointing are all in the direction of the previous rotation and can be correlated with the persistent direction of endolymphatic flow. The patient experiences a sense of vertigo opposite to that of the prior rotation.

Lesions of the MLF rostral to the abducens nuclei produce a disturbance of conjugate horizontal eye movements known as *anterior internuclear ophthalmoplegia*. A unilateral lesion in the MLF rostral to the abducens nucleus results in (1) paresis of ipsilateral ocular adduction on attempted lateral gaze to the opposite side, (2) monocular horizontal nystagmus in the contralateral abducted eye, and (3) no impairment of ocular convergence. The paresis of ocular adduction on attempted lateral gaze to the opposite side occurs ipsilateral to a unilateral lesion of the MLF (Fig. 6.17). Bilateral lesions of the MLF rostral to the abducens nuclei result in dissociated horizontal eye movements on attempted lateral gaze to both the right and left. In the bilateral syndrome no ocular adduction is seen on attempted lateral gaze to either side. An adequate explanation for the monocular horizontal nystagmus seen in the abducting eye has eluded clinicians and investigators. This syndrome has been produced in the monkey and occurs in humans, mainly as a consequence of brain stem vascular lesions or in association with demyelinating disease (i.e., multiple sclerosis). The paresis of ocular adduction on attempted lateral gaze to the opposite side results from interruption of ascending fibers from abducens internuclear neurons after they have crossed from the opposite side (Fig. 6.17).

Mechanisms governing equilibrium (i.e., maintenance of appropriate body position) and orientation in three-dimensional space are largely reflex in character and depend on afferent inputs from several sources. The most important of these are (1) kinesthetic sense conveyed by the posterior column-medial lemniscal system from receptors in joints and joint capsules, (2) impulses conveyed centrally by spinocerebellar systems from stretch receptors in muscles and tendons, (3) the suprasegmental kinesthetic sense provided by the vestibular end organ, and (4) visual input from the retina. The labyrinth is a highly specialized receptor stimulated by the change of position, or changes in the position of the head. When the head is moved, the cristae are stimulated and effect compensatory reflexes of the eyes and limbs. Sustaining or static reflexes are initiated by gravitational forces acting upon the macular hair cells.

The vestibulospinal tracts and descending fibers from the pontine reticular formation exert strong excitatory influences upon muscle tone, particularly extensor muscle tone. Normally, muscle tone is maintained by a balance of inhibitory and facilitatory influences, a large part of which are mediated by the brain stem reticular formation. If the influences of higher centers acting upon brain stem structures are removed by transection of the brain stem at the intercollicular level (i.e., between the superior and inferior colliculi), a condition known as *decerebrate rigidity* develops. This condition is characterized by tremendously increased tone in the antigravity muscles, due to an increased firing rate of muscle spindles by gamma (γ) motor neurons. The increased firing rate of the muscle

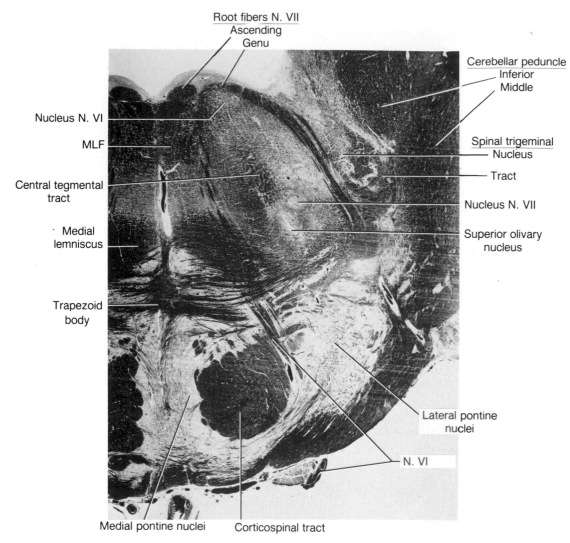

Figure 6.18. Photomicrograph of the right half of the pons showing the intramedullary course of the abducens and facial nerves (Weigert's myelin stain).

spindle afferents activates alpha (α) motor neurons that maintain the tonic state (Fig. 3.23). In this experimental preparation, facilitatory pathways from the reticular formation of the pons and from the lateral vestibular nucleus (vestibulospinal tract) remain active, while inhibitory elements of the medullary reticular formation no longer function. Inhibitory regions of the reticular formation are considered to be dependent on descending impulses from higher levels, while facilitating regions of the reticular formation remain active. Midbrain transection removes the input essential to the reticular inhibitory system but has little effect upon brain stem facilitating mechanisms. Decerebrate rigidity can be abolished, or diminished, by a variety of different lesions, including section of the vestibular nerve, destruction of the vestibular nuclei, or section of the vestibulospinal tract. Surgical section of several successive dorsal or ventral spinal roots will abolish the phenomenon segmentally because either will interrupt the γ loop.

FACIAL NERVE

The facial nerve and the intermediate nerve usually are discussed together although they subserve separate functions (Figs. 6.1, 6.2, 6.5,

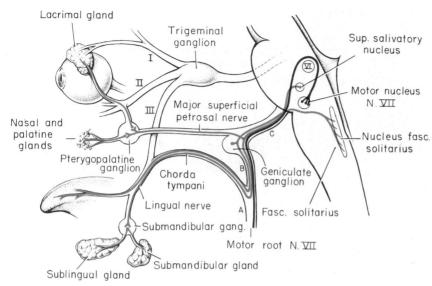

Figure 6.19. Diagram showing the functional components, organization, and peripheral distribution of the facial nerve. *Special visceral efferent* (SVE) fibers (motor) are shown in *red*. *General visceral efferent* (GVE) fibers (parasympathetic) are in *green*, and *special visceral afferent* (SVA) fibers (taste) are in *blue*. A, B, and C denote lesions of the facial nerve at the stylomastoid foramen, distal to the geniculate ganglion, and proximal to the geniculate ganglion. Disturbances resulting from lesions at these locations are described in the text (pp. 172–173). (From Carpenter and Sutin, *Human Neuroanatomy*, 1983; courtesy of Williams & Wilkins.)

and (6,18). Functional components of these nerves include (1) *special visceral efferent* (SVE, branchiomotor) fibers, (2) *general visceral efferent* (GVE, parasympathetic) fibers, (3) *special visceral afferent* (SVA, taste) fibers, and (4) a few *general somatic afferent* (GSA, sensory) fibers.

Special visceral efferent (SVE) *fibers* of the motor component innervate the muscles of facial expression, the platysma, the buccinator, and the stapedius muscles. The motor nucleus of N. VII forms a column of cholinergic multipolar neurons in the ventrolateral tegmentum dorsal to the superior olivary nucleus and ventromedial to the spinal trigeminal nucleus (Figs. 6.1, 6.2, 6.3, and 6.4). Several distinct cell groups that innervate specific muscles have been recognized: (1) dorsomedial (auricular and occipital muscles), (2) ventromedial (platysma), (3) intermediate (orbicularis oculi and upper mimetic facial muscles), and (4) lateral (buccinator and buccolabial muscles). Efferent fibers, emerging from the dorsal surface of the nucleus, project dorsomedially into the floor of the fourth ventricle. These fibers ascend longitudinally medial to the abducens nucleus and dorsal to the MLF (Figs. 6.5 and 6.18), but near the rostral pole of the abducens nucleus they make a sharp lateral bend and project ventrolaterally. In their emerging course these fibers pass medial to the spinal trigeminal complex and exit from the brain stem near to caudal border of the pons, at the cerebellopontine angle (Figs. 6.2, 6.5, and 6.18).

The *intermediate nerve*, which emerges at the cerebellopontine angle between the facial motor root and the vestibular nerve (Fig. 6.2), contains afferent and general visceral efferent fibers. Afferent fibers (SVA and GSA) arise from cells of the geniculate ganglion, located at the external genu of the facial nerve (Fig. 6.19). *Special visceral afferent* (SVA) *fibers* convey gustatory sense (taste) from the anterior two-thirds of the tongue. Centrally these fibers enter the solitary fasciculus and terminate upon cells in the rostral part of the solitary nucleus, referred to as the gustatory

Figure 6.20. Dark-field photomicrographs of [³H] amino acids injected into the right abducens nucleus in a monkey showing transport via abducens root fibers and the contralateral medial longitudinal fasciculus (MLF) (*A*). Isotope transported from abducens internuclear neurons via the MLF terminates in the medial rectus subdivision of the opposite oculomotor complex (*B*). The medial rectus subdivisions in the caudal oculomotor complex are represented by cell groups designated *a* and *b*. (From Carpenter and Carleton, 1983. Brain Res., **274**: 114–149.)

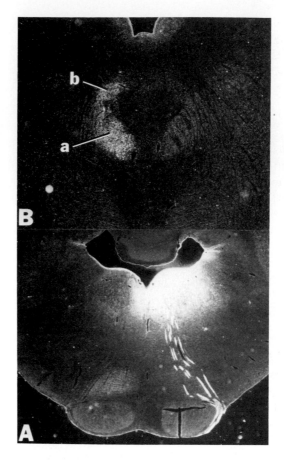

nucleus. *General somatic afferent* (GSA) *fibers* convey cutaneous sensation from the external auditory meatus and the region back of the ear; centrally these fibers enter the dorsal part of the spinal trigeminal tract.

General visceral efferent (GVE) *fibers* in the intermediate nerve arise from the superior salivatory nucleus, which consists of scattered cholinergic neurons in the dorsolateral reticular formation (Fig. 6.19). Preganglionic parasympathetic fibers from these cells pass peripherally as a component of the intermediate nerve, but near the external genu of the facial nerve they divide so that (1) one group passes to the pterygopalatine ganglion via the major superficial petrosal nerve, and (2) another group projects via the chorda tympani and branches of the lingual nerves to the submandibular ganglion. Synapses with postganglionic neurons occur in the pterygopalatine and submandibular ganglia. Postganglionic fibers from the pterygopalatine ganglion give rise to secretory and vasomotor fibers that innervate the lacrimal gland and the mucous membranes of the nose and mouth. Postganglionic parasympathetic fibers from the submandibular ganglion pass to the submandibular and sublingual salivary glands.

Lesions of the Facial Nerve

Lesions of the facial nerve (Bell's palsy) produce paralysis of the ipsilateral facial muscles and other sensory and autonomic disturbances that depend upon the location and extent of the peripheral lesion. A complete lesion of the motor part of the facial nerve as it emerges from the stylomastoid foramen (*A*, Fig. 6.19) results in a complete paralysis of the ipsilateral facial muscles. On the side of the lesion, the patient is unable to wrinkle the forehead, close the eye, show the teeth, or purse the lips. The palpebral fissure is widened, the nasolabial fold is flattened, and the corner of the mouth droops. The corneal reflex is abolished on the side of the lesion, but corneal sensation remains. A lesion distal to the geniculate ganglion (*B*, Fig. 6.19) produces the deficits associated with a lesion at *A* but in addition produces impairment of sublingual and submandibular salivary secretions, hyperacusis, and frequently loss of taste in the anterior two-thirds of the tongue ipsilaterally. Salivary secretions are impaired due to interruption of preganglionic parasympathetic fibers, and loss of taste is due to interruption of SVA fibers. Hyperacusis results from paralysis of the stapedius muscle, which serves to dampen the oscillations of the ear ossicles and causes sounds to be abnormally loud on the affected side. Lesions of the facial nerve proximal to the geniculate ganglion (*C*, Fig. 6.19) produce all of the disturbances described for lesions at *A* and *B* and in addition invariably result in loss of taste over the anterior two-thirds of the tongue and impairment of ipsilateral lacrimation. This lesion interrupts all SVA fibers as they course centrally and all preganglionic parasympathetic (GVE) fibers en route to both the pterygopalatine and submandibular ganglia. Following complete lesions proximal to the geniculate ganglion, taste is permanently lost and no regeneration of sensory fibers takes place. Preganglionic parasympathetic fibers may regenerate, but this frequently occurs in an aberrant manner. Fibers that previously projected to the submandibular ganglion may regrow and enter the major superficial petrosal nerve. As a consequence of this aberrant regeneration a salivary stimulus may produce lacrimation (syndrome of *crocodile tears*).

Central type facial palsies involve corticobulbar and corticoreticular fibers that directly and indirectly convey impulses to cells of the facial nucleus. Two types of central facial paralysis are recognized: (1) voluntary and (2) mimetic. Voluntary central type facial palsy occurs contralateral to a lesion involving corticobulbar fibers and affects only the muscles of the lower half of the face, especially those in the perioral region (Fig. 5.25). The accepted explanation is that corticobulbar fibers projecting to cell groups of the facial nucleus innervating muscles in the upper part of the face and forehead are distributed bilaterally; those projecting to cell groups that innervate the lower part of the face are only crossed. Thus a unilateral lesion interrupting corticobulbar pathways results in paralysis only of the lower facial muscles contralaterally. A lesion involving corticobulbar and corticospinal fibers in the internal capsule produces a contralateral voluntary central type facial paralysis and a contralateral hemiplegia. Such a lesion never impairs taste, salivary or lacrimal secretions, or the corneal reflex.

Mimetic or emotional innervation of the muscles of facial expression may be preserved even in the presence of a voluntary central type facial palsy. In response to a genuine emotional stimulus, the muscles of the lower part of the face will contract symmetrically. Mimetic facial innervation is involuntary and is mediated by pathways that are independent of those arising from the cerebral cortex. While it is recognized that these pathways are separate from those mediating voluntary facial expression, their origin and course are unknown. Thus certain neural lesions can produce a mimetic facial paralysis without impairing voluntary facial contractions. More extensive lesions can produce combined voluntary and mimetic facial palsies.

ABDUCENS NERVE

The abducens nerve arises from a collection of typical motor cells in the floor of the fourth ventricle that are within the complicated loop formed by fibers of the facial nerve (Figs. 6.1, 6.2, 6.3, 6.5, and 6.18). This motor nerve (GSE) innervates the lateral rectus muscle, which serves to abduct the eye. Root fibers emerge from the medial aspect of the nucleus, pass ventrally through the pontine tegmentum, and emerge from the brain stem at the caudal border of the pons lateral to the corticospinal tract (Figs. 5.2, 5.26, and 6.18). This slender nerve has a long intracranial course and traverses the cavernous sinus and superior orbital fissure en route to the lateral rectus muscle. In the cavernous sinus the abducens nerve lies close to the internal carotid artery (Fig. 14.4). The abducens nucleus is unique among motor cranial nerve nuclei in that it contains two populations of neurons: (1) typical motor neurons that project fibers via the nerve root to innervate the ipsilateral lateral rectus muscle and (2) internuclear neurons whose axons (retained within the brain stem) cross the midline, ascend in the contralateral MLF, and terminate upon cells of the oculomotor complex that innervate the medial rectus muscle of the opposite side (Fig. 6.20). Abducens internuclear neurons, constituting 25–50% of the nucleus, are distributed throughout the nucleus and are virtually impossible to distinguish from motor neurons in common stains. Abducens motor neurons are immunocytochemically reactive to choline acetyltransferase (ChAT) (Fig. 6.16).

The abducens nucleus receives inputs from the medial vestibular nucleus, the reticular formation, and the nucleus prepositus. Afferents from the medial vestibular nucleus are predominantly ipsilateral and both populations of abducens neurons are considered to receive the same profile of disynaptic excitation and inhibition from the labyrinth. Afferents to the abducens nucleus from the paramedian pontine reticular formation (PPRF) and the nucleus prepositus hypoglossi are uncrossed. Cortico-bulbar fibers convey impulses bilaterally to the abducens nuclei via intercalated neurons in the reticular formation.

Lesions of the Abducens Nerve

Lesions of the abducens nerve produce a paralysis of the ipsilateral lateral rectus muscle that results in horizontal diplopia (double vision), maximal on attempted lateral gaze to the side of the lesion (Fig. 6.17). Because of the unopposed action of the medial rectus muscle, the affected eye maintains a strongly adducted position. Diplopia is the phenomenon that results when light reflected by an object in the visual field does not fall upon corresponding points of the two retinae. The abducens nerve is the most frequently injured cranial nerve. An isolated lesion of the sixth nerve has no neurological localizing value because of its long intracranial course. If the lesion produces ipsilateral horizontal diplopia and a contralateral hemiparesis, the lesion can be localized to the medial pons where it involves root fibers of the abducens nerve and parts of the corticospinal tract (i.e., middle alternating hemiplegia). Ipsilateral horizontal diplopia combined with a facial paralysis (same side) indicates a lesion in the caudal pontine tegmentum involving root fibers of the sixth and seventh cranial nerves.

Lesions of the Abducens Nucleus

Discrete unilateral lesions of the abducens nucleus produce a paralysis of lateral gaze to the side of the lesion (Fig. 6.17). The syndrome of *lateral gaze paralysis* differs from paralysis of the lateral rectus muscle in that neither eye can be directed laterally toward the side of the lesion and both eyes tend to be forcefully and conjugately deviated to the opposite side. Ocular convergence usually is not affected. Thus the abducens nerve appears unique in that it is the only cranial nerve in which lesions of the root fibers and nucleus do not produce the same effects.

Lateral gaze paralysis, due to discrete lesions in the abducens nucleus, is caused by (1) destruction of motor neurons in the abducens nucleus, which results in paralysis of the ipsilateral lateral rectus muscle, and (2) destruction of internuclear neurons within the abducens nucleus, that give rise to ascending fibers that project via the opposite MLF to the medial rectus subdivision (see p. 203) of the contralateral oculomotor complex (Fig. 6.20). The paresis of ocular adduction in the contralateral eye, which forms part of the syndrome of lateral gaze paralysis, appears to be due to destruction of abducens internuclear neurons that are intermingled with cells whose axons form the abducens nerve root.

Horizontal and Vertical Eye Movements

While the general somatic efferent (GSE) cranial nerves innervating the extraocular muscles are regarded the simplest of all the cranial nerves, this simplicity applies only to their peripheral activities. Because the nuclei of the extraocular muscles are widely separated and function bilaterally and synergistically to produce a full range of precise conjugate eye movements, a central neural mechanism must control activities of the abducens, trochlear, and oculomotor nuclei. The observation that paralysis of vertical or horizontal eye movements can occur independently implies separate anatomical sites at some distance from each other that generate vertical and horizontal eye movements. However, many conjugate eye movements have precisely synchronized vertical and horizontal components, suggesting that centers controlling vertical and horizontal eye movements must be functionally connected and coordinated. Considerable evidence suggests that the pontine "center for lateral gaze" and the abducens nucleus probably constitute a single entity.

The localized region most concerned with vertical eye movements lies in the tegmental area rostral to the oculomotor complex in the zone of transition between diencephalon and mesencephalon, referred to as the *rostral interstitial nucleus of the MLF* (RiMLF). Centers for horizontal (i.e., the abducens nucleus) and vertical (i.e., RiMLF) gaze are interrelated by a collection of physiologically defined neurons in the paramedian reticular formation rostral to the abducens nucleus, called the *paramedian pontine reticular formation* (PPRF). Stimulation of caudal regions of the PPRF produces conjugate horizontal deviation of the eyes, while stimulation in rostral regions produces vertical eye movements. Caudal parts of the PPRF project fibers to the ipsilateral abducens nucleus: rostral regions of the PPRF project uncrossed fibers to the RiMLF, which ascend outside of the MLF. The RiMLF in turn project to the ipsilateral oculomotor nuclear complex. Lesions in the PPRF may cause paralysis of horizontal eye movements (caudal part), paralysis of vertical eye movements (rostral part), or both if extensive.

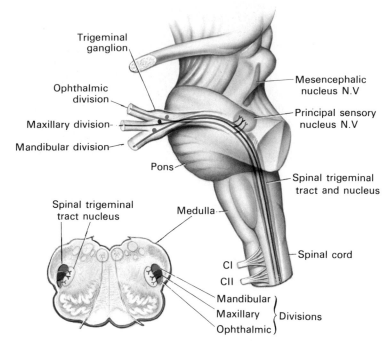

Figure 6.21. Diagram of the topographical arrangement of fibers in the different divisions of the trigeminal nerve and their rearrangement and terminations in the brain stem. As the trigeminal nerve root enters the brain stem, it rotates so that fibers in the mandibular division become most dorsal. This inverted arrangement persists throughout the spinal trigeminal tract and is also present in the principal sensory nucleus of N. V.

TRIGEMINAL NERVE

The trigeminal, the largest cranial nerve, contains both sensory and motor components. *General somatic afferent* (GSA) components convey both exteroceptive and proprioceptive impulses. Exteroceptive impulses (i.e., pain, thermal, and tactile sense) are transmitted from (1) the face and forehead, (2) mucous membranes of the nose and mouth, (3) the teeth, and (4) large portions of the cranial dura. Deep pressure and kinesthesis are conveyed from the teeth, periodontium, hard palate, and temporomandibular joint. In addition impulses are transmitted centrally from stretch receptors in the muscles of mastication. *Special visceral efferent* (SVE) fibers (branchiomotor) innervate the muscles of mastication, the tensor tympani, and the tensor veli palatini.

Trigeminal Ganglion

Afferent fibers, except for those associated with pressure and stretch receptors, have their cell bodies in the trigeminal ganglion. This ganglion, composed of typical unipolar cells, lies on the petrous bone in the middle cranial fossa (Fig. 1.3). Peripheral processes of these cells form the ophthalmic, maxillary, and mandibular divisions of the trigeminal nerve, which innervate distinctive regions of the face, head, and intraoral structures without overlap. All three divisions of the trigeminal nerve contribute sensory fibers to the dura.

Central processes of trigeminal ganglion cells form the large sensory root of this nerve, which traverses the lateral part of the rostral pons, to enter the pontine tegmentum and terminate upon sensory relay nuclei in

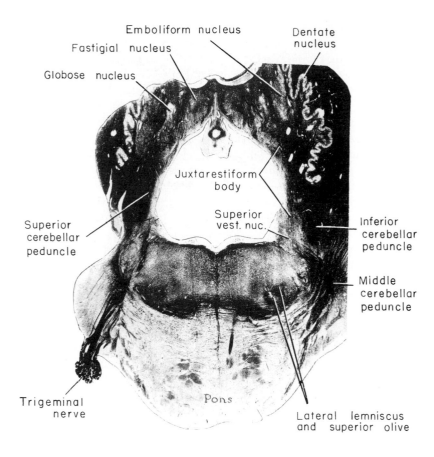

Emboliform nucleus

Fastigial nucleus

Globose nucleus

Dentate nucleus

Juxtarestiform body

Superior vest. nuc.

Superior cerebellar peduncle

Inferior cerebellar peduncle

Middle cerebellar peduncle

Trigeminal nerve

Pons

Lateral lemniscus and superior olive

Figure 6.22. Section of pons, pontine tegmentum, and part of cerebellum through the trigeminal nerve root. One-month-old infant. Weigert's myelin stain. Photograph. (From Carpenter and Sutin, *Human Neuroanatomy*, 1983; courtesy of Williams & Wilkins.)

the pons and medulla (Figs. 2.22, 6.21, and 6.22). Many sensory root fibers bifurcate into short ascending and long descending branches; other fibers ascend or descend without branching. Ascending fibers terminate upon cells of the principal sensory nucleus, while descending fibers form the spinal trigeminal tract (Fig. 6.25).

Spinal Trigeminal Tract and Nucleus

Root fibers entering the spinal trigeminal tract have a definite topographical organization. Fibers of the ophthalmic division are most ventral, fibers of the mandibular division are most dorsal, and those of the maxillary division are intermediate (Fig. 6.21). This inverted laminar arrangement of fibers results from medial rotation of the trigeminal sensory root as it enters the brain stem and persists throughout the length of the tract. The tract extends from the level of the trigeminal root entry in the pons to the uppermost cervical spinal segments. Fibers of the spinal trigeminal tract terminate upon cells of the spinal trigeminal nucleus, which form a long laminated cell column medial to the tract. Rostrally the nucleus merges with the principal sensory nucleus, while caudally it blends into the substantia gelatinosa of the first two cervical spinal segments (Figs. 6.21 and 6.25). Fibers of the spinal trigeminal tract project into that part of the spinal trigeminal nucleus immediately adjacent to it. There is a sharp segregation of terminal fibers within parts of the nucleus and virtually no overlap of fibers from the different divisions of the nerve. The spinal trigeminal tract also contains small groups of GSA fibers from the facial, glossopharyngeal, and vagus nerves, which occupy dorsomedial regions.

Cytoarchitecturally the spinal trigeminal nucleus consists of three parts: (1) a *pars oralis*, (2) a *pars interpolaris*, and (3) a *pars caudalis*. The laminar configurations within caudal parts of the spinal trigeminal nucleus consist of four layers (Fig. 5.9) and resemble those of the posterior gray horn at spinal levels. Cells in lamina I respond to nociceptive and thermal stimuli; lamina II corresponds to the substantia gelatinosa, and laminae III and IV (magnocellular layers) correspond to the proper sensory nucleus. Fibers containing substance P terminate in lamina I and the outer part of lamina II in the pars caudalis; cells positive for enkephalin are found in deep parts of lamina II (Fig. 5.10). Throughout the nucleus the face is represented in an upside down fashion, with the jaw dorsal and the forehead ventral (Fig. 6.21). The pars oralis receives impulses predominantly from internal structures of the nose and mouth. The pars interpolaris is related mainly to cutaneous facial regions, while the pars caudalis has large receptive fields over the forehead, cheek, and jaw.

Lesions of the spinal trigeminal tract result in a loss or diminution of pain and thermal sense in areas innervated by the trigeminal nerve. Such lesions do not abolish tactile sense, because some neurons at all levels of the nucleus respond to tactile stimuli. Tactile sense may be mediated by fibers that bifurcate and send branches to both the spinal trigeminal nucleus and the principal sensory nucleus (Fig. 6.25). Virtually no overlap exists between cutaneous areas supplied by the three peripheral divisions of the trigeminal nerve, in contrast to the extensive overlap seen for spinal nerves. Trigeminal tractotomy (i.e., sectioning of the spinal trigeminal tract) can relieve various forms of facial pain, including trigeminal neuralgia (tic douloureux). This procedure eliminates or greatly reduces pain and thermal sense without abolishing tactile sense. Corneal sensation remains, as does the corneal reflex, though it may not be as brisk.

Principal Sensory Nucleus

This nucleus lies lateral to the entering trigeminal root fibers in the upper pons (Figs. 6.21, 6.22, 6.23, and 6.25). Root fibers conveying impulses for tactile and pressure sense enter the principal sensory nucleus and are distributed in a manner similar to that described for the spinal trigeminal nucleus. Fibers of the ophthalmic division terminate ventrally, fibers of the maxillary division are intermediate, and fibers of the mandibular division are most dorsal. Cells of the principal sensory nucleus have large receptive fields, show high spontaneous activity, and respond to a wide range of pressure stimuli with little adaptation.

Mesencephalic Nucleus

This trigeminal nucleus forms a slender cell column near the lateral margin of the central gray of the upper fourth ventricle and cerebral aqueduct. The nucleus, composed of large unipolar neurons, extends from the level of the motor nucleus of N.V to the rostral midbrain (Figs. 6.21, 6.22, 6.23, and 6.25). Cells resemble those of the dorsal root ganglion but are not encapsulated and lie within the central nervous system. The principal processes of these cells form the sickle-shaped *mesencephalic tract of the trigeminal nerve* (Figs. 5.20, 6.21, 6.22, and 6.23), which descends to the level of the motor nucleus of N.V. Collaterals of these processes enter the motor nucleus, while the main fibers emerge as part of the motor root. Cells of this nucleus are considered to be primary sensory neurons that have been "retained" within the central nervous

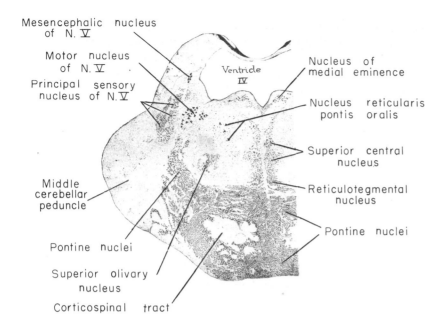

Mesencephalic nucleus
of N. V

Motor nucleus
of N. V

Principal sensory
nucleus of N. V

Ventricle
IV

Nucleus of
medial eminence

Nucleus reticularis
pontis oralis

Superior central
nucleus

Reticulotegmental
nucleus

Pontine nuclei

Middle
cerebellar
peduncle

Pontine nuclei

Superior olivary
nucleus

Corticospinal tract

Figure 6.23. Section through the pons of a 1-month-old infant at about same level as Figure 6.22. Cresyl violet. Photograph, with cell groups schematically blocked in. (From Carpenter and Sutin, *Human Neuroanatomy,* 1983; courtesy of Williams & Wilkins.)

system. Afferent fibers of the mesencephalic nucleus of the trigeminal nerve convey pressure and kinesthesis sense from the teeth, periodontium, hard palate, and joint capsules. This nucleus is concerned with mechanisms that control the force of the bite. It also receives impulses from stretch receptors in the muscles of mastication. While afferent fibers of the mesencephalic nucleus travel with fibers of the motor root, some fibers from this nucleus pass peripherally with all three divisions of the trigeminal nerve.

Motor Nucleus

The *motor nucleus of the trigeminal nerve* forms an oval column of typical large motor neurons medial to the motor root and the principal sensory nucleus (Figs. 6.22 and 6.23). Fibers from this nucleus exit from the brain stem medial to the entering sensory root, pass underneath the trigeminal ganglion, and become incorporated in the mandibular division. The motor nucleus receives collaterals from the mesencephalic root, which form a two-neuron reflex arc. Secondary trigeminal fibers, both crossed and uncrossed, establish reflex connections between the muscles of mastication and cutaneous regions as well as with lingual and oral mucous membranes. Some corticobulbar fibers terminate directly and bilaterally upon trigeminal motor neurons, while others pass to reticular neurons, which in turn project to the motor nucleus (Fig. 5.25).

Secondary Trigeminal Pathways

These pathways originate from cells in the principal sensory and spinal trigeminal nuclei and project to higher levels of the brain stem, the cerebellum, and the spinal cord. Collaterals of these fibers provide numerous projections to motor nuclei of the brain stem involved in complex reflexes (Fig. 6.25).

Trigeminothalamic projections arise largely from cells in laminae I and IV of the pars caudalis and interpolaris of the spinal trigeminal nucleus. Axons from these cells in the spinal trigeminal nucleus project ventromedially into the reticular formation, cross the median raphe, and

Figure 6.24. Schematic diagram of trigeminothalamic pathways. The three divisions of the trigeminal sensory root are shown in *black* entering the pons at the level of the principal sensory nucleus. Many of these fibers give collaterals to the principal sensory nucleus and descend as part of the spinal trigeminal tract. At various levels primary sensory fibers synapse upon cells of the spinal trigeminal nucleus, which give rise to fibers (*red*) that cross and ascend in association with the medial lemniscus. Ventral portions of the principal sensory nucleus also give rise to crossed fibers that ascend together with those from lower levels. These crossed *trigeminothalamic fibers* (*red*) terminate in the ventral posteromedial nucleus (VPM) of the thalamus. Cells in dorsal portion of the principal sensory nucleus give rise to uncrossed fibers, which form the *dorsal trigeminal tract* (*blue*). This tract also terminates in the ventral posteromedial nucleus of the thalamus. Abbreviations: CM, centromedian nucleus; IC, internal capsule; LD, lateral dorsal nucleus; LP, lateral posterior nucleus; LPS, lateral pallidal segment; MD, mediodorsal nucleus; ML, medial lemniscus; MPS, medial pallidal segment; VPL, ventral posterolateral nucleus; V_1, V_2, and V_3 ophthalmic, maxillary, and mandibular divisions of the trigeminal nerve.

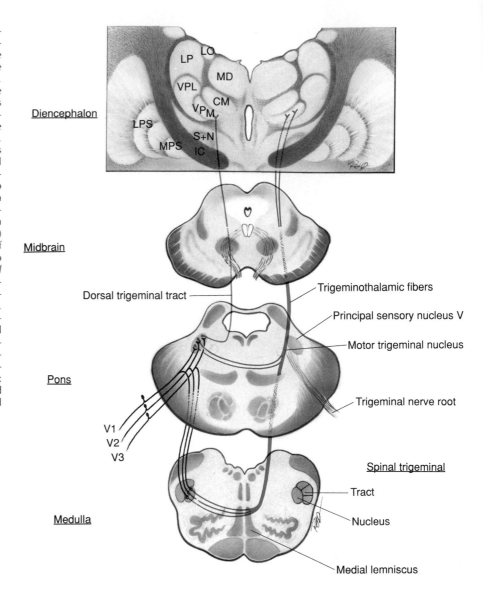

Diencephalon

Midbrain

Dorsal trigeminal tract

Pons

V1
V2
V3

Medulla

Trigeminothalamic fibers

Principal sensory nucleus V

Motor trigeminal nucleus

Trigeminal nerve root

Spinal trigeminal

Tract

Nucleus

Medial lemniscus

ascend in close association with the contralateral medial lemniscus (Fig. 6.24). These secondary trigeminal fibers terminate in a selective manner about cells of the ventral posteromedial (VPM) nucleus of the thalamus. Crossed axons from cells of the spinal trigeminal nucleus that ascend in the brain stem with the contralateral medial lemniscus form the ventral trigeminal tract (*ventral trigeminothalamic tract*).

Secondary trigeminal fibers from the principal sensory nucleus are both crossed and uncrossed. Cells in the dorsomedial part of the nucleus give rise to a small bundle of uncrossed fibers that ascend close to the central gray of the mesencephalon and enter the ipsilateral ventral posteromedial (VPM) nucleus of the thalamus. These fibers form the *dorsal trigeminal tract* and appear to be associated in a unique way with the mandibular division of the trigeminal nerve (Fig. 6.24).

Cells in the ventral part of the principal sensory nucleus of N. V give rise to a larger, entirely crossed bundle of trigeminothalamic fibers, which ascends in association with the contralateral medial lemniscus, in a manner similar to that described for the ventral trigeminal tract. These crossed secondary trigeminal fibers terminate in the VPM nucleus of the thalamus.

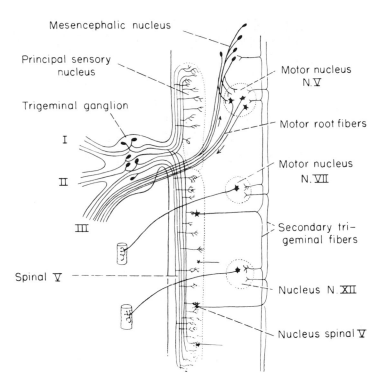

Mesencephalic nucleus

Principal sensory
nucleus

Trigeminal ganglion

I

II

III

Spinal V

Motor nucleus
N.V

Motor root fibers

Motor nucleus
N.VII

Secondary tri-
geminal fibers

Nucleus N.XII

Nucleus spinal V

Figure 6.25. Diagram of the trigeminal nuclei and some of the pathways involved in trigeminal reflexes. *I*, Ophthalmic division; *II*, maxillary division; *III*, mandibular division. (From Carpenter and Sutin, *Human Neuroanatomy*, 1983; courtesy of Williams & Wilkins.)

Trigeminocerebellar fibers arise from cells in lamina IV in all parts of the spinal trigeminal nucleus with the largest number originating from rostral parts of the nucleus. Additional trigeminocerebellar fibers come from cells in ventral portions of the principal sensory nucleus. These portions of the trigeminal nuclei project uncrossed fibers to the paramedian lobule, the simple lobule, and posterior parts of crus II (Fig. 8.1). A large number of these fibers enter the cerebellum via the inferior cerebellar peduncle.

The central connections of the mesencephalic nucleus of the trigeminal nerve are not established, although it has been suggested that they may project to the cerebellum.

Trigeminospinal projections arise from cells in laminae I and III in all subdivisions of the spinal trigeminal nucleus. Fibers from the pars caudalis and interpolaris are ipsilateral while those from pars oralis are bilateral in distribution. These descending projections may modulate incoming sensory information in the posterior horn, contribute to a variety of reflexes, and link receptors in the trigeminal distribution with somatic and visceral effectors in the spinal cord.

Trigeminal Reflexes

Although secondary trigeminal fibers are involved in a large number of reflexes, the *corneal reflex* is one of the most important (Fig. 6.25). Stimulation of the cornea with a wisp of cotton produces bilateral blinking and closing of the eyes. The blinking and closing of the eyes is effected by impulses reaching the facial nuclei on both sides. This reflex is effected by secondary trigeminal fibers projecting bilaterally to the facial nuclei. Following an injury to the ophthalmic division of the trigeminal nerve, corneal sensation and the corneal reflex are lost on that side because the afferent limb of the reflex arc has been destroyed. However, corneal sensation remains on the opposite side, and stimulation of that cornea will produce bilateral blinking and eye closure, indicating that the efferent limb (facial nucleus and nerve) of the reflex arc is intact. In patients with peripheral facial palsies, corneal sensation will be present on both sides, but no corneal reflex can be elicited on the side of the lesion because the efferent limb of the reflex arc has been destroyed. However, stimulation of the cornea on the side of the lesion will cause blinking and closure of the opposite eye (consensual response).

Secondary trigeminal fibers ascending and descending in dorsolateral regions of the brain stem reticular formation give off collaterals to various motor nuclei that mediate specific reflexes (Fig. 6.25). These reflexes include (1) the *tearing reflex*, in which corneal irritation initiates impulses via trigeminal nerve fibers that synapse upon neurons of the superior salivatory nucleus (parasympathetic) resulting in lacrimation; (2) *sneezing*, in which trigeminal impulses pass to the nucleus ambiguus, to respiratory centers in the reticular formation, and to cell groups of the spinal cord (i.e., phrenic nerve nuclei and anterior horn cells innervating the intercostal muscles), which are paroxysmally activated; (3) *vomiting*, in which trigeminal impulses pass to vagal nuclei; and (4) *salivary reflexes* in which secondary trigeminal fibers project to the inferior salivatory nuclei. Secondary trigeminal fibers probably also pass to the hypoglossal nuclei and mediate reflex movements of the tongue in response to stimulation of the tongue and the mucous membranes of the mouth.

The *jaw jerk*, or masseter reflex, a monosynaptic reflex, is elicited by gently tapping the patient's chin (with mouth open slightly). The response is bilateral contractions of the masseter and temporal muscles. This myotatic reflex involves stretch receptors in the muscles of mastication, the mesencephalic nucleus, and collaterals from that nucleus that terminate in the motor trigeminal nucleus. The jaw reflex is absent in peripheral lesions of the trigeminal nerve.

PONTINE TEGMENTUM

Transverse sections through the pons at the level of the trigeminal nerve root (Figs. 5.2, 6.22, and 6.23) reveal significant changes when compared with lower pontine levels. These changes include the following: (1) the fourth ventricle is narrower, (2) fibers of the superior cerebellar peduncle form the dorsolateral wall of the fourth ventricle, (3) fibers of the inferior and middle cerebellar peduncles can be seen entering the cerebellum, and (4) portions of the cerebellum dorsal to the pons contain parts of all the deep cerebellar nuclei. The ventral portion of the pons is larger than at lower levels, and the mass of pontine nuclei is greater.

In the dorsal part of the pons the medial lemniscus is located ventrally and is traversed in part by fibers of the trapezoid body. Portions of the superior olivary nuclei retain their same position. Dorsomedial to the superior olivary complex is the central tegmental tract. The spinothalamic and anterior spinocerebellar tracts are located lateral to the medial lemniscus, and the MLF is located dorsally on each side of the median raphe. The central part of the pontine tegmentum contains the pontine reticular formation.

Pontine Reticular Formation

Two relatively large nuclear masses, the *nucleus reticularis pontis caudalis* and *oralis*, compose the bulk of the pontine reticular formation. The pars caudalis, which replaces the gigantocellular reticular nucleus of the medulla, extends rostrally to levels of the trigeminal motor nucleus

(Figs. 6.1 and 6.3). The pars oralis extends rostrally into the caudal mesencephalon where its precise boundary is indistinct (Fig. 6.23). Cells of the pontine reticular formation give rise to uncrossed reticulospinal fibers, which in the brain stem descend as a component of the MLF. Other cells give rise to fibers that ascend as part of the central tegmental tract (Figs. 6.5 and 6.26). Many cells have dichotomizing axons that project branches both rostrally and caudally. Ascending pontine reticular fibers project via the central tegmental fasciculus to parts of the intra-laminar thalamic nuclei. Impulses passing to these thalamic nuclei profoundly influence the electrical activity of broad areas of the cerebral cortex.

Other reticular nuclei present at pontine levels are the reticuloteg-mental and the superior central nuclei (Figs. 6.23 and 6.27). The reti-culotegmental nucleus lies near the median raphe dorsal to the medial lemniscus and is regarded as a tegmentally displaced pontine nuclear group. The superior central nucleus develops in the median raphe, en-larges at isthmus levels, and is known as the median nucleus of the raphe (Figs. 5.13 and 6.27).

ISTHMUS OF THE HINDBRAIN

The *isthmus rhombencephali*, the narrowest portion of the hind-brain, is situated rostral to the cerebellum and immediately caudal to the midbrain (Figs. 6.26 and 6.27). As in other parts of the brain stem three regions are recognized, namely, a roof plate, a tegmental region, and a ventral cortically dependent part. The roof is formed by a thin membrane, the *superior medullary velum*. This membrane, containing the decussating fibers of the trochlear nerve, forms the roof of the most rostral part of the fourth ventricle (Fig. 6.26).

The tegmental region, ventral to the fourth ventricle, is smaller than at caudal levels. The more abundant central gray resembles that seen at mesencephalic levels. The lateral border of the central gray contains the mesencephalic nucleus and tract of the trigeminal nerve. Ventral and medial to these structures is the relatively large collection of pigmented cells (melanin) that form the *locus ceruleus*. Lateral to the central gray are the fibers of the *superior cerebellar peduncle* that have passed into the tegmentum and are shifting ventromedially to undergo a complete decussation (Fig. 6.26). Fibers of the superior cerebellar peduncle arise from the dentate, emboliform, and globose nuclei and constitute the largest and most important cerebellar efferent system. Cells of the *para-brachial nuclei* lie adjacent to the superior cerebellar peduncle.

The *lateral lemniscus* forms a well-defined bundle near the lateral surface of the tegmentum (Fig. 6.26). Groups of cells situated among the fibers of this tract constitute the *nuclei of the lateral lemniscus* (Fig. 6.27). Most of the fibers in the lateral lemniscus project rostrally and enter the inferior colliculus. The medial lemniscus is a flattened band of ascending fibers in the ventrolateral tegmentum; fibers of the spinothalamic tract are located laterally near the junction of the medial and lateral lemnisci. At this level the principal ascending sensory pathways form a peripheral shell of fibers that encloses most of the pontine tegmentum.

The ventral part of the pons at this level is larger than the tegmental part, but it is not as massive as at midpontine levels. Corticospinal and corticopontine tracts are broken up into numerous small bundles sur-rounded by pontine nuclei (Fig. 6.26).

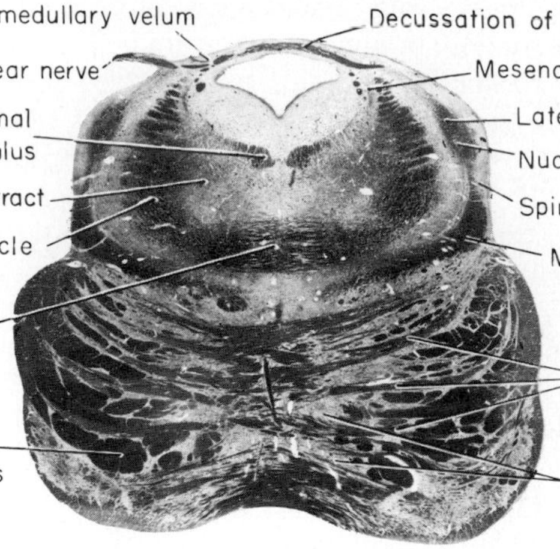

Figure 6.26. Section of the isthmus of an adult brain at the level of the decussation and exit of the trochlear nerve. Weigert's myelin stain. Photograph. (From Carpenter and Sutin, *Human Neuroanatomy*, 1983; courtesy of Williams & Wilkins.)

Parabrachial Nuclei

These nuclei consist of distinct groups of neurons that surround medial and lateral regions of the superior cerebellar peduncle. The *lateral parabrachial nuclei* receive inputs mainly from general visceral nuclei in caudal regions of the nucleus solitarius. The *medial parabrachial nuclei* receive afferents from gustatory parts of the nucleus solitarius. Afferents from the nucleus solitarius ascend uncrossed in the brain stem (Fig. 5.24). The medial parabrachial nuclei project to the thalamus, the hypothalamus, and amygdala. The lateral parabrachial nuclei innervate nuclei in the hypothalamus and amygdala. One group of large cells, ventral to the lateral parabrachial nuclei, the Kölliker-Fuse nucleus, projects to the nucleus of the solitary tract. These neurons are associated with the central control of respiration.

Locus Ceruleus

Near the periventricular gray of the upper part of the fourth ventricle is an irregular collection of pigmented cells known as the locus ceruleus (Figs. 6.27, 6.28, and 6.29). Cells of this nucleus are partially intermingled with those of the mesencephalic nucleus of the trigeminal nerve, but the large globular neurons of the mesencephalic nucleus extend further dorsally and rostrally at the margin of the central gray (Fig. 6.28). Cells of the locus ceruleus are of two types: (1) medium-sized cells with eccentric nuclei containing clumps of melanin pigment granules and (2) small oval cells with scant cytoplasm and no pigment. Ventrolateral to the locus ceruleus is a diffuse collection of similar cells known as the nucleus subceruleus.

Although the locus ceruleus is a relatively small structure, it can be identified readily in gross sections of the brain stem. The significance of this small pigmented nucleus was unknown until it was demonstrated by a sensitive fluorescence technic that its cells contain catecholamines, nearly all of which was norepinephrine (Fig. 6.29). Unlike other brain stem norepinephrine cells found as scattered neurons in the lateral tegmentum, the locus ceruleus is a compact nucleus that projects fibers widely to portions of the telencephalon, diencephalon, midbrain, cerebellum, pons, medulla, and spinal cord. Information concerning the wide-

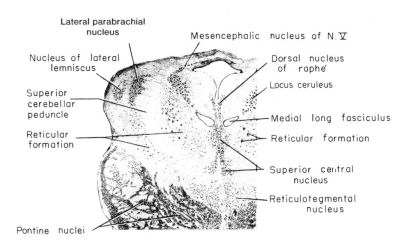

Lateral parabrachial
nucleus

Mesencephalic nucleus of N. Ⅴ

Nucleus of lateral
lemniscus

Dorsal nucleus
of raphe

Locus ceruleus

Superior
cerebellar
peduncle

Reticular
formation

Medial long fasciculus

Reticular formation

Superior central
nucleus

Reticulotegmental
nucleus

Pontine nuclei

Figure 6.27. Section through isthmus of a 3-month-old infant. Cresyl violet. Photograph, with cell groups schematically blocked in. (From Carpenter and Sutin, *Human Neuroanatomy*, 1983; courtesy of Williams & Wilkins.)

spread projections of locus ceruleus and the nucleus subceruleus has been developed through a combination of different anatomical, histochemical, biochemical, and immunocytochemical methodologies.

Major ascending projections from the locus ceruleus pass rostrally to and through the lateral hypothalamus (Fig. 10.12). Near the level of the anterior commissure, the pathway divides into bundles that respectively innervate telencephalic and diencephalic structures. Noradrenergic fibers are distributed widely in the cerebral cortex and the hippocampal formation. In the thalamus noradrenergic terminals are distributed to specific nuclear groups, including the lateral geniculate body.

Variable percentages (more than 10%) of cells in the locus ceruleus innervate both the cerebral and cerebellar cortex. Noradrenergic neurons in the locus ceruleus project to the inferior and superior colliculus and the cerebellar cortex, where fibers terminate around Purkinje cell somata. In the brain stem the locus ceruleus innervates primary sensory and association nuclei, as well as portions of the pontine nuclei. Both the locus ceruleus and the subceruleus project fibers to spinal cord via the anterior and lateral funiculi, which innervate portions of the anterior and intermediate gray at all levels; a high percentage of these fibers cross at segmental levels.

Noradrenergic neurons in the lower brain stem consist of smaller collections of cells and scattered neurons in the lateral tegmentum of the pons and medulla (Figs. 4.16 and 5.15). These cell groups have projections to regions of the central nervous system that do not receive fibers from the locus ceruleus. Ipsilateral projections from the pontine cell group descend to all thoracic spinal levels where fibers are distributed bilaterally to the intermediolateral cell columns. The remarkable feature of this central noradrenergic system (locus ceruleus and lateral tegmental cell groups) is the widespread distribution of its projections throughout the neuraxis. Projections of the locus ceruleus and the lateral tegmental groups appear complementary and specific. The locus ceruleus and its efferent projections have been considered to play a role in paradoxical sleep, facilitation and inhibition of sensory neurons, and control of cortical activation.

Raphe Nuclei

Both the pons and medulla contain cell groups in the median raphe that properly belong to the reticular formation but appear to be the source of serotonergic fiber systems widely distributed in the central nervous

Figure 6.28. Photograph of the cell groups surrounding the periventricular gray at isthmus levels. Cells of the locus ceruleus contain melanin pigment granules and high concentrations of norepinephrine. Globular cells of the mesencephalic nucleus of N. V, present along the dorsal border of the locus ceruleus, extend dorsally and rostrally at the margin of the central gray. (From Carpenter and Sutin, *Human Neuroanatomy,* 1983; courtesy of Williams & Wilkins.)

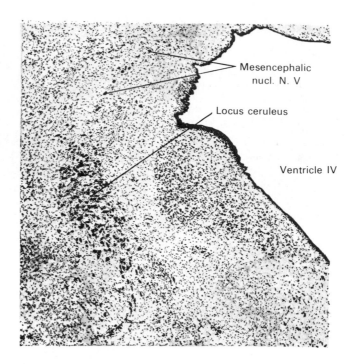

Mesencephalic nucl. N. V

Locus ceruleus

Ventricle IV

system. The raphe nuclei of the medulla are smaller and less conspicuous than those seen in the pons (Fig. 5.13). The *inferior central nucleus* appears in the median raphe at the junction of pons and medulla (Fig. 5.26) and represents the rostral part of the nucleus raphe magnus (Fig. 5.13). The *nucleus raphe pontis* consists of several cell groups dorsal and rostral to the inferior central nucleus. The rostral extension of the pontine raphe nuclei is the *superior central nucleus*, also known as the *median nucleus of the raphe* (Fig. 6.27). Decussating fibers of the superior cerebellar peduncle pass through portions of the superior central nucleus (Fig. 6.26). The *dorsal nuclei of the raphe* are paired and lie on each side of the raphe within the anterior periaqueductal gray, dorsal to the medial longitudinal fasciculi (Figs. 6.27 and 6.30).

Serotonergic (5-hydroxytryptamine, 5-HT) neurons, identified by histofluorescence and immunocytochemical technics, are widely distributed in the raphe nuclei. The highest percentage of 5-HT neurons are found in the dorsal nucleus of the raphe (79%) and the lowest percentages in the smaller raphe nuclei of the pons and medulla (10–25%). Some of the nuclei of the raphe also contain noradrenalin, dopamine, and cholecystokinin. Substance P or enkephalin may coexist with 5-HT in some cells with the raphe.

The principal ascending fibers arise from serotonin-containing cell bodies located in the dorsal nucleus of the raphe and in the superior central nucleus. The major ascending pathway from the rostral raphe nuclei passes through the ventral tegmental area (Tsai) and joins the medial forebrain bundle in the lateral hypothalamus (Fig. 10.12). Fibers leaving this main ascending bundle enter the substantia nigra, the intralaminar thalamic nuclei, the stria terminalis, the septum, and the internal capsule. The most rostral projections terminate mainly in the frontal lobe, although some fibers are distributed throughout the neocortex. The dorsal nucleus of the raphe selectively innervates the substantia nigra, the lateral geniculate body, the neostriatum, the pyriform lobe, the olfactory bulb, and the amygdaloid nuclear complex. The superior central nucleus is particularly associated with serotonergic fibers projecting to the inter-

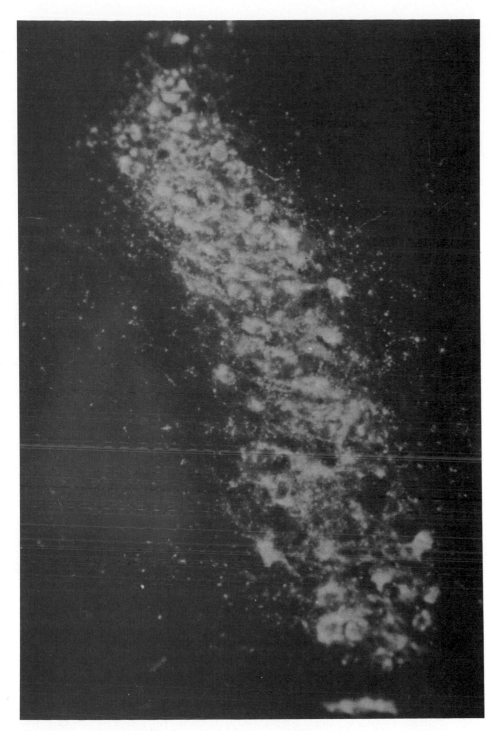

Figure 6.29. Photomicrograph of neurons containing norepinephrine in the locus ceruleus of the rat. The norepinephrine-containing cells were reacted with glyoxylic acid, which converts norepinephrine into a fluorescent chemical derivative. (Courtesy of Drs. Jacqueline McGinty and Floyd Bloom, Salk Institute, La Jolla, California.) (From Carpenter and Sutin, *Human Neuroanatomy*, 1983; courtesy of Williams & Wilkins.)

peduncular nucleus, the mammillary bodies, and the hippocampal formation. Ascending projections from the caudal raphe nuclei are less numerous and distributed to the superior colliculus, the pretectum, and the nuclei of the posterior commissure. Ascending serotonergic pathways from the superior central nucleus project mainly to mesolimbic structures, such as the hippocampus and the septal nuclei, while the dorsal nucleus

Figure 6.30. Nuclei of the raphe at isthmus levels in the monkey. In *A*, cells of the dorsal nucleus of the raphe (DNR) on the left are retrogradely labeled with horseradish peroxidase (HRP) from an injection in the substantia nigra. In *B*, cells of the dorsal nucleus of the raphe and the medial nucleus of the raphe (MNR) demonstrate immunoreactivity to serotonin (5-HT). Cells of these raphe nuclei also contain cholecystokinin (CCK).

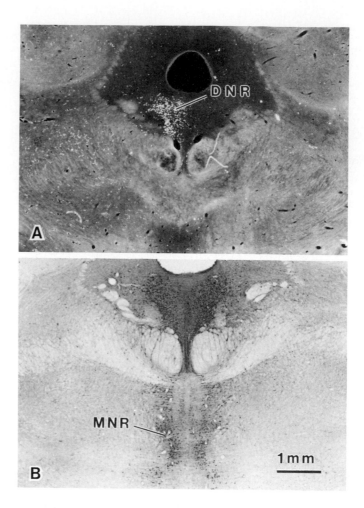

of the raphe has major projections to the neostriatum and substantia nigra (Fig. 6.30). Ascending projections of cells in the raphe nuclei are mainly ipsilateral, but axons give rise to abundant collaterals with different terminations.

Descending projections of the dorsal nucleus of the raphe are modest but include the locus ceruleus. The superior central nucleus gives rise to descending projections to (1) the cerebellum via the middle cerebellar peduncle, (2) the locus ceruleus, and (3) large regions of the pontine reticular formation. Autoradiographic studies of the nucleus raphe magnus suggest that descending fibers project primarily to structures concerned with nociceptive and/or visceral afferent input (Fig. 5.14). Structures receiving efferents from the nucleus raphe magnus include the dorsal motor nucleus of the vagus, the solitary nucleus, and the spinal trigeminal nucleus (pars caudalis). Spinal projections of this nucleus are bilateral and descend in the lateral funiculus. These fibers terminate in the marginal zone (lamina I), the substantia gelatinosa (lamina II), and in parts of laminae V, VI, and VII. Evidence suggests that this nucleus is linked to endogenous analgesic mechanisms. Serotonin and the raphe nuclei have been implicated in the regulation of diverse physiological processes such as the regulation of sleep, mood, aggressive behavior, and a variety of neuroendocrine functions.

Structurally, the serotonin molecule is similar to a portion of the larger D-lysergic acid diethylamide (LSD) molecule in that both contain an indole nucleus. LSD is a hallucinogenic drug considered to be the prototype of a psychotomimetic drug (i.e., a drug whose effects mimic psychosis). Some data suggest that LSD produces a specific depression of activity in raphe neurons that contain serotonin, but its mode of action remains unknown. Serotonin may serve to modulate and maintain behavior within specific limits, either directly or by its action upon cells with other neurotransmitters. Studies indicate that as the overall level of motor activity or arousal increases, so does the activity of serotonin-containing cells. As an animal becomes quiescent and drowsy, the activity of these cells diminishes. Neurons of the raphe fire slowly as an animal enters sleep, and during rapid eye movement (REM) sleep, the cells stop firing.

Both serotonin- and norepinephrine-containing neurons in the reticular formation have been considered to play active roles in the mechanisms that control sleep states. Inhibition of serotonin synthesis or destruction of serotonin-containing neurons in the raphe system leads to insomnia. Serotonin may be involved in the neural mechanism related to so-called *slow sleep*, a state characterized by an electroencephalogram (EEG) with slow waves and spindles. In addition, serotonin may have effects upon cells of the locus ceruleus that trigger what is called *paradoxical sleep*. Paradoxical sleep is characterized by (1) abolition of antigravity muscle tone; (2) reductions in blood pressure, bradycardia, and irregular respirations; (3) bursts of REM; and (4) an EEG that resembles the waking state. Bilateral lesions of the locus ceruleus in animals cause a selective suppression of paradoxical sleep for about 2 weeks, after which it returns to nearly the normal range.

SUGGESTED READINGS

AGHAJANIAN, G. K., HAIGLER, H. J., AND BENNETT, J. L. 1975. Amine receptors in the CNS. III. 5-Hydroxytryptamine in the brain. In L. L. IVERSON, S. D. IVERSON, AND S. H. SNYDER (Editors), *Handbook of Psychopharmacology*, Ed. 6. Plenum Press, New York, pp. 63–96.

BASBAUM, A. I. 1976. Opiate and stimulus-produced analgesia: Functional anatomy of a medullospinal pathway. Proc. Natl. Acad. Sci., USA, **73**: 4685–4688.

BASBAUM, A. I., RALSTON, D. D., AND RALSTON, H. J. 1986. Bulbospinal projections in the primate: A light and electron microscopic study of a pain modulating system. J. Comp. Neurol., **250**: 311–323.

BÉKÉSY, G. VON. 1960. *Experiments in Hearing*. McGraw-Hill, New York.

BÜTTNER-ENNEVER, J. A. 1977. Pathways from the pontine reticular formation to structures controlling horizontal and vertical eye movements in the monkey. In A. BERTHOZ AND R. BAKER (Editors), *Control of Gaze by Brain Stem Neurons*. Developments in Neuroscience, Vol. 1. Elsevier/North-Holland, Amsterdam, pp. 89–98.

CAJAL, S. RAMÓN y. 1909, 1911. *Histologie due système nerveux de l'homme et des vertébres*. Norbert Maloine, Paris. 2 vols.

CARLETON, S. C., AND CARPENTER, M. B. 1983. Afferent and efferent connections of the medial, inferior and lateral vestibular nuclei in the cat and monkey. Brain Res., **278**: 29–51.

CARLETON, S. C., AND CARPENTER, M. B. 1984. Distribution of primary vestibular fibers in the brain stem and cerebellum of the monkey. Brain Res., **294**: 281–298.

CARPENTER, M. B., AND BATTON, R. R. III. 1982. Connections of the fastigial nucleus in the cat and monkey. Exp. Brain Res (Suppl. 6), : 250–295.

CARPENTER, M. B., AND CARLETON, S. C. 1983. Comparison of vestibular and abducens projections to the medial rectus subdivision of the oculomotor complex in the monkey. Brain Res., **274**: 144–149.

CARPENTER, M. B., CHANG, L., PEREIRA, A. B., HERSH, L. B., BRUCE, G., AND WU, J. Y. 1987. Vestibular and cochlear efferent neurons in the monkey identified by immunocytochemical methods. Brain Res., **408**: 275–280.

CARPENTER, M. B., AND COWIE, R. J. 1985. Connections and oculomotor projections of the superior vestibular nucleus and cell group "y." Brain Res., **336**: 265–287.

CARPENTER, M. B., McMASTERS, R. E., AND HANNA, G. R. 1963. Disturbances of conjugate horizontal eye movements in the monkey. I. Physiological effects and anatomical degeneration resulting from lesions of the abducens nucleus and nerve. Arch. Neurol., **8**: 231–247.

CARPENTER, M. B., AND STROMINGER, N. L. 1965. The medial longitudinal fasciculus and disturbances of conjugate horizontal eye movements in the monkey. J. Comp. Neurol., **125**: 41–66.

CHU, N. S., AND BLOOM, F. E. 1973. Norepinephrine-containing neurons: Changes in spontaneous discharge patterns during sleeping and waking. Science, **179**: 908–910.

COOPER, J. R., BLOOM, F. E., AND ROTH, R. H. 1986. *The Biochemical Basis of Neuropharmacology*. Oxford University Press, New York.

FIELDS, H. L. 1981. An endorphin-mediated analgesia system: Experimental and clinical observations. In J. B. MARTIN, S. REICHLIN, AND K. L. BICK (Editors), *Neurosecretion and Brain Peptides*. Raven Press, New York, pp. 199–212.

FIELDS, H. L., BASBAUM, A. I., CLANTON, C. H., AND ANDERSON, S. D. 1977. Nucleus raphe magnus inhibition of spinal cord dorsal horn neurons. Brain Res., **126**: 441–454.

FULWILER, C. E., AND SAPER, C. B. 1984. Subnuclear organization of the efferent connections of the parabrachial nucleus in the rat. Brain Res. Rev., **7**: 229–259.

GALAMBOS, R. 1956. Suppression of auditory nerve activity by stimulation of efferent fibers to cochlea. J. Neurophysiol., **19**: 424–437.

GOBEL, S. 1978. Golgi studies of the neurons in layer I of the dorsal horn of the medulla (trigeminal nucleus caudalis). J. Comp. Neurol., **180**: 375–394.

GOBEL, S. 1978. Golgi studies of the neurons in layer II of the dorsal horn of the medulla (trigeminal nucleus caudalis). J. Comp. Neurol., **180**: 395–414.

GOLDBERG, J. M., AND FERNÁNDEZ, C. 1980. Efferent vestibular system in the squirrel monkey: Anatomical location and influence on afferent activity. J. Neurophysiol., **43**: 986–1025.

GUINAN, J. J., WARR, W. B., AND NORRIS, B. E. 1983. Differential olivocochlear projections from the lateral versus medial zones of the superior olivary complex. J. Comp. Neurol., **221**: 358–370.

HAIGLER, H. J., AND AGHAJANIAN, G. K. 1974. Lysergic acid diethylamine and serotonin: A comparison of effects on serotonergic neurons and neurons receiving serotonergic input. J. Pharmacol. Exp. Ther., **188**: 688–699.

JACOBS, B. L., AND TRULSON, M. E. 1979. Mechanisms of action of LSD. Am. Sci., **67**: 396–404.

KEVETTER, G. A., AND PERACHIO, A. A. 1986. Distribution of vestibular afferents that innervate the sacculus and posterior canal in the gerbil. J. Comp. Neurol., **254**: 410–424.

LEVITT, P., AND MOORE, R. Y. 1979. Origin and organization of brainstem catecholamine innervation in the rat. J. Comp Neurol., **186**: 505–528.

LINDVALL, O., AND BJÖRKLUND, A. 1983. Dopamine- and norepinephrine-containing neuron systems: Their anatomy in the rat brain. In P. EMSON (Editor), *Chemical Neuroanatomy*. Raven Press, New York, pp. 229–255.

MANTYH, P. W., AND HUNT, S. P. 1984. Neuropeptides are present in projection neurones at all levels in visceral and taste pathways: From periphery to sensory cortex. Brain Res., **299**: 297–311.

MASON, S. T., AND FIBIGER, H. C. 1979. Regional topography within noradrenergic locus coeruleus as revealed by retrograde transport of horseradish peroxidase. J. Comp. Neurol., **187**: 703–724.

MCGEER, P. L., ECCLES, J. C., AND MCGEER, E. G. 1987. *Molecular Neurobiology of the Mammalian Brain*, Ed. 2. Plenum Press, New York.

OLSZEWSKI, J. 1950. On the anatomical and functional organization of the spinal trigeminal nucleus. J. Comp. Neurol., **92**: 401–413.

OSEN, K. K. 1969. The intrinsic organization of the cochlear nuclei in the cat. Acta Otolaryngol. (Stockh.) **67**: 352–359.

PRECHT, W. 1978. *Neuronal Operations in the Vestibular System*. Springer-Verlag, Berlin.

RASMUSSEN, G. L. 1960. Efferent fibers of the cochlear nerve and cochlear nucleus. In G. L. RASMUSSEN AND W. F. WINDLE (Editors), *Neural Mechanisms of the Auditory and Vestibular Systems*. Charles C Thomas, Springfield, IL, Ch. 8, pp. 105–115.

RAYMOND, J., NIECULLON, A., DÊMEMES, D., AND SANS, A. 1984. Evidence for glutamate as a neurotransmitter in the cat vestibular nerve: Radioautographic and biochemical studies. Exp. Brain Res., **56**: 523–531.

ROSE, J. E. 1960. Organization of frequency sensitive neurons in the cochlear complex of the cat. In G. L. RASMUSSEN AND W. F. WINDLE (Editors), *Neural Mechanisms of the Auditory and Vestibular Systems*. Charles C Thomas, Springfield, IL, Ch. 9, pp. 116–136.

SIEGBORN, J., AND GRANT, G. 1983. Brain stem projections of different branches of the vestibular nerve. An experimental study by transganglionic transport of horseradish peroxidase in the cat. I. The horizontal ampullar and utricular nerves. Arch. Ital, Biol., **121**: 237–248.

STEIGER, H. J., AND BÜTTNER-ENNEVER, J. A. 1978. Relationship between motoneurons and internuclear neurons in the abducens nucleus: A double retrograde tracer study in the cat. Brain Res., **148**: 181–188.

STEIN, B. M., AND CARPENTER, M. B. 1967. Central projections of portions of the vestibular ganglia innervating specific parts of the labyrinth in the rhesus monkey. Am. J. Anat., **120**: 281–318.

STEINBUSCH, H. W. M., AND NIEUWENHUYS, R. 1983. The raphe nuclei of the rat brain stem: A cytoarchitectonic and immunohistochemical study. In P. C. EMSON (Editor), *Chemical Neuroanatomy*. Raven Press, New York, pp. 131–207.

STRONG, O. S. 1915. A case of unilateral cerebellar agenesia. J. Comp. Neurol., **25**: 361–391.

WHITE, J. S., AND WARR, W. B. 1983. The dual origins of the olivocochlear bundle in the albino rat. J. Comp. Neurol., **219**: 203–214.

WIKLUND, L., LÉGER, L., AND PERSSON, M. 1981. Monamine cell distribution in the cat brain stem. A fluorescence histochemical study with quantification of indolaminergic and locus coeruleus cell groups. J. Comp. Neurol., **203**: 613–647.

WILSON, V. J., AND MELVILL JONES, G. 1979. *Mammalian Vestibular Physiology*. Plenum Press, New York.

The Mesencephalon

The midbrain, representing the smallest and least differentiated segment of the infratentorial brain stem, lies rostral to the pons. Like other parts of the brain stem, the midbrain can be divided into three parts: (1) the *tectum* or *quadrigeminal* plate dorsal to the cerebral aqueduct; (2) a central part, the *tegmentum*, representing the rostral continuation of the pontine reticular formation; and (3) a ventral part, the massive *crura cerebri*, containing descending cortical projections (Fig. 7.1). The *substantia nigra*, a darkly pigmented nucleus, separates the midbrain tegmentum from the crus cerebri. Two cranial nerve nuclei, the trochlear and the oculomotor, lie in the midline, ventral to the periaqueductal gray. The midbrain contains important relay nuclei of the auditory and visual systems, represented by the inferior and superior colliculi.

INFERIOR COLLICULAR LEVEL

The transition from isthmus to midbrain is associated with changes mainly in the tectum and tegmentum (Figs. 6.26 and 7.2). Comparison of these levels reveals that (1) the rostral fourth ventricle narrows and becomes the cerebral aqueduct, (2) the superior medullary velum is replaced by two rounded eminences, the inferior colliculi, (3) fibers of the superior cerebellar peduncles move ventromedially and begin to decussate, and (4) the tegmentum is reduced in size. The ventral part of the pons becomes smaller and at more rostral levels undergoes a reorganization as the massive crura cerebri appear (Figs. 7.2 and 7.3). Fibers of the lateral lemniscus, located near the lateral surface of the tegmentum, migrate dorsally and enter the inferior colliculus.

Inferior Colliculi

The distinctive paired ovoid cellular masses of the caudal tectum can be divided into three parts (1) an ovoid cell mass called the central nucleus; (2) a thin dorsal cellular layer, the pericentral nucleus, referred to as the cortex; and (3) an external nucleus that surrounds the central nucleus laterally and ventrally.

The *central nucleus* of the inferior colliculus in Nissl and Myelin sheath preparations appears fairly homogeneous. In Golgi preparations it can be divided into a smaller dorsomedial division composed of large cells and a larger ventrolateral division of medium and small cells with a laminar arrangement (Fig. 7.4). Laminae in the ventrolateral division form an overlapping onionlike series of concentric shells, most of which are incomplete. The thickness of the laminae is determined by the dendritic ramifications of fusiform and bitufted cells that compose the layers. These laminae provide the basis for the tonotopic organization of neurons

192

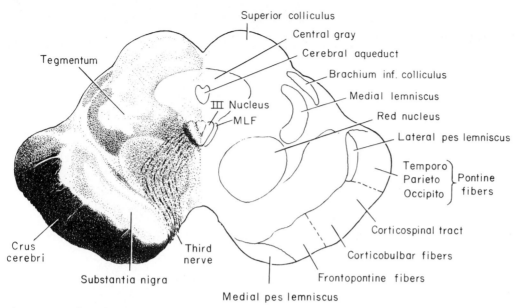

Figure 7.1. Schematic transverse section through the rostral midbrain. (From Carpenter and Sutin, *Human Neuroanatomy*, 1983; courtesy of Williams & Wilkins.)

in the central nucleus. Each of these cellular laminae corresponds to an isofrequency contour. Large numbers of GABAergic neurons are found in the central nucleus.

The *pericentral nucleus* is a thin sheet of densely packed cells extending over the dorsal and caudal surfaces of the inferior colliculus that overlies both divisions of the central nucleus (Fig. 7.4). This nucleus is composed of spiny and aspiny neurons. Large aspiny neurons project axons in the brachium of the inferior colliculus.

The *external nucleus*, ventral and lateral to the pericentral nucleus, is traversed by fibers entering and leaving the inferior colliculus.

The inferior colliculus serves as the major brain stem auditory relay nucleus, transmitting signals received from the lateral lemniscus to the medial geniculate body. Ascending auditory fibers in the lateral lemniscus project to both dorsomedial and ventrolateral divisions of the central nucleus of the inferior colliculus. Fibers entering the ventrolateral division of the inferior colliculus course along the length of each lamina following its curvature. As fibers traverse these laminae they establish synaptic contacts with collicular neurons. The dorsomedial division of the central nucleus receives commissural connections from the corresponding region of the opposite inferior colliculus (Fig. 7.2) and bilateral projections from the auditory cortex. The pericentral nucleus also receives bilateral inputs from the auditory cortex and ascending projections from the dorsal nucleus of the lateral lemniscus. Cells of the pericentral nucleus project fibers into the central nucleus, which course parallel to its laminae.

Most cells of the inferior colliculus respond to binaural stimulation, and many cells encode sound localization with spatiotemporal discharge patterns. A definite tonotopic localization is present within the central and pericentral nuclei of the inferior colliculus. Neurons in the central nucleus of the inferior colliculus are arranged in a laminar pattern that represents different frequency bands. Isofrequency contours parallel the cellular laminae, which are tilted ventrally, laterally, and down rostrally. Most units respond to binaural stimuli. Advancement of an electrode from dorsal to ventral in the inferior colliculus consistently gives a se-

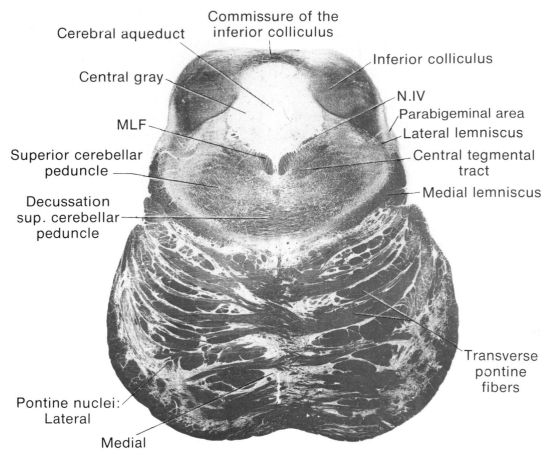

Cerebral aqueduct

Commissure of the
inferior colliculus

Inferior colliculus

Central gray

N.IV

Parabigeminal area

MLF

Lateral lemniscus

Superior cerebellar
peduncle

Central tegmental
tract

Decussation
sup. cerebellar
peduncle

Medial lemniscus

Transverse
pontine
fibers

Pontine nuclei:
Lateral

Medial

Figure 7.2.   Transverse section of midbrain through the inferior colliculus. Large fascicles of corticospinal and corticopontine fibers (unlabeled), cut in cross section, are located among the bundles of transverse pontine fibers. Photograph. Weigert's myelin stain. (From Carpenter and Sutin, *Human Neuroanatomy*, 1983; courtesy of Williams & Wilkins.)

quence of frequencies from low to high in the central nucleus. The disc-shaped laminae representing the lowest frequencies (i.e., dorsal regions) are not as thick as those representing middle and high frequencies (i.e., ventral region). The frequency representation in the central nucleus reflects the proportional representation of frequencies along the cochlear partition, in which low frequencies are perceived at the apex of the cochlea and high frequencies at the base. The central nucleus of the inferior colliculus is a tightly organized structure bearing specific relationships to the cochlea with elements sharply tuned to different frequencies. Small sections of the basilar membrane of approximately equal lengths are represented across individual anatomically defined cellular laminae within the nucleus. This tonotopic organization applies only to the ventrolateral division of the central nucleus.

In the tonotopic organization of the pericentral nucleus high frequencies are located externally and low frequencies are found near the margins of the central nucleus. This nucleus contains units with broad tuning characteristics, the majority of which receive only a contralateral monaural input. The overall behavior of units in the pericentral nucleus and their monaural input suggests that cells in this nucleus may serve to direct auditory attention. The external nucleus probably is not an auditory relay nucleus like the central nucleus of the inferior colliculus; this nucleus is related primarily to acousticomotor reflexes.

Efferent fibers from the ventrolateral division of the central nucleus

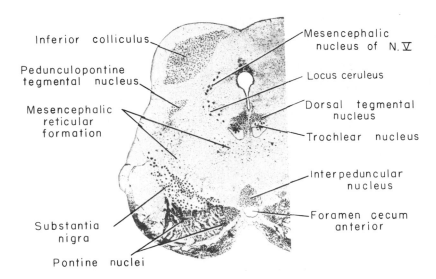

Inferior colliculus

Pedunculopontine
tegmental nucleus

Mesencephalic
reticular
formation

Substantia
nigra

Pontine nuclei

Mesencephalic
nucleus of N. Ⅴ

Locus ceruleus

Dorsal tegmental
nucleus

Trochlear nucleus

Interpeduncular
nucleus

Foramen cecum
anterior

Figure 7.3. Section through inferior colliculi of midbrain. Three-month-old infant. Cresyl violet. Photograph, with schematic representation of main cell groups. (From Carpenter and Sutin, *Human Neuroanatomy*, 1983; courtesy of Williams & Wilkins.)

of the inferior colliculus project via the brachium of the inferior colliculus to the ventral laminated part of the medial geniculate body (Figs. 7.15 and 9.19). Cells in the dorsal division of the central nucleus and in the pericentral nucleus send fibers to the dorsal part of the medial geniculate body. Thus, the dorsal division of the central nucleus and the pericentral nucleus of the inferior colliculus, which receive fibers from the auditory cortex, ultimately send signals back to the secondary auditory cortex. Cells of the ventral part of the medial geniculate body project tonotopically, via the auditory radiation, upon the primary auditory cortex.

Parabigeminal Area

Ventrolateral to the inferior colliculus and lateral to the lateral lemniscus is a cellular region known as the parabigeminal area (Fig. 7.2). This small oval-shaped nucleus on the lateral surface of the midbrain contains cholinergic neurons and receives a substantial projection from the superficial layers of the superior colliculus, which has a visuotopic organization. Cells of each parabigeminal nucleus project bilaterally upon superficial layers of the superior colliculi and show a regional organization. Cells of the parabigeminal nucleus respond briskly and consistently to visual stimuli, can be activated by both moving and stationary light spots, and have receptive fields similar to those of the superficial layers of the superior colliculus. The parabigeminal nucleus functions with the superior colliculus in processing visual information.

Trochlear Nerve

The nucleus of the trochlear nerve appears as a small compact cell group at the ventral border of the periaqueductal gray at levels through the inferior colliculus (Figs. 7.3 and 7.5). The nucleus (GSE) is a small caudal appendage to the oculomotor complex that indents the dorsal margin of the medial longitudinal fasciculus (MLF). Root fibers from the nucleus curve dorsolaterally and caudally near the margin of the central gray, decussate completely in the superior medullary velum (Fig. 6.26), and emerge from the dorsal surface of the brain stem caudal to the inferior colliculi (Figs. 2.21 and 2.22). Peripherally the nerve root curves around the lateral surface of the midbrain; passes between the superior cerebellar and posterior cerebral arteries (Figs. 14.3 and 14.7), as do fibers of the

Figure 7.4. Drawings of transverse (*A, B*) and sagittal (*C, D*) sections through the inferior colliculus outlining the nuclear subdivisions. The pericentral nucleus is indicated in *red* and the external nucleus is *blue*. The central nucleus in *white* shows contours of cellular laminae. *Black dots* indicate the division of the central nucleus into the large-celled dorsomedial part and the ventrolateral laminated part. Laminae in the central nucleus represent a given frequency band across the width of the nucleus and form the basis for the tonotopic organization of neurons. The disc-shaped laminae in dorsal regions are not as thick and represent the lower frequencies; high frequencies are represented ventrally. (From Carpenter and Sutin, *Human Neuroanatomy*, 1983; courtesy of Williams & Wilkins.)

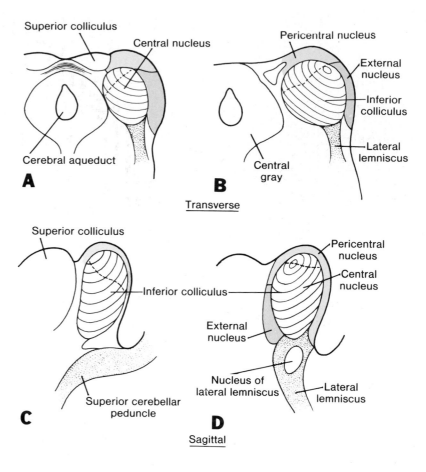

oculomotor nerve; and enters the cavernous sinus (Fig. 14.4). This nerve innervates the superior oblique muscle that serves to (1) intort the eye when abducted and (2) depress the eye when adducted. Although isolated lesions of the trochlear nerve are unusual, and detection of resulting disturbances by inspection is difficult, vertical diplopia results. Vertical diplopia is maximal on attempted downward gaze to the opposite side. Inability to intort the affected eye causes the patient to tilt the head laterally to the opposite side. Patients with trochlear nerve lesions complain of difficulty in walking down stairs.

Tegmental Nuclei

The periaqueductal gray surrounding the cerebral aqueduct contains several nuclear groups. The mesencephalic nucleus of the trigeminal nerve and the pigmented cells of the locus ceruleus occupy lateral regions at isthmus levels (Figs. 6.27 and 7.3). The raphe region contains the *dorsal nucleus of the raphe* and is flanked laterally by the *dorsal tegmental nuclei* (Figs. 5.13 and 7.3). This dorsal nucleus of the raphe, composed mainly of small cells dorsomedial to, and between, the trochlear nuclei, has been called the supratrochlear nucleus (Fig. 6.30). Although the dorsal nucleus of the raphe and the dorsal tegmental nucleus are adjacent to each other, only cells in the dorsal nucleus of the raphe synthesize and transport serotonin (5-HT) and cholecystokinin (CCK). Ventral to the medial longitudinal fasciculus and lateral to the raphe are the cells of the *ventral tegmental nucleus*. These cells appear as a rostral continuation of the *superior central nucleus* (Fig. 6.27).

The dorsal nucleus of the raphe and the median nucleus of the raphe

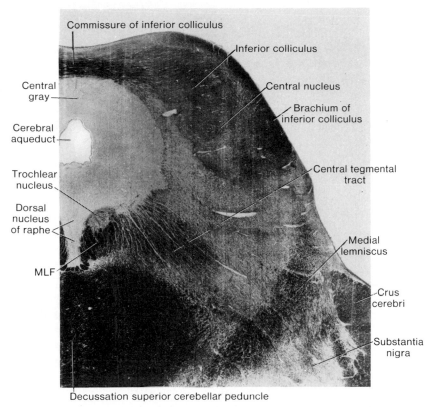

Commissure of inferior colliculus

Inferior colliculus

Central nucleus

Brachium of inferior colliculus

Central gray

Cerebral aqueduct

Central tegmental tract

Trochlear nucleus

Dorsal nucleus of raphe

Medial lemniscus

MLF

Crus cerebri

Substantia nigra

Decussation superior cerebellar peduncle

Figure 7.5.   Photograph of the right dorsal quadrant of a section through the rostral part of the inferior colliculus. Weigert's myelin stain. (From Carpenter and Sutin, *Human Neuroanatomy*, 1983; courtesy of Williams & Wilkins.)

(i.e., the superior central nucleus) give rise to ascending serotonergic pathways. Ascending projections from the dorsal nucleus of the raphe project to both the substantia nigra and the putamen. Projections from the median raphe nucleus form the mesolimbic system, which projects to the midbrain reticular formation, the hypothalamus, the septal area, the entorhinal cortex, and the hippocampal formation. Descending fibers from the median raphe nucleus project to the cerebellum, the locus ceruleus, the reticular formation of the lower brain stem, and the raphe nuclei of the pons and the medulla. Serotonin conveyed by these systems is believed to act as an inhibitory neurotransmitter.

The midbrain periaqueductal gray (PAG) consists of a dense collection of relatively small cells surrounding the cerebral aqueduct, which is functionally heterogeneous. This region has been implicated in central analgesic mechanisms, vocalization, control of reproductive behavior, aggressive behavior, and mechanisms of upward gaze. Afferents to the PAG arise from the hypothalamus, the brain stem reticular formation, the raphe nuclei, the locus ceruleus, and the spinal cord; many of these regions receive reciprocal projections from the PAG. Neurons in the PAG are immunoreactive to enkephalin, substance P, cholecystokinin, neurotensin, serotonin, dynorphin, and somatostatin, and single cells often contain several neuropeptides. The role of the PAG in brain stem analgesic mechanisms has received considerable attention. Ventrolateral regions of the PAG appear to be the most effective sites for stimulation-produced analgesia. Microinjections of morphine in the ventral PAG produce pronounced analgesia in rodents.

The *interpeduncular nucleus* lies dorsal to the interpeduncular fossa (Fig. 7.3). This nucleus receives fibers from the habenular nucleus via the fasciculus retroflexus (Figs. 9.4 and 10.11); large numbers of cholinergic fibers terminate in the interpeduncular nucleus. Fibers of the fascicular retroflexus bypassing the interpeduncular nucleus are distributed to the superior central nucleus, the dorsal tegmental nucleus, and the PAG. The dorsal tegmental nucleus also receives fibers from the mammillary bodies via the mammillotegmental tract and is closely related to the dorsal longitudinal fasciculus (of Schütz), a small pathway in ventromedial PAG. These pathways constitute part of a system by which signals related to the limbic system, concerned with visceral and behavioral functions, are projected to midbrain nuclei.

SUPERIOR COLLICULAR LEVEL

Transverse sections of the rostral midbrain appear strikingly different from those through the inferior colliculus in that (1) the flattened superior colliculi form the tectum; (2) the oculomotor nuclei form a V-shaped complex ventral to the periaqueductal gray and root fibers of the nerve emerge from the interpeduncular fossa; (3) the red nuclei, surrounded by fibers of the superior cerebellar peduncle, occupy the central tegmental region; and (4) the substantia nigrae achieve their maximum size ventral to the tegmentum and dorsal to the crura cerebri (Fig. 7.6). Fibers of the brachium of the inferior colliculus lie on the lateral surface of the tegmentum at this level. The medial lemniscus appears as a curved bundle dorsal to the substantia nigra and lateral to the red nucleus. The spinothalamic and spinotectal tracts lie together medial to the most dorsal fibers of the medial lemniscus.

Superior Colliculi

The superior colliculi are flattened, laminated eminences that form the rostral half of the tectum. In organization these structures resemble the cerebral cortex. Each colliculus consists of alternate gray and white layers. From the surface inward these layers are (1) the *stratum zonale* (mainly fibrous), (2) the *stratum cinereum* (outer gray layer), (3) the *stratum opticum* (superficial white layer), and (4) the *stratum lemnisci* consisting of middle and deep gray and white layers (Fig. 7.7). The superficial layers of the superior colliculus, which receive most of their input from the retina and visual cortex, are concerned with the detection of movement of objects in the visual field. The deep layers of the superior colliculus, which receive inputs from multiple sources (i.e., somesthetic and auditory systems, neurons concerned with motor activities, and various regions of the reticular formation), have anatomical and physiological characteristics of the brain stem reticular formation. Despite morphological, connectional, and biochemical differences, the superficial and deep layers of the superior colliculus are intimately linked with each other in a spatial registration. Efferent fibers arising from the superficial layers of the superior colliculus project primarily to vision related nuclei. In contrast, intermediate and deep laminae of the superior colliculus project to diverse regions related to head and eye movements.

Afferents to the Superior Colliculus

The superior colliculus receives afferents from the retina, the cerebral cortex, brain stem nuclei, and the spinal cord.

Retinotectal fibers leave the optic tract rostral to its principal termination in the lateral geniculate body and project to the superior col-

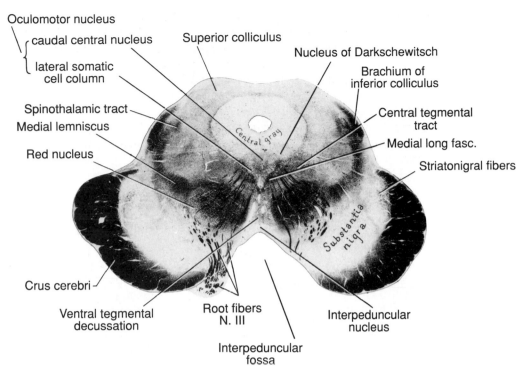

Figure 7.6. Transverse section of adult midbrain through the level of the oculomotor nerve. Weigert's myelin stain. Photograph. (From Carpenter and Sutin, *Human Neuroanatomy,* 1983; courtesy of Williams & Wilkins.)

liculus via its brachium. Fibers come from homonymous portions of the retina of each eye, but crossed fibers are most numerous. Thus, the contralateral homonymous halves of the visual field are represented in each superior colliculus (Fig. 7.8). Optic tract fibers project to all parts of the superior colliculus. The upper quadrants of the contralateral visual field are represented in medial parts of the superior colliculus; the lower quadrants are related to lateral regions of this structure. The contralateral peripheral visual field is represented in the caudal two-thirds of the superior colliculus, while central regions of the visual field are represented rostrally. The region of the retina corresponding to the optic disc (the blind spot) has been identified near the center of the superior colliculus. Retinal ganglion cells projecting to the superior colliculus are the Y and W cell types (see p. 284). In the superior colliculus, representation of the contralateral eye is dominant, a finding that contrasts with the equal representation of the two eyes in the lateral geniculate body and the striate cortex.

Corticotectal fibers arise from portions of the frontal, temporal, parietal, and occipital lobes. The most substantial and highly organized projection arises from the visual cortex and reaches the superior colliculus via the brachium of the superior colliculus (Fig. 7.8). These fibers enter the stratum opticum and pass into the superficial and middle gray layers. Fibers from the retina enter via the same route and appear to terminate in the same layers. Although retinal and visual cortical projections to the superior colliculus are similar, there are important differences: (1) retinal projections are bilateral and greatest contralaterally, while (2) striate cortical projections are unilateral. Anatomical data indicate that portions of the visual cortex and superior colliculus related to particular regions of the retina are interconnected. Thus, essentially the same cells of the superior colliculus receive distinct, but related, inputs from the ganglion

Figure 7.7. Drawing of the myelinated structure of the superior colliculus based on Weigert-stained sections. (From Carpenter and Sutin, *Human Neuroanatomy*, 1983; courtesy of Williams & Wilkins.)

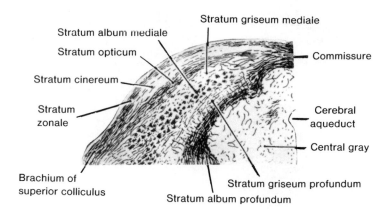

cells of the retina and cells of the striate cortex. Afferents to the superficial laminae also arise from the parabigeminal nucleus.

Corticotectal fibers from the frontal lobe (Brodmann's area 8) terminate in the middle gray layer, the stratum opticum, and the stratum zonale. These fibers reach the superior colliculus via a transtegmental approach and are thought to participate in motor mechanisms related to conjugate eye movements. Cells in the superficial layers respond to visual stimuli, while cells in the middle gray layer discharge prior to saccadic eye movements. The auditory cortex projects to deeper layers of the superior colliculus that receive no visual input.

Brain stem afferents to the superior colliculus arise from the inferior colliculus and a number of auditory relay nuclei. Most of these fibers project to deep layers of caudal parts of the superior colliculus. Commissural connections (Figs. 7.7 and 7.12) primarily relate deep and intermediate gray layers in the rostral halves of the superior colliculi. The pars reticulata of the substantia nigra projects fibers to the deep and intermediate layers of the caudal two-thirds of the superior colliculus. Many of these GABAergic neurons have dichotomizing axons that also project to the thalamus. These connections appear related to motor functions, since all brain stem and spinal afferents arise from deep layers.

Spinotectal fibers projecting to the deep layers of the superior colliculus are not numerous. Although some somatosensory input to the superior colliculus arises from cells in spinal lamina IV, the major inputs are from the nucleus cuneatus and all parts of the spinal trigeminal nucleus. These inputs are topographically organized with the head represented rostrally.

As the preceding discussion indicates, the superior colliculus can be partitioned into two zones: (1) the superficial layers, which receive primary visual afferents, and (2) deep layers, which receive heterogeneous multimodal inputs. Although the superficial layers of the superior colliculus have projections distinct from that of all deeper layers, they also project to the deep layers.

Efferents from the Superior Colliculus

In general the superficial layers give rise to ascending fibers and the deep layers project descending fibers to nuclei in the brain stem and spinal cord.

Tectothalamic fibers, arising from superficial layers of the superior colliculus, project ipsilaterally to the pulvinar, the dorsal lateral geniculate nuclei, and the pretectum. The pulvinar receives the most extensive projection from the superficial layers of the colliculus and in turn projects

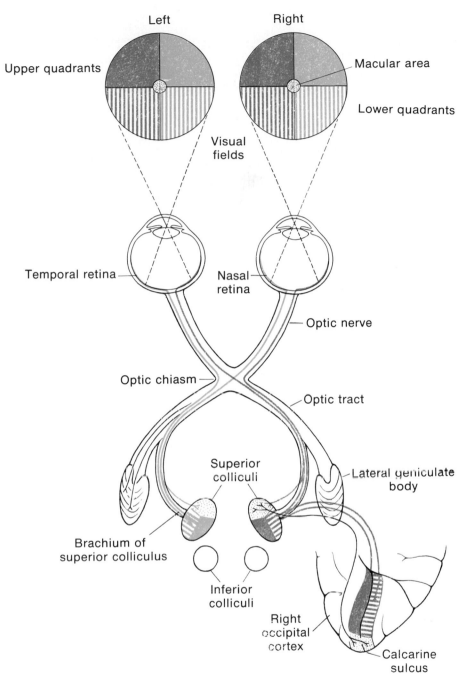

Figure 7.8.   Diagrammatic representation of the projections of the retinae and striate cortex upon the superior colliculi in the monkey. Retinotectal fibers from the ipsilateral temporal and contralateral nasal halves of the retinae, which subserve the contralateral homonymous visual field, project to the superior colliculus. Cells in portions of the retinae concerned with the contralateral peripheral visual field project to the posterior two-thirds of the superior colliculus. Upper quadrants of the contralateral peripheral visual field (*solid blue* and *red*) are represented in medial region of caudal parts of the superior colliculus, while lower quadrants of the contralateral peripheral visual field (*blue* and *red stripes*) are represented in lateral regions. Portions of the retinae concerned with central vision (i.e., within 10° of the fovae centralis; *blue* and *red dots*) are represented in the rostral third of the superior colliculus. Although retinotectal fibers arise from all portions of the retina of each eye, crossed fibers are most numerous. Corticotectal fibers from the striate cortex, shown on the right, project to all parts of the superior colliculus via its brachium. There is a correspondence in the superior colliculus of retinotectal and corticotectal terminations that represent both central and peripheral parts of the visual field. (From Carpenter and Sutin, *Human Neuroanatomy*, 1983; courtesy of Williams & Wilkins.)

upon extrastriate cortical areas (areas 18 and 19). Thus the superficial layers of the superior colliculus give rise to tectothalamic fibers, part of which convey visual information to the extrastriate cortex via the pulvinar. Cells in the most superficial layers of the superior colliculus also project upon the dorsal lateral geniculate body and the parabigeminal nucleus. Some tectogeniculate fibers terminate in intralaminar geniculate regions. Thus, visual pathways to the cortex via the superior colliculus and the lateral geniculate body are not entirely separate. The intermediate and deep collicular neurons project to both motor and sensory nuclei. These collicular projections include the pretectum, the paramedian pontine reticular formation (PPRF), and the rostral interstitial nucleus of the MLF (RiMLF), involved in subcortical control of eye movements.

Descending tectofugal fibers arising from intermediate and deep laminae of the superior colliculus can be grouped into uncrossed tectopontine and tectobulbar tracts, and crossed tectobulbar and tectospinal projections.

Uncrossed tectopontine and tectobulbar fibers project to the ipsilateral dorsolateral pontine nuclei, the lateral part of the reticulotegmental nucleus, and to the nucleus reticularis pontis oralis. The dorsolateral region of the pontine nuclei, which receives fibers from the superior colliculus, also receives inputs from the visual and auditory cortex; this collection of pontine nuclei projects to lobules VI and VII of the cerebellar vermis (Fig. 8.14).

Tectoreticular fibers project profusely and bilaterally to dorsal regions of the midbrain reticular formation. None of these projections enter the oculomotor complex.

Tectospinal and *tectobulbar fibers* cross in the dorsal tegmental decussation at midbrain levels and descend near the median raphe; at medullary levels these fibers become incorporated within the medial longitudinal fasciculus (Fig. 4.11). Tectospinal fibers continuing to cervical spinal segments ramify primarily within laminae VII and VIII.

Functional Considerations

Each superior colliculus receives a retinal input related to the contralateral visual field. In addition it receives an ipsilateral projection from the visual cortex concerning only the contralateral visual field. These two systems are precisely and topographically organized. Unilateral lesions of the superior colliculus in a variety of animals produce (1) relative neglect of visual stimuli in the contralateral visual field, (2) deficits in perception involving spatial discriminations and tracking of moving objects, (3) heightened responses to stimuli in the ipsilateral visual field, and (4) no impairment of eye movements. These disturbances suggest that the superior colliculus contributes to head and eye movements used to localize and follow visual stimuli. Physiological studies indicate that collicular receptive fields are two to four times larger than receptive fields in the visual cortex. The receptive field in the visual system is defined as that region of the retina (or visual field) over which one can influence the firing of a particular ganglion cell. The receptive field consists of a central circular region (excitatory) and a concentric surround (inhibitory), or the reverse. Most collicular cells respond only to moving stimuli, and three-fourths of these cells show a directional selectivity. These cells respond well to movement in one direction, poorly, or not at all, to movement in the opposite direction, and are nonresponsive to stationary stimuli flashed on and off. In the superior colliculus the preferred directional selectivity is parallel to the horizontal meridian of the visual field and toward the periphery of the visual field. Thus, units in the left superior colliculus have receptive fields in the right visual field and respond best to stimuli moving from left to right.

Stimulation of the superior colliculus results in contralateral conjugate deviations of the eyes, even though this structure has no direct projections to the nuclei of the extraocular muscles. These responses may be mediated by collicular projections to (1) the rostral interstitial nucleus of the MLF (RiMLF), which projects to specific subdivisions of the ipsilateral oculomotor complex, or (2) the pontine paramedian reticular formation (PPRF), which projects to the ipsilateral abducens nucleus and the RiMLF. Electrical stimulation of the superior colliculus in alert monkeys also elicits short-latency saccadic eye movements. The amplitude and direction of these saccades are a function of the site stimulated within the superior colliculus. The superior colliculus is involved in coding the location of an object in the visual field relative to the fovea and in eliciting saccadic eye movements that produce foveal acquisition of the object. The superficial laminae of the superior colliculus also play an important role in extrageniculate visual pathways related to depth perception.

OCULOMOTOR NERVE

Oculomotor Nuclear Complex

This complex is a collection of cell columns and discrete nuclei that (1) innervate the inferior oblique and the superior, medial, and inferior recti muscles; (2) supply the levator palpebrae muscle; and (3) provide preganglionic parasympathetic fibers to the ciliary ganglion (Figs. 7.6 and 7.9). Functional components of the nerve are categorized as *general somatic efferent* (GSE) and *general visceral efferent* (GVE). This complex lies ventral to the periaqueductal gray in the midline in a V-shaped trough formed by the diverging fibers of the MLF; it extends from the rostral pole of the trochlear nucleus to the upper limit of the midbrain (Figs. 7.1, 7.6, and 7.9). The complex consists of paired lateral somatic cell columns, midline and dorsal visceral nuclei, and a somatic midline dorsal cell group called the caudal central nucleus (Figs. 7.9 and 7.10).

The *lateral somatic cell columns*, composed of large motor type neurons, innervate the extraocular muscles. The dorsal cell column (or nucleus) innervates the inferior rectus muscle, the intermediate cell column innervates the inferior oblique muscle, and the ventral cell column supplies fibers to the medial rectus muscle. Although major representation of the medial rectus muscle is in the ventral cell column, a discrete collection of cells in dorsal regions also innervates this muscle (Fig. 6.20). Root fibers arising from these cell columns are uncrossed. A cell column medial to both the dorsal and intermediate cell columns, referred to as the medial cell column, provides crossed fibers that innervate the superior rectus muscle (Fig. 7.10).

The *caudal central nucleus* is a midline somatic cell group found only in the caudal third of the complex. This nucleus gives rise to crossed and uncrossed fibers that innervate the levator palpebrae muscle (Figs. 7.9 and 7.10).

Visceral nuclei of the oculomotor nuclear complex consist of two distinct nuclear groups, which are in continuity rostrally. The *Edinger-Westphal* nucleus consists of two slender columns of small cells dorsal to the rostral three-fifths of the somatic cell columns. In transverse sections through the middle third of the complex each of these paired columns

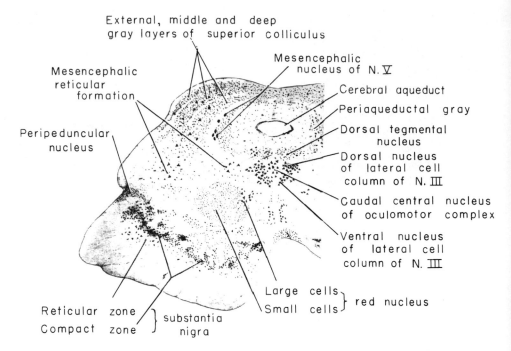

Figure 7.9. Section of the midbrain through the superior colliculi. Three-month-old infant. Cresyl violet. Photograph in which the main cell groups have been schematically blocked in. (From Carpenter and Sutin, *Human Neuroanatomy*, 1983; courtesy of Williams & Wilkins.)

divides into two smaller cell columns, which taper and gradually disappear. Rostrally the cell columns of the Edinger-Westphal nucleus merge in the midline dorsally and become continuous with the visceral cells of the *anterior median nucleus* (Fig. 7.10). Cells of the anterior median nucleus lie in the raphe between portions of the rostral lateral somatic cell columns. Both the Edinger-Westphal and anterior median nuclei give rise to uncrossed preganglionic parasympathetic fibers that emerge with somatic root fibers and project to the ciliary ganglion. Although the visceral nuclei have been considered to supply preganglionic parasympathetic fibers only to the ciliary ganglion, retrograde transport studies demonstrate that these visceral neurons also project to the lower brain stem and spinal cord (Fig. 4.15).

The so-called *central nucleus of Perlia* has been regarded as a midline cell group concerned with convergence. There has been great difficulty in identifying this nucleus in humans and monkeys, and its function remains in doubt.

Root fibers of the oculomotor nerve pass ventrally in numerous small bundles, some of which traverse the red nucleus. The rootlets converge and emerge from the brain stem in the interpeduncular fossa (Figs. 5.2 and 7.6).

Accessory Oculomotor Nuclei

Grouped under this designation are three nuclei closely associated with the oculomotor complex. These nuclei are the interstitial nucleus of Cajal, the nucleus of Darkschewitsch, and the nuclei of the posterior commissure.

The *interstitial nucleus* is a small collection of multipolar neurons situated among, and lateral to, the fibers of the MLF in the rostral midbrain (Fig. 7.11). This nucleus receives projections from the superior and medial vestibular nuclei, the pretectum, the frontal eye fields, and the

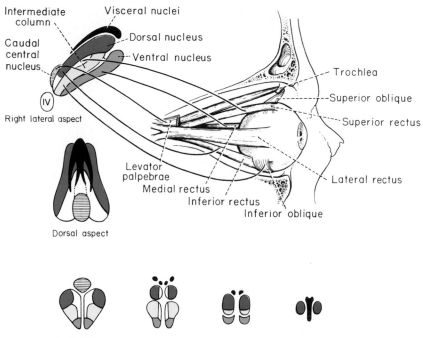

Figure 7.10. Schematic representation of the localization of the extraocular muscles within the oculomotor nuclear complex, based on studies in the rhesus monkey. Cell columns composing the complex are shown in lateral, dorsal, and transverse views through various levels. The visceral motor (parasympathetic) cell columns are shown in *black*. The ventral nucleus (*blue*) innervates the medial rectus muscle. The dorsal nucleus (*red*) innervates the inferior rectus muscle. The intermediate cell column (*yellow*) innervates the inferior oblique muscle. The cell column (*white*) medial to the dorsal and intermediate cell columns innervates the superior rectus muscle. The caudal central nucleus (*lined*) supplies fibers to the levator palpebrae superioris. Fibers innervating the medial rectus, inferior rectus, and inferior oblique muscles are uncrossed; fibers supplying the levator palpebrae muscle are both crossed and uncrossed, while those to the superior rectus muscle are crossed. The *drawing in the upper right* shows the positions of the extraocular muscles in relation to the globe and the bony orbit. (From Carpenter and Sutin, *Human Neuroanatomy*, 1983; courtesy of Williams & Wilkins.)

fastigial nucleus. Efferent fibers from the interstitial nucleus cross in the ventral part of the posterior commissure and are distributed to all somatic cell columns of the contralateral oculomotor complex, except the ventral (Fig. 7.14). In addition, the nucleus projects fibers bilaterally to the trochlear nuclei and ipsilaterally to the medial vestibular nucleus and spinal cord (i.e., interstitiospinal tract). This nucleus is concerned with slow rotatory and vertical eye movements and smooth pursuit eye patterns. This nucleus also plays a role in control of head movements and posture.

The *nucleus of Darkschewitsch* is formed by small cells that lie inside the ventrolateral border of the central gray, dorsal and lateral to the somatic cell columns of the oculomotor complex (Fig. 7.11). The nucleus projects to the nuclei of the posterior commissure but does not project fibers into the oculomotor complex or to lower brain stem.

The *nuclei of the posterior commissure* consist of collections of cells intimately associated with fibers of the posterior commissure (Figs. 7.11 and 7.13). Cells of these nuclei lie dorsolateral and dorsal to the central gray and have connections with the pretectal and posterior thalamic nuclei. In the monkey, interruption of fibers in the posterior commissure in the midline does not impair the pupillary light reflex, but lesions involving the nuclei of the posterior commissure and crossing fibers from the interstitial nuclei of Cajal produce bilateral eyelid retraction and impairment of vertical eye movements.

Pretectal Region

This region lies immediately rostral to the superior colliculus at levels of the posterior commissure (Figs. 7.11 and 7.12). Several distinctive cell groups found in this region all appear related to the visual system. Some, but not all, of these nuclei receive fibers from the optic tract, the visual cortex, and the lateral geniculate body. The nucleus of the optic tract consists of a plate of large cells along the dorsolateral border of the

Figure 7.11. Outline drawing of a brain stem section through the most compact portion of the posterior commissure (*PC*). At this level, the nucleus of the optic tract (*NOT*), the sublentiform nucleus (*SL*), the nucleus of the pretectal area (*NPA*), and the nuclei of the posterior commissure (*NPC*) are well developed. The anterior median nuclei (*AM*) are present, but the dorsal visceral nuclei (*VN*) of the oculomotor complex have not separated into medial and lateral cell columns. Additional abbreviations: *INC*, interstitial nucleus of Cajal; *ND*, nucleus of Darkschewitsch; *NPCm*, nucleus of posterior commissure, pars magnocellularis; *NPCp*, nucleus of posterior commissure, pars principalis; III N. oculomotor nerve. (From Carpenter and Sutin, *Human Neuroanatomy*, 1983; courtesy of Williams & Wilkins.)

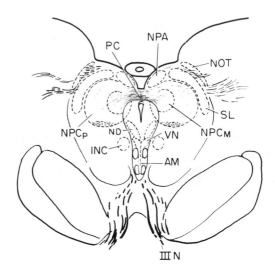

pretectum at its junction with the pulvinar (Fig. 7.11). The pretectal olivary nucleus, which forms a sharply delimited cell group at levels through caudal parts of the posterior commissure, receives crossed and uncrossed fibers of the optic tract and projects bilaterally to the visceral nuclei of the oculomotor complex (Figs. 7.12 and 7.13). These fiber systems are involved in the direct and consensual pupillary light reflex.

Posterior Commissure

The transition from midbrain to diencephalon is marked dorsally by the posterior commissure (Figs. 2.23, 2.24, 7.11, and 7.12). This small commissure lies dorsal to the periaqueductal gray and rostral to the superior colliculi at the point of transition between cerebral aqueduct and third ventricle. As fibers of this commissure fan out laterally, they are surrounded by cells that collectively form the *nuclei of the posterior commissure*. Identified elements in the commissure include fibers from (1) the pretectal nuclei, (2) the nuclei of the posterior commissure, (3) the interstitial nucleus, and (4) the nucleus of Darkschewitsch. Fibers involved in the pupillary light reflex partially cross in the posterior commissure.

The ependyma of the cerebral aqueduct beneath the posterior commissure consists of tall columnar cells with cilia. These modified ependymal cells form the *subcommissural organ*, which is considered to have a secretory function and is recognized as a circumventricular organ (Fig. 1.18). The subcommissural organ is the only midbrain structure not included in the blood-brain barrier.

Afferents of the Oculomotor Complex

Although no direct corticobulbar fibers reach the oculomotor complex, impulses from the cerebral cortex are conveyed to reticular neurons, which relay these impulses to the complex. Direct projections to the oculomotor nuclear complex arise from parts of the vestibular nuclei, the interstitial nucleus of Cajal (Fig. 7.14), abducens internuclear neurons, parts of the perihypoglossal nuclei, the rostral interstitial nucleus of the MLF (RiMLF), and the pretectal olivary nucleus. The superior colliculus does not project directly to the oculomotor complex, but it projects to parts of the periaqueductal gray close to the oculomotor nuclei. Secondary fibers from the medial and superior vestibular nuclei project to the oc-

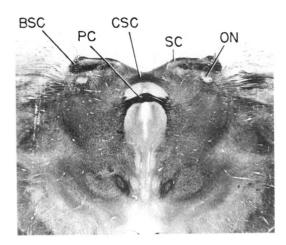

Figure 7.12. Photomicrograph of a myelin-stained section at the junction of pretectum and superior colliculus in the rhesus monkey. Abbreviations: *BSC*, brachium of the superior colliculus; *CSC*, commissure of the superior colliculus; *ON*, pretectal olivary nucleus; *PC*, posterior commissure; *SC*, superior colliculus. Weil stain. (From Carpenter and Sutin, *Human Neuroanatomy*, 1983; courtesy of Williams & Wilkins.)

ulomotor complex via the MLF. Projections from the medial vestibular nuclei via the MLF are bilateral while those from the superior vestibular nucleus via this bundle are ipsilateral. Fibers from peripheral parts of the superior vestibular nucleus, not contained in the MLF, cross in the caudal midbrain and project to the superior rectus and inferior oblique subdivisions of the oculomotor complex. Abducens internuclear neurons give risc to axons that ascend in the contralateral MLF and terminate selectively upon cells of the opposite medial rectus subdivision of the oculomotor complex. The nucleus prepositus, which receives an input from the flocculus, projects ipsilaterally to the oculomotor complex and may be concerned with vertical eye movements. The rostral interstitial nucleus of the MLF (RiMLF), situated among fibers of the MLF rostral to the oculomotor complex at the junction of mesencephalon and diencephalon, appears uniquely concerned with vertical eye movements, particularly in a downward direction. Cells in the RiMLF are activated in short bursts before vertical eye movements occur in response to vestibular or optokinetic stimuli. The RiMLF receives inputs from the superior vestibular nucleus via the MLF and uncrossed projections from the paramedian pontine reticular formation (PPRF), which ascend outside of the MLF. Cells of the RiMLF project ipsilaterally to the oculomotor complex and terminate mainly in the inferior rectus subdivision. Thus the PPRF projects fibers to both the principal center for conjugate horizontal eye movements, the abducens nucleus, and the established center for vertical eye movements, the RiMLF. These data indicate that paralysis of conjugate horizontal or vertical eye movements can occur independently, yet a mechanism exists that integrates horizontal and vertical components of conjugate eye movements.

Pupillary Reflexes

Light shone on the retina of one eye causes both pupils to constrict. The response in the eye stimulated is called the *direct pupillary light reflex*, while that in the opposite eye is known as the *consensual pupillary light reflex*. Pathways involved in the pupillary light reflex are not entirely known but involve (1) axons of retinal ganglion cells that pass via the optic nerve, optic tract, and brachium of the superior colliculus to the pretectal area; (2) axons of pretectal neurons that partially cross in the posterior commissure and terminate bilaterally in visceral nuclei of the oculomotor complex; (3) preganglionic fibers from the visceral nuclei that course with fibers of the third nerve and synapse in the ciliary ganglion; and (4) postganglionic

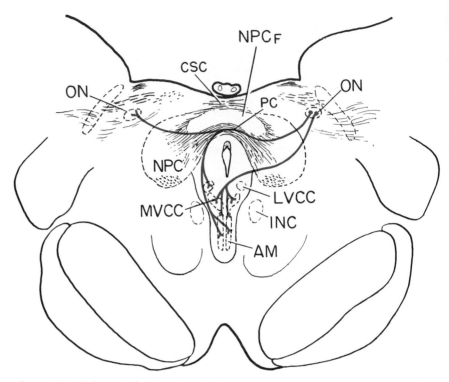

Figure 7.13.   Schematic drawing of the brain stem through the posterior commissure, showing the course and terminations of afferents projecting to the visceral nuclei of the oculomotor complex. The pretectal olivary nucleus (ON) receives direct bilateral retinal projections. Projections of the pretectal olivary nucleus (*red*) partially cross ventral to the cerebral aqueduct and terminate in the medial visceral cell columns (MVCC) and the anterior median nuclei (AM). Other efferents from the pretectal olivary nuclei cross in the posterior commissure and end in the lateral visceral cell column (LVCC) and the anterior median nuclei. Commissural connections interrelate the pretectal olivary nuclei. Abbreviations: CSC, commissure of the superior colliculus; INC, interstitial nucleus of Cajal; NPC, nuclei of the posterior commissure; NPC_F, nucleus of posterior commissure, pars infracommissuralis.

fibers from the ciliary ganglion that project to the sphincter of the iris. Cells of the pretectal olivary nucleus receive fibers of the optic tract and project bilaterally to the visceral nuclei of the oculomotor complex. In humans direct and consensual pupillary light reflexes are equal. The term *anisocoria* is used to denote pupillary inequality. The principal central lesions producing anisocoria involve efferent pathways from the oculomotor complex.

The *accommodation-convergence* reaction occurs when gaze is shifted from a distant object to a near one. This reaction involves (1) contractions of both medial recti muscles for convergence; (2) contraction of the ciliary muscle, which relaxes the suspensory ligament of the lens and causes the lens to assume a more convex shape; and (3) pupillary constriction. In this reflex retinal impulses must first reach the visual cortex and be relayed via corticofugal fibers to brain stem centers. Corticofugal fibers involved in this response reach the superior colliculus and pretectal region and are relayed to the oculomotor complex. Although under normal circumstances accommodation always is accompanied by pupillary constriction, certain central nervous system lesions can impair or abolish the pupillary light reflex without affecting accommodation. Such lesions occur with central nervous system syphilis (tabes dorsalis) in which the pupils are small (miosis) and do not react to light but react to accommodation. This is the *Argyll-Robertson pupil*. The precise location of the responsible lesion is unknown.

The central pathways for pupillary dilatation are not entirely known,

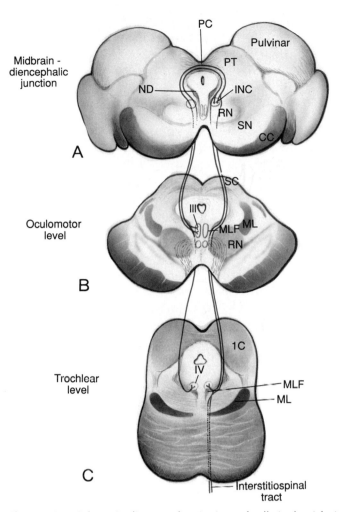

Figure 7.14. Schematic diagram of projections of cells in the right interstitial nucleus of Cajal (INC). *A*, Cells in the INC project fibers which cross in the ventral part of the posterior commissure (PC) and traverse the opposite INC. *B*, Most of the crossed projections of the INC terminate in all lateral somatic cell columns of the contralateral half of the oculomotor complex (III), except for the ventral cell column which innervates the medial rectus muscle. *C*, In the caudal midbrain crossed fibers from the INC terminate in the trochlear nucleus (IV). *A, B, and C*, Uncrossed fibers from the INC descending in the MLF terminate in the ipsilateral trochlear nucleus (IV). Remaining uncrossed fibers project to the medial vestibular nucleus (not shown) and descend to all spinal levels, as the *interstitiospinal tract*. Abbreviations: CC, crus cerebri; IC, inferior colliculus; ML, medial lemniscus; ND, nucleus of Darkschewitsch; PT, pretectum; RN, red nucleus; SN, substantia nigra.

but dilatation occurs reflexly on shading the eyes, scratching the side of the neck, and in association with severe pain and extreme emotion. Impulses related to pain probably reach cells of the intermediolateral cell column in upper thoracic spinal segments that give rise to preganglionic sympathetic fibers that convey impulses to the superior cervical ganglion. Postganglionic fibers from the superior cervical ganglion pass via blood vessels to dilator muscle fibers in the iris.

A *Horner's syndrome* usually results from interruption of descending autonomic pathways that course in the dorsolateral tegmentum at all brain stem levels caudal to the hypothalamus. This syndrome may also occur as a consequence of interrupting descending autonomic fibers in the brain stem or cervical spinal cord and with lesions involving either preganglionic or postganglionic sympathetic fibers of the superior cervical ganglion. The syndrome is characterized by miosis, pseudoptosis, apparent enophthalmos, and dryness of the skin over the face. If Horner's syndrome is the result of a brain stem lesion, the pupil shows relatively little dilatation to adrenaline. If the provocative lesion involves postganglionic sympathetic fibers, adrenaline produces mydriasis and eyelid retraction on the affected side due to denervation sensitivity.

Lesions of the Oculomotor Nerve

Complete lesions of the third nerve produce an ipsilateral lower neuron paralysis of the muscles supplied by that nerve. There is a complete ptosis (drooping) of the eyelid, due to paralysis of the levator palpebrae muscle. The eye is deviated laterally (external strabismus) due to paralysis of the oculomotor-innervated muscles and the unopposed action of the intact lateral rectus muscle. The pupil is fully dilated (mydriasis), and there is a loss of the pupillary light reflex as well as a loss of lens accommodation. Loss of the pupillary light reflex and accommodation results from interruption of visceral efferent fibers. Lesions involving the oculomotor nerve and corticospinal fibers in the ventral part of the midbrain result in an ipsilateral oculomotor paralysis and a contralateral hemiplegia, which clinically are known as *Weber's syndrome*. This syndrome, also known as *superior alternating hemiplegia*, is the midbrain equivalent of similar syndromes occurring from lesions in the pons (i.e., middle alternating hemiplegia) with involvement of the VI nerve and the corticospinal tract and in the medulla (i.e., inferior alternating hemiplegia) with involvement of the XII nerve and the pyramid.

MESENCEPHALIC TEGMENTUM

The midbrain tegmentum contains the reticular formation, the red nucleus, and many smaller cell groups in addition to the oculomotor and trochlear nuclei.

Red Nucleus

The most conspicuous structure in the midbrain tegmentum is the red nucleus, a part of the reticular formation characterized by its pinkish-yellow color, its central position, and its "capsule" formed by fibers of the superior cerebellar peduncle (Figs. 7.6, 7.9, and 7.15). The nucleus is an oval column of cells extending from the caudal margin of the superior colliculus into the caudal diencephalon (Fig. 9.2). In transverse sections the nucleus has a circular configuration. Cytologically the nucleus consists of a caudal magnocellular part and a rostral parvicellular part. Between the cells of the nucleus there are small bundles of myelinated fibers of the superior cerebellar peduncle. Root fibers of the oculomotor nerve partially traverse the nucleus en route to the interpeduncular fossa (Fig. 7.6).

Afferent fibers projecting to the red nucleus are derived from two principal sources, the deep cerebellar nuclei and the cerebral cortex. Fibers from both sources terminate somatotopically within the red nucleus. Fibers of the superior cerebellar peduncle undergo a complete decussation in the caudal midbrain and enter and surround the contralateral red nucleus (Figs. 7.2 and 8.15). Fibers and collaterals from the dentate nucleus terminate in the rostral third of the opposite red nucleus (parvicellular part), while those from the emboliform and globose nuclei (anterior and posterior interposed nuclei) project somatotopically upon cells in the caudal two-thirds of the nucleus (Figs. 8.15 and 8.16). The

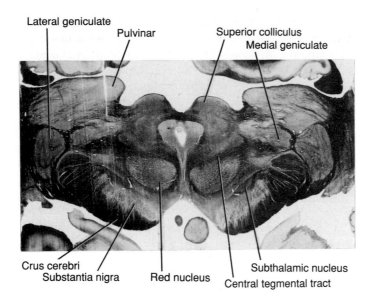

Lateral geniculate
Pulvinar
Superior colliculus
Medial geniculate

Crus cerebri
Substantia nigra
Red nucleus
Subthalamic nucleus
Central tegmental tract

Figure 7.15. Transverse section through the rostral mesencephalon demonstrating the manner in which diencephalic nuclei surround dorsal and lateral portions of the mesencephalon. Weigert's myelin stain. Photograph. (From Carpenter and Sutin, *Human Neuroanatomy*, 1983; courtesy of Williams & Wilkins.)

latter connection links paravermal regions of the cerebellar cortex to the magnocellular part of the red nucleus that in turn projects somatotopically to spinal levels (Fig. 8.16). Two decussations are involved, that of the superior cerebellar peduncle and that of the rubrospinal tract. Somatotopical projections from the magnocellular part of the red nucleus terminate primarily to cervical and lumbar spinal segments.

Corticorubral projections arise from precentral and premotor cortex; both of these areas project somatotopically upon cells in the red nucleus. Projections from the medial part of area 6 (the supplementary motor area, MII) are crossed and end in the magnocellular region of the nucleus. Projections from the precentral motor cortex to the magnocellular part of the red nucleus are ipsilateral and correspond to the somatotopic origins of rubrospinal fibers. These fibers have a somatotopic linkage and, together with the rubrospinal tract (crossed), constitute a pathway by which impulses can be conveyed from the "motor" cortex to spinal levels.

Descending rubral efferent fibers cross in the *ventral tegmental decussation* and project to (1) the interposed nuclei of the cerebellum; (2) the principal sensory and spinal trigeminal nuclei; (3) parts of the facial nucleus; (4) several medullary relay nuclei; and (5) the spinal cord (Fig. 4.11). Uncrossed descending rubral efferents from the parvicellular part of the nucleus enter the central tegmental tract and project to the dorsal lamella of the principal inferior olivary nucleus (Fig. 6.18); these fibers are referred to a *rubroolivary* and constitute part of a feedback system to the cerebellum. No fibers from the red nucleus project to thalamic nuclei.

Stimulation of the red nucleus in the decerebrate cat results in (1) excitatory postsynaptic potentials in contralateral flexor alpha motor neurons, and (2) inhibitory postsynaptic potentials in contralateral extensor alpha motor neurons. These observations suggest that the rubrospinal tract transmits impulses that facilitate flexor muscle tone. Because of somatotopic relationships between the interposed nuclei of the cerebellum and the red nucleus, stimulation of these nuclei in decerebrate animals produces flexion in the ipsilateral limb muscles (Fig. 8.16). These responses are ipsilateral because both fiber systems involved are crossed (i.e, the superior cerebellar peduncle and the rubrospinal tract).

Lesions involving the midbrain tegmentum and the red nucleus unilaterally produce a syndrome characterized by (1) ipsilateral oculomotor disturbances, and (2) contralateral motor disturbances of an involuntary nature (i.e., tremor, ataxia, or choreiform movements). This combination of disturbances is known as the *syndrome of Benedikt*. Experimental evidence suggests that the contralateral abnormal involuntary motor activity is due primarily to involvement of crossed fibers of the superior cerebellar peduncle.

Mesencephalic Reticular Formation

The midbrain reticular formation is less extensive than that of the pons. Although the red nucleus is part of the reticular formation, this term usually is used to designate structures dorsal and lateral to the red nucleus. Three principal reticular nuclei are recognized: (1) cuneiformis, (2) subcuneiformis, and (3) tegmenti pedunculopontinus (pedunculopontine nucleus).

The *pedunculopontine nucleus* lies in the lateral tegmentum ventral to the inferior colliculus (Figs. 7.3 and 7.18). Fibers of the superior cerebellar peduncle traverse this nucleus as they course ventromedially toward their decussation. The pedunculopontine nucleus receives inputs from multiple sources that include (1) the cerebral cortex; (2) the medial pallidal segment; and (3) the pars reticulata of the substantia nigra (Fig. 7.18). Cells of the compact part of the pedunculopontine nucleus are strongly cholinergic, but adjacent cells have other neurotransmitters. Cells immunoreactive to choline acetyltransferase (ChAT) in the pedunculopontine nucleus are considered to project to the thalamus, although some project to the pars compacta of the substantia nigra. This nucleus lies in a region from which walking movements can be elicited on stimulation. This region is referred to as the "locomotor center."

The *cuneiform* and *subcuneiform nuclei* lie ventral to the tectum and dorsal to the pedunculopontine nucleus and extend rostrally. Fibers of the central tegmental tract lie medial to these reticular nuclei. The *interpeduncular nucleus*, composed of small cells, lies in the midline dorsal to the interpeduncular fossa (Figs. 7.3, 7.6, and 7.9). This nucleus receives fibers from the habenular nuclei via the fasciculus retroflexus (Figs. 9.4 and 10.11).

FUNCTIONAL CONSIDERATIONS OF THE RETICULAR FORMATION

The anatomical organization of the brain stem reticular formation has been described regionally. In the medulla and pons four zones are recognized: (1) a median zone containing nuclei of the raphe, (2) the paramedian reticular nuclei, (3) a medial zone regarded as an "effector" area, and (4) a smaller lateral zone referred to as the "sensory" part because it receives collaterals from secondary sensory pathways. In the medulla the paramedian reticular nuclei project mainly to the cerebellum. The effector zone, which is coextensive with the giant cell area of the reticular formation, gives rise to both ascending and descending fibers. The "sensory" zone, coextensive with the parvicellular area, projects its axons medially into the "effector" area. The pontine reticular formation has essentially the same zones, although the "sensory" part is smaller.

Electrical stimulation of the caudal and medial "effector" zone of the medullary reticular formation inhibits most forms of motor activity (e.g., myotatic reflexes, flexion reflex, extensor muscle tone, and cortically induced movements). Regions of the medullary reticular formation from which inhibitory responses are obtained correspond roughly to the area of the gigantocellular part that gives rise to medullary reticulospinal fibers. Stimulation of the rostral and dorsal part of the nucleus reticularis gigantocellularis produces monosynaptic excitatory postsynaptic potentials in motor neurons supplying axial muscles in the neck and back.

A far larger region of the brain stem reticular formation facilitates reflex activity and cortically induced movements. The facilitatory area extends rostrally from the upper medulla into the caudal diencephalon. Bilateral facilitatory effects can be evoked throughout this extensive region of the reticular formation.

Descending influences of the brain stem reticular formation are not limited to inhibition and facilitation of somatic motor functions. Inspiratory and vasodepressor effects can be obtained from the gigantocellular region in the medulla, while expiratory effects are obtained from the parvicellular region. Vasopressor effects are evoked from lateral reticular regions that project noradrenergic fibers to spinal levels (Fig. 5.15). Although nearly all parts of the central nervous system are capable of exerting detectable influences upon the heart and blood vessels, the primary vasomotor control center is located laterally in the reticular formation of the pons and medulla. Transections of the brain stem as far caudal as the lower third of the pons have little effect upon arterial pressure. Successively more caudal transections produce (1) a drop in blood pressure and (2) a reduction in the discharge of cardiac accelerator impulses. The bulbar pressor and depressor areas constitute a central cardiovascular mechanism that reflexly regulates blood pressure and the parameters of the heart rate. In the intact animal, a normal arterial pressure is dependent on the bulbar pressor area. A group of noradrenergic neurons located in the caudal pons and rostral medulla (Figs. 4.16 and 5.15) sends axons to the nucleus of the solitary tract, the nucleus ambiguus, and preganglionic sympathetic neurons in the intermediolateral cell column of the thoracic spinal cord. These noradrenergic neurons are part of a neural network related to the regulation of the cardiovascular system.

The region surrounding the nucleus of the solitary tract is coextensive with the physiologically defined dorsal medullary respiratory "center." A ventral medullary respirator "center" includes the nucleus ambiguus and the surrounding reticular formation. Additional brain stem regions important in the control of respiration are the "pneumotaxic center" found in the pons near the medial parabrachial nucleus and an "apneustic center," which remains poorly defined. The parabrachial nuclei receive input from nucleus of the solitary tract and in turn project to both dorsal and ventral respiratory "centers" in the medulla (Fig. 6.27). The "pneumotaxic center" periodically releases the inhibition of the "apneustic center."

Stimulation of inhibitory and facilitatory regions of the reticular formation can decrease or increase the rates of discharge from the muscle spindles via gamma efferent fibers. A part of the effects exerted upon alpha motor neurons may result from the firing of gamma efferents, which indirectly influence these neurons through the gamma loop (Fig. 3.23). The reticular formation also is thought to modify the transmission of other sensory impulses by facilitation and inhibition exerted at the second neuronal level.

Ascending influences of the reticular formation exert powerful influences upon the electrical activity of the cerebral cortex. Wakefulness, alertness, and sleep are characterized by strikingly different electroencephalographic patterns. Alertness is characterized by low voltage fast activity, while sleep is associated with high voltage slow activity. Fundamental insight into the underlying brain mechanisms was provided by comparing the electroencephalograms (EEG) of animals following high spinal transections (*encéphale isolé*) and decerebration (i.e., transection of the midbrain at the intercollicular level, *cerveau insolé*). In the encéphale isolé preparation the EEG displayed the waking pattern, while the cerveau isolé preparation exhibited an EEG pattern characteristic of the sleeping state. These experiments pointed to a potent electrotonic influence, associated with the awake state, generated in the lower brain stem. While it was well known that a variety of different stimuli could change the EEG from a synchronized pattern (i.e., sleep state) to a desynchronized one (i.e., alert state), the puzzling feature was how impulses channeled in the classic pathways exerted such broad and diffuse electronic changes in the cerebral cortex. The observation that stimulation of the brain stem reticular formation could activate and desynchronize the EEG and produce behavioral arousal without discharging the classic lemniscal pathways suggested the concept of a second ascending system. This second ascending system with powerful influences upon broad regions of the cerebral cortex is known as the *ascending reticular activating system* (ARAS).

Interruption of the long ascending sensory pathways in the brain stem does not prevent impulses ascending in the reticular formation from provoking their characteristic EEG arousal response. Lesions in the rostromedial midbrain reticular formation abolish the EEG arousal response elicited by sensory stimulation, even though long ascending sensory pathways are intact. Thus two functionally distinct ascending sensory pathways must project to the diencephalon: (1) long ascending pathways, the *lemniscal systems*, concerned with specific sensory modalities (i.e., medial lemniscus, lateral lemniscus, spinothalamic tracts, and secondary trigeminothalamic pathways) that end upon specific thalamic nuclei, and (2) the *ascending reticular activating system*, which receives collaterals from surrounding specific systems and conveys impulses via the reticular core. Physiologically, the ascending reticular activating system is considered to be a multineuronal, polysynaptic system conveying impulses of a nonspecific nature related to wakefulness and arousal. Although physiologically the reticular formation behaves as if it consisted of chains of neurons that fire successively, the reticular formation does not contain short-axoned Golgi type II cells. The main ascending pathway in the reticular formation appears to be the *central tegmental tract* (Figs. 6.1, 6.4, 6.26, and 7.15). Ascending components of this bundle arise from effector regions of the reticular core and give rise to long axons with numerous collaterals that project laterally. Rapid conduction in the reticular core is via the long central axons, while slowly conducted impulses pass via collaterals and involve multiple synapses. The central tegmental tract projects to the rostral intralaminar nuclei of the thalamus. Ascending projections from medial regions of the midbrain reticular formation projecting to the hypothalamus are distinct from those contained in the central tegmental tract. Although there has been agreement that the intralaminar nuclei influence electrical activity in broad cortical regions, it is mainly cells in the rostral intralaminar thalamic that project directly to cortex.

In humans, lesions of the brain stem often produce disturbances of consciousness that range from fleeting unconsciousness to sustained coma. As Magoun has stated, "It is not easy for the physiologist to put his finger upon consciousness, though it is present abundantly and for long periods of time." In all forms of disturbed consciousness due to brain stem lesions, there is a loss of crude awareness. With lesions of the lower brain stem, unconsciousness is accompanied by respiratory and cardiovascular disturbances. The loss of consciousness frequently is sudden, and depression of vital functions leads to extreme states. Lesions of the upper brain stem most commonly produce hypersomnia characterized by muscular relaxation, slow respiration, and an EEG pattern showing large amplitude slow waves. The level of unconsciousness may not be deep and some patients can be aroused briefly. If the patient develops decerebrate rigidity, there is usually coma. A variant of hypersomnia seen with upper brain stem lesions is referred to as *akinetic mutism* (coma vigil). In this variant the EEG pattern mainly resembles that associated with slow sleep, but eye movements remain normal.

At all levels of the brain stem liability to unconsciousness is related to the rapidity with which lesions develop. Lesions associated with hemorrhage usually produce sudden coma; slowly developing lesions, such as tumors, may not disturb consciousness for a considerable period of time. Although there is no center particularly concerned with consciousness, the functional integrity of the brain stem reticular formation is essential for its maintenance. A healthy cerebral cortex cannot by itself maintain the conscious state.

Major serotonergic neurons in the midbrain lie in the dorsal (supratrochlear) and median (superior central) raphe nuclei (Fig. 5.13). Ascending pathways from these nuclei pass through the ventral tegmental area and join the medial forebrain bundle (Figs. 7.16 and 10.11). Fibers of this bundle project medially into the hypothalamus and laterally into the striatum. Ascending fibers continuing in the medial forebrain bundle divide into several components that pass to (1) the thalamus, (2) amygdala, (3) the hippocampus, (4) the cortex on the medial aspect of the hemisphere, and (5) the olfactory bulb. The raphe nuclei of the midbrain have ascending fiber systems with functional relationships to the ascending reticular activating system and the limbic system. The general inhibitory action of serotonin in the central nervous system serves to modulate and maintain behavior within certain limits. Hallucinogenic drugs, such as LSD, depress the serotonergic system, and the release of inhibition results in a hypersensitivity to environmental stimuli and hyperactivity in a brain otherwise behaving as if it were asleep.

SUBSTANTIA NIGRA

The substantia nigra lies dorsal to the crus cerebri, ventral to the midbrain tegmentum, and extends throughout the length of the mesencephalon (Figs. 7.1, 7.6, 7.9, and 7.15). Descriptively, the substantia nigra is divided into two parts: (1) the *compact part* (SNC), a cell-rich region composed of large, pigmented cells, and (2) a *reticular part* (SNR), which is a cell-poor region close to the crus cerebri. Three types of nigral neurons have been described: (1) large neurons distributed exclusively in the reticular part, (2) medium-sized and large neurons containing melanin pigment in the compact part, and (3) short-axoned (Golgi type II) cells found in both the compact and reticular parts.

Golgi studies demonstrate that nigral neurons give rise to long,

Figure 7.16. Neurons in the pars compacta of the substantia nigra (SNc) in the monkey immunoreactive to dopamine (DA) antiserum. In rostral parts of the SNc dopaminergic neurons occupy a dorsomedial location (A). In more caudal parts of the SNc, dopaminergic neurons extend in columns, or trabeculae, into the pars reticulata (SNr) (B). Cells of the ventral tegmental area (VTA) also are dopaminergic (B). Abbreviations: CP, cerebral peduncle; FR, fasciculus retroflexus; OT, optic tract; STN, subthalamic nucleus; III, oculomotor nerve rootlets. (Published with the permission and courtesy of Arsenault et al., 1988. J. Comp. Neurol., **267**: 489–506.)

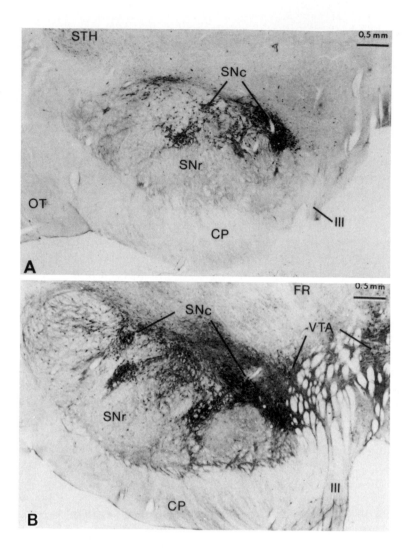

smooth radiating dendrites with few branches oriented in two main directions. Dendrites of cells in the SNR and in the caudal SNC are oriented primarily rostrocaudally. Dendrites of most cells in the SNC have a dorsoventral orientation. Thus the dendritic fields of cells in the pars compacta and pars reticulata overlap extensively in the pars reticulata.

Dorsomedial to the substantia nigra is a region containing scattered cells of various sizes, many of which are pigmented. This tegmental region, which appears similar to the pars compacta, is referred to as the *ventral tegmental area* (VTA) (Tsai) (Fig. 7.16). Lateral to the substantia nigra the small cells of the *peripeduncular nucleus* cap the dorsal margin of the crus cerebri (Fig. 7.9).

Neurotransmitters

Cells of the pars compacta contain high concentrations of dopamine (Fig. 7.16) and are recognized as the principal source of striatal (i.e., caudate nucleus and putamen) dopamine. Immunocytochemical studies based on highly specific antiserum raised against dopamine (DA) have provided precise data concerning the disposition of DA-containing cells in the pars compacta of the substantia nigra (SNC) and the ventral tegmental area (VTA) in the primate. Almost all DA-containing cells were found in the SNC (Fig. 7.16). In rostral parts of the substantia nigra, large DA-containing cells were localized to a ventromedial region; in more caudal regions distinct columns of DA-containing cells extended into the underlying pars reticulata (SNR). Dopamine immunoreactive neurons in the VTA formed a triangular zone dorsal to the interpeduncular nucleus, medial to the substantia nigra, and ventral to the oculomotor nuclear complex. In a rat a high percentage of DA-containing neurons in the SNC and the VTA also contained the peptide cholecystokinin (CCK). Neurons containing both DA and CCK project to the striatum, the nucleus accumbens, the amygdala, and the prefrontal cortex. The enzyme glutamate decarboxylase (GAD) utilized in the synthesis of gamma (γ)-aminobutyric acid (GABA) is found in high concentrations in the pars reticulata. In the rodent, GAD-immunoreactive cells constituted about 90% of the neurons in the SNR. In the monkey less numerous GABA-positive cells are present largely in the lateral part of the SNR. Terminals immunoreactive for GABA were present in all parts of the SNR. The SNR also contains serotonin (5-HT) fibers and terminals. The dorsal nucleus of the raphe is the principal source of this serotonergic pathway. Stimulation of the dorsal nucleus of the raphe produces inhibition of spontaneous activity in single neurons of the substantia nigra.

Fibers in the substantia nigra also contain substance P (SP), characterized as an undecapeptide. The highest concentration of SP in any brain region is found in the substantia nigra where the substance is concentrated in nerve endings within both the SNR and the SNC. The pars reticulata also contains enkephalinergic (ENK) fibers and terminals. Striatonigral fibers arising from spiny neurons within the caudate nucleus and the putamen contain GABA, SP, and ENK. These fibers arise from a different population of spiny neurons than striatopallidal fibers, but the major neurotransmitters are the same.

The substantia nigra is implicated in the metabolic disturbances that underlie parkinsonism (paralysis agitans), and it may be involved in Huntington's disease and other forms of dyskinesia characterized by abnormal involuntary movements and alterations of muscle tone. In parkinsonism the synthesis and transport of dopamine (DA) from the substantia nigra to the striatum is greatly impaired. In Huntington's disease striatal dopamine may be at normal, but GABA is greatly reduced.

Nigral Afferent Fibers

Afferent fibers to the substantia nigra arise from the neostriatum (caudate nucleus and putamen), the lateral segment of the globus pallidus, the subthalamic nucleus, the dorsal nucleus of the raphe, and the pedunculopontine nucleus. Quantitatively the largest number of nigral afferents arise from the caudate nucleus and the putamen and are known as striatonigral fibers (Fig. 7.17).

Striatonigral fibers are topographically organized in that fibers from the head of the caudate nucleus project to the rostral third of the substantia nigra while the putamen projects to all other parts of the nigra. Virtually all of the striatonigral fibers end upon dendrites of neurons in the pars reticulata. Striatonigral fibers arise from medium-sized, spiny striatal neurons.

Pallidonigral projections have been identified in a number of animals by retrograde transport studies. These fibers are considered GABAergic and arise from the lateral pallidal segment. GABA-immunoreactive terminals are most abundant in the SNR, but a few are present in the SNC.

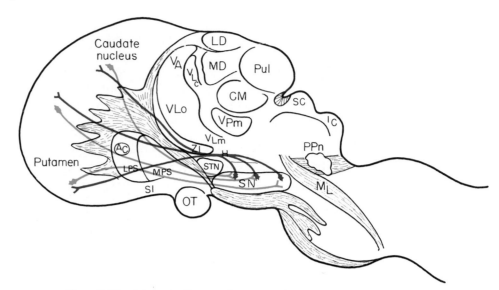

Figure 7.17. Schematic diagram of striatonigral and nigrostriatal feedback system in a sagittal plane. Striatonigral fibers (*blue*) arise from spiny striatal neurons; project to the pars reticulata (SNR); and have γ-aminobutyric acid (GABA), substance P (SP), and enkephalin (ENK) as neurotransmitters. Intermingled clusters of cells in the pars compacta of the substantia nigra (SNC) project nigrostriatal fibers (*red*) to either the caudate nucleus or the putamen, but not to both. Cells of the SNC synthesize and convey dopamine to terminals in the striatum. Abbreviations: AC, anterior commissure; CM, centromedian nucleus; IC, inferior colliculus; LD, lateral dorsal nucleus; LPS, lateral segment of the globus pallidus; MD, mediodorsal nucleus; ML, medial lemniscus; MPS, medial pallidal segment; OT, optic tract; PPn, pedunculopontine nucleus; Pul, pulvinar; SC, superior colliculus; SI, substantia innominata; SN, substantia nigra; STN, subthalamic nucleus; VA, ventral anterior nucleus; VLc, VLo, and VLm, ventral lateral nucleus, pars caudalis, pars oralis, and pars medialis; VPM, ventral posteromedial nucleus; ZI, zona incerta.

In comparison to the striatonigral projection, the number of pallidonigral fibers appears small.

Subthalamonigral fibers have been demonstrated by both anterograde and retrograde transport studies in a number of species. These fibers terminate in patchy areas in the pars reticulata. Fluorescent double-labeling studies suggest that in the rat virtually all cells in the subthalamic nucleus project axons to both the globus pallidus and the substantia nigra. Similar studies in the monkey indicate that only 10% of subthalamic nucleus neurons project to both the SNR and the globus pallidus. The neurotransmitter of subthalamic nucleus neurons is unknown.

Tegmentonigral fibers consist of projections from midbrain raphe nuclei that have serotonin (5-HT) and cholecystokinin (CCK) as their neurotransmitters and projections from the pedunculopontine nucleus. The bulk of the serotonergic projections to the substantia nigra rise from the dorsal nucleus of the raphe. Projections of the pedunculopontine nucleus appear to be mainly ascending; the largest number of ascending fibers project to the substantia nigra, although smaller numbers of fibers project to the medial pallidal segment and other structures. Neurons in the compact part of the pedunculopontine nucleus are cholinergic. Some morphological evidence indicates that large numbers of these cells terminate upon neurons in the SNC.

Nigral Efferent Projections

Efferent fibers arising from the pars compacta and pars reticulata of the substantia nigra have distinctive neurotransmitters and projections (Figs. 7.17 and 7.18).

Nigrostriatal fibers arise from dopaminergic neurons in the pars

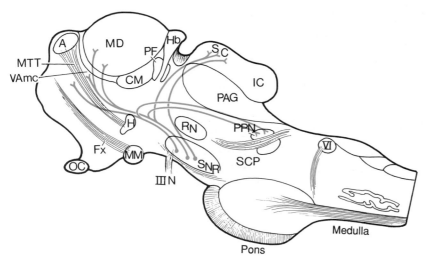

Figure 7.18. Schematic drawing of efferent projections from the substantia nigra, pars reticulata (SNR). These GABAergic neurons give rise to *nigrothalamic*, *nigrotectal*, and *nigrotegmental projections (blue)*. Collectively these fibers represent part of the output system of the corpus striatum by virtue of their input from spiny striatal neurons. Nigrothalamic fibers project to medial parts of the ventral lateral nucleus (VLm) (not shown), the magnocellular part of the ventral anterior nucleus (VAmc), which surrounds the mammillothalamic tract (MMT), and parts of the mediodorsal thalamic nucleus (MD). Of the fibers projecting to the middle and deep layers of the superior colliculus (SC), 20–30% represent collaterals of nigrothalamic fibers. About 60% of the cells in the SNR projecting to the thalamus have collaterals that project to the pedunculopontine nucleus (PPN). Abbreviations: A, anterior thalamic nuclei; CM, centromedian nucleus; CS, superior colliculus; Fx, fornix; H, Forel's field H; Hb, habenular nucleus; IC, inferior colliculus; MD, mediodorsal thalamic nucleus; MM, mammillary body; OC, optic chiasm; PAG, periaqueductal gray; PF, parafascicular nucleus; RN, red nucleus; SCP, superior cerebellar peduncle; VI, abducens nucleus; III N, oculomotor nerve.

compacta and project topographically to different parts of the striatum (Figs. 7.16 and 7.17). Intermingled clusters of cells in the SNC project to either the caudate nucleus or the putamen, but not to both. These fibers traverse parts of the globus pallidus en route to the caudate nucleus and putamen. Data based upon histofluorescence indicated that dopamine is stored in varicosities in nerve terminals. Varicosities, both terminal and nonterminal, in the striatum are fine, densely packed, and exhibit a diffuse green fluorescence. Dopaminergic fibers form a matrix of fine varicose axons around both small and large striatal neurons. Striatonigral neurons identified by retrograde transport of horseradish peroxidase receive symmetrical synaptic contacts from terminals immunoreactive for tyrosine hydroxylase (indicative of dopamine). Nerve terminals containing dopamine have small granular vesicles about 50 nm in diameter. Dopamine is considered to have an inhibitory action upon striatal neurons. Biochemical data distinguish two types of dopamine receptors, designated as D_1 and D_2. Activation of D_1 receptors produces a reduction in membrane excitability, while activation of the D_2 receptors causes a decrease in release of neurotransmitter at synaptic terminals. In the striatum these different types of receptors function synergistically.

Striatonigral and nigrostriatal fibers appear to form a closed feedback loop in which striatonigral fibers form the afferent limb and nigrostriatal fibers constitute the efferent limb (Fig. 7.17). This reciprocal arrangement is evident in that HRP injected into the striatum is transported (1) retrograde from axon terminals to cells of the pars compacta and (2) anterograde via striatal neurons to terminals in the pars reticulata of the substantia nigra. Spiny striatal neurons transport GABA, substance P, and enkephalin to terminals in the pars reticulata of the substantia

Figure 7.19. Dark-field photomicrograph of an autoradiograph demonstrating nigrotectal terminations. Nigrotectal fibers arise from cells in the pars reticulata (SNR) and terminate in the deep and middle gray layers of the superior colliculus.

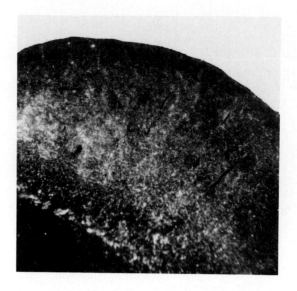

nigra. GABA appears to be inhibitory, while substance P is considered to be excitatory. The precise role of the opioid peptide enkephalin remains to be defined.

Following lesions in the substantia nigra, dopamine in nigrostriatal nerve terminals is greatly reduced. In patients with paralysis agitans, there is a virtual absence of dopamine in the striatum and the substantia nigra. An effective treatment for this metabolic disorder is L-hydroxyphenyl-alanine (L-dopa), a precursor of dopamine, which passes the blood-brain barrier. This therapy is essentially a replacement of striatal dopamine, which is not synthesized in sufficient quantities by cells of the pars compacta.

Nigrothalamic fibers arise from GABAergic cells of the pars reticularis and project to (1) the large-celled part of the ventral anterior nucleus (VAmc) and (2) parts of the mediodorsal nucleus (MD_{Pl}) (Fig. 7.18). Cells of the SNR constitute an important component of the output system of the corpus striatum by virtue of their linkage with striatonigral projections. Nigrothalamic fibers terminate in thalamic nuclei, which do not receive afferents from any other part of the corpus striatum. Fluorescent double-labeling studies indicate that nigrothalamic fibers have significant numbers of collaterals that project to the superior colliculus and to nuclei in the midbrain tegmentum (Figs. 7.18 and 7.19). *Nigrotectal fibers* arise only from cells of the pars reticulata, project to the middle gray layers of the caudal two-thirds of the ipsilateral superior colliculus, and appear topographically organized (Fig. 7.19). Projections of nigrotectal fibers are to portions of the superior colliculus that receive inputs not related to the visual system (Fig. 7.19). Fluorescent double retrograde labeling technics indicate that about 20% of the cells in the SNR projecting to the superior colliculus also project to the thalamus. Nigrocollicular projections are considered to play a role in initiating saccadic (rapid) eye movements.

Nigrotegmental fibers arise from GABAergic neurons of the pars reticulata and project to the pedunculopontine nucleus (Fig. 7.18). Cells of the pedunculopontine nucleus (Fig. 7.3) also receive inputs from multiple sources including the cerebral cortex and the medial pallidal segment. A large proportion of SNR neurons, up to 60%, project collaterals to both thalamic nuclei and the pedunculopontine nucleus. Cells in the pedunculopontine nucleus are cholinergic. Although opinion differs concerning the projections of cells in the pedunculopontine nucleus, electron microscopic evidence suggests that part of the fibers from this nucleus terminate upon cells of the SNC.

The substantia nigra is the brain stem nucleus most closely related to the largest part of the corpus striatum, the caudate nucleus and the putamen, and is the only brain nucleus that projects back to that structure in a massive reciprocal fashion. The pars reticulata receives its major input from the caudate nucleus and putamen. These striatonigral fibers have GABA and substance P and the opioid peptide enkephalin as their neurotransmitters. Cells in the pars compacta of the substantia nigra convey dopamine to terminals within the striatum. GABAergic cells of the pars reticulata constitute an important output component of the corpus striatum that is different from that arising from the medial pallidal segment. Although both the pars reticulata and medial pallidal segment project to the pedunculopontine nucleus at midbrain levels, only the pars reticulata has projections to the superior colliculus. Nigrothalamic and pallidothalamic projections collectively constitute the output systems of the corpus striatum complex.

The substantia nigra is the principal site of the pathological process that underlies the metabolic disturbances associated with paralysis agitans. Discrete electrolytic lesions of the substantia nigra in the monkey do not produce tremor, alterations of muscle tone, or impairment of associated movements, although they interfere with a variety of neurotransmitters. Meperdine analogues, such as MPTP, produce severe degeneration in the substantia nigra in humans and monkeys and many features of Parkinson's disease.

CRUS CEREBRI

The most ventral part of the midbrain contains a massive bundle of corticofugal fibers, the crus cerebri. Classically the medial two-thirds of the crus are thought to contain *corticospinal* and *corticobulbar fibers* (Fig. 7.1); the most lateral of these fibers in the crus are related to the lower extremity, the most medial to the musculature of the face and larynx, and the intermediate fibers to the upper extremity. Extreme medial and lateral portions of the crus contain corticopontine fibers. Frontopontine fibers are medial, while corticopontine fibers from the temporal, parietal, and occipital areas are located laterally. More recent data indicate that corticospinal fibers in the internal capsule are largely confined to a compact region in the caudal part of the posterior limb of the internal capsule. Somatotopical organization of fibers destined for particular segmental levels appears relatively crude. These data suggest that the somatotopic arrangement of corticospinal fibers in the crus cerebri probably is much less precise than commonly depicted. In humans, corticospinal fibers probably account for only 1 million of the 20 million fibers in the crus cerebri; the remaining fibers are largely corticopontine.

SUGGESTED READINGS

AITKIN, L. M., WEBSTER, W. R., VEALE, J. L., AND CROSBY, D. C. 1975. Inferior colliculus. I. Comparison of response properties of neurons in central, pericentral and external nuclei of adult cat. J. Neurophysiol., **38**: 1196–1207.

ANDÉN, N. E., DAHLSTRÖM, A., FUXE, K., LARSSON, K., OLSON, L., AND UNGERSTEDT, U. 1966. Ascending monoamine neurons to the telencephalon and diencephalon. Acta Physiol. Scand., **67**: 313–326.

ARSENAULT, M.-Y., PARENT, A., SÉQUELA, P., AND DESCARRIES, L. 1988. Distribution and morphological characteristics of dopamine-immunoreactive neurons in the midbrain of the squirrel monkey (*Saimiri sciureus*). J. Comp. Neurol., **267**: 489–506.

BECKSTEAD, R. M., DOMESICK, V. B., AND NAUTA, W. J. H. 1979. Efferent connections of the substantia nigra and ventral tegmental area in the rat. Brain Res., 175: 191–217.

BEITZ, A. J. 1985. The midbrain periaqueductal gray in the rat. I. Nuclear volume, cell number, density, orientation and regional subdivisions. J. Comp. Neurol., 237: 445–459.

BEITZ, A. J., AND SHEPARD, R. D. 1985. The midbrain periaqueductal gray in the rat. II. A Golgi analysis. J. Comp. Neurol., 237: 460–475.

BENTIVOGLIO, M., VAN DER KOOY, D., AND KUYPERS, H. G. J. M. 1979. The organization of the efferent projections of the substantia nigra in the rat: A retrograde fluorescent double labeling study. Brain Res., 175: 1–17.

CARLETON, S. C., AND CARPENTER, M. B. 1983. Afferent and efferent connections of the medial, inferior and lateral vestibular nuclei in the cat and monkey. Brain Res., 278: 29–51.

CARPENTER, M. B., CARLETON, S. C., KELLER, J. T., AND CONTE, P. 1981. Connections of the subthalamic nucleus in the monkey. Brain Res., 224: 1–29.

CARPENTER, M. B., CHANG, L., PEREIRA, A. B., HERSH, L. B., BRUCE, G., AND WU, J. Y. 1987. Vestibular and cochlear efferent neurons in the monkey identified by immunocytochemical methods. Brain Res., 408: 275–280.

CARPENTER, M. B., AND COWIE, R. J. 1985. Connections and oculomotor projections of the superior vestibular nucleus and cell group "y." Brain Res., 336: 265–287.

CARPENTER, M. B., HARBISON, J. W., AND PETER, P. 1970. Accessory oculomotor nuclei in the monkey: Projections and effects of discrete lesions. J. Comp. Neurol., 140: 131–154.

CARPENTER, M. B., AND PETER, P. 1972. Nigrostriatal and nigrothalamic fibers in the rhesus monkey. J. Comp. Neurol., 144: 93–116.

CARPENTER, M. B., AND McMASTERS, R. E. 1964. Lesions of the substantia nigra in the rhesus monkey: Efferent fiber degeneration and behavioral observations. Am. J. Anat., 114: 293–320.

CARPENTER, M. B., NAKANO, K., AND KIM, R. 1976. Nigrothalamic projections in the monkey demonstrated by autoradiographic technics. J. Comp. Neurol., 165: 401–416.

CARPENTER, M. B., AND PIERSON, R. J. 1973. Pretectal region and the pupillary light reflex: An anatomical analysis in the monkey. J. Comp. Neurol., 149: 271–300.

DiFIGLIA, M., ARONIN, N., AND LEEMAN, S. E. 1981. Immunoreactive substance P in the substantia nigra of the monkey: Light and electron microscopic localization. Brain Res., 233: 381–388.

DiFIGLIA, M., ARONIN, N., AND MARTIN, J. B. 1982. Light and electron microscopic localization of immunoreactive leu-enkephalin in monkey basal ganglia. J. Neurosci., 2: 303–320.

EDWARDS, S. B., AND HENKEL, C. K. 1978. Superior colliculus connections with the extraocular motor nuclei in the cat. J. Comp. Neurol., 179: 451–467.

FREUND, T. F., POWELL, J. F., AND SMITH, A. D. 1984. Tyrosine hydroxylase-immunoreactive synaptic boutons in contact with identified strionigral neurons, with particular reference to dendritic spines. Neuroscience, 13: 1189–1215.

FUKUSHIMA, K. 1987. The interstitial nucleus of Cajal and its role in the control of movements of head and eyes. Prog. Neurobiol., 29: 107–192.

GARCIA-RILL, E. 1986. The basal ganglia and the locomotor regions. Brain Res., 11: 46–63.

GENIEC, P., AND MOREST, D. K. 1971. The neuronal architecture of the human posterior colliculus. Acta Otolaryngol. [Suppl.] (Stockh.), 295: 1–33.

GRAYBIEL, A. M. 1978. A satellite system of the superior colliculus: The parabigeminal nucleus and its projection to the superficial collicular layers. Brain Res., 145: 365–374.

HARTING, K. J., HALL, W. C., DIAMOND, I. T., AND MARTIN, G. F. 1973. Anterograde degeneration study of the superior colliculus in Tupaia glis: Evidence for a subdivision between superficial and deep layers. J. Comp. Neurol., 148: 361–386.

HARTMANN-VON MONAKOW, K., AKERT, K., AND KÜNZLE, H. 1979. Projections of the precentral and premotor cortex to the red nucleus and other midbrain areas in Macaca fascicularis. Exp. Brain Res., 34: 91–105.

HUERTA, M. F., AND HARTING, J. K. 1984. The mammalian superior colliculus: Studies of its morphology and connections. In H. VANEGAS (Editor), Comparative Neurology of the Optic Tectum. Plenum Press, New York.

HUTCHINS, B., AND WEBER, J. T. 1985. The pretectal complex of the monkey: A reinvestigation of the morphology and retinal terminations. J. Comp. Neurol., 232: 425–442.

JAYARAMAN, A., BATTON, R. R., III, AND CARPENTER, M. B. 1977. Nigrotectal projections in the monkey: An autoradiographic study. Brain Res., 135: 147–152.

MAGOUN, H. W. 1954. The ascending reticular system and wakefulness. In J. B. DELAFRESNAYE (Editor), Brain Mechanisms and Consciousness. Blackwell Scientific Publications, Oxford, pp. 1–20.

McGEER, P. L., ECCLES, J. C., AND McGEER, E. G. 1987. Molecular Neurobiology of the Mammalian Brain, Ed. 2. Plenum Press, New York.

MERZENICH, M. M., AND REID, M. D. 1974. Representation of the cochlea within the inferior colliculus of the cat. Brain Res., 77: 397–415.

PARENT, A., BOUCHARD, C., AND SMITH, Y. 1984. The striatopallidal and striatonigral projections: Two distinct systems in primate. Brain Res., 303: 385–390.

PARENT, A., MACKEY, A., AND DeBELLEFEUILLE, L. 1983. The subcortical afferents to caudate nucleus and putamen in primate: A fluorescence retrograde double labeling study. Neuroscience, 10: 1137–1150.

PARENT, A., MACKEY, A., SMITH, Y., AND BOUCHER, R. 1983. The output organization of the substantia nigra in primate as revealed by a retrograde double labeling method. Brain Res. Bull., **10**: 529–537.

PIERSON, R. J., AND CARPENTER, M. B. 1974. Anatomical analysis of pupillary reflex pathways in the rhesus monkey. J. Comp. Neurol., **158**: 121–143.

RICHFIELD, E. K., YOUNG, A., AND PENNY, J. B. 1987. Comparative distribution of dopamine D_1 and D_2 receptors in the basal ganglia of turtles, pigeons, rats, cats and monkeys. J. Comp. Neurol., **262**: 446–463.

ROBERTS, R. C., AND RIBAK, C. E. 1987. GABAergic neurons and axon terminals in the brainstem auditory nuclei of the gerbil. J. Comp. Neurol., **258**: 267–280.

ROBINSON, F. R., HOUK, J. C., AND GIBSON, A. R. 1987. Limb specific connections of the cat magnocellular red nucleus. J. Comp. Neurol., **257**: 553–577.

ROCKEL, A. J., AND JONES, E. G. 1973. The neuronal organization of the inferior colliculus of the adult cat. I. The central nucleus. J. Comp. Neurol., **147**: 11–60.

ROCKEL, A. J., AND JONES, E. G. 1973. The neuronal organization of the inferior colliculus of the adult cat. II. The pericentral nucleus. J. Comp. Neurol., **149**: 301–334.

SEROOGY, K. B., DANGARAN, K., LINN, S., HAYCOCK, J. W., AND FALLON, J. H. 1989. Ventral mesencephalic neurons containing both cholecystokinin- and tyrosine hydroxylase-like immunoreactivities project to forebrain regions. J. Comp. Neurol., **279**: 397–414.

STEIGER, H. J., AND BÜTTNER-ENNEVER, J. A. 1979. Oculomotor nucleus afferents in the monkey demonstrated with horseradish peroxidase. Brain Res., **160**: 1–15.

STERLING, P., AND WICKELGREN, B. G. 1969. Visual receptive fields in the superior colliculus of the cat. J. Neurophysiol., **32**: 1–15.

STRONG, O. S. 1915. A case of unilateral cerebellar agenesia. J. Comp. Neurol., **25**: 587–594.

TOKANO, H., MORIIZAMI, T., KUDO, M., AND NAKAMURA, Y. 1988. A morphological evidence for monosynaptic projections from the nucleus tegmenti pedunculopontine pars compacta (TPC) to nigrostriatal projection neurons. Neurosci. Lett., **85**: 1–4.

8

The Cerebellum

The cerebellum is derived from ectodermal thickenings about the cephalic borders of the fourth ventricle, known as the rhombic lip. Although the cerebellum is derived from portions of the embryonic neural tube dorsal to the sulcus limitans and receives sensory inputs from virtually all types of receptors, it is not concerned with conscious sensory perception. Sensory information transmitted to the cerebellum is used in the automatic coordination of somatic motor function, the regulation of muscle tone and the maintenance of equilibrium. This metencephalic derivative functions in a suprasegmental manner in that its integrative influences affect activities at all levels of the neuraxis. The major influences of the cerebellum on segmental levels of the neuraxis are mediated indirectly by relay nuclei of the brain stem.

Structurally the cerebellum consists of (1) a superficial gray mantle, the *cerebellar cortex*; (2) an internal white mass, the *medullary substance*; and (3) four pairs of *intrinsic nuclei* embedded in the white matter. The cerebellum is divided into a median portion, the *cerebellar vermis*, and two lateral lobes, referred to as the *cerebellar hemispheres*.

The cerebellar cortex is composed of numerous narrow *laminae* or *folia*, most of which are oriented transversely. Five deep fissures divide the cerebellum into lobes and lobules (Fig. 8.1). All of these fissures can be identified in gross specimens as well as in midsagittal section (Figs. 2.28, 2.29, 2.30, and 2.31). The cerebellar fissures are (1) the *primary*, (2) the *posterior superior*, (3) the *horizontal*, (4) the *prepyramidal*, and (5) the *posterolateral* (prenodular). The primary fissure is the deepest of all cerebellar fissures. These fissures form the basis for all subdivisions of the cerebellum (Fig. 8.1). Portions of the cerebellar vermis in Figure 8.1 are labeled by name and by serial *Roman numerals*. The portion of the lateral lobe between the primary and the posterior superior fissures is known as the *simple lobule*. The *ansiform lobule* lies between the posterior superior fissure and the gracile lobule and is divided by the horizontal fissure into *crus I* (superior semilunar lobule) and *crus II* (inferior semilunar lobule). The *biventer lobule* and the *cerebellar tonsil* lie between the prepyramidal and posterolateral fissures in the cerebellar hemisphere (Fig. 2.30). The posterolateral fissure separates the nodulus from the uvula in the cerebellar vermis.

Embryologically and functionally the cerebellum can be divided into three parts: the archicerebellum, the paleocerebellum, and the neocerebellum.

The *archicerebellum*, represented by the *nodulus*, the paired *flocculi* and their peduncular connections (i.e., the *flocculonodular lobule*), is phylogenetically the oldest part. This division of the cerebellum is most

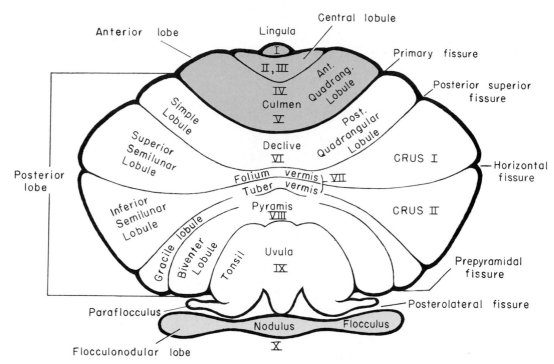

Figure 8.1.   Schematic diagram of the fissures and lobules of the cerebellum rolled flat in a single plane. Portions of the cerebellum caudal to the posterolateral fissure (*blue*) represent the flocculonodular lobule (archicerebellum), while portions of the cerebellum rostral to the primary fissure (*red*) constitute the anterior lobe (paleocerebellum). The neocerebellum lies between the primary and the posterolateral fissures. *Roman numerals*, referring to portions of the cerebellar vermis, are used to indicate lobules.

closely related to the vestibular system and is separated from the posterior lobe of the cerebellum by the posterolateral fissure (*blue* in Fig. 8.1).

The *paleocerebellum* (i.e., the anterior lobe of the cerebellum) lies rostral to the primary fissure (*red* in Fig. 8.1). This division of the cerebellum receives impulses from stretch receptors via the spinocerebellar tracts and is the part most concerned with the regulation of muscle tone.

The *neocerebellum* is the largest and phylogenetically newest part of the cerebellum. This part of the cerebellum lies between the primary and posterolateral fissures and constitutes the posterior lobe (Fig. 8.1). The neocerebellum receives inputs from the contralateral cerebral cortex via relays in the pontine nuclei, and is the part of the cerebellum most concerned with coordination of somatic motor function.

The gross anatomy of the cerebellum is described in Chapter 2, pages 52–54. The cerebellum is attached to the medulla, pons, and midbrain by three paired cerebellar peduncles. These peduncles serve to connect the cerebellum with the spinal cord, brain stem and higher levels of the neuraxis (Figs. 2.21 and 2.30).

CEREBELLAR CORTEX

The cerebellar cortex is uniformly structured in all parts and extends across the midline without evidence of a median raphe (Fig. 2.28). The cortex is composed of three well-defined layers containing five different types of neurons. These layers from the surface are (1) the molecular layer, (2) the Purkinje cell layer, and (3) the granular layer (Figs. 8.2, 8.3, and 8.4).

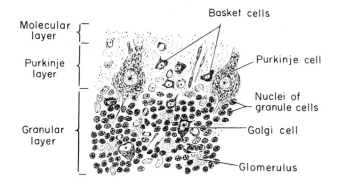

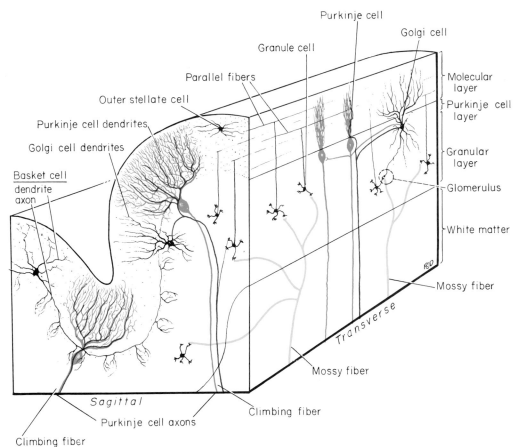

Figure 8.3. Schematic diagram of the cerebellar cortex in sagittal and transverse planes showing cell and fiber arrangements. Purkinje cells and cell processes (i.e., axons and dendrites) are shown in *blue*. Mossy fibers are in *yellow*; climbing fibers are shown in *red*. Golgi cells, basket cells, and outer stellate cells are in *black*. While the dendritic arborizations of Purkinje cells are oriented in a sagittal plane, dendrites of the Golgi cells show no similar arrangement. Layers of the cerebellar cortex are indicated. (From Carpenter and Sutin, *Human Neuroanatomy*, 1983; courtesy of Williams & Wilkins.)

Molecular Layer

The molecular layer contains two types of neurons, dendritic arborizations of cells in deeper layers, and numerous thin axons coursing parallel to the long axis of the folia. Cells found in the molecular layer are the basket cell and the outer stellate cell (Figs. 8.3 and 8.4). Dendrites of these cells are confined to the molecular layer, as are the axons of the outer stellate cells. Processes of both cells are oriented in a sagittal plane (transversely to the long axis of the folia). Axons of *outer stellate cells*

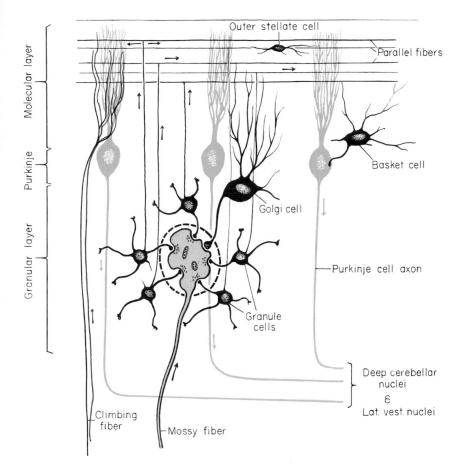

Molecular layer

Purkinje

Granular layer

Outer stellate cell

Parallel fibers

Basket cell

Golgi cell

Purkinje cell axon

Granule
cells

Deep cerebellar
nuclei
&
Lat. vest. nuclei

Climbing
fiber

Mossy fiber

Figure 8.4. Schematic diagram of the cellular and fiber elements of the cerebellar cortex in the longitudinal axis of a folium. Excitatory inputs to the cerebellar cortex are conveyed by the mossy fibers (*yellow*) and the climbing fibers (*red*). The *broken line* represents a glia lamella ensheathing a glomerulus, containing (1) a mossy fiber rosette, (2) several granule cell dendrites, and (3) one Golgi cell axon. Axons of granule cells ascend to the molecular layer, bifurcate, and form an extensive system of parallel fibers which synapse on the spiny processes of the Purkinje cells. Purkinje cells and their processes are shown in *blue*. Climbing fibers traverse the granular layer and ascend the dendrites of the Purkinje cells where they synapse on smooth branchlets. *Arrows* indicate the directions of impulse conduction. Outer stellate and basket cells are shown in the molecular layer, but the axons of the basket cells which ramify about Purkinje cell somata are not shown. (From Carpenter and Sutin, *Human Neuroanatomy*, 1983; courtesy of Williams & Wilkins.)

make synaptic contacts with Purkinje cell dendrites. *Basket cells*, located in deep parts of this layer near Purkinje cell bodies, give rise to dendrites that ascend in the molcular layer and elaborate unmyelinated axons that form intricate terminal arborizations about the somata of many Purkinje cells in a sagittal plane (Fig. 8.3). A single basket cell may establish synaptic relationships with 10 Purkinje cells in a plane transverse to the folia. In addition to the relatively few cells, the molecular layer contains the dendrites of Purkinje and Golgi type II cells and the transversely oriented axons of granule cells (i.e., parallel fibers) (Fig. 8.4).

Purkinje Cell Layer

This layer consists of great numbers of large flask-shaped cells uniformly arranged along the upper margin of the granular layer (Figs. 8.2, 8.3, 8.4, 8.5, and 8.6). Purkinje cells have a clear vesicular nucleus with a deep-staining nucleolus and irregular Nissl granules. Each cell gives rise to an elaborate flattened, fanlike dendritic tree oriented at right angles to the long axis of the folia. The full extent of the dendritic arborization can be appreciated only in sagittal sections (Figs. 8.3, 8.5, and 8.6). Primary and secondary dendritic branches are smooth, but tertiary dendritic branches have spines that are short, thick, and rough. These thick dendritic spines are referred to as *spiny branchlets* or *gemmules* (Fig. 8.5). Larger dendritic processes bear stubbier spines known as *smooth branchlets*. Purkinje cell axons are myelinated, pass through the granular layer and white matter, and establish synaptic contacts with the deep cerebellar nuclei (Fig. 8.4). Purkinje cell axons project to the deep cerebellar nuclei by the shortest direct route. The unique feature of Purkinje

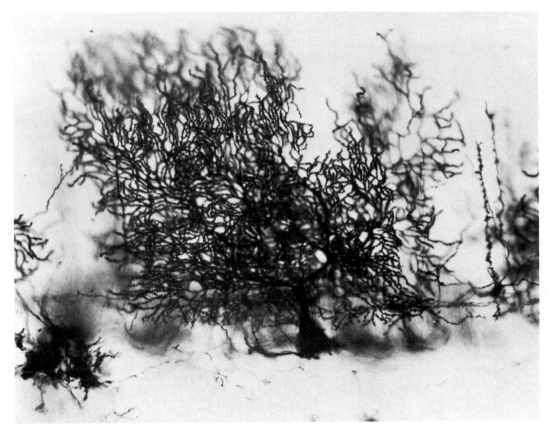

Figure 8.5.   Photograph of a single Purkinje cell and its rich dendritic arborizations in the molecular layer (× 300). (Courtesy of the late Dr. C. A. Fox, School of Medicine, Wayne State University.) (From Carpenter and Sutin, *Human Neuroanatomy*, 1983; courtesy of Williams & Wilkins.)

cells is their pericular monoplanar shape (Figs. 8.3 and 8.4). Both the dendritic arbors and the axonal projections of Purkinje cells lie in a single plane perpendicular to the major axis of the folia. Purkinje cell axons represent the discharge pathway from the cerebellar cortex. Purkinje cell collaterals make synaptic contact with Golgi type II cells in the granular layer (Fig. 8.3). Histochemical studies indicate that most Purkinje cells contain γ-aminobutyric acid (GABA), which acts as the principal neurotransmitter. Purkinje cells of the cerebellum were the first neurons to be identified (1837) and the first neurons to be analyzed in microscopic detail. They are also the first class of neurons for which a specific immunological marker, not related to the biosynthesis of a neurotransmitter, has been identified. Guanosine 3′:5′-phosphate-dependent protein kinase (cGK) antiserum is a specific immunohistochemical marker for Purkinje cells. This marker labels Purkinje cell cytoplasm, dendrites, and axonal ramifications (Fig. 8.6).

Granular Layer

This layer is composed of closely packed chromatic nuclei that in Nissl-stained sections resemble lymphocytes (Fig. 8.2). Granule cells are so tightly packed (3 to 7 million cells per cubic millimeter) that residual space seems insufficient to accommodate their processes and fibers of passage. These cells are round or oval, 5–8 μm in diameter, with aggregated chromatin granules near the nuclear membrane. Granule cell nuclei appear as naked nuclei because of the thinness of the rimming cytoplasm and the absence of discrete Nissl granules. Granule cells are immuno-

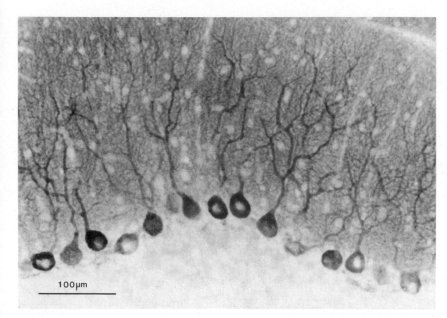

Figure 8.6.   Sagittal section of the rat cerebellar cortex immunoreacted with antiserum to guanosine 3′ : 5′ phosphate-dependent protein kinase (cGK), a specific immunohistochemical marker for Purkinje cells. This immunological marker is not related to the biosynthesis of any neurotransmitters, but specifically labels all parts of the Purkinje cell. With this immunohistochemical marker the Purkinje cell somata, dendrites, axons, axon collaterals, and terminals can be imaged. (Courtesy of Dr. P. De Camilli, Department of Cell Biology, School of Medicine, Yale University.)

reactive for glutamate. Each granule cell gives rise to four or five short dendrites with clawlike endings which terminate in the "glomeruli" (Fig. 8.7). The so-called cerebellar islands or glomeruli are irregularly dispersed spaces free of granule cells (Figs. 8.2 and 8.3). Axons of granule cells are unmyelinated fibers that ascend vertically into the molecular layer and bifurcate into branches which run parallel to the long axis of the folium (Figs. 8.3 and 8.4). These fibers, referred to as *parallel fibers*, are found throughout the molecular layer where they are oriented perpendicular to the sagittal fan-shaped dendritic expansions of the Purkinje cells. In a descriptive sense, they resemble telegraph wires strung through the branches of a bushy tree. Granule cell axons make synaptic contacts with the spiny processes of Purkinje cells. This synaptic contact between the parallel fibers and the Purkinje cell dendrites is called the "crossover" synapse (Figs. 8.3 and 8.4).

   Golgi type II cells, found mainly in the upper parts of the granular layer, have vesicular nuclei, definite chromophilic bodies, and are strongly GABAergic (Figs. 8.2, 8.3, 8.4, and 8.10). Dendrites of these cells extend throughout all layers of the cerebellar cortex, and arborizations are not restricted to one plane (Figs. 8.3 and 8.4). Golgi cell dendrites are contacted by parallel fibers in the molecular layer, while axonal arborizations are dense within the granular layer beneath the cell body. Axons of these cells terminate within the cerebellar "glomeruli."

Cortical Input

   Afferents to the cerebellum convey impulses primarily to the cerebellar cortex. These tracts enter the cerebellum mainly via the inferior and middle cerebellar peduncles and include the spinocerebellar, cuneocerebellar, olivocerebellar, vestibulocerebellar, and pontocerebellar tracts, as well as numerous smaller bundles. Within the cerebellar cortex

Figure 8.7. Photomicrograph of granule cells in the cerebellar cortex showing short dendrites with clawlike endings. Golgi preparation (× 200). (Courtesy of Dr. Donald B. Newman, Uniformed Services University.)

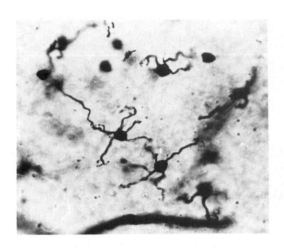

these fibers lose their myelin sheath and end either as mossy fibers or climbing fibers.

Mossy fibers bifurcate repeatedly in the white matter, enter the granular layer and often provide branches to adjacent folia (Fig. 8.3). In the granular layer fibers lose their myelin sheath and give off many fine collaterals. Fine lobulated enlargements occur along the course of the branches and at their terminals; these are referred to as *mossy fiber rosettes*. A single mossy fiber may have as many as 44 mossy fiber rosettes along its many branches. Each mossy fiber rosette forms the center of a cerebellar glomerulus. In Golgi preparations under oil immersion, mossy fiber rosettes appear as coiled, convoluted fibers (Fig. 8.8). Electron micrographs also reveal synaptic vesicles, concentrations of mitochondria neurofilaments, and neurotubules.

A cerebellar *glomerulus* is a complex synaptic structure contained within the "cerebellar islands" of the granular layer (Figs. 8.3, 8.4, and 8.9). The glomerular complex is a nodular structure formed by (1) one mossy fiber rosette, (2) the dendritic terminals of numerous granule cells, (3) the terminals of Golgi cell axons, and (4) proximal parts of Golgi cell dendrites (Fig. 8.9). The center of the glomerulus contains a single mossy fiber rosette (Fig. 8.8) with which dendrites of about 20 different granule cells interdigitate (Figs. 8.4, 8.7, and 8.9). Axons of Golgi cells form a plexus on the outer surface of the granule cell dendrites. The entire structure is ensheathed in a single glial lamella. In the glomerulus the mossy fiber-granule cell synapse is excitatory, while the Golgi axon-granule cell junction is inhibitory. Thus a cerebellar glomerulus is a synaptic cluster in which two types of presynaptic fibers enter into a complex relationship with one postsynaptic element. The granule cell dendrites constitute the postsynaptic element. Golgi cells function as a negative feedback to the mossy fiber-granule cell relay. Mossy fibers constitute the principal mode of termination of most cerebellar afferent systems. The spinocerebellar, pontocerebellar, and vestibulocerebellar systems terminate as mossy fibers.

Climbing fibers pass from the white matter through the granular and Purkinje cell layer to reach the dendrites of the Purkinje cells (Figs. 8.3 and 8.4). These nonmyelinated fibers divide into numerous branches and climb the dendritic arborizations of the Purkinje cells. Climbing fibers contact only the smooth branches of Purkinje cell dendrites. Many climbing fibers form infraganglionic plexuses immediately beneath the Purkinje cell layer before turning toward the surface to be displayed over the dendritic arbor of a single Purkinje cell (Figs. 8.3 and 8.4). Collaterals

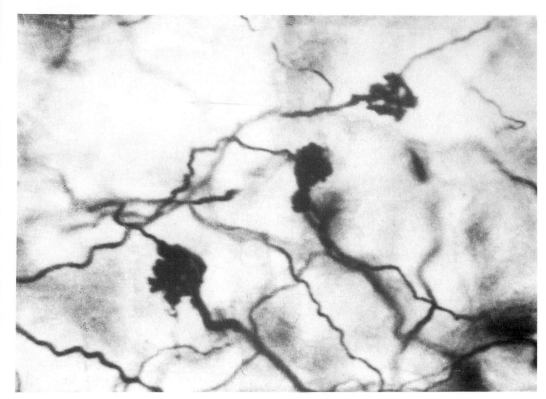

Figure 8.8.   Mossy fiber rosettes in the granular layer of the monkey cerebellum as seen in a Golgi preparation. Although mossy fiber rosettes appear as solid structures under low magnifications, under oil immersion the rosettes appear as coiled convoluted fibers (× 850). (Courtesy of the late Dr. C. A. Fox, School of Medicine, Wayne State University.) (From Carpenter and Sutin, *Human Neuroanatomy*, 1983; courtesy of Williams & Wilkins.)

of climbing fibers may establish synaptic contact with adjacent Purkinje cells.

Physiologically the climbing fiber system is remarkably specific. Each climbing fiber possesses an extensive all-or-none excitatory connection with Purkinje cell dendrites. When a climbing fiber discharges, the Purkinje cell also discharges. Stimulation of a climbing fiber not only excites a single Purkinje cell, but it also excites a number of granule cells whose axons (parallel fibers) in turn excite Purkinje cells arranged in the long axis of a folium. Climbing fibers originate from the inferior olivary complex, are crossed and appear to have glutamate as their neurotransmitter. Olivocerebellar fibers terminate in a pattern of thin sagittal strips that interdigitate with unlabeled strips. Because it has been shown that olivary neurons distribute fibers to different regions of the cerebellar cortex, it has been postulated that the empty strips receive climbing fibers from other unlabeled regions of the inferior olivary nucleus, rather than from extraolivary sources.

Fluorescence microscopy has revealed a hitherto unrecognized fiber system in the cerebellar cortex that contains norepinephrine. These fibers, detectable by their green fluorescence, are present in all layers of the cortex, are not restricted to any particular plane, and are moderately concentrated in the Purkinje cell layer. These fibers are considered to arise from the locus ceruleus (Figs. 6.27, 6.28, and 6.29) and establish synaptic contacts with Purkinje cells somata. Cells in the caudal half of the locus ceruleus project to the entire cerebellar vermis, the flocculus, and the ventral paraflocculus.

Figure 8.9. Schematic reconstruction of a cerebellar glomerulus based upon electron microscopic studies. A cerebellar glomerulus is formed by one mossy fiber rosette, the dendritic terminals of numerous granule cells (*red*), and terminals of Golgi cell axons (*yellow*). Proximal parts of Golgi dendrites (*blue*) also enter the glomerulus and establish broad synaptic contacts with the mossy fiber rosette. The entire nodular structure is ensheathed in a glial capsule. In this reconstruction the glomerulus is shown in horizontal section, and in a schematic three-dimensional view. (From Carpenter and Sutin, *Human Neuroanatomy*; courtesy of Williams & Wilkins.)

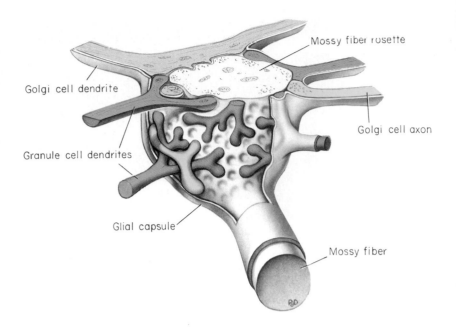

The raphe nuclei, which synthesize and transmit serotonin (5-hydroxytryptamine; 5-HT) to various parts of the central nervous system, project fibers to the cerebellum, presumably via periventricular routes. The largest number of serotonergic fibers appear to arise from the raphe nuclei of the pons and medulla (Fig. 5.13). All parts of the cerebellar cortex receive afferents from the raphe nuclei, with the most profuse projections passing to lobules VII and X of the vermis and to crus I and II. Axons of raphe neurons terminate as mossy fiber rosettes in the granular layer and end diffusely throughout all cortical layers. Serotonergic fibers differ from noradrenergic afferents in that they do not synapse upon Purkinje cells.

Structural Mechanisms

Geometric relationships of elements within the cerebellar cortex have furnished many hypotheses concerning the functions of individual neurons. Physiological studies indicate that (1) climbing fibers exert powerful excitatory synaptic drives on Purkinje cell dendrites; (2) parallel fiber systems excite Purkinje cells via "cross-over" synapses; and (3) outer stellate cells, basket cells, and Golgi type II cells are inhibitory interneurons in the cerebellar cortex. Outer stellate cells exert inhibitory influences on dendrites of Purkinje cells. Basket cell inhibition is effected by axo-somatic synapses on many Purkinje cells in a sagittal plane. Golgi type II cells inhibit afferent input to the cerebellar cortex at the mossy fiber-granule cell relay in the glomeruli (Figs. 8.4, 8.9, and 8.10). Because Golgi cell axons reach glomeruli throughout the depth of the cerebellar cortex, they can inhibit mossy fiber input to parallel fibers (Fig. 8.4).

The entire output of the cerebellar cortex is represented by the discharge of Purkinje cells. Every Purkinje cell is subject to two distinct excitatory inputs via (1) climbing fibers and (2) mossy fibers. Climbing fibers have powerful, direct, all-or-none, excitatory action on a single Purkinje cell. The same climbing fiber has synaptic articulations with inhibitory interneurons, the Golgi type II, stellate, and basket cells. Excitation of basket cells results in inhibition of Purkinje cells on both sides

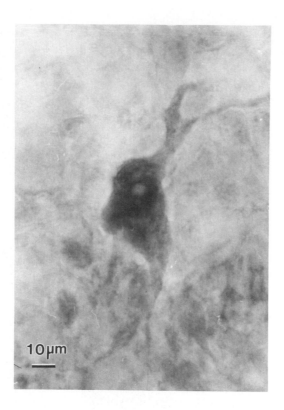

Figure 8.10. Golgi type II neuron in the superficial granular layer of the cerebellar cortex immunoreacted with GABA. These cells show more intense immunostaining with antiserum to GABA than Purkinje cells.

of the single Purkinje cell receiving the main branches of a climbing fiber. A single basket cell theoretically could inhibit 7 rows of about 10 Purkinje cells. The excitation of Golgi cells via climbing fibers results in the inhibition of impulses through all glomeruli reached by the ramifications of the Golgi cell axon. This mechanism depresses the activity in Purkinje cells on both sides of the single Purkinje cell excited by the climbing fiber. The widespread inhibitory influence exerted by a single climbing fiber via interneurons appears to be a device to silence the background for a single Purkinje cell activated by a climbing fiber volley.

Mossy fiber impulses exert their synaptic excitatory action solely within the cerebellar glomerulus, where they excite granule cells whose axons (the parallel fibers) excite all cells with dendrites in the molecular layer (i.e., Purkinje, basket, stellate, and Golgi cells). Impulses conveyed to dendrites in the molecular layer by parallel fibers result in excitation of (1) a narrow band of Purkinje and Golgi cells in the longitudinal axis of the folia, and (2) basket and outer stellate cells whose axons extend sagittally (transverse to the folia) on each side of the excited band of parallel fibers. This geometric configuration results in excitation of a narrow band of Purkinje cells, flanked on each side by Purkinje cells inhibited by basket and stellate cells.

The entire output of the cerebellar cortex, conveyed by Purkinje cell axons, is inhibitory. Thus, axons of Purkinje cells exert inhibitory influences on cells with which they synapse, namely the deep cerebellar nuclei and portions of the vestibular nuclei. The neurotransmitter responsible for Purkinje cell inhibition is γ-aminobutyric acid (GABA). Purkinje cell collaterals taking origin from proximal portions of the axon (Fig. 8.3) exert inhibitory influences on Golgi cells, which in turn inhibit granule cells; this disinhibition tends to release granule cells whose axons excite Purkinje cells.

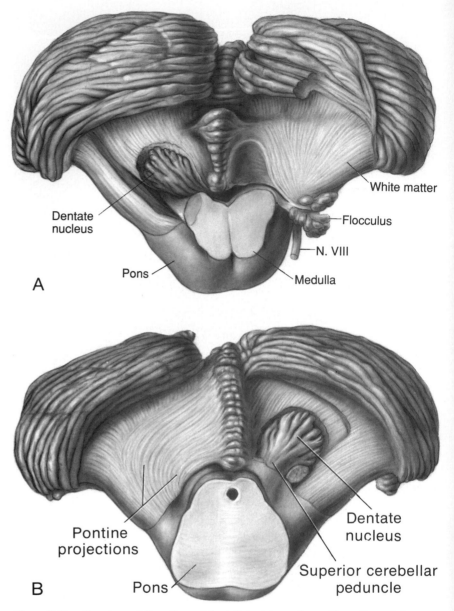

Figure 8.11. Drawings of dissections of the left dentate nucleus with portions of the cerebellar cortex and vermis intact. *A*, Dissection of the posterior surface of the cerebellum exposing the dentate nucleus. *B*, Dissection of the superior surface of the cerebellum from above showing the left dentate nucleus in relationship to the isthmus of the pons. (From Mettler's *Neuroanatomy*, 1948.)

DEEP CEREBELLAR NUCLEI

The corpus medullare is a compact mass of white matter, continuous from hemisphere to hemisphere. The four paired deep cerebellar nuclei are imbedded in the white matter of the cerebellum. From medial to lateral these nuclei are the fastigial, the globose, the emboliform and the dentate.

Dentate Nucleus

This nucleus, the largest of the deep cerebellar nuclei, lies in the white matter of the cerebellar hemisphere (Figs. 8.11, 8.12, and 8.13). In transverse section this large nucleus appears as a convoluted band of

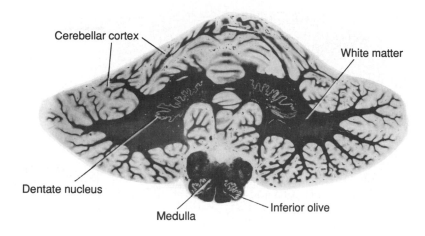

Cerebellar cortex

White matter

Dentate nucleus

Medulla

Inferior olive

Figure 8.12. Transverse Weigert-stained section through the cerebellum and medulla. This photomicrograph provides a comparison of the size and shape of the dentate nucleus and the inferior olivary nuclear complex.

gray, having the shape of a folded bag with the opening or hilus directed medially. Its resemblance to the inferior olivary complex is obvious (Fig. 8.12). The nucleus is composed mainly of large multipolar neurons with branching dendrites.

Emboliform Nucleus

This is a wedge-shaped cell mass situated close to the hilus of the dentate nucleus, composed of cells similar to those found in the dentate nucleus and often difficult to delimit from the latter (Figs. 6.22 and 8.13).

Globose Nucleus

This nucleus consists of one or more rounded cell groups lying medial to the emboliform nucleus and lateral to the fastigial nucleus (Figs. 6.22 and 8.13). This nucleus contains both large and small multipolar neurons.

In lower mammals the emboliform and globose nuclei appear continuous and collectively are referred to as the *nucleus interpositus*. Cytological differences and distinctive connections make it possible to divide this complex into two parts: (1) the anterior interposed nucleus, considered to be the homologue of the emboliform nucleus, and (2) the posterior interposed nucleus, which is homologous to the globose nucleus.

Fastigial Nucleus

The most medial of the deep cerebellar nuclei, the fastigial nucleus, lies near the mid-line in the roof of the fourth ventricle (Fig. 6.22). There are cytological differences within the fastigial nucleus, in that smaller cells are found in ventral regions. Cell strands emerging from the lateral border of the nucleus extend ventrolaterally toward the vestibular nuclei. Both large and small cells have dendrites radiating in all directions which bear spines on distal branches. Dendritic fields of neurons within the nucleus show extensive overlap, but there are no Golgi type II cells. Unlike the other deep cerebellar nuclei, cells of the fastigial nucleus give rise to both crossed and uncrossed axons; axons crossing to the opposite side are most numerous in rostral regions of the nucleus. Unlike Purkinje cells, cells of the deep cerebellar nuclei are excitatory and project beyond the cerebellum. Immunocytochemical data suggest that glutamate and aspartate may be the excitatory neurotransmitter of all cells in the deep cerebellar nuclei. Thus, Purkinje cells, which provide the only output from the

Figure 8.13. Horizontal section through adult cerebellum showing portions of the deep cerebellar nuclei and the corpus medullare (Cm). Weigert's myelin stain. Photograph. (From Carpenter and Sutin, *Human Neuroanatomy*, 1983; courtesy of Williams & Wilkins.)

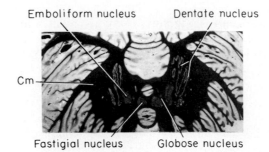

Emboliform nucleus   Dentate nucleus

Cm

Fastigial nucleus   Globose nucleus

cerebellar cortex, project in an orderly systematic fashion to the deep cerebellar nuclei. Purkinje cells inhibit the excitatory output system, which originates from the nuclear masses within the white matter of the cerebellum.

CONNECTIONS OF THE DEEP CEREBELLAR NUCLEI

Corticonuclear Projections

The largest number of afferents to the deep cerebellar nuclei arise from Purkinje cells and have GABA as their neurotransmitter. All parts of the cerebellar cortex project fibers to the deep cerebellar nuclei. Cerebellar cortical projections to the deep cerebellar nuclei form three rostrocaudal longitudinal zones: (1) a medial or vermal zone projecting to the fastigial nucleus, (2) a paravermal zone projecting to the interposed nuclei, and (3) a lateral or hemispheric zone projecting to the dentate nucleus.

The *medial cortical zone*, constituting the vermis proper, projects to the fastigial nucleus and is strictly unilateral. Fibers from the lobules of the vermis project to the nearest region of the fastigial nucleus which results in a sequential representation of the cerebellar vermis in the fastigial nucleus. Each fastigial nuclus receives afferents from a narrow band of Purkinje cells in the ipsilateral cerebellar vermis in folia of lobules I through X. Information concerning the *paravermal* and *lateral longitudinal cerebellar zones* is less precise, but the same principle appears to apply. Studies based upon anterograde transport technics support the concept of three rostrocaudal zones projecting, respectively, to the fastigial, interposed and dentate nuclei. Other data indicate that nucleocortical fibers from the deep cerebellar nuclei project collaterals back to their specific cortical zones. Corticonuclear and nucleocortical fibers have reciprocal relationships.

Nucleocortical Projections

The conceptional division of the cerebellum into three sagittal zones, each consisting of a longitudinal strip of cerebellar cortex and the deep cerebellar nucleus to which its Purkinje cells project, has been strengthened by the observation that cells in the deep cerebellar nuclei project recurrent collaterals to the cortex in a specific manner. Tracer substances injected into a localized region of the cerebellar cortex results in retrograde transport to cells of a single deep cerebellar nucleus, and injections of [³H]amino acids into the deep cerebellar nuclei can be traced anterograde into the cerebellar cortex. Nucleocortical and corticonuclear projections are reciprocally organized, so that neurons in the deep cerebellar nuclei project back to regions of the cerebellar cortex from which they receive input. Axons of the deep cerebellar nuclei projecting to the cerebellar cortex arise from a heterogenous population of cells, similar to those that project fibers to the thalamus and brain stem. Some cells in the dentate and interposed nuclei have collateral axons that project via the superior cerebellar peduncle to the thalamus and inferior olive, as well as to the cerebellar cortex. Nucleocortical collaterals terminate in the granular layer of the cerebellar cortex. Since the nucleocortical projection arises from axon collaterals of deep cerebellar neurons, the same signals projected to brain stem nuclei are fed back to the cerebellar cortex. These collateral projections from the deep cerebellar nuclei represent a major afferent system to the cerebellar cortex.

Extracerebellar Inputs

Although the Purkinje cells exert inhibitory influences on the deep cerebellar nuclei, these nuclei maintain a high-frequency excitatory discharge. It is presumed that excitatory inputs from extracerebellar sources overcome the tonic inhibitory output from the cerebellar cortex. The current thesis is that extracerebellar inputs to the deep cerebellar nuclei provide the tonic facilitation which at times predominates over the cortical inhibition and maintains the discharge of impulses directed toward brain stem nuclei.

The dentate nucleus receives afferents from (1) the pontine nuclei, (2) the principal inferior olivary nucleus, (3) the trigeminal sensory nuclei, (4) the reticulotegmental nucleus, (5) the locus ceruleus, and (6) the raphe nuclei. The largest number of afferent fibers appear to arise from the pontine nuclei, the inferior olivary nucleus and the reticulotegmental nucleus. Both ipsilateral and contralateral pontine nuclei project to the dentate nucleus, but the larger number of fibers arise from the opposite side. Olivocerebellar fibers pass to all parts of the cerebellar cortex and to the deep cerebellar nuclei. Afferent projections to the dentate nucleus are crossed and arise from cells of the principal inferior olivary nucleus. The interposed nuclei receive crossed fibers from the medial and dorsal accessory olivary nuclei, and the fastigial nucleus receives fibers from subdivisions of the medial accessory olive. These projections to the deep cerebellar nuclei probably are collaterals of climbing fibers. The anterior interposed nucleus (i.e., the emboliform nucleus) receives a projection from the red nucleus that is crossed, and is reciprocal to the major projection from this nucleus.

SOMATOTOPIC LOCALIZATION

Afferent systems conveying sensory information from various kinds of receptors in different parts of the body are localized to particular parts of the cerebellum.

Exteroceptive impulses, such as tactile sense, audition, and vision, give rise to action potentials in specific regions of the cerebellum which are somatotopically organized (Fig. 8.14). Tactile stimulation evokes potentials ipsilaterally in the anterior lobe and simple lobule, and bilaterally in the paramedian lobules. The leg area is represented in the central lobule, the arm in the culmen, and the head and face in the simple lobule. The somatotopic localization is the reverse in the paramedian lobules with the leg represented caudally and the head represented rostrally. Responses in this pattern were most easily obtained from skin receptors or cutaneous nerves. The head area was found to partially overlap the middle region of the vermis (i.e., simple lobule, folium and tuber, and

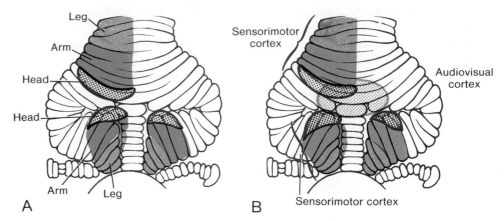

Figure 8.14. Schematic diagrams of somatotopic localization in the cerebellar cortex of the monkey. *A*, diagram of the tactile receiving areas of the cerebellum mapped by potentials recorded in response to movement of hairs on the left side of the body. *B*, diagram of cerebellar cortical areas responding to stimulation of the sensorimotor, auditory, and visual cortex in the right hemisphere. The leg (*red*), arm (*blue*), and head (*black stipple*) are represented ipsilaterally in the anterior lobe and bilaterally in reversed fashion in the paramedian lobules. The auditory and visual cortex (*blue stipple*) are represented in the simple lobule, folium, tuber, and adjacent cortex. (From Carpenter and Sutin, *Human Neuroanatomy*, 1983; courtesy of Williams & Wilkins.)

adjacent areas) where action potentials were recorded following auditory and visual stimuli (Fig. 8.14). The same somatotopic regions of the cerebellum can be activated by stimulating corresponding areas of the sensorimotor cortex contralaterally. Stimulation of the auditory and visual cortex in cerebrum likewise produced potentials in the audiovisual representation in the cerebellum.

CEREBELLAR CONNECTIONS

Afferent Fibers

The cerebellum receives inputs generated in virtually all kinds of receptors in all parts of the body. Most afferents enter the cerebellum via the inferior and middle cerebellar peduncles. Afferent fibers exceed efferent fibers by an estimated ratio of about 40:1.

The *inferior cerebellar peduncle* consists of a larger entirely afferent portion, the restiform body and a smaller medial juxtarestiform portion containing both afferent and efferent fibers. The juxtarestiform body (Fig. 6.22) contains primary and secondary vestibulocerebellar fibers and cerebellovestibular originating from the nodulus, uvula, and the fastigial nuclei. Brain stem afferents to the cerebellar cortex are relayed by the inferior olive and a number of smaller nuclei located in the medulla. Nuclei in the brain stem that project to the cerebellum are collectively referred to as *precerebellar nuclei*.

The pontine nuclei represent the most massive collection of precerebellar nuclei, and they constitute the most important relay in the conduction of impulses from the cerebral cortex to the cerebellum. Corticopontine fibers arise from the cortex of the four major lobes of the cerebrum and terminate upon ipsilateral pontine nuclei. Cortical projections from the primary motor and sensory cortex and portions of the visual cortex give rise to the major corticopontine fibers. Although projections from the motor and somatosensory areas are somatotopically organized they are separated from each other. All fibers from the pontine nuclei project into the *middle cerebellar peduncle*. Projections to the cortex of the cerebellar hemisphere are crossed, while those to the vermal cortex are bilateral. The nodulus appears to be the only part of the cerebellum that does not receive a pontine projection. Pontocerebellar fibers terminate as mossy fibers, and most cerebellar lobules receive afferents from two or more different sites within the pontine nuclei.

Efferent Fibers

Cerebellar efferent fibers arise from all of the deep cerebellar nuclei and from specific regions of the cerebellar cortex. Direct projections from the cortex of the vermis and from the vestibulocerebellum (i.e., regions of the cerebellar cortex receiving vestibular inputs) pass to the ipsilateral vestibular nuclear complex and collectively constitute the cerebellovestibular projection. The largest and most widely distributed efferent fibers from the cerebellum arise from the deep cerebellar nuclei. Cerebellar efferent fibers from the deep cerebellar nuclei are organized into two main systems contained in three separate bundles. The major efferent systems are the superior cerebellar peduncle and the fastigial efferent projections.

Superior Cerebellar Peduncle

The largest cerebellar efferent bundle, the superior cerebellar peduncle, is formed by fibers arising from cells in the dentate, emboliform, and globose nuclei (Figs. 2.21, 2.22, 6.22, and 6.26). These fibers emerge from the hilus of the dentate nucleus and pass rostrally into the upper pons where they form a compact bundle along the dorsolateral wall of the fourth ventricle (Fig. 8.11). At isthmus levels, fibers of the superior cerebellar peduncle sweep ventromedially into the tegmentum and all fibers decussate at levels through the inferior colliculus (Figs. 6.26 and 7.2). Most of these crossed fibers ascend to enter and surround the contralateral red nucleus. A relatively small part of the fibers from the dentate nucleus terminate in the rostral third of the red nucleus. The bulk of these fibers project to the thalamus and end in parts of the ventral lateral and ventral posterolateral thalamic nuclei (Fig. 8.15). Fibers from the dentate nucleus terminate somatotopically in the ventral posterolateral (pars oralis, VPLo) and the ventral lateral (pars caudalis, VLc) thalamic nuclei. Although somatotopical features of the deep cerebellar nuclei are not compelling, the pattern of terminations of these fibers in thalamic nuclear subdivisions appears similar to that of somatosensory relay nuclei (Fig. 9.15). In this arrangement the head is represented medially and caudal parts of the body are lateral; the extremities lie ventrally and the back lies dorsally. A small number of fibers from the dentate nucleus project to the rostral intralaminar thalamic nuclei, mainly the central lateral (CL) nucleus. The ventral lateral (VLc) and the ventral posterolateral (VPLo) nuclei of the thalamus project on the primary motor cortex (Fig. 9.16). Thus impulses from the dentate nucleus are conveyed via contralateral thalamic nuclei to the motor cortex. In this manner, signals from the dentate nucleus can influence activity of motor neurons in the cerebral cortex; impulses from the motor cortex are transmitted to spinal levels via the corticospinal tract. This system, concerned primarily with the coordination of somatic motor function, also provides the explanation for occurrence of ipsilateral asynergic disturbances with unilateral cerebellar lesions.

Fibers from the interposed nuclei (i.e., the emboliform and globose nuclei) project primarily to cells in the caudal two-thirds of the red nucleus

Figure 8.15. Schematic diagram of the efferent fibers from the dentate nucleus. These fibers emerge as the major constituent of the superior cerebellar peduncle (*blue*) and decussate completely in the caudal mesencephalon. Ascending fibers project to rostral parts of the contralateral red nucleus and to the cell sparse zone of the thalamus [i.e., ventral lateral nucleus, pars caudalis (VLc) and the ventral posterolateral nucleus, pars oralis (VPLo)]. Fibers from the dentate nucleus terminate somatotopically in these thalamic nuclei, which in turn project upon the primary motor cortex (area 4, Fig. 9.16). Fibers forming the descending division of the superior cerebellar peduncle project to reticular nuclei and the inferior olivary nucleus (*blue*), which project back to the cerebellar cortex of the opposite hemisphere.

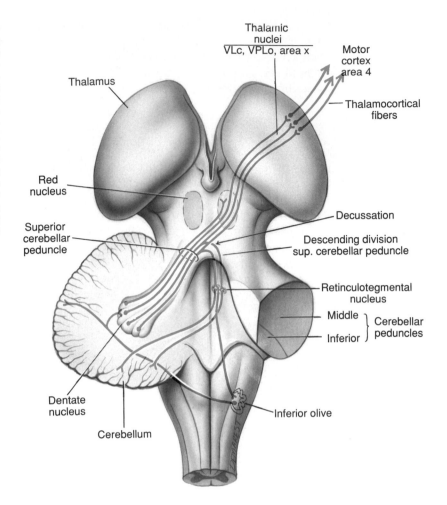

(Fig. 8.16); a smaller number of these fibers pass beyond the red nucleus to the same thalamic nuclei as fibers from the dentate nucleus. Fibers from the interposed nuclei end in an interdigitating fashion in VPLo and VLc but do not overlap those from the dentate nucleus. Fibers from the interposed nuclei projecting somatotopically on cells of the red nucleus form part of a somatotopic linkage extending from the paravermal cortex to spinal levels. In this pathway fibers from the paravermal cortex pass to the interposed nuclei; fibers from the interposed nuclei project via the superior cerebellar peduncle to the opposite red nucleus. Somatotopically organized rubrospinal fibers cross in the midbrain and descend to spinal levels. This small system involves two decussations, that of the superior cerebellar peduncle and that of the rubrospinal tract (Fig. 8.16). Thus, impulses conveyed from paravermal cortex to the spinal cord end on the same side. This system appears to be primarily concerned with mechanisms that facilitate ipsilateral flexor muscle tone.

The deep cerebellar nuclei not only receive inputs from the contralateral inferior olivary nucleus but have reciprocal connections with specific parts of the inferior olivary nuclear complex. The dentate nucleus projects primarily to the principal olive, while the anterior interposed nucleus (equivalent to the emboliform nucleus) projects to the dorsal accessory olive and the posterior interposed nucleus (equivalent to the globose nucleus) distributes fibers to the medial accessory olivary nucleus. These fibers reach parts of the contralateral inferior olivary nucleus via the descending limb of the superior cerebellar peduncle.

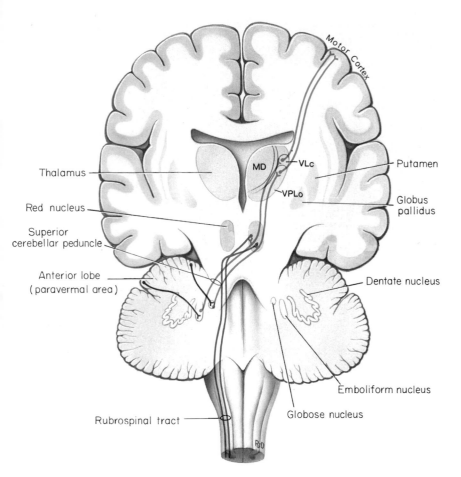

Figure 8.16. Schematic diagram of the projections from the interposed nuclei of the cerebellum (i.e., emboliform and globose nuclei) via the superior cerebellar peduncle (*blue*). The interposed nuclei receive afferents from the paravermal cortex (*black*) and project somatotopically (*blue*) upon cells in caudal portions of the contralateral red nucleus. Cells in caudal portions of the red nucleus give rise to the crossed rubrospinal tract (*red*), which influences flexor muscle tone. Thalamic projections from the interposed nuclei (*blue*) terminate in the cell sparse zone of the thalamus (VLc and VPLo) contralaterally. Thalamic terminations interdigitate with those of the dentate nucleus without overlap. Thalamic neurons receiving input from the interposed nuclei project to the primary motor cortex (*blue*).

Fastigial Efferent Projections

Efferent projections of the fastigial nucleus are unique in that (1) they do not emerge via the superior cerebellar peduncle, (2) a large part of the efferent fibers cross within the cerebellum, and (3) they project to nuclei at all levels of the brain stem. Crossed fibers from the fastigial nucleus emerge from the cerebellum via the *uncinate fasciculus (Russell)*, which arches around the superior cerebellar peduncle (Fig. 8.17 and 8.18). Uncrossed fastigial efferent fibers project to the brain stem in the *juxtarestiform body* (Figs. 6.22 and 8.17). Crossed efferent fibers contained in the uncinate fasciculus arise from cells in all parts of the fastigial nucleus and outnumber uncrossed efferents in the juxtarestiform body. The largest number of fastigial efferent fibers project to structures in the lower brain stem. Fastigial projections to the vestibular nuclei are bilateral, symmetrical, and terminate in ventral parts of the lateral and inferior vestibular nuclei. Fastigioreticular fibers arise predominantly from rostral parts of the nucleus, are mainly crossed, and project to (1) medial regions of the nucleus reticularis gigantocellularis, (2) parts of the caudal pontine reticular formation, (3) the dorsal paramedian reticular nucleus, and (4) portions of the lateral reticular nucleus. Crossed fastigiopontine fibers separate from the uncinate fasciculus and pass ventrally to terminations in the dorsolateral pontine nuclei (Fig. 8.18). A small number of crossed fastigiospinal fibers descend into the upper cervical spinal cord where they contact anterior horn cells (Fig. 8.18).

Small numbers of fastigial efferent fibers ascending in dorsolateral regions of the brain stem provide collaterals to the superior colliculus and the nuclei of the posterior commissure and terminate bilaterally in the

Figure 8.17. Dark-field photomicrograph of [³H] amino acids transported by fibers of the uncinate fasciculus as seen in an autoradiograph. (From Carpenter and Sutin, *Human Neuroanatomy*, 1983; courtesy of Williams & Wilkins.)

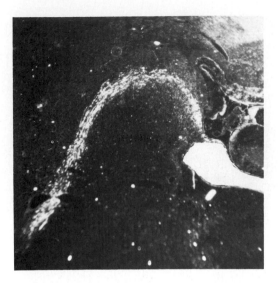

cell sparse zone of the thalamus (VLc and VPLo). These terminations do not overlap those from the dentate and interposed nuclei.

Cerebellovestibular Projections

Certain regions of the cerebellar cortex project directly to the vestibular nuclei (Fig. 8.19). These fibers, representing axons of Purkinje cells, arise from the cerebellar vermis and the vestibulocerebellum (i.e., the flocculonodular lobule). Thus, the vestibular nuclei receive cerebellar afferents bilaterally from the fastigial nucleus and ipsilaterally from specific cortical regions. Direct projections from the cerebellar vermis terminate in dorsal regions of the ipsilateral lateral and inferior vestibular nucleus, are somatotopically organized, and have GABA as their neurotransmitter (Fig. 8.19). Stimulation of the anterior lobe vermis of the cerebellum produces a monosynaptic inhibition of neurons of the lateral vestibular nucleus.

The regions of the cerebellum that receive primary and secondary vestibular fibers constitute the "vestibulocerebellum." This designation includes ventral parts of the uvula in addition to the flocculonodular lobule. All parts of the "vestibulocerebellum" project fibers to the vestibular nuclei. The flocculus projects to the superior and medial vestibular nuclei; the nodulus and uvula projects fibers to the superior, medial, and inferior vestibular nuclei. All of these cerebellovestibular projections are ipsilateral.

CEREBELLAR ORGANIZATION

On the basis of cortical projections to the deep cerebellar nuclei and projections from the deep nuclei to the cerebellar cortex, the cerebellum has been divided into three sagittal zones of cortex with their connecting deep nuclei. This concept provides an elementary view of the functional organization of the cerebellum. In this simplified scheme cerebellar efferent systems are related to three longitudinal (sagittal) zones referred to as vermal, paravermal and lateral.

The *vermal zone* is the midline, unpaired portion of the cerebellum related to the fastigial nuclei and concerned primarily with mechanisms that can modify muscle tone (Fig. 8.18). Direct projections from the cerebellar vermis exert inhibitory influences on the vestibular nuclei which can result in a reduction of extensor muscle tone (Fig. 8.19). The pro-

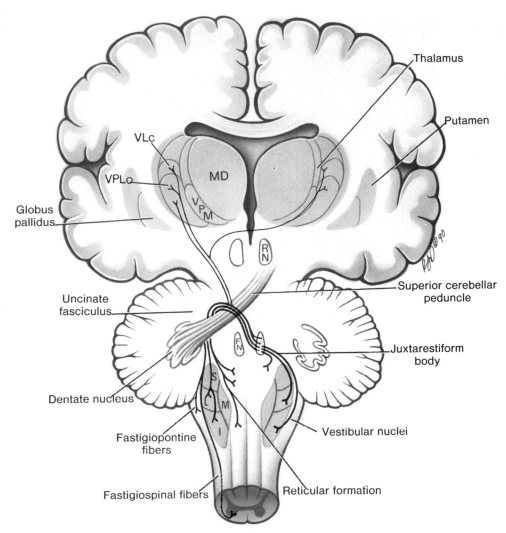

Figure 8.18.   Schematic diagram of fastigial efferent projections. Crossed fastigial efferent fibers (*red*), contained in the uncinate fasciculus, arise from cells in all parts of the fastigial nucleus (FN) and outnumber uncrossed efferents that emerge via the juxtarestiform body (*red*). The largest number of fastigial efferent fibers project to structures in the lower brain stem. Fastigiovestibular fibers project bilaterally and symmetrically upon ventral portions of the lateral and inferior vestibular nuclei. Fastigioreticular fibers are largely crossed, as are fastigiopontine fibers. A small number of fastigial efferents terminate on motor neurons in the upper cervical spinal cord. Ascending fastigial efferents project collateral to the superior colliculus and the nuclei of the posterior commissure and terminate bilaterally in the ventral lateral (VLc) and ventral posterolateral (VPLo) thalamic nuclei; crossed projections to the thalamus predominate. *Abbreviations*: MD, mediodorsal thalamic nucleus; vestibular nuclei: I, inferior; L, lateral; M, medial; S, superior.

jections of the fastigial nucleus, which receive strictly ipsilateral afferents from the vermis, are bilateral, although crossed fibers are more numerous. These excitatory fibers pass to terminations in the vestibular nuclei, and to broad regions of the reticular formation of the pons and medulla (Fig. 8.18). A small number of crossed fastigiospinal fibers descending directly to the upper cervical spinal have excitatory influences on motoneurons. Ascending fastigial efferents projecting to thalamic nuclei bilaterally make a contribution to coordinated somatic motor activity. The vermal zone of the cerebellum is particularly concerned with control of posture, muscle tone, locomotion, and equilibrium for the entire body.

The *paravermal zone* relates the paravermal cortex with the emboliform and globose nuclei which have connections predominantly with

Figure 8.19. Schematic diagram of cerebellovestibular projections from the anterior and posterior vermis. Purkinje cell axons from the anterior vermis project somatotopically on dorsal regions of the lateral vestibular nucleus and exert inhibitory influences. Similar direct projections from the pyramis and parts of the uvula which are not somatotopically arranged are shown by *arrows*. (From Carpenter and Sutin, *Human Neuroanatomy*, 1983; courtesy of Williams & Wilkins.)

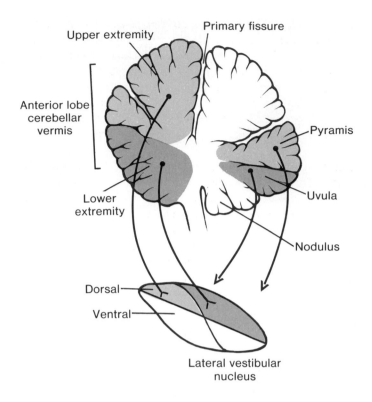

the contralateral red nucleus. The interposed nuclei project somatotopically on the caudal two-thirds of the contralateral red nucleus. This somatotopically organized system is concerned with mechanisms that can facilitate ipsilateral flexor muscle tone via the rubrospinal tract (Fig. 8.16). In addition the interposed nuclei have modest projections to the contralateral thalamic nuclei.

The *lateral zone* relates the cortex of the cerebellar hemisphere with the dentate nucleus which has the most extensive thalamic projections. These efferent fibers project somatotopically on the cell sparse zone of the thalamus (VLc and VPLo) (Figs. 8.15 and 9.16). This, the largest of all cerebellar efferent systems, appears to be concerned with the coordination of ipsilateral somatic motor activity. Neurons in the cell sparse zone of the thalamus project somatotopically upon the primary motor cortex.

FUNCTIONAL CONSIDERATIONS

The cerebellum is concerned with the coordination of somatic motor activity, the regulation of muscle tone, and mechanisms that influence and maintain equilibrium. Afferent cerebellar pathways convey impulses from a wide variety of different receptors, including the organs of special sense. Among these afferent systems, the input from stretch receptors (i.e., muscle spindle and Golgi tendon organ) is especially large. These impulses are conveyed by the spinocerebellar and cuneocerebellar tracts. The principal function of stretch receptors appears to be the unconscious neural control of muscle tone. The cerebellum, which receives the major afferent input from stretch receptors, provides part of the neural mechanism that (1) effects gradual alterations of muscle tensions for proper maintenance of equilibrium and posture, and (2) assures the smooth and orderly sequence of muscular contractions that characterize skilled voluntary movement.

Each movement requires the coordinated action (synergy) of a group of muscles. The *agonist* is the muscle that provides the actual movement of the part; the *antagonist* is the opposing muscle that must relax to permit movement. Other muscles must fix, or stabilize, certain joints in order to produce the desired movement. Such synergistic motor activity requires not only complex reciprocal innervation but coordinated control of muscle tone and movement. The cerebellum provides this control for the somatic motor system in an efficient, automatic manner without our being aware of it.

There are certain general principles that pertain to most of the disturbances resulting from cerebellar lesions. The principles are (1) cerebellar lesions produce ipsilateral disturbances, (2) cerebellar disturbances occur as a constellation of intimately related phenomena, (3) cerebellar disturbances due to nonprogressive pathology undergo gradual attenuation with time, and (4) disturbances resulting from cerebellar lesions are the physiological expression of intact neural structures deprived of controlling and regulating influences. Lesions involving the dentate nucleus or the superior cerebellar peduncle produce the most severe and enduring cerebellar disturbances.

Neocerebellar Lesions

Lesions involving the cerebellar hemispheres and the dentate nucleus affect primarily skilled voluntary and associated movements (i.e., movements related to the corticospinal system). The muscles become *hypotonic* (flabby) and tire easily. The deep tendon reflexes tend to be sluggish and often have a pendular quality. There are severe disturbances of coordinated movement referred to as *asynergia* in which the range, direction, and force of muscle contractions are inappropriate. Cerebellar asynergia can be demonstrated by many tests. Among these are tests of precise movements to a point; distances frequently are improperly gauged (*dysmetria*) and fall short of the mark or exceed it (*past-pointing*). Rapid successive movements, such as alternately, supinating and pronating the hands and forearms are poorly performed (*dysdiadochokinesis*). The patient is unable to adjust to changes of muscle tension. When the forearm is flexed at the elbow and held flexed against resistance, a sudden release of resistance causes the forearm to strike the chest. This is an example of the *rebound phenomenon*. These patients also demonstrate a *decomposition of movement* in which phases of complex movements are performed as a series of successive single simple movements.

The *tremor* seen in association with neocerebellar lesions occurs primarily during voluntary and associated movements. This tremor is referred to as "*intention tremor*" because it is not present at rest. It involves especially the proximal appendicular musculature but is transmitted mechanically to distal parts of the extremities.

Ataxia is an asynergic disturbance associated with neocerebellar lesions which results in a bizarre distortion of voluntary and associated movements. It involves particularly the axial muscles, and groups of muscle around the shoulder and pelvic girdles. This disturbance is evident during walking and is characterized by muscle contractions that are highly irregular in force, amplitude, and direction, and that occur asynchronously in different parts of the body. There frequently is unsteadiness in standing, especially if the feet are close together. The gait is broadbased and the patient reels, lurches, and stumbles.

Nystagmus commonly is seen in association with cerebellar disease;

it is most pronounced when the patient deviates the eyes laterally toward the side of the lesion. This disturbance consists of an oscillatory pattern in which the eyes slowly drift in one direction and then rapidly move in the opposite direction to correct the drift. Although nystagmus seen in association with cerebellar disease has been considered as an expression of asynergic phenomena in the extraocular muscles, many pathological processes which affect the cerebellum also involve the underlying brain stem and the vestibular nuclei in the floor of the fourth ventricle.

Speech disturbances are common in association with cerebellar lesions of long standing. Speech often is slow, monotonous, and some syllables are unnaturally separated. There is a slurring of speech and some words are uttered in an explosive manner.

Archicerebellar Lesions

Lesions involving portions of the posterior cerebellar vermis (i.e., nodulus and uvula) and probably portions of the flocculus produce what has been called the *archicerebellar syndrome*. These lesions produce disturbances of locomotion and equilibrium bilaterally. The patient is unsteady in the standing position and shows considerable swaying of the body. When attempts are made to walk, there is staggering and a tendency to fall to one side or backwards. The gait is jerky, uncoordinated, and resembles that of a drunken individual. Muscle tone is not significantly altered and no tremor or asynergic disturbances are seen in the extremities. This syndrome, primarily a trunkal ataxia frequently occurs in children with tumors in the posterior cerebellar vermis.

Anterior Lobe of the Cerebellum

There is no established paleocerebellar syndrome in humans, but lesions of the anterior lobe of the cerebellum in the dog produce severe disturbances of posture and greatly increased extensor muscle tone. These animals exhibit many of the features seen in association with decerebration, but in time regain the ability to walk and perform voluntary movements.

Sherrington in a classic experiment demonstrated that electrical stimulation of the anterior lobe of the cerebellum could inhibit extensor muscle tone in a decerebrate animal. Subsequent studies showed that both inhibitory and facilitory effects upon muscle tone could be obtained by stimulating the anterior lobe of the cerebellum, depending on the parameters of stimulation. Stimulation with low repetitive rates (2–10 cycles/sec) cause a slow increase in ipsilateral extensor muscle tone, while rapid stimulation (30–300 cycles/sec) produce a relaxation of muscle tone. Inhibitory influences obtained by stimulating the anterior lobe appear to be mediated by (1) cerebellovestibular fibers of cortical origin which project to the lateral vestibular nucleus, and (2) fastigial efferent projections to the reticular formation. Facilitatory influences obtained from stimulating the anterior lobe of the cerebellum are mediated by projections from the fastigial nucleus acting on the lateral vestibular nucleus.

Other cerebellar mechanisms that can influence muscle tone involve the paravermal cortex, the interposited nuclei and the contralateral red nucleus. All of the above structures are somatotopically interconnected. Stimulation of the rostral part of the interposed nuclei in the cat produces flexion of the ipsilateral hindlimb; stimulation of the caudal part of these nuclei produces flexion in the ipsilateral forelimb. These responses are ipsilateral because fibers of the superior cerebellar peduncle and the rubrospinal tract both are crossed. Crossed projections of the interposed nuclei excite rubral neurons which exert facilitatory influences on flexor muscle tone via the rubrospinal tract.

Computer Functions

The functional organization of the cerebellar cortex suggests that the cerebellum may function as a special kind of computer in the regulation and control of movement. The cerebellum organizes and integrates information flowing to it via numerous neural pathways. The cerebellar output participates in the control of motor function by transmitting impulses to (1) brain stem nuclei (i.e., the lateral vestibular and red nuclei) that in turn project to spinal levels, and (2) thalamic relay nuclei which can modify the activity of cortical neurons directly concerned with motor function.

Every part of the cerebellar cortex receives two different inputs, that of the mossy fibers and that of the climbing fibers. Although these inputs differ in structural characteristics, they appear to convey similar "sensory" information. The only output of the cerebellar cortex is conveyed by Purkinje cell axons. This output, entirely inhibitory, is exerted on the deep cerebellar nuclei and the lateral vestibular nucleus. The output of the deep cerebellar nuclei is excitatory, which implies that both excitatory and inhibitory impulses must reach these nuclei. Excitatory input to the deep cerebellar nuclei, derived from extracerebellar sources, is conveyed by collaterals of climbing and mossy fibers.

The observation that the cerebellar cortex transforms all input into inhibition, suggests that there is probably no dynamic storage of information. Thus, the cerebellum processes its input information rapidly, conveys its output indirectly to specific brain stem nuclei, and has virtually no short-term dynamic memory. These qualities enhance the performance of the cerebellum as a special kind of computer in that it can provide a quick and clear response to any "sensory" input.

SUGGESTED READINGS

ASANUMA, C., THACH, W. T., AND JONES, E. G. 1983. Distribution of cerebellar terminations and their relation to other afferent terminations in the ventral lateral thalamic region of the monkey. Brain Res. Rev., **5**: 237–265.

ASANUMA, C., THACH, W. T., AND JONES, E. G. 1983a. Anatomical evidence for segregated focal groupings of efferent cells and their terminal ramifications in the cerebellothalamic pathway of the monkey. Brain Res. Rev., **5**: 267–297.

BENTIVOGLIO, M., AND KUYPERS, H. G. J. M. 1982. Divergent axon collaterals from rat cerebellar nuclei to diencephalon, mesencephalon, medulla oblongata and cervical cord. Exp. Brain Res., **46**: 339–356.

BRODAL, A. 1976. The olivocerebellar projection in the cat as studied with the method of retrograde axonal transport of horseradish peroxidase. II. The projection of the uvula. J. Comp. Neurol., **166**: 417–426.

BRODAL, A., AND HODDEVIK, G. H. 1978. The pontocerebellar projection to the uvula in the cat. Exp. Brain Res., **32**: 105–116.

BRODAL, P. 1978. Principles of organization of the monkey corticopontine projection. Brain Res., **148**: 214–218.

BRODAL, P. 1978a. The corticopontine projection in the rhesus monkey: Origin and principles of organization. Brain, **101**: 251–283.

BROOKS, V. B., AND THACH, W. T. 1981. Cerebellar control of posture and movement. In V. B. BROOKS (Editor), *Handbook of Physiology*, Sect. I: The Nervous System. Vol. II: *Motor Control*. American Physiological Society, Washington, D.C., pp. 877–946.

CAJAL, S. RAMÓN Y. 1909, 1911. *Histologie due système nerveux de l'homme et des vertébres*. Norbert Maloine, Paris. 2 vols.

CARLETON, S. C., AND CARPENTER, M. B. 1983. Afferent and efferent connections of the medial, inferior and lateral vestibular nuclei in the cat and monkey. Brain Res., **278**: 29–51.

CARPENTER, M. B. 1988. Vestibular nuclei: Afferent and efferent projections. In O. POMPEIANO AND J. H. J. ALLUM (Editors), *Vestibulospinal Control of Posture and Movement.* Progress in Brain Research, Elsevier Science Publishers, Amsterdam, **76:** 5–15.

CARPENTER, M. B. 1989. Connectivity patterns of thalamic nuclei implicated in dyskinesia. Stereotact. Funct. Neurosurg., **58:** 79–119.

CARPENTER, M. B., AND BATTON, R. R. 1982. Connections of the fastigial nucleus in the cat and monkey. In S. L. PALAY AND V. CHAN-PALAY (Editors), *The Cerebellum—New Vistas.* Springer-Verlag, Berlin, pp. 250–295.

CARPENTER, M. B., AND COWIE, R. J. 1985. Connections and oculomotor projections of the superior vestibular nucleus and cell group "y." Brain Res., **336:** 265–287.

CHAN-PALAY, V. 1977. *Cerebellar Dentate Nucleus.* Springer-Verlag, Berlin, 548 pp.

CHAN-PALAY, V., NILAVER, G., PALAY, S., BEINFELD, M. C., ZIMMERMAN, E. A., WU, J.-Y., AND DONOHUE, T. L. 1981. Chemical heterogeneity in cerebellar Purkinje cells: Existence and coexistence of glutamic acid decarboxylase-like and motlin-like immunoreactivities. Proc. Natl. Acad. Sci. USA, **78:** 7787–7791.

CORVAJA, N., AND POMPEIANO, O. 1979. Identification of cerebellar cortico-vestibular neurons retrogradely labeled with horseradish peroxidase. Neuroscience, **4:** 507–515.

COURVILLE, J. 1966. Somatotopical organization of the projection from the nucleus interpositus anterior of the cerebellum to the red nucleus: An experimental study in the cat with silver impregnation methods. Exp. Brain Res., **2:** 191–215.

COURVILLE, J. 1975. Distribution of olivocerebellar fibers demonstrated by a radioautographic tracing method. Brain Res., **95:** 253–263.

COURVILLE, J., AUGUSTINE, J. R., AND MARTEL, P. 1977. Projections from the inferior olive to the cerebellar nuclei in the cat demonstrated by retrograde transport of horseradish peroxidase. Brain Res., **130:** 405–419.

COURVILLE, J., AND DIAKIW, N. 1976. Cerebellar corticonuclear projection in the cat: The vermis of the anterior and posterior lobes. Brain Res., **110:** 1–20.

COURVILLE, J., AND FARACO-CANTIN, F. 1978. On the origin of the climbing fibers of the cerebellum: An experimental study in the cat with an autoradiographic tracing method. Neuroscience, **3:** 797–809.

DE CAMILLI, P., MILLER, P. E., LEVITT, W. V., AND GREENGARD, P. 1984. Anatomy of cerebellar Purkinje cells in the rat determined by a specific immunohistochemical marker. Neuroscience, **11:** 761–817.

DOW, R. S., AND MORUZZI, G. 1958. Albation experiments. In R. S. DOW AND G. MORUZZI (Editors), *The Physiology and Pathology of the Cerebellum.* University of Minnesota Press, Minneapolis, pp. 8–102.

ECCLES, J. C., ITO, M., AND SZENTÁGOTHAI, J. 1967. *The Cerebellum as a Neuronal Machine.* Springer-Verlag, New York, 335 pp.

FONNUM, F., AND WALBERG, F. 1973. An estimate of the concentration of γ-aminobutyric acid and glutamate decarboxylase in the inhibitory Purkinje axon terminals in the cat. Brain Res., **54:** 115–127.

FOX, C. A., HILLMAN, D. E., SIEGESMUND, K. A., AND DUTTA, C. R. 1967. The primate cerebellar cortex. A Golgi and electron microscopic study. In C. A. FOX AND R. S. SNIDER (Editors), *The Cerebellum, Progress in Brain Research.* Elsevier, Amsterdam, Vol. 25, pp. 174–225.

GOULD, B. B. 1980. Organization of afferents from the brain stem nuclei to the cerebellar cortex in the cat. Adv. Anat. Embryol. Cell Biol., **62:** 1–90.

GOULD, B. B., AND GRAYBIEL, A. M. 1976. Afferents to the cerebellar cortex in the cat: Evidence for an intrinsic pathway leading from the deep nuclei to the cortex. Brain Res., **110:** 601–611.

GRAY, E. G. 1961. The granule cells, mossy synapses and Purkinje spinal synapses of the cerebellum: Light and electron microscopic observations. J. Anat., **95:** 345–356.

HAINES, D. E. 1977. Cerebellar corticonuclear and corticovestibular fibers of the flocculonodular lobe in a prosimian primate (*Galago senegalensis*). J. Comp. Neurol., **174:** 607–630.

HOUSER, C. R., BARBER, R. P., AND VAUGHN, J. E. 1984. Immunocytochemical localization of glutamic acid decarboxylase in the dorsal lateral vestibular nucleus: Evidence for an intrinsic and extrinsic GABAergic innervation. Neurosci. Lett., **47:** 213–220.

KALIL, K. 1981. Projections of the cerebellar and dorsal column nuclei upon the thalamus of the rhesus monkey. J. Comp. Neurol., **195:** 25–50.

MONAGHAN, P. L., BEITZ, A. J., LARSON, A. A., ALTSCHULER, R. A., MADL, J. E., AND MULLETT, M. A. 1986. Immunocytochemical localization of glutamate-, glutaminase- and aspartate aminotransferase-like immunoreactivity in the rat deep cerebellar nuclei. Brain Res., **363:** 364–370.

MUGNAINI, E. 1972. The histology and cytology of the cerebellar cortex. In O. LARSELL AND J. JANSEN (Editors), *The Comparative Anatomy and Histology of the Cerebellum. The Human Cerebellum, Cerebellar Connections, and Cerebellar Cortex.* University of Minnesota Press, Minneapolis, pp. 201–264.

ORIOLI, P. J., AND STRICK, P. L. 1989. Cerebellar connections with the motor cortex and the arcuate premotor area: An analysis employing retrograde transneuronal transport of WGA-HRP. J. Comp. Neurol., **288:** 612–626.

OTTERSEN, O. P., AND STORM-MATHISEN, J. 1984. Glutamate- and GABA-containing neurons in the mouse and rat brain, as demonstrated with a new immunocyto-chemical technique. J. Comp. Neurol., **229**: 374–392.

PERCHERON, G. 1977. The thalamic territory of cerebellar afferents and the lateral region of the thalamus of the macaque in stereotaxic ventricular coordinates. J. Hirnforsch., **18**: 375–400.

PURKINJE, J. E. 1837. Neueste untersuchungen aus der nerven—und Hirn—Anatomie. In K. STERNBERG AND J. V. KROMBHOLTZ (Editors), *Bericht über die versammlung deutsches Naturforscher und Ärzte in Prag.*, pp. 177–180.

SCHULMAN, J. A. 1983. Chemical neuroanatomy of the cerebellar cortex. In P. C. EMSON (Editor), *Chemical Neuroanatomy*. Raven Press, New York, pp. 209–227.

SHERRINGTON, C. S. 1898. Decerebrate rigidity and reflex coordination of movements. J. Physiol., **22**: 319–332.

SNIDER, R. S. 1950. Recent contributions to the anatomy and physiology of the cerebellum. Arch. Neurol. Psychiatry, **64**: 196–219.

SOMANA, R., AND WALBERG, F. 1978. Cerebellar afferents from the paramedian reticular nucleus studied with retrograde transport of horseradish peroxidase. Anat. Embryol. (Berl.), **154**: 353–368.

THACH, W. T., AND JONES, E. G. 1979. The cerebellar dentatothalamic connection: terminal field, lamellae, rods and somatotopy. Brain Res., **169**: 168–172.

TOLBERT, D. L., BANTLI, H., AND BLOEDEL, J. R. 1978. Organization features of the cat and monkey cerebellar nucleocortical projection. J. Comp. Neurol., **182**: 39–56.

TRACEY, D. J., ASANUMA, C., JONES, E. G., AND PORTER, R. 1980. Thalamic relay to motor cortex: Afferent pathways from brain stem, cerebellum and spinal cord in monkeys. J. Neurophysiol., **44**: 532–554.

VAN DER WANT, J. J. L., AND WOOGD, J. 1987. Ultrastructural identification and localization of climbing fiber terminals in the fastigial nucleus of the cat. J. Comp. Neurol., **258**: 81–90.

WILSON, V. J., UCHINO, Y., MAUNZ, R. A., SUSSWEIN, A., AND FUKUSHIMA, K. 1978. Properties and connections of cat fastigiospinal neurons. Exp. Brain Res., **32**: 1–17.

YAGINUMA, H., AND MATSUSHITA, M. 1989. Spinocerebellar projections from the upper lumbar segments in the cat, as studied by anterograde transport of wheat germ agglutinin-horseradish peroxidase. J. Comp. Neurol., **281**: 298–319.

9

The Diencephalon

Although the entire diencephalon constitutes less than 2% of the neuraxis, it has long been regarded as the key to the understanding of the organization of the central nervous system. The diencephalon extends from the region of the posterior commissure rostrally to the region of the interventricular foramen. Laterally it is bounded by the posterior limb of the internal capsule, the tail of the caudate nucleus, and the stria terminalis (Figs. 9.1 and 9.6). The third ventricle separates the diencephalon into two symmetrical parts, except in the region of the interthalamic adhesion where the medial surfaces of the thalami may be in continuity (Fig. 9.10). The diencephalon is divisible into four major parts: the epithalamus, the thalamus, the hypothalamus, and the subthalamus or ventral thalamus (Fig. 2.27). The medial and lateral geniculate bodies, constituting the metathalamus, are partially separated from the more rostral parts of the thalamus by fibers of the internal capsule.

MIDBRAIN–DIENCEPHALIC JUNCTION

Several nuclear masses of the caudal thalamus closely surround the posterior and lateral surfaces of the mesencephalon. These structures include the *medial* (MGB) and *lateral geniculate bodies* (LGB) and the *pulvinar*. External to all of these is the *retrolenticular* portion of the internal capsule (Fig. 9.2). The pineal body lies dorsally between the superior colliculi, while portions of the mammillary bodies can be seen in the interpeduncular fossa (Figs. 9.2 and 9.3). Projections from thalamic nuclei pass laterally into the internal capsule, through which they are distributed to various parts of the cerebral cortex. The internal capsule also contains corticofugal fibers projecting to thalamic nuclei (Fig. 9.24).

The pulvinar is a large nuclear mass dorsal to the medial and lateral geniculate bodies. Its dorsal surface is covered by a thin plate of fibers, the *stratum zonale*. Fibers passing laterally from the pulvinar contribute to the retrolenticular portion of the internal capsule (Figs. 9.2 and 9.3). The innermost portion of the internal capsule, wedged between the pulvinar and lateral geniculate body, forms an area known as the *zone of Wernicke* (Fig. 9.2).

CAUDAL DIENCEPHALON

Transverse sections through the habenular nuclei and the mammillary bodies (Figs. 9.1 and 9.4) reveal the structural organization of the caudal diencephalon. The habenular nuclei are two small gray masses forming triangular eminences on the dorsomedial surface of the thalami. Some fibers cross to the opposite side in the *habenular commissure*. Axons from the habenular nuclei form the *fasciculus retroflexus*, which passes

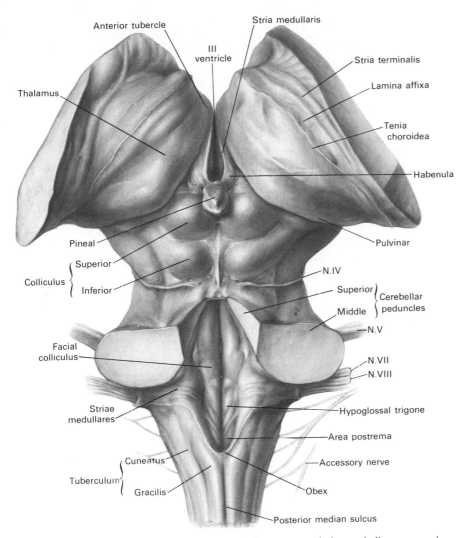

Figure 9.1. Drawing of the posterior aspect of the brain stem with the cerebellum removed, showing the epithalamus and the pulvinar. (From Mettler's *Neuroanatomy*, 1948.)

ventrally and caudally to terminate in the interpeduncular nuclei and nuclei in the midbrain raphe (Figs. 9.3 and 9.4).

The third ventricle appears enlarged, and parts of it are seen in two locations (Fig. 9.4). The main part of the third ventricle is present dorsally, where it is covered by a thin membrane extending between the habenular nuclei and the striae medullares. The margins of this attachment (not shown in Fig. 9.4) on each side constitute the *tenia thalami*. A small part of the third ventricle, referred to as the infundibular recess, is present ventral to the mammillary bodies and dorsal to the infundibulum. The mammillary bodies, tuber cinereum, and infundibulum are parts of the hypothalamus.

EPITHALAMUS

The epithalamus comprises the pineal body, the habenular trigones, the striae medullares, and the epithelial roof of the third ventricle (Figs. 9.1, 9.3, 9.4, 9.5, and 9.6). The habenula in humans consists of a smaller medial and a larger lateral nucleus. These nuclei receive terminals of the stria medullaris (Figs. 9.1, 9.4, and 9.6) and give rise to the fasciculus retroflexus, which terminates in the interpeduncular nucleus and nuclei

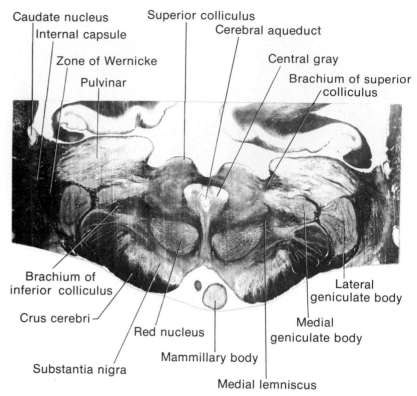

Caudate nucleus   Superior colliculus
Internal capsule   Cerebral aqueduct
Zone of Wernicke   Central gray
Pulvinar   Brachium of superior colliculus
Brachium of inferior colliculus   Lateral geniculate body
Crus cerebri   Medial geniculate body
Red nucleus
Substantia nigra   Mammillary body
Medial lemniscus

Figure 9.2.   Transverse section through the rostral midbrain and caudal thalamus demonstrating relationships of the pulvinar and the geniculate bodies. Weigert's myelin stain. Photograph.

Figure 9.3.   Transverse section of the brain stem at the junction of the mesencephalon and diencephalon. This junction is at levels through the posterior commissure, but portions of the pulvinar and the geniculate bodies extend further caudally. The posterior thalamic zone lies medial to the medial geniculate body and caudal to the ventral posterior thalamic nucleus (Figs. 9.4 and 9.18). Weigert's myelin stain. Photograph.

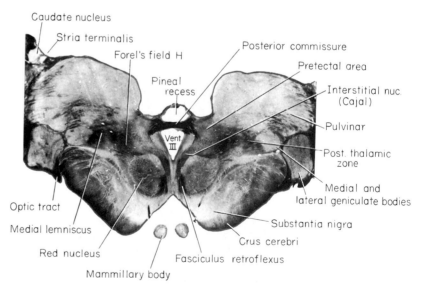

Caudate nucleus
Stria terminalis
Forel's field H
Pineal recess
Posterior commissure
Pretectal area
Interstitial nuc. (Cajal)
Pulvinar
Vent. III
Post. thalamic zone
Optic tract
Medial and lateral geniculate bodies
Medial lemniscus
Substantia nigra
Red nucleus
Crus cerebri
Fasciculus retroflexus
Mammillary body

of the midbrain raphe. The *stria medullaris* is a complex bundle composed of fibers arising from (1) the septal nuclei, (2) lateral preoptic region, and (3) the anterior thalamic nuclei. Both the hippocampal formation and the amygdaloid nuclear complex project fibers to the septal nuclei (Fig. 10.12).

The lateral habenular nucleus receives afferents from the globus pallidus, the lateral hypothalamus, the substantia innominata, and the lateral preoptic area, as well as from the ventral tegmental area and the midbrain raphe nuclei. The smaller medial habenular nucleus contains

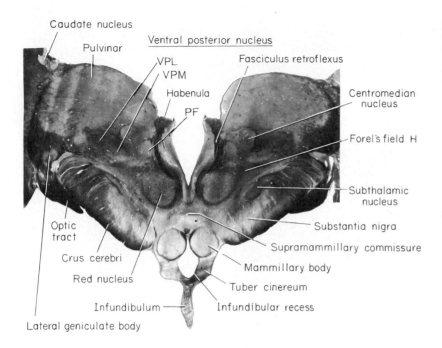

Caudate nucleus
Pulvinar
Ventral posterior nucleus
VPL
VPM
Fasciculus retroflexus
Habenula
PF
Centromedian nucleus
Forel's field H
Subthalamic nucleus
Substantia nigra
Supramammillary commissure
Mammillary body
Tuber cinereum
Infundibular recess
Optic tract
Crus cerebri
Red nucleus
Infundibulum
Lateral geniculate body

Figure 9.4. Transverse section of the diencephalon through the habenula, the fasciculus retroflexus, the mammillary bodies, and the infundibulum. *VPL* and *VPM* indicate the ventral posterolateral and ventral posteromedial thalamic nuclei, respectively. The parafascicular nucleus (*PF*) surrounds the fasciculus retroflexus. Weigert's myelin stain. Photograph.

cholinergic neurons that receive afferents from posterior parts of the septal nuclei and the midbrain raphe nuclei. Serotonergic projections from the raphe nuclei and adrenergic innervation from the superior cervical ganglion reach the medial habenular nucleus. The habenular nuclei are sites of convergence of limbic pathways that convey impulses to rostral portions of the midbrain.

Pineal Gland

The pineal body or epiphysis is a small, cone-shaped body attached to the roof of the third ventricle in the region of the posterior commissure (Figs. 9.1 and 9.6). It appears as a rudimentary gland consisting of a network of richly vascular connective tissue containing glia cells and *pinealocytes* or *epiphysial cells*. Pinealocytes in the monkey contain serotonin (5-HT) and cholecystokinin (CCK). Mammalian pinealocytes are phylogenetically related to neurosensory photoreceptor elements that become predominantly secretory cells, but they remain indirectly photosensitive. The club-shaped endings of these processes terminate close to perivascular spaces.

The best-known pineal secretions are the biogenic amines serotonin, norepinephrine, and melatonin, but the gland also contains significant concentrations of identified hypothalamic peptides such as thyrotropin-releasing hormone (TRH), luteinizing hormone-releasing hormone (LHRH), and somatostatin (SRIF). Serotonin is synthesized in the pinealocyte and released into the extracellular space. Norepinephrine is synthesized in sympathetic neurons which terminate on pineal parenchymal cells.

The pineal gland synthesizes melatonin from serotonin by the action of two enzymes sensitive to variations of diurnal light, *N*-acetyltransferase, and hydroxyindole-*o*-methyltransferase. Daily fluctuations in melatonin synthesis are rhythmic and directly related to the daily cycle of photic input. Light entrains the circadian rhythm to the environmental light cycle and also acts by an unidentified pathway to rapidly block the transmission of neural signals to the pineal gland. *N*-Acetyltransferase

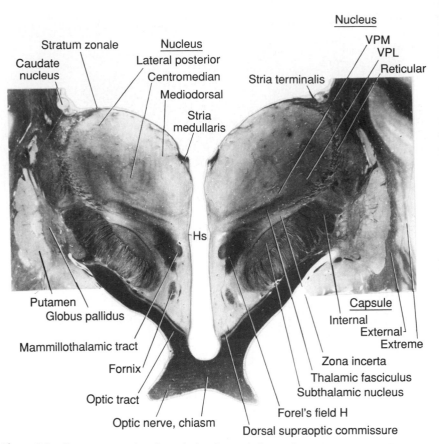

Figure 9.5. Transverse section through the diencephalon and corpus striatum at the level of the subthalamic nucleus. *HS* indicates the hypothalamic sulcus in the wall of the third ventricle. *VPM* and *VPL* refer to the ventral posteromedial and the ventral posterolateral thalamic nuclei, respectively. Weigert's myelin stain. Photograph.

activity is elevated during the night, but exposure to light turns off the enzyme activity. Bilateral lesions of the suprachiasmatic nucleus (Figs. 10.1 and 10.6) of the hypothalamus, which receives the retinohypothalamic tract, abolish the rhythm in pineal *N*-acetyltransferase activity and result in low levels of hydroxyindole-*o*-methyltransferase activity. Such lesions abolish the circadian rhythms of spontaneous locomotor activity and of both feeding and drinking. In female rats the normal estrous cycle is abolished by lesions of the suprachiasmatic nuclei. The retinohypothalamic projection alters pineal function by directly interacting with structures in the suprachiasmatic nucleus. Environmental light can be regarded as having an entraining function and a transmission function. The effect of light in entraining the endogenous oscillator to the light cycle is slow, but the effect of light on signal transmission is rapid and probably accounts for the rapid ''turn off'' of *N*-acetyltransferase by light and the blocking of circadian rhythm by constant light.

Although a single neural pathway from the suprachiasmatic nucleus regulates both enzymes involved in the formation of melatonin by the pineal, details concerning these connections are not known. Indirect evidence suggests that the pathway from the suprachiasmatic nucleus to the pineal involves relays to the tuberal region of the hypothalamus, the medial forebrain bundle, and spinal pathways that reach the intermediolateral cell column and cells of the superior cervical ganglion. Thus the pineal gland appears to be a neuroendocrine transducer that converts neural signals into an endocrine output, melatonin.

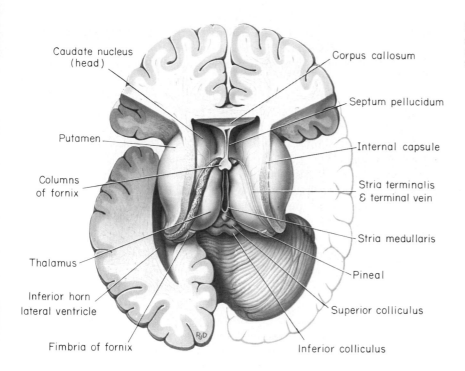

Figure 9.6. Drawing of a brain dissection showing the gross relationships of the thalamus, internal capsule, corpus striatum, and the ventricular system.

Pineal secretions that alter hypothalamic functions do so after they enter the general circulation or the cerebrospinal fluid. Daily fluctuations in pineal serotonin and melatonin are rhythmic in response to the cycle of photic input. These rhythmic changes in pineal activity, suggest that this gland functions as a biological clock delivering signals that regulate both physiological and behavioral processes. Fluctuations, called *circadian rhythms*, have a period of exactly 24 hours in the presence of environmental cues, while in the absence of such cues they only approximate the 24-hour cycle.

Parenchymatous pinealomas are associated with depression of gonadal function and delayed pubescence, while lesions which destroy the pineal frequently are associated with precocious puberty. These observations are consistent with experimental studies indicating that the pineal gland exerts an inhibitory influence on the gonads and the reproductive system.

THALAMUS

Transverse sections through the central part of the diencephalon demonstrate three major divisions of the diencephalon: (1) the thalamus, (2) the hypothalamus, and (3) the subthalamic region (Fig. 2.27).

The narrow third ventricle, extending from the region immediately ventral to the striae medullares to the optic chiasm, completely separates the thalami. A shallow groove on the ventricular surface, the hypothalamic sulcus (Figs. 2.23, 2.24, 2.27, and 9.5), separates the dorsal thalamus from the hypothalamus. The dorsal surface of the thalamus is covered by the *stratum zonale*. At the junction of the dorsal and medial thalamic surfaces, fibers of the striae medullares are cut transversely and appear as small bundles of myelinated fibers (Fig. 9.5). The dorsal thalamus is divided into medial and lateral nuclear groups by a band of myelinated fibers, the *internal medullary lamina* of the thalamus, which contains several different cell groups (Figs. 2.27, 9.9, 9.10, and 9.11). The lateral nuclear group, between the internal and external medullary laminae, is further divided into ventral and lateral (dorsal) nuclear masses (Fig. 9.5).

The ventral nuclear mass, extending nearly the entire length of the thalamus, is divisible into three separate nuclei: (1) a caudal, *ventral posterior nucleus* (VP); (2) an intermediate, *ventral lateral nucleus* (VL); and (3) a rostral, *ventral anterior nucleus* (VA). The ventral posterior nucleus is subdivided into a ventral posterolateral nucleus, located laterally, and a ventral posteromedial nucleus, located medially (Figs. 2.27, 9.5, 9.10, and 9.11).

The lateral nuclear mass of the thalamus, located dorsal to the ventral nuclear mass discussed above, also is divided into three separate nuclei: (1) a greatly expanded caudal part, the *pulvinar*; (2) an intermediate part, the *lateral posterior nucleus*; and (3) a smaller encapsulated rostral part, the *lateral dorsal nucleus* (Figs. 9.3, 9.4, 9.7, 9.8, and 9.12).

The medial nuclear group of the thalamus, located medial to the internal medullary lamina, contains the *mediodorsal nucleus*, a nuclear mass intimately related to the cortex of the frontal lobe. Wedged between the mediodorsal nucleus and the ventral nuclei caudally is the *centromedian nucleus*, the largest of the intralaminar thalamic nuclei (Figs. 9.4, 9.5, 9.11, and 9.12). The internal medullary lamina partially splits to surround this large nucleus.

Along the lateral border of the thalamus, near the internal capsule, is a narrow band of myelinated fibers, the *external medullary lamina* of the thalamus. Cells located external to the lamina form a thin outer nuclear envelope, the *reticular nucleus* (RN) of the thalamus (Figs. 9.5, 9.10, 9.11, and 9.12). Ventrally the reticular nucleus becomes continuous with the zona incerta (Fig. 9.5).

SUBDIVISIONS OF THE THALAMUS

The thalamic nuclei, many of which are microscopic subdivisions, are particularly difficult to visualize in three dimensions (Fig. 9.12). The nomenclature of the thalamus is complex, and in some instances the fiber connections and the significance of the smaller thalamic nuclei are unknown. In a general way, depending upon their fiber connections, most of the major thalamic nuclei can be classified either as specific relay nuclei, or as association nuclei. Specific relay nuclei receive recognized ascending pathways and project to well defined cortical areas that are related to specific functions. Association nuclei of the thalamus do not receive direct fibers from ascending systems but project to association areas of the cortex. Other thalamic nuclei have predominantly, or exclusively, subcortical connections. Physiological and anatomical studies indicate that certain thalamic nuclei have diffuse cortical connections.

The gross appearance of the dorsal surface of the diencephalon is shown in different dissections in Figures 9.1 and 9.6. These figures illustrate the relationships of the thalamus and epithalamus to surrounding structures and the infratentorial brain stem. Two important levels of the thalamus in transverse section in Figures 9.10 and 9.11 show portions of major thalamic nuclei as they appear in Nissl-stained sections. Major nuclear subdivisions of the thalamus are shown schematically together with established afferent and efferent connections in Figure 9.12. Cortical projection areas of major thalamic nuclei are represented diagrammatically in Figure 9.13. The same color coding is used in Figures 9.12 and 9.13. Several ascending thalamic afferent systems have been diagrammed in earlier chapters. Ascending spinal pathways are shown in Figures 4.1,

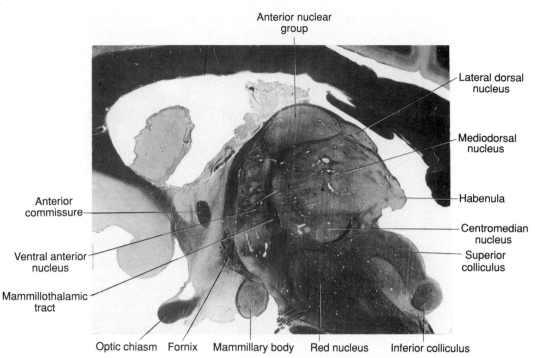

Anterior nuclear group

Lateral dorsal nucleus

Mediodorsal nucleus

Habenula

Centromedian nucleus

Superior colliculus

Anterior commissure

Ventral anterior nucleus

Mammillothalamic tract

Optic chiasm   Fornix   Mammillary body   Red nucleus   Inferior colliculus

Figure 9.7. Sagittal section through medial parts of the thalamus showing the anterior tubercle (anterior nuclear group), the mammillothalamic tract, and the fornix. Also seen are the relationship of the anterior thalamic nuclei to the lateral dorsal nucleus. The centromedian nucleus, the largest of the intralaminar thalamic nuclei, lies ventral to the mediodorsal nucleus. Weigert's myelin stain. Photograph.

4.2, and 4.3, while pathways originating in the brain stem are diagrammed in Figures 5.24, 6.9, 6.24, and 7.18. Cerebellar pathways projecting to the thalamus are shown in Figures 8.15, 8.16, and 8.18. These schematic diagrams and those in Chapter 11 (Figs. 11.17 and 11.21) supplement information contained in Figures 9.12 and 9.13.

Anterior Nuclear Group

The anterior nuclear group lies beneath the dorsal surface of the most rostral part of the thalamus, where it forms the anterior tubercle (Figs. 9.7, 9.8, and 9.12). It consists of a large principal nucleus, the *anteroventral* (AV), and accessory nuclei, the *anterodorsal* (AD) and *anteromedial* (AM). Cells composing these nuclei are of medium size, they have little chromophilic substance, a moderate amount of yellow pigment, and are surrounded by a capsule of myelinated fibers. The anterior nuclei receive the mammillothalamic tract. Fibers from the medial mammillary nucleus project to the ipsilateral anteroventral and anteromedial nuclei, while the lateral mammillary nucleus projects bilaterally to the anterodorsal nucleus. The lateral mammillary nucleus projects fibers to both AD and the midbrain tegmentum. The anterior nuclei of the thalamus receive as many direct fibers from the fornix as from the mammillothalamic tract. The cortical projections of the anterior nuclei are to the cingulate gyrus (areas 23, 24, and 32) via the anterior limb of the internal capsule (Fig. 9.13). The bulk of the projections from these cortical areas are to the entorhinal cortex via the cingulum (Fig. 2.15).

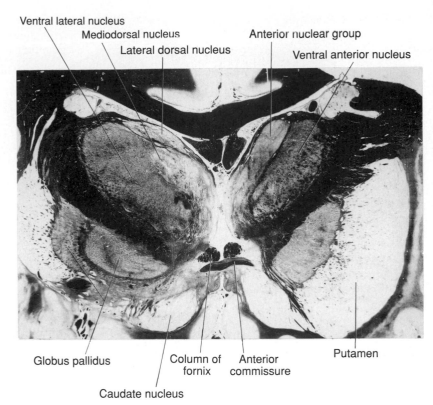

Ventral lateral nucleus
Mediodorsal nucleus
Lateral dorsal nucleus
Anterior nuclear group
Ventral anterior nucleus

Globus pallidus
Column of fornix
Anterior commissure
Putamen
Caudate nucleus

Figure 9.8. Photograph of an asymmetrical transverse section through rostral portions of the thalamus and the corpus striatum. On the right side the anterior nuclear group and the ventral anterior nucleus are seen. The more caudal level on the left is through the dorsomedial nucleus, ventral lateral, and lateral dorsal thalamic nuclei. Weigert's myelin stain.

Mediodorsal Nucleus

The mediodorsal nucleus (MD), or dorsomedial nucleus, occupies most of the area between the internal medullary lamina and the periventricular gray (Figs. 9.5, 9.7, 9.8, 9.9, 9.10, 9.11, 9.12, and 9.14). Three major regions of the nucleus are recognized: (1) a magnocellular portion (MDmc), located rostrally and dorsomedially, (2) a larger dorsolateral and caudal parvicellular portion (MDpc), and (3) a paralaminar portion (MDpl, pars multiformis) characterized by large cells forming a band adjacent to the internal medullary lamina. The nucleus has extensive connections with intralaminar and lateral thalamic nuclear groups. The medial magnocellular division of the mediodorsal nucleus receives fibers from the amygdaloid complex, the temporal neocortex, and the caudal orbitofrontal cortex. Most of these fibers constitute components of the *ansa peduncularis*. The ansa peduncularis consists of the inferior thalamic peduncle, plus fibers interconnecting the amygdaloid complex and the preopticohypothalamic region (Fig. 9.9).

The larger parvicellular portion of this nucleus is connected by a massive projection with practically the entire frontal cortex rostral to areas 6 and 32 (Fig. 9.13). After extensive prefrontal cortical lesions, or lesions interrupting fibers from this region (i.e., prefrontal lobotomy), nearly all small cells of the mediodorsal nucleus degenerate. No cells of the mediodorsal nucleus project to the precentral motor cortex. There are reciprocal connections between the mediodorsal nucleus and the granular frontal cortex (i.e., prefrontal cortex). Particularly profuse reciprocal connections exist between area 8 (frontal eye field) and the paralaminar

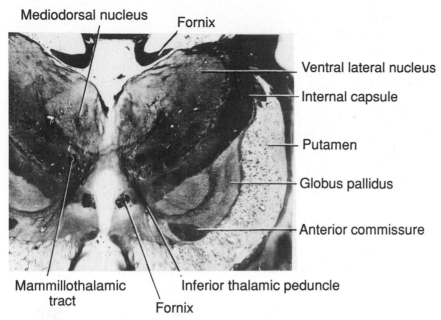

Mediodorsal nucleus   Fornix

Ventral lateral nucleus

Internal capsule

Putamen

Globus pallidus

Anterior commissure

Mammillothalamic tract   Inferior thalamic peduncle

Fornix

Figure 9.9.   Transverse section through the diencephalon and corpus striatum demonstrating fibers of the inferior thalamic peduncle. The inferior thalamic peduncle consists of fibers from the amygdaloid nuclear complex, temporal neocortex, and possibly the substantia innominata that project to the mediodorsal nucleus of the thalamus. Weigert's myelin stain. Photograph.

part of the mediodorsal nucleus. The paralaminar part of the mediodorsal nucleus also receives a substantial projection from the pars reticulata of the substantia nigra. Although the magnocellular division of the dorsomedial nucleus receives projections from the amygdala, this connection is not reciprocal.

The mediodorsal nucleus is thought to be concerned with integration of somatic and visceral activities. Impulses relayed to the prefrontal cortex may enter consciousness and influence various feeling tones. Psychosurgical studies (i.e., prefrontal lobotomy) suggest that the mediodorsal nucleus and large regions of the frontal association cortex are concerned with aspects of affective behavior.

Midline Nuclei

The midline nuclei are less distinct cell clusters which lie in the periventricular gray matter of the dorsal half of the ventricular wall and in the interthalamic adhesion (Figs. 9.10 and 9.11). These nuclei are small and difficult to delimit in humans. Efferent fibers from the paraventricular nucleus, the central nuclear complex, and the nucleus reuniens project to the amygdaloid nuclear complex. Some of the midline thalamic nuclei may also project to the anterior cingulate cortex. Fine myelinated and unmyelinated fibers are thought to relate these nuclei to the hypothalamus.

Intralaminar Nuclei

The intralaminar nuclei (Figs. 9.4, 9.5, 9.7, 9.10, 9.11, 9.12, and 9.14) are cell groups within the internal medullary lamina, which separates the medial and the lateral subdivisions of the thalamus. Cells vary in size in the different nuclei, are fusiform and dark staining, and resemble those of the midline nuclei.

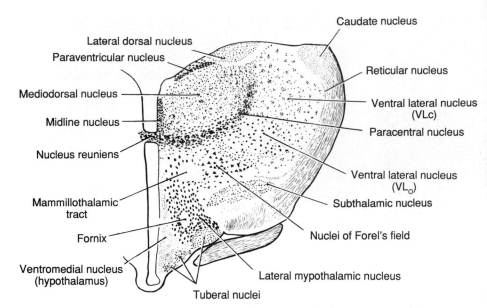

Figure 9.10.   Drawing of a transverse Nissl section of the diencephalon at the level of the tuber cinereum showing nuclear subdivisions of the thalamus and hypothalamus. (Modified from Malone, 1910.)

Centromedian Nucleus

This nucleus, the largest and most easily identified of the intralaminar thalamic nuclei (Figs. 9.4, 9.5, 9.11, 9.12, and 9.14), is located in the caudal third of the thalamus between the mediodorsal nucleus and the ventral posterior nucleus (Figs. 9.7, 9.11, 9.12, and 9.14). It is almost completely surrounded by fibers of the internal medullary lamina, except along its medial border, where it merges with the parafascicular nucleus (Figs. 9.4 and 9.14). It is composed of ovoid or round cells, some of which contain a yellow pigment (lipofuscin). Cells in the lateral portion of the nucleus are small, while those in more medial regions bordering the mediodorsal nucleus are larger and more densely arranged.

Parafascicular Nucleus

This nucleus lies medial to the centromedian nucleus and ventral to the caudal part of the dorsomedial nucleus (Figs. 9.4 and 9.14). The most distinguishing feature of the parafascicular nucleus is that its cells surround the dorsomedial part of the fasciculus retroflexus.

Rostral Intralaminar Nuclei

The paracentral, central lateral, and central medial nuclei lie within the rostral internal medullary lamina of the thalamus (Figs. 9.10 and 9.11). The paracentral nucleus (PCN) lies in the internal medullary lamina adjacent to the rostral part of the mediodorsal nucleus. Cells are large, dark, multipolar, and grouped into clusters. Caudally the paracentral nucleus appears to fuse with the central lateral nucleus (CL) which lies dorsal to the centromedian nucleus and lateral to the mediodorsal nucleus (Figs. 9.10, 9.11, and 9.14). The central lateral nucleus is broader than the paracentral nucleus and composed of similar cells. The central medial nucleus lies adjacent to the medial part of the paracentral nucleus.

The brain stem reticular formation is regarded as one of the principal sources of afferent impulses to the intralaminar thalamic nuclei. Fibers from broad regions of the brain stem reticular formation ascending in the

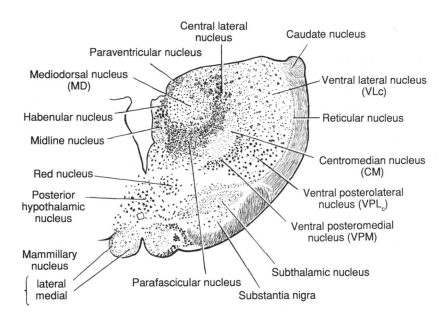

Central lateral
nucleus

Caudate nucleus

Paraventricular nucleus

Mediodorsal nucleus
(MD)

Ventral lateral nucleus
(VLc)

Habenular nucleus

Reticular nucleus

Midline nucleus

Centromedian nucleus
(CM)

Red nucleus

Posterior
hypothalamic
nucleus

Ventral posterolateral
nucleus (VPL$_o$)

Ventral posteromedial
nucleus (VPM)

Mammillary
nucleus

lateral
medial

Parafascicular nucleus

Subthalamic nucleus

Substantia nigra

Figure 9.11. Drawing of a transverse Nissl section of the diencephalon at the level of the habenular nuclei and the mammillary bodies. (Modified from Malone, 1910.)

central tegmental tract (Figs. 6.1, 6.5, 6.18, 7.2, and 7.4) have been traced into (1) the paracentral and central lateral nuclei and (2) the subthalamic region. These projections are chiefly ipsilateral. Because potentials in the brain stem reticular formation have been recorded following stimulation of virtually every type of receptor, it has been presumed that activation of the ascending reticular system was a consequence of "collateral" excitation derived from specific sensory pathways (Chapter 7).

The centromedian (CM) and parafascicular (PF) nuclei receive afferent fibers mainly from forebrain derivatives. Area 4 projects fibers that are distributed throughout the centromedian nucleus, while area 6 projects to the lateral part of the parafascicular nucleus. Substantial cortical projections to the intralaminar thalamic nuclei arise from broad regions of the frontal lobe. The precentral motor cortex (area 4) projects terminals to the paracentral, central lateral, and centromedian thalamic nuclei. The cortical projection to the centromedian nucleus is massive and some of these fibers cross the midline to corresponding parts of the same nucleus on the opposite side. The premotor area (area 6) sends afferents to parts of the central lateral nucleus and to the parafascicular nucleus. Although most corticothalamic and thalamocortical projection systems are reciprocal, this generalization does not pertain to the intralaminar thalamic nuclei which have diffuse cortical projections that are in no sense reciprocal.

The centromedian nucleus (CM) also receives pallidal efferent fibers that separate from the thalamic fasciculus. These fibers are collaterals of pallidofugal fibers passing to the ventral anterior and ventral lateral thalamic nuclei (Figs. 11.20 and 11.21).

While all of the efferent projections of the intralaminar nuclei are not known, the principal projections of the centromedian-parafascicular nuclear complex (CM-PF) are to the striatum. Cells in the centromedian nucleus (CM) project to the putamen where they terminate in a mosaiclike fashion. Cell in the parafascicular nucleus (PF) project to the caudate nucleus; few, if any, thalamostriate fibers project to both the caudate nucleus and the putamen. The intralaminar nuclei of the thalamus were long regarded as having no cortical projections. This conclusion was based on the apparent absence of retrograde cell changes in these nuclei following virtually complete decortication and the absence of degeneration

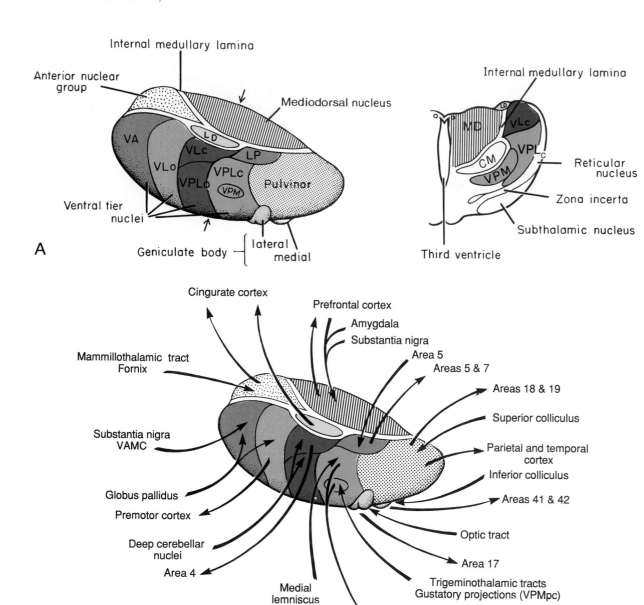

Figure 9.12. Schematic diagrams of the major thalamic nuclei. *A,* an oblique dorsolateral view of the thalamus and its major subdivisions. *Arrows* indicate the level of the transverse section of the thalamus on the right, which shows relationships between VPM and VPLc and the location of the largest of the intralaminar thalamic nucleus, the centromedian (CM). In *B,* the principal afferent and efferent connections of the major thalamic nuclei are indicated. *Abbreviations: LD,* lateral dorsal nucleus; *LP,* lateral posterior nucleus; *MD,* mediodorsal nucleus; *VA,* ventral anterior nucleus; *VAmc,* magnocellular part; *VLc,* ventral lateral nucleus, pars caudalis; *VLo,* pars oralis of VL; *VPLc,* ventral posterolateral nucleus, pars caudalis; *VPLo,* pars oralis of VPL; *VPM,* ventral posteromedial nucleus; *VPMpc,* ventral posteromedial nucleus, parivcellular part.

traceable to any part of the cortex. Retrograde transport of the enzyme horseradish peroxidase (HRP) suggested that thalamostriate fibers give rise to collateral systems that project diffusely to broad cortical regions. The rostral intralaminar thalamic nuclei (central lateral and paracentral) contain cells that receive fibers from the midbrain reticular formation and project directly to widespread cortical regions. These neurons in CL and PCN do not have bifurcating axons and conduction velocities of fibers projecting to cortex and to the striatum are different. Thus some pathways from the midbrain reticular formation to the cerebral cortex are mono-

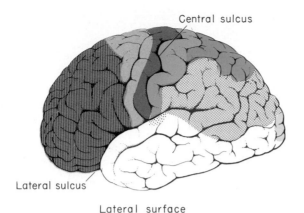

Central sulcus

Lateral sulcus

Lateral surface

Figure 9.13. Diagram of the left cerebral hemisphere showing the cortical projection areas of the major thalamic nuclei. Color coding is the same as in Figure 9.12. Diffuse projections of the ventral anterior nucleus (*VApc*) to the frontal lobe largely overlap those of the mediodorsal nucleus (*MD*).

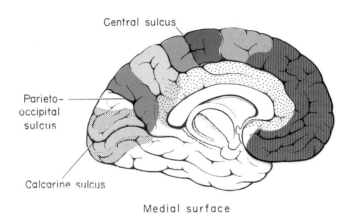

Central sulcus

Parieto-
occipital
sulcus

Calcarine sulcus

Medial surface

synaptic with relays in the central lateral and paracentral nuclei (CL-PCN). Monosynaptic relays in CL-PCN convey impulses from the midbrain reticular formation to many separate cortical areas, as well as to the caudate nucleus. Cortical projecting intralaminar thalamic neurons that relay activity from the midbrain reticular formation to the cerebral cortex play an important role in processes that characterize wakefulness and desynchronized sleep.

The intralaminar thalamic nuclei show a striking development in primates and man, in relation to thalamic relay nuclei, suggesting that they constitute a complex intrathalamic regulating mechanism concerned with diverse functions. The intralaminar thalamic nuclei have been considered to serve as the thalamic pacemaker controlling electrocortical activities. The large CM-PF nuclear complex appears most closely related to motor functions in that it receives inputs from the motor and premotor cortex and from the globus pallidus; this nuclear complex projects mainly to the striatum.

Lateral Nuclear Group

The lateral nuclear group begins as an oblique narrow strip on the dorsomedial surface of the thalamus caudal to the anterior nuclear group (Figs. 9.7 and 9.12). This group consists of three nuclear masses arranged in rostrocaudal sequence: the lateral dorsal nucleus, the lateral posterior nucleus, and the pulvinar (Figs. 9.3 and 9.12).

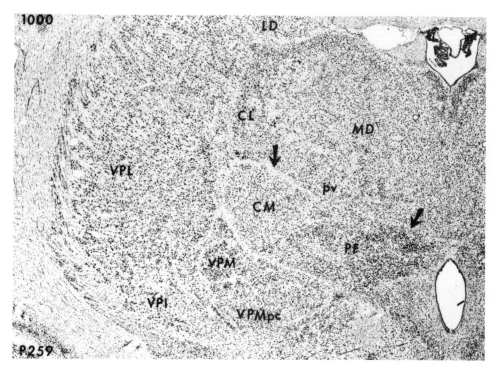

Figure 9.14. Photomicrograph of a transverse section of the monkey thalamus through the ventrobasal complex and the intralaminar nuclei in monkey. *Abbreviations*: *CL*, central lateral nucleus; *CM*, centromedian nucleus; *LD*, lateral dorsal nucleus; *MD*, mediodorsal nucleus; *PF*, parafascicular nucleus; *pv*, ventral paralaminar part of the mediodorsal nucleus; *VPI*, ventral posterior inferior nucleus; *VPL*, ventral posterolateral nucleus; *VPM*, ventral posteromedial nucleus; *VPMpc*, ventral posteromedial nucleus, parvicellular part. *Arrows* define the superior border of the internal medullary lamina that splits to enclose the centromedian nucleus. Cresyl violet (× 22). (From Roberts and Akert, 1963; courtesy of Prof. Konrad Akert, Zurich.)

Lateral Dorsal Nucleus

This nucleus, which lies on the dorsal surface of the thalamus, extends along the upper margin of the internal medullary lamina and is surrounded by a myelin fiber capsule, similar to that of the anterior nuclear group (Figs. 9.7, 9.8, 9.10, and 9.12). The nucleus achieves its largest size dorsal to the paracentral (PCN) and central lateral nuclei (Fig. 9.7) and has been considered as a caudal extension of the anterior thalamic nuclei. Projections from the lateral-dorsal nucleus (LD) are mainly to the posterior parts of the cingulate gyrus, but it also sends fibers to the supralimbic cortex of the parietal lobe (Fig. 9.13).

Lateral Posterior Nucleus

This nucleus lies caudal, lateral, and ventral to the lateral dorsal nucleus and is composed of medium-sized cells evenly distributed (Fig. 9.12). The irregularly shaped nucleus lies dorsal to the ventral posterolateral nucleus and adjacent to the lateral medullary lamina. Caudally the nucleus merges with the oral and medial parts of the pulvinar, from which it is not easily distinguished. Unlike the lateral dorsal nucleus it has no myelin capsule. The input to this thalamic nucleus is poorly understood, but it may receive inputs from adjacent primary relay nuclei, especially the ventral posterior nucleus. Degeneration studies in the cat indicate that the superior and inferior parietal lobules project upon the lateral posterior nucleus (LP). Area 5 of the parietal cortex, constituting part of the superior parietal lobule, has been demonstrated to transport isotope to laminar arrays distributed throughout the lateral posterior nucleus. Some of the these thalamic neurons appear to have reciprocal cortical connections. Retrograde transport studies indicate that the lateral posterior nucleus projects upon areas 5 and 7.

Pulvinar

This large nuclear mass, forming the posterior and dorsolateral portion of the thalamus, overhangs the geniculate bodies and dorsolateral surface of the midbrain (Figs. 9.1, 9.3, 9.4, and 9.12). Because the pulvinar exhibits considerable cytologic uniformity it is subdivided on a topographic basis. The pulvinar is composed of lightly stained, medium-sized, multipolar cells, whose density and arrangement varies in the different subdivisions. Cells in the oral division of the pulvinar are small, light-staining, and loosely arranged. The pars inferior, separated from the main body of the pulvinar by fibers of the brachium of the superior colliculus, is composed of scattered dark-staining cells. The lateral pulvinar is traversed by oblique fiber bundles extending from the external medullary lamina.

The nuclei of the pulvinar do not receive inputs from long ascending sensory pathways, but the inferior division receives a projection from the superficial layers of the superior colliculus. Topographically this projection represents the contralateral visual hemifield. Both the inferior pulvinar and the adjacent portion of the lateral pulvinar have reciprocal connections with occipital cortex, including striate cortex. The inferior pulvinar and the adjacent lateral pulvinar each contain a representation of the contralateral visual hemifield and project retinotopically on (1) cortical areas 18 and 19 and (2) the striate cortex (area 17) where fibers terminate on the supragranular layers. These findings indicate three visuotopically organized inputs from the thalamus (lateral geniculate body, inferior pulvinar, and adjacent lateral pulvinar) to the primary visual cortex that terminate upon different layers. Projections from the inferior pulvinar to cortical areas 17, 18, and 19 constitute the final link in an extrageniculate visual pathway.

The lateral nucleus of the pulvinar (other than portions adjacent to the inferior pulvinar) projects to temporal cortex and receives reciprocal projections from the same region. The medial pulvinar appears to project to the superior temporal gyrus.

Ventral Nuclear Mass

The ventral nuclear mass of the thalamus is divided into three nuclei: the *ventral anterior*, the *ventral lateral*, and the *ventral posterior*. The ventral anterior nucleus is the most rostral and the smallest subdivision (Figs. 9.7, 9.8, and 9.12). The ventral posterior nucleus, the largest and most posterior nucleus of this group, is further subdivided into the *ventral posterolateral* and *ventral posteromedial nuclei* (Figs. 9.5 and 9.12). Although the *medial* and *lateral geniculate bodies* together constitute the *metathalamus*, these well-defined nuclear masses may be considered as a caudal continuation of the ventral nuclear mass. The ventral nuclear group and the metathalamus constitute the largest division of the thalamus concerned with relaying impulses from other portions of the neuraxis to specific parts of the cerebral cortex. Caudal parts of this complex are concerned with relaying impulses of specific sensory systems to cortical regions, while more rostral nuclei (ventral anterior and ventral lateral and rostral parts of the ventral posterolateral nuclei) relay impulses from the corpus striatum, the substantia nigra and the contralateral deep cerebellar nuclei.

Ventral Anterior Nucleus

This subdivision lies in the extreme rostral part of the ventral nuclear mass where it is bounded anteriorly and ventrolaterally by the reticular nucleus. Rostrally the ventral anterior nucleus (VA) occupies the entire thalamic region lateral to the anterior nuclear group (Figs. 9.8 and 9.12), but caudally it becomes restricted to a more medial region. The mammillothalamic tract passes through the ventral anterior nucleus but does not form its medial border. The nucleus is composed of large and medium-sized multipolar cells arranged in clusters. Thick myelinated fiber bundles course longitudinally within the nucleus.

Parts of the nucleus adjacent to the mammillothalamic tract and along the ventral border of the nucleus are composed of large, dark, densely arranged cells. This subdivision, called the magnocellular part (VAmc), extends further caudally than the principal part of the ventral anterior nucleus (VApc) (Fig. 9.7). Thus, there are two distinctive cytological subdivisions of the ventral anterior nucleus. Each of these subdivisions receives fibers from different sources without overlap. Afferent fibers to the ventral anterior nucleus (VApc) arise from the medial segment of the globus pallidus (Figs. 9.12 and 11.20). The magnocellular part of the ventral anterior nucleus (VAmc) receives fibers from the pars reticulata of the substantia nigra (Fig. 7.18).

Cortical area 6 projects primarily to VApc while fibers from area 8 terminate in VAmc; fibers from primary motor area do not reach any part of the nucleus. Afferent fibers, arising from the intralaminar and midline nuclei, may account for some of the characteristics of the nonspecific thalamic system exhibited by this nucleus.

Information concerning the efferent projections of the ventral anterior nucleus is incomplete and conflicting. Efferent fibers from this nucleus are distributed to the intralaminar nuclei and to widespread areas of the frontal cortex (Fig. 9.13). Rostrally projecting fibers from VAmc have been described as terminating in localized regions of the caudal and medial orbitofrontal cortex.

Physiological data indicate that the ventral anterior nucleus may be functionally related to the intralaminar nuclei of the thalamus, in that recruiting responses in widespread cortical areas can be evoked by repeated low frequency stimulation of the nucleus. The *recruiting response* is a surface negative response evoked by repetitive low frequency stimulation of the ventral anterior, the midline or the intralaminar thalamic nuclei that waxes and wanes and can be recorded over broad areas of the cerebral cortex. The ventral anterior nucleus appears to be the preeminent site among thalamic nuclei for the production of the recruiting response.

Ventral Lateral Nucleus

This nucleus, caudal to the ventral anterior nucleus, is composed of small and large neurons that show considerable differences in various parts of the nucleus (Figs. 9.8, 9.9, and 9.10). The nucleus has been subdivided into two main parts: (1) pars oralis (VLo) and (2) pars caudalis (VLc) (Fig. 9.12). The largest subdivision (VLo) consists of numerous deep staining cells arranged in clusters. The pars caudalis (VLc) is less cellular but formed of scattered large cells. A crescent-shaped thalamic area in the monkey caudal to VAmc and medial to VLo, designated as "area x," appears on the basis of connectivity to be an integral part of the ventral lateral nuclear complex. Nuclear subdivisions designated as VLc, "area x" and the oral part of the ventral posterolateral nucleus (VPLo) have been referred to as the "cell-sparse" zone and cytologically are distinct from VLo, VPLc, and VPM.

Pallidofugal fibers arising from the medial pallidal segment project to the ventral lateral nucleus of the thalamus via the thalamic fasciculus. The major projection from the globus pallidus is to the pars oralis, VLo. Pallidofugal fibers also project rostrally to ventral anterior nucleus (VApc) and give off collateral fibers to the centromedian nucleus (CM) (Figs. 11.19 and 11.21). These pallidal projections are topographically organized.

Efferent fibers, originating from the deep cerebellar nuclei and ascending beyond the contralateral red nucleus, enter the thalamic fasciculus and project to nuclei composing the "cell sparse" zone of the ventral lateral thalamus (VLc, VPLo, and area x) (Figs. 8.15, 8.16, and 8.18). Single-unit recordings have not revealed a sharp somatotopic organization within the deep cerebellar nuclei, but thalamic nuclei receiving these efferents have a somatotopic representation similar to that of thalamic somatosensory relay nuclei. Different parts of the body are systematically represented with rostral body regions medial and caudal parts of the body lateral; the extremities are represented ventrally (Fig. 9.15). Although dentatothalamic and interpositothalamic fibers appear to end in the same region, terminations are in an interdigitating pattern without overlap. Fastigothalamic projections are bilateral with fibers crossing in the region of the posterior commissure and/or the internal medullary lamina of the thalamus.

The ventral lateral nucleus of the thalamus receives a considerable number of fibers from the precentral cortex. Studies in the monkey demonstrate that area 4 projects to VLo, VLc, and VPLo as well as to CM, the paracentral nucleus (PCN) and the central lateral nucleus (CL). The projection from area 4 to VLc is not as impressive as that from area 6, which also projects to "area x." A systematic analysis indicates that the "cell-sparse" zone of the ventral lateral thalamic region, consisting of VPLo and VLc, projects topographically upon area 4 (Fig. 9.16). Medial parts of the nucleus send fibers to the face area, lateral parts send fibers to the leg area, and fibers from intermediate portions of the nucleus pass to cortical regions representing the arm and trunk. Thus the thalamic termination zones for the dentate, interposed and fastigial nuclei are nearly identical and relay impulses to the primary motor area.

The cortical projection zone for VLo, which receives input from the medial pallidal segment, appears different in that VLo projects to the supplementary motor area and to the lateral premotor area. The distinctive cytoarchitectural subdivisions of the ventral lateral thalamic region project to separate cortical areas concerned with different aspects of motor function.

Ventral Posterior Nucleus

This nuclear complex, whose cells are among the largest in the thalamus, is composed of two main portions, the *posteromedial* and the *posterolateral* (Figs. 9.5, 9.11, and 9.12). The VP is the largest primary somatic sensory relay nucleus of the thalamus and is referred to as the ventrobasal complex.

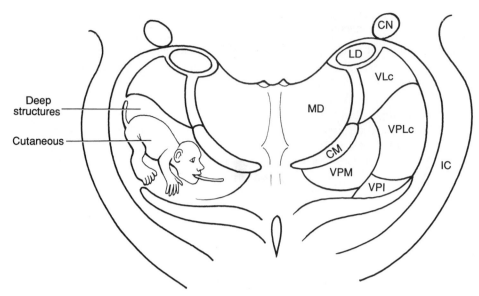

Figure 9.15. Schematic diagram of the ventrobasal complex in the monkey indicating the cutaneous somatotopic representation of the body surface on the *left*. Neurons responsive to stimulation of deep receptors lie in a dorsal outer shell. Areas representing the head, face, and tongue lie in the ventral posteromedial nucleus (*VPM*). The body is represented in the ventral posterolateral nucleus (*VPLc*) with the trunk dorsal and the extremities ventral. Nuclear subdivisions of the thalamus are shown on the *right*. *Abbreviations*: *CM*, centromedian nucleus; *CN*, caudate nucleus; *IC*, internal capsule; *LD*, lateral dorsal nucleus; *VLc*, ventral lateral nucleus, pars caudalis; *VPI*, ventral posterior inferior nucleus. (Based on Jones and Friedman, 1982.)

Ventral Posterolateral Nucleus (VPL)

This nucleus has been subdivided into a pars oralis (VPLo), characterized by very large cells sparsely distributed, and a pars caudalis (VPLc), containing large evenly dispersed cells and a high density of small cells. Both divisions of the nucleus contain medium-sized fiber bundles radiating in an oblique dorsal direction.

As described above, VPLo constitutes a distinctive part of the "cell sparse" zone of the ventral lateral thalamic region which receives inputs from the contralateral deep cerebellar nuclei and projects to the primary motor cortex.

Thalamic inputs to VPLc convey somesthetic impulses from the spinal cord and somatosensory relay nuclei in the medulla via (1) the medial lemniscus and (2) the spinothalamic tracts. Fibers of the medial lemniscus course through the brain stem, without supplying collateral or terminal fibers to the reticular formation, and terminate exclusively in the ventral posterolateral nucleus, pars caudalis (VPLc) (Fig. 4.1). Fibers arising from the nucleus gracilis terminate lateral to those of the nucleus cuneatus (Fig. 9.15). Terminals of the medial lemniscus establish predominantly axodendritic contacts throughout VPLc.

Single-unit studies of the ventral posterior nucleus in a large number of species have revealed somatotopic features in which the contralateral limbs, trunk, and tail are represented in VPLc, and the head, face, and intraoral structures in VPM (Fig. 9.15). Each large body part was represented by a curved lamella with adjacent lamellae related to neighboring body parts. Lamellae representing large divisions of the body contain labeled axons or terminals arising from cell groups in the dorsal column nuclei, or retrograde labeling of thalamic neurons projecting to parts of the somesthetic cortex. Representation of the body in the ventral posterior nucleus (VP) is continuous but distorted in a fashion that reflects the

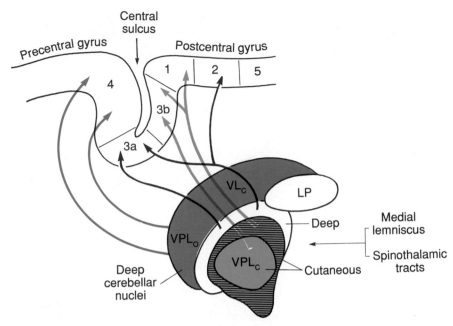

Figure 9.16. Schematic diagram in a sagittal plane showing projections of thalamic subdivisions to the sensorimotor cortex. Neurons in the ventral posterolateral (*VPLc*) and ventral posteromedial (*VPM*) nuclei (not shown) form a central core (*blue*) consisting of two parts (one represented by *solid blue* and another by *lined blue*) responsive to cutaneous stimuli and an outer shell (*white*) composed of neurons responsive to deep stimuli. Input to VPLc is via the medial lemniscus and the spinothalamic tracts; input to VPM (not shown) is via trigeminothalamic projections. Cell in the the outer shell project to cortical area 3a (muscle spindles) and to area 2 (deep receptors). Cells in the central core (*blue*) project to areas 3b and 1(cutaneous). These projections are somatotopic. Input to the ventral posterolateral nucleus, pars oralis (*VPLo*), and the ventral lateral nucleus, pars caudalis (*VLc*) (*red*) is from the contralateral deep cerebellar nuclei. Cerebellar input to these thalamic nuclei is considered to be somatotopically organized in nearly the same way as in VPLc and VPM. VPLo and VLc project somatotopically on the primary motor area (area 4). (Based on Jones and Friedman, 1982.)

greater innervation density of receptors in peripheral parts of the extremities and in the oral region. The distribution of individual, medial lemniscus axons in VPLc suggests that all axons have terminal ramifications at one level, are focal, and none are sufficiently long to occupy more than one half of the anteroposterior extent of the nucleus. Terminal ramifications are compressed into narrow sagittal slabs 200 to 300 μm wide. Axonal ramifications end in either an anterodorsal shell or in the central core of VPLc. Cells in the anterodorsal shell respond to stimulation of deep tissue and largely terminate in cortical areas 3a and 2, while neurons in the central core respond to cutaneous stimulation and largely project to cortical areas 3b and 1.

The spinothalamic tracts form a far less discrete ascending sensory pathway than the medial lemniscus. The spinothalamic tract, and fiber systems ascending with it, contributes a large number of projections and collaterals to the brain stem reticular formation at all levels.

Physiological studies indicate the precise and orderly fashion in which the contralateral body surface is represented in the ventral posterolateral nucleus (VPLc; external portion of the ventrobasal complex). There is a complete, though distorted, image of the body; volume representation of a given part of the body is related to its effectiveness as a tactile organ (i.e., to its innervation density). Cervical segments are represented most medially and sacral segments most laterally. The thoracic and lumbar regions are represented only dorsally, while the regions concerned with the distal parts of the limbs extend ventrally. Each neuron

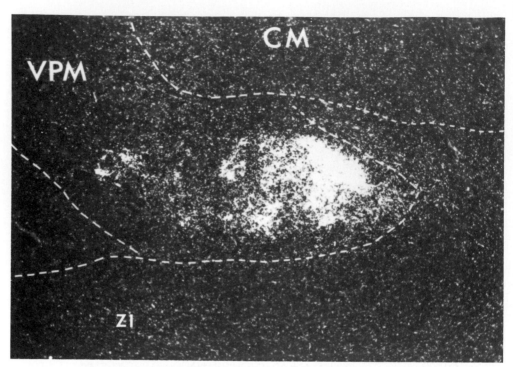

Figure 9.17. Photomicrograph of an autoradiograph demonstrating transport of isotope from the nucleus solitarius to the ipsilateral ventral posteromedial nucleus, pars parvicellaris (VPMpc). See Figure 5.24. *Abbreviations*: *CM*, centromedian nucleus:; *VPM*, ventral posteromedial nucleus; *ZI*, zona incerta. (From Beckstead et al., 1980; courtesy of Dr. Norgren and Alan R. Liss, Inc., New York.)

of this complex is related to a restricted, specific and unchanging receptive field on the contralateral side of the body. These neurons are regarded as place specific, modality specific, and concerned, almost exclusively, with the perception of tactile sense and position sense (kinesthesis). Only a few cells of the ventrobasal complex appear to be activated by noxious stimuli. The inner portion of the ventrobasal complex is known as the ventral posteromedial nucleus.

Ventral Posteromedial Nucleus (VPM)

This crescent-shaped nucleus with a relatively light-staining neuropil lies medial to the ventral posterolateral nucleus and lateral to the curved boundary of the centromedian nucleus (Figs. 9.4, 9.5, 9.11, and 9.14). The ventral posteromedial nucleus (VPM) consists of two distinct parts: (1) a principal part composed of both small and large cells, designated simply as VPM, and (2) a small celled, lighter staining part, which occupies the medial apex of this arcuate-shaped nucleus, referred to as the pars parvicellularis (VPMpc). The principal part of VPM receives somatic afferent fibers from receptors in the head, face, and intraoral structures, while VPMpc is concerned with taste (Figs. 5.24, 9.14, and 9.17). Ascending secondary trigeminal fibers terminating in VPM include (1) crossed fibers from the spinal and principal sensory trigeminal nuclei, which ascend in association with the medial lemniscus, and (2) uncrossed fibers of the dorsal trigeminal tract (Fig. 6.24). Tactile impulses from the face and intraoral structures are transmitted bilaterally to parts of the ventral posteromedial nucleus.

Secondary gustatory fibers arising from the nucleus solitarius ascend ipsilaterally in the central tegmental tract to terminate in VPMpc (Figs.

5.24 and 9.17). VPMpc also receives ipsilateral gustatory fibers from the parabrachial nuclei that also receive projections from the nucleus solitarius.

Ventral Posterior Inferior Nucleus (VPI)

This smallest subdivision of the ventral posterior nucleus lies ventrally between VPL and VPM. The ventral border of the nucleus is adjacent to the reticular nucleus and the thalamic fasciculus. Inputs to VPI are not understood, but cells in this nucleus appear to provide the major projection to somatic sensory area II (SS II) (Fig. 13.11). It has been suggested that a population of sensory neurons of VP with projections to SS II have become segregated in VPI.

Cortical Connections of the Ventral Posterior Nucleus

The ventral posterior nucleus has a precise topical projection to the cortex of the postcentral gyrus. Portions of the gyrus high on the lateral convexity receive fibers from VPLc while inferior portions of the gyrus near the lateral sulcus are supplied by fibers from VPM (Fig. 9.13). This thalamocortical projection forms a large part of the superior thalamic radiation. Neurons in the large central core of VPLc, responsive to cutaneous stimuli, project to cortical areas 3b on the posterior surface of the central sulcus and to area 1 on the lip of the sulcus. Cells in the thinner peripheral shell of VPLc, responsive to stimulations of deep tissues, project to cortical area 3a in the depths of the central sulcus and to area 2, which forms the posterior part of the postcentral gyrus (Fig. 9.16). Collectively VPLc and VPM project somatotopically upon the primary somesthetic cortex with a modality segregation. Cells of VPMpc that receive ascending gustatory fibers project fibers upon the parietal operculum, area 43.

Posterior Thalamic Nuclear Complex

Caudal to the ventral posterior nucleus there is a transitional diencephalic zone with a complex and varied cellular morphology (Fig. 9.18). The posterior nuclear complex lies caudal to VPLc, medial to the rostral part of the pulvinar, and dorsal to the medial geniculate body (Figs. 9.3 and 9.18). The posterior nucleus is of particular interest because it receives spinothalamic fibers and possibly some fibers of the medial lemniscus. The medial part of the posterior nucleus may also receive projections from the primary (S I) somatosensory cortex.

Studies in the cat and monkey indicate that cells in the medial division of the posterior thalamic nucleus (Fig. 9.18) project to the retroinsular cortex and cells in the lateral division of this nucleus project to postauditory cortex. Neither of these cortical projections overlap recognized somatosensory or auditory areas.

Medial Geniculate Body

The medial geniculate body (MGB) lies on the caudal ventral aspect of the thalamus, medial to the lateral geniculate body (LGB) and dorsal to the crus cerebri (Figs. 9.2, 9.3, and 9.19). This nuclear mass, the thalamic auditory relay nucleus, receives fibers from the inferior colliculus and gives rise to the auditory radiation (Fig. 9.24). Unlike auditory relay nuclei at lower brain stem levels, there are no commissural connections between the medial geniculate bodies. The medial geniculate nucleus

Figure 9.18. Outline drawings through two levels of the caudal thalamus in the cat showing relationships of the nuclei of the posterior complex to other thalamic nuclei. Two divisions of the posterior thalamic nuclei are recognized, medial (*PO~m~*) and lateral (*PO~l~*). In *B* the posterior thalamic nuclei lie medial and dorsal to the magnocellular part of the medial geniculate body (*MGm*); the medial nucleus (*PO~m~*) appears continuous with the suprageniculate nucleus (*SG*). In (*A*), *PO~m~* and *PO~l~* lie dorsal and lateral to the ventral posteromedial nucleus (*VPM*) and immediately caudal to the ventral posterolateral nucleus (*VPL*). *Abbreviations*: *CC*, crus cerebri; *CM*, centromedian nucleus; *DM*, mediodorsal nucleus; *Hb*, habenula; *LG*, lateral geniculate body; *MGp*, medial geniculate body, parvicellular part; *NR*, red nucleus; *OT*, optic tract; *Pt*, pretectum; *Pul*, pulvinar; *RN*, reticular nucleus of the thalamus; *SN*, substantia nigra; *ZI*, zona incerta. (Modified from Jones and Powell, 1971.)

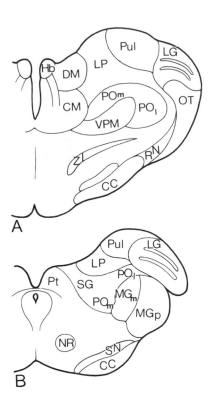

consists of several subdivisions with distinctive cytoarchitecture and connections. The three main divisions of the medial geniculate body are referred to as medial, dorsal, and ventral (Fig. 9.19). These subdivisions of the medial geniculate nucleus, not easily distinguished in ordinary histological preparations, become apparent in Golgi preparations.

The ventral nucleus extends throughout the rostrocaudal length of the MGB and is bounded medially by the brachium of the inferior colliculus. Unlike all other major subdivisions of the MGB, the ventral nucleus has a distinct laminar organization. Cells of the ventral division are fairly constant in size and shape and have tufted dendrites. The lamination, produced by the dendrites of tufted cells and fibers of the brachium of the inferior colliculus, is in the form of spirals or curved vertical sheets (Fig. 9.19). Afferent fibers from the inferior colliculus enter particular laminae and remain continuously associated with the same layers. The lamination in the ventral division of the MGB is similar to that in the lateral geniculate body (LGB), except the cellular laminae are not separated by bands of myelinated fibers. Physiological mapping of ventral division of the MGB reveals that the cellular laminae are related to the tonotopic organization, in which high frequencies are represented medially and low frequencies laterally. Neurons in the ventral division of the MGB give rise to the auditory radiation, which terminates in the primary auditory cortex (Figs. 9.13, 9.24, and 13.23), where there is a spatial representation of tonal frequencies. The primary auditory cortex gives rise to reciprocal corticothalamic fibers that terminate in the ventral division of the MGB. Both geniculocortical and cortiogeniculate fibers are ipsilateral.

In humans, the principal cortical projection of the medial geniculate body is to the superior temporal convolution (transverse superior temporal convolution (transverse gyrus of Heschl) via the geniculotemporal or auditory radiation (Figs. 2.4, 2.9, 6.9, 9.13, and 9.24). This cortical projection area (area 41) has a tonotopic localization in which high tones

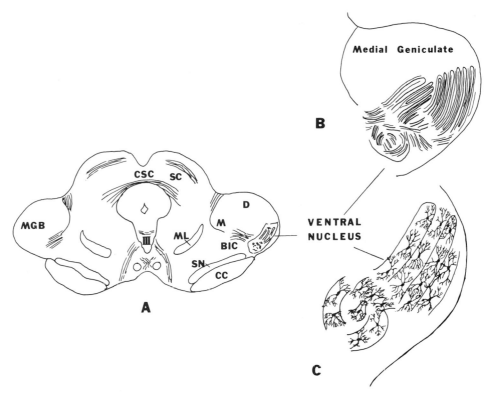

Figure 9.19. Transverse reconstructions of the fibrodendritic laminations in the ventral nucleus of the medial geniculate body in the cat based on Golgi preparations. *A*, Transverse section of the midbrain through the medial geniculate body (*MGB*); *M* and *D* indicate the magnocellular and dorsal nuclei, respectively. The lamination in the ventral nucleus of the MGB (*A, B,* and *C*) is produced by the arrangement of dendrites of geniculate neurons and fibers of the brachium of the inferior colliculus. Abbreviations: *BIC*, brachium of the inferior colliculus; *CC*, crus cerebri; *CSC*, commissure of the superior colliculus; *SC*, superior colliculus; *SN*, substantia nigra; III, oculomotor nucleus. (Based on Morest, 1965.)

are appreciated medially and low tones are represented laterally and anteriorly.

The dorsal division of the MGB contains several nuclei, among which are the suprageniculate and the dorsal nuclei. The dorsal nucleus, prominent at caudal levels of the MGB (Fig. 9.19), receives projections from a lateral tegmental area, extending from the deep layers of the superior colliculus to the area adjacent to the lateral lemniscus. The medial magnocellular division of the MGB receives inputs from the inferior colliculus, the lateral tegmentum and spinal cord (Fig. 9.19). Nonlaminated portions of the MGB send fibers ipsilaterally to a cortical belt surrounding the primary auditory area (Figs. 13.22 and 13.23).

Lateral Geniculate Body

The lateral geniculate body (LGB), the thalamic relay nucleus for the visual system, lies rostral and lateral to the medial geniculate body (MGB), lateral to the crus cerebri, and ventral to the pulvinar (Figs. 9.2, 9.3, 9.12, and 9.20). This laminated cellular structure in transverse sections has a horseshoe-shaped configuration with the hilus directed ventromedially. Crossed and uncrossed fibers of the optic tract enter via the hilus and are distributed in precise pattern. In humans and primates the LGB consists of six cellular layers or laminae arranged in two subdivisions. The six concentric cell layers, separated by intervening fiber bands, customarily are numbered from 1 to 6, beginning from the hilar region (Fig.

Figure 9.20. Drawing of the cellular lamination in the lateral geniculate body with laminae numbered from the hilus. The magnocellular laminae (*1* and *2*) and the parivcellular laminae (*3* through *6*) constitute the dorsal nucleus of the lateral geniculate. Crossed fibers in the optic tract terminate in laminae *1*, *4*, and *6*; uncrossed optic fibers terminate in the other laminae.

Dorsolateral

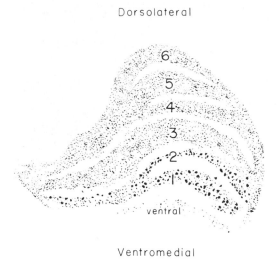

Ventromedial

9.20). Subdivisions of the dorsal nucleus of the LGB are magnocellular (layers 1 and 2) and parvicellular (layers 3 to 6). Both divisions of the dorsal lateral geniculate nucleus receive afferents from the ganglion cells of the retina.

The parvicellular layers of LGB, consisting of layers 3, 4, 5, and 6 in ventrodorsal sequence, are easily distinguished. As these layers are traced laterally they fuse in pairs: layer 4 with layer 6, and layer 3 with layer 5. The projection from the retina onto the lateral geniculate body is precise and crossed and uncrossed fibers in the optic tract end upon separate layers. Crossed fibers of the optic tract end upon layers 1, 4, and 6, while uncrossed fibers terminate in layers 2, 3, and 5 (Figs. 9.20 and 9.21).

Two unique features related to crossed retinogeniculate fibers are reflected in structure. The monocular crescent of the visual field is subserved by receptor elements in the most medial part of the nasal retina (Fig. 9.23). Ganglion cells in this part of the retina project crossed fibers to the bilaminar segment (Fig. 9.21) of opposite LGB, located laterally where parts of layers 4 and 6 fuse. The optic disc, located in the nasal half of the retina and representing optic nerve fibers, has no photoreceptors; it is responsible for the blind spot detectable on perimetry. The optic disc, represented in the contralateral LGB by cellular discontinuities in layers 4 and 6, is a constant feature (Fig. 9.21).

Nissl preparations through the human lateral geniculate nucleus reveal a linear cellular organization in which the long axis of the cells is oriented perpendicular to the axis of the laminae. Perikarya in different layers are aligned to form "lines of projection," which indicate identical points in the visual field (Fig. 9.22).

The topographic representation of the retinal surface within the LGB is highly organized and precise. The contralateral half of the binocular visual field is represented in each of the six layers of the LGB, even though crossed and uncrossed fibers end in different layers (Fig. 9.23). The projection locales in the six layers lie in perfect register so that any small area in the contralateral binocular visual field can be shown to correspond to a dorsoventral column of cells extending radially through all six layers in the "lines of projection" (Figs. 9.22 and 9.23). The LGB consists of six sheets of cells bent in a horseshoe configuration, but in exact registration, so that columns of cells in the "lines of projection" receive inputs from corresponding points in the retina of each eye related

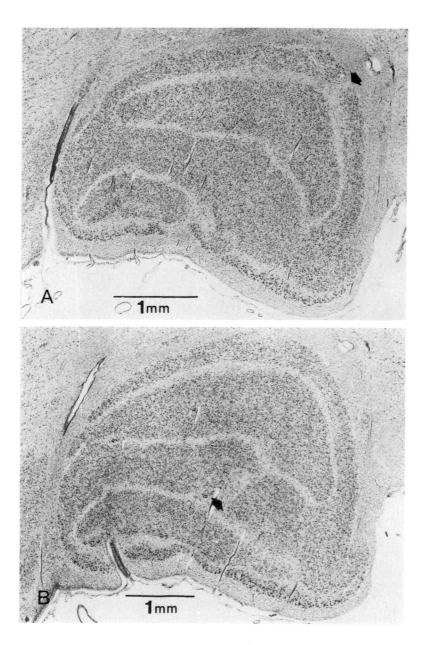

Figure 9.21. Photomicrographs of sections of the human lateral geniculate body. The blind spot is represented by discontinuities in laminae 6 (*A, arrow*) and 4 (*B, arrow*). Laminae 4 and 6 fuse laterally (*right*) in both *A* and *B* producing the bilaminar segment ventrally. The bilaminar segment receives input from the most medial contralateral nasal retina that subserves the monocular visual field (i.e., the monocular crescent.) See Figure 9.23. (From Hickey and Guillery, 1979; courtesy of the Wistar Institute Press.)

to the contralateral binocular visual field (Fig. 9.23). Binocular fusion does not occur in the LGB because retinogeniculate fibers end on different layers. Following section of the optic nerve, anterograde degeneration or transneuronal degeneration (after long survivals) occurs in three layers of the LGB on each side. The layers in which degeneration of fibers or cells occur differs in accordance with the disposition of crossed (layers 1, 4, and 6) and uncrossed (layers 2, 3, and 5) retinal fibers. Small lesions of the retina produce transneuronal degeneration in localized clusters of cells in three different layers on each side aligned according to the "lines of projection." The contralateral monocular visual field (monocular crescent), related to receptor elements in the most medial nasal retina, is represented by crossed fibers terminating in the only bilaminar segment (Figs. 9.21 and 9.23).

The "lines of projection" in the lateral geniculate body also can be demonstrated by retrograde cell degeneration in the LGB following a small lesion in the striate cortex (Fig. 9.22). Since one half of the visual

Figure 9.22. Photomicrography of the lateral geniculate body (*LGB*) of a baboon that sustained several lesions in the striate cortex. Retrograde degeneration in a large V-shaped sector of the *LGB* demonstrates the lines of projection. *Lines of projection* represent points of isorepresentation in the visual field. (From Kaas, Guillery, and Allman, 1972 with permission.)

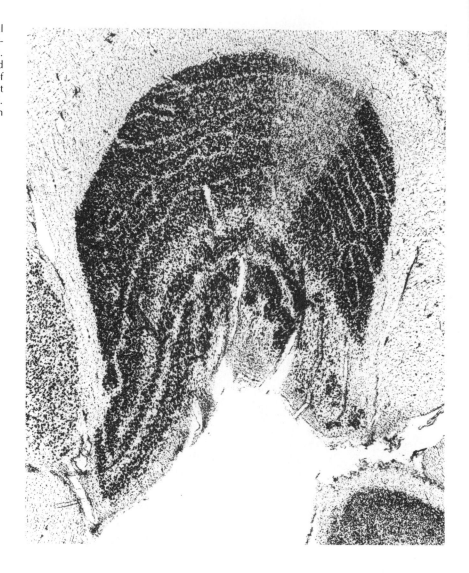

field is represented topographically in the striate cortex of each hemisphere, the zone of retrograde cell degeneration in the LGB would be bounded on each side by lines of projections.

In the LGB the horizontal meridian of the visual field corresponds to an oblique dorsoventral plane that divides the nucleus into medial and lateral segments. Fibers from superior retinal quadrants of both eyes project to the medial half of the LGB; the inferior retinal quadrants send fibers to the lateral half of the nucleus. The retinal projection from the macula is represented in a wedge-shaped sector in the caudal part of the LGB on both sides of the plane representing the horizontal meridian. The macular representation accounts for about 12% of the total volume of the LGB. The vertical meridian of the visual field, corresponding to the line separating temporal and nasal parts of the retina, is represented along the caudal margin of the nucleus from its medial to lateral borders.

The lateral geniculate nucleus is the main end station of the optic tract. It projects to the calcarine cortex (area 17) via the geniculocalcarine tract or visual radiation, and it receives corticogeniculate fibers from the same area (Figs. 2.9, 9.24, 9.27, and 9.28). Its internuclear connections are with the pulvinar.

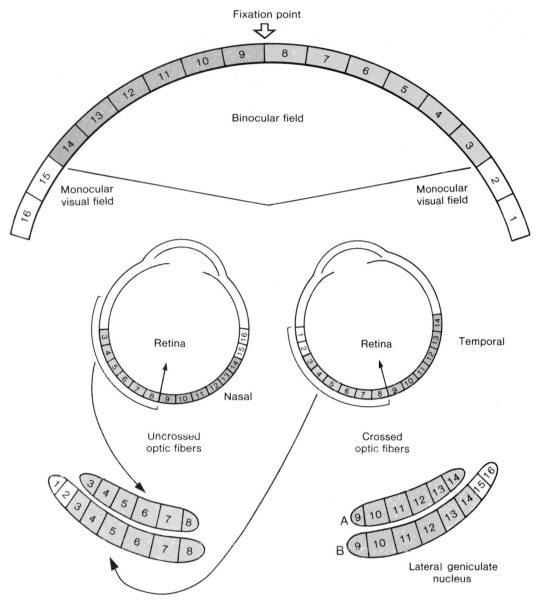

Figure 9.23. Schematic diagram of the representation of the visual field in the retinae and in the laminae of the lateral geniculate nucleus. Portions of the binocular visual field are shown in *red* (*left*) and *blue* (*right*), while the monocular visual fields are *white*. Light from numbered sectors of both the binocular and monocular visual fields falls on correspondingly numbered sectors of the retinae. Crossed and uncrossed retinofugal fibers project on columns of cells in different laminae of the lateral geniculate nucleus in exact registration, represented by corresponding numbers. *A* represents laminae receiving uncrossed fibers (i.e., laminae 2, 3, and 5). *B* represents laminae receiving crossed fibers (i.e., 1, 4, and 6). Light from the right monocular visual field (sectors 1 and 2) falls on retinal receptors of the corresponding numbers in the most medial ipsilateral nasal retina. Crossed retinal fibers from sectors 1 and 2 project to cell columns of the same number in the left lateral geniculate. Sectors 1 and 2 in the lateral geniculate body form the bilaminar segment in which cells of laminae 4 and 6 are fused (see Fig. 9.21). (Modified from Kass et al., 1972.)

Thalamic Reticular Nucleus

The thalamic reticular nucleus (RN) is a thin neuronal shell which surrounds the lateral, superior, and rostroinferior aspects of the dorsal thalamus (Figs. 9.5, 9.10, 9.11, and 9.12). This thalamic nuclear envelope is a derivative of the ventral thalamus which has migrated dorsally and lies between the external medullary lamina of the thalamus and the internal capsule. Cells in this nucleus are heterogeneous in type, ranging from very small cells in dorsal regions to quite large cells in ventral and caudal regions. Golgi studies of the reticular nucleus reveal neurons similar to those of the brain stem reticular formation. Long dendrites of these cells exhibit no specific orientation. The main axons of the cells project medially into the principal thalamic nuclei, although some axons run entirely within the reticular nucleus.

Inputs to the reticular nucleus are derived from the principal thalamic nuclei and from the cerebral cortex. Fibers emanating from a nucleus of the dorsal thalamus and destined for a specific cortical area give collateral branches that terminate in a particular part of the reticular nucleus. Corticothalamic fibers passing toward a particular nucleus of the dorsal thalamus give collaterals to the same portions of the reticular nucleus as the target nucleus of the thalamus. Cells in restricted parts of the reticular nucleus project back to the thalamic nucleus from which it receives an input. Both the intralaminar and relay nuclei of the dorsal thalamus project to the reticular nucleus and both receive fibers from it. The reticular nucleus is situated so as to sample neural activity passing between the cerebral cortex and nuclei of the dorsal thalamus, but it has no projection to the cerebral cortex. Cortical projections to portions of the reticular nucleus arise from the entire cerebral cortex and are topographically organized. Since the major projections of the thalamic reticular nucleus are to specific and nonspecific thalamic nuclei, it probably serves to integrate and "gate" activities of thalamic neurons.

NEUROCHEMICAL FEATURES OF THE THALAMUS

Cholinesterase-staining of the thalamus has revealed no cholinesterase-positive cells in the thalamus, but certain regions of the neuropil, positive for acetylcholinesterase (AChE), appear to correspond to locations of cholinergic receptors. AChE staining is present in the anterior nuclei of the thalamus (AD,AV), the internal medullary lamina, the reticular nucleus, and in parts of the midline nuclei. The significance of these regional concentrations of AChE is not clear, since it does not necessarily imply cholinergic neurotransmission. The only unquestioned diencephalic cholinergic neurons are in the medial habenular nuclei. Studies based on choline acetyltransferase (ChAT), the synthesizing enzyme for acetylcholine (ACh), suggest that cholinergic neurons in the pedunculopontine nucleus provide the major tegmental innervation of the ventral lateral thalamic region in the rat. These cholinergic thalamic projections have been regarded as playing a role in the reticular activating system. ChAT-immunoreactive terminals in the thalamic reticular have been shown to originate from the basal nuclei of Meynert (substantia innominata), the pedunculopontine nucleus, and the lateral dorsal tegmental nucleus, the three major collections of cholinergic neurons in the central nervous system.

γ-Aminobutyric acid (GABA) is the best-documented thalamic neurotransmitter. Virtually all cells in the thalamic reticular nucleus are strongly GABAergic. In the lateral geniculate nucleus GABAergic neurons have been identified in all laminae but were most abundant in the magnocellular laminae. GABA-immunoreactive neurons in the thalamus, other than those in the reticular nucleus, appear more numerous in the primate than in other forms. Most of these GABAergic neurons in the monkey are small and have been regarded as interneurons. The major projections of the medial pallidal segment to VApc and VLo and the projections from the pars reticulata of the substantia nigra to VAmc and MDpl are GABAergic. These projections are considered to play a cardinal role in aspects of motor function.

Transmitter substances of the major afferent pathways to the thalamus are not presently known. Glutamate and/or aspartate are considered to be the neurotransmitter of the deep cerebellar nuclei. Among the long ascending pathways from the spinal cord, the spinothalamic tract is involved in mechanisms concerned with pain perception. Immunocytochemical studies of neuropeptides in the thalamus have not revealed cells positive for substance P (SP), somatostatin (SRIF), cholecystokinin (CCK), neuropeptide Y (NPY), or enkephalin (ENK). Fibers staining positive for these substances have been identified in the reticular nucleus of thalamus and in parts of the intralaminar nuclei. SP-immunoreactive fibers and terminals appeared particularly dense in the ventral posteromedial nucleus VPM, but were absent in the centromedian nucleus (CM). Fibers containing neuropeptides appeared to enter the thalamus from the hypothalamus and from the midbrain tegmentum.

Glutamate and aspartate appear to be the principal neurotransmitters in corticothalamic projection systems. Combined retrograde transport technics and immunocytochemical methods clearly reveal that corticothalamic neurons in lamina VI are positive for these neurotransmitters. Approximately 90% of corticothalamic neurons are positive for either glutamate or aspartate and about 25% of these neurons are immunopositive for both. These massive cortical afferents have excitatory actions on thalamic neurons.

CLAUSTRUM

This thin plate of gray matter lies in the white matter of the hemisphere between the lentiform nucleus and the insular cortex; it is separated from these structures by the external capsule medially and the extreme capsule laterally (Figs. 2.11, 2.16, 2.17, and 11.5). Although the claustrum is situated close to the striatum, its principal connections are with the cerebral cortex and it bears striking resemblances to the thalamus. Two distinct parts of the claustrum are recognized: (1) an insular part composed of large cells underlying the insular cortex and (2) a temporal part located between the putamen and the temporal lobe. The claustrum has widespread reciprocal connections with the sensory cortex; it also receives inputs from the lateral hypothalamus, the centromedian nucleus of the thalamus, and the locus ceruleus. However, the sensory nuclei of the thalamus do not project to the claustrum. The major afferents to claustrum arise from the cerebral cortex; corticoclaustral projections arise from pyramidal cells in layer VI, the same layer that projects to the thalamus. Fibers from numerous cortical areas each terminate in distinct zones within the claustrum. Thus, the claustrum contains discrete somesthetic, visual and auditory zones. The claustrum has no subcortical projections.

THALAMIC RADIATIONS AND THE INTERNAL CAPSULE

Fibers that reciprocally connect the thalamus and the cortex constitute the thalamic radiations. Thalamocortical and corticothalamic fibers form a continuous fan that emerges along the whole lateral extent of the caudate nucleus. Fiber bundles, radiating forward, backward, upward, and downward, form large portions of various parts of the internal capsule (Figs. 2.10, 2.11, 2.16, 2.17, 9.2, 9.5, 9.7, 9.8, 9.24, 9.25, and 9.28).

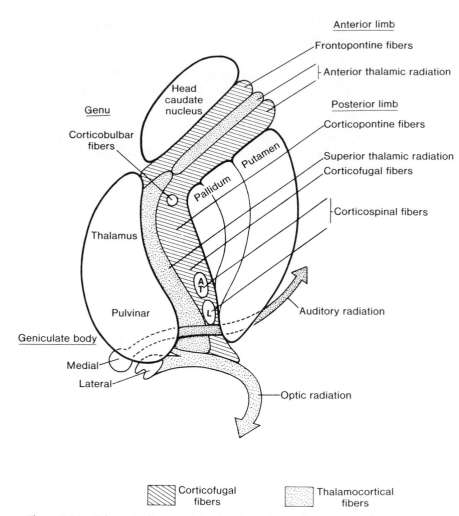

Figure 9.24. Schematic diagram of the right internal capsule as seen in a horizontal section similar to that in Figure 9.25. Corticospinal fibers in humans are in the caudal third of the posterior limb of the internal capsule.

Though the radiations connect with practically all parts of the cortex, the richness of connections varies in different cortical areas. Most abundant are the projections to the frontal granular cortex, the precentral and postcentral gyri, the calcarine area, and the gyrus of Heschl. The posterior parietal region and adjacent portions of the temporal lobe also have rich thalamic connections, but relatively scanty radiations go to other cortical areas.

The thalamic radiations are grouped into four subradiations designated as the thalamic peduncles (Figs. 9.24 and 9.25). The *anterior* or *frontal peduncle* connects the frontal lobe with the medial and anterior thalamic nuclei. The *superior* or *centroparietal peduncle* connects the Rolandic area and adjacent portions of the frontal and parietal lobes with the ventral tier thalamic nuclei. Fibers, carrying general somatic sensory signals from the body and head, form part of this radiation and terminate in the postcentral gyrus (Figs. 9.14 and 9.24). The *posterior* or *occipital peduncle* connects the occipital and posterior parietal convolutions with the caudal portions of the thalamus. It includes the optic radiation from the lateral geniculate body and claustrocortical projections to the calcarine cortex (Fig. 9.28). The *inferior* or *temporal peduncle* is relatively small and includes the connections of the thalamus with the temporal lobe and

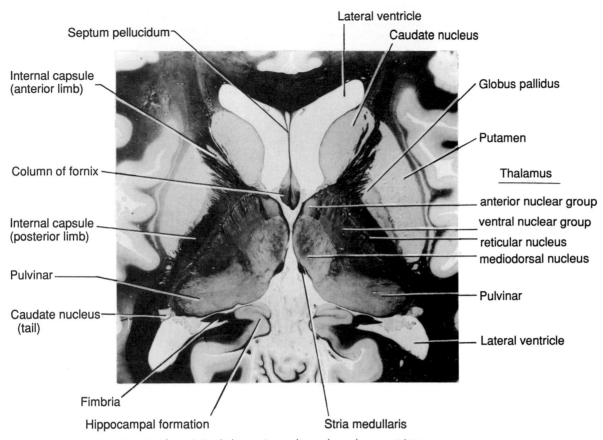

Septum pellucidum

Lateral ventricle

Caudate nucleus

Internal capsule
(anterior limb)

Globus pallidus

Putamen

Column of fornix

Thalamus

anterior nuclear group

ventral nuclear group

Internal capsule
(posterior limb)

reticular nucleus

mediodorsal nucleus

Pulvinar

Pulvinar

Caudate nucleus
(tail)

Lateral ventricle

Fimbria

Hippocampal formation

Stria medullaris

Figure 9.25.   Horizontal section through the thalamus, internal capsule, and corpus striatum. Weigert's myelin stain. Photograph.

the insula (Fig. 9.9). Included in this peduncle is the auditory radiation from the medial geniculate body to the transverse temporal gyrus of Heschl (Figs. 2.9 and 9.24).

The cerebral hemisphere is connected with the brain stem and spinal cord by an extensive system of projection fibers. These fibers arise from the whole extent of the cortex, enter the white substance of the hemisphere, and appear as a radiating mass of fibers, the *corona radiata*, which converges toward the brain stem (Figs. 2.9 and 2.10). On reaching the latter they form a broad, compact fiber band, the *internal capsule*, flanked medially by the thalamus and caudate nucleus and laterally by the lentiform nucleus (Figs. 2.11, 2.16, 2.17, 9.6, 9.24, and 9.25). Thus the internal capsule is composed of all the fibers, afferent and efferent, which go to, or come from, the cerebral cortex. A large part of the capsule is composed of the thalamic radiations described above. The rest is composed mainly of cortical efferent fiber systems (i.e., corticofugal fibers), which descend to the brain stem and to the spinal cord. These include the corticospinal, corticobulbar, corticoreticular and corticopontine tracts.

The internal capsule, as seen in a horizontal section, is composed of *anterior* and *posterior limbs*, which meet at an obtuse angle; the junctional zone is known as the *genu* (Figs. 2.11, 9.24, and 9.25). The anterior limb lies between the lentiform and caudate nuclei. The posterior limb of the internal capsule (*lenticulothalamic portion*), lies between the lentiform nucleus and the thalamus. A *retrolenticular part* of the internal capsule extends caudally behind the lentiform nucleus for a short distance (Fig. 9.2). Fibers passing beneath the lentiform nucleus to reach the

Pigment
epithelium

External limiting
membrane

Plexiform layers

Ganglion cell layer

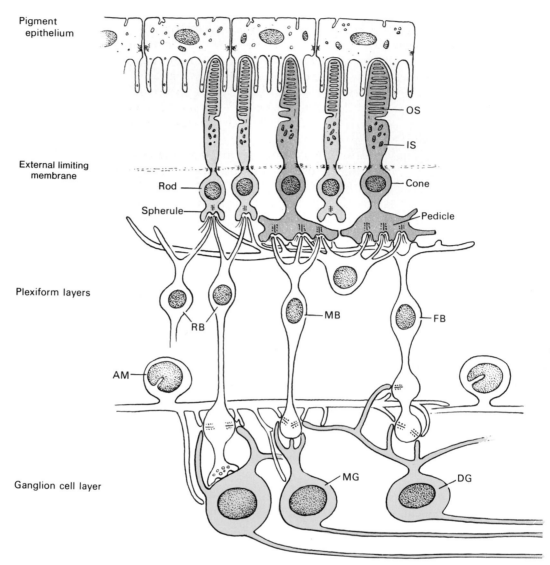

Figure 9.26.   Schematic diagram of the ultrastructural organization of the retina. Rods (*blue*) and cones (*red*) arc composed of outer (*OS*) and inner (*IS*) segments, cell bodies, and synaptic bases. Photopigments are present in laminated discs in the outer segments. The synaptic base of a rod cell is called a *spherule*; the synaptic base of a cone cell is known as a *pedicle*. In the plexiform layers *RB* denotes rod bipolar cells, *MB* a midget bipolar cell, and *FB* a flat bipolar cell. *AM* indicates an amacrine cell. Ganglion cells (*MG*, midget ganglion cell; *DG*, diffuse ganglion cell) and retinal afferents are in *yellow*. (Modified from Dowling and Boycott, 1966.)

temporal lobe collectively form the *sublenticular* portion of the internal capsule (Fig. 9.24).

The *anterior limb* of the internal capsule contains the anterior thalamic radiation and the prefrontal corticopontine tract. The *genu* contains corticobulbar and corticoreticular fibers.

The *posterior limb* of the internal capsule contains (1) corticospinal fibers, (2) frontopontine fibers, (3) the superior thalamic radiation, and (4) relatively smaller numbers of corticotectal, corticorubral and corticoreticular fibers (Fig. 9.24). Corticospinal fibers in man classically have been considered to lie in the posterior limb of the internal capsule relatively close to the genu. Recent data suggest that corticospinal fibers are largely confined to compact region in the caudal half of the posterior limb of the internal capsule. Fibers of the corticospinal tract are somatotopically arranged in this part of the internal capsule, with those destined for cervical, thoracic, lumbar, and sacral spinal arranged in a rostrocaudal sequence. The classic view that corticospinal fibers occupy the medial three-fifths of the crus cerebri appears unreasonable on the basis of the number of fibers in the crus cerebri. The somatotopic arrangement of corticospinal fibers in the crus cerebri is much less precise than commonly depicted (Fig. 7.1). Fibers of the superior thalamic radiation, located caudal to the corticospinal fibers, project signals concerned with general somatic sense to the postcentral gyrus (Fig. 9.24).

The *retrolenticular portion* of the posterior limb contains the posterior thalamic radiations, including the optic radiation, parietal and occipital corticopontine fibers, and fibers from the occipital cortex to the superior colliculi and pretectal region (Figs. 9.2 and 9.3). The *sublenticular* portion, difficult to separate from the retrolenticular, contains the *inferior thalamic peduncle* (Fig. 9.9), the auditory radiation, and corticopontine fibers from the temporal and the parieto-occipital area.

Thalamocortical and *corticofugal* fibers within the internal capsule occupy a small, compact area (Fig. 9.24). Lesions in this area produce more widespread disturbances than lesions in any other region of the nervous system. Thrombosis or hemorrhage of the anterior choroidal, striate, or capsular branches of the middle cerebral arteries (Figs. 14.9 and 14.10) are responsible for most of the lesions in the internal capsule. Vascular lesions in the posterior limb of the internal capsule result in contralateral hemianesthesia due to injury of thalamocortical fibers. There is also a contralateral hemiplegia due to injury of corticospinal fibers. If the genu of the internal capsule is included in the injury, corticobulbar fibers may be destroyed. Lesions in the most posterior region of the posterior limb may include the optic and auditory radiations. In such instances there may be a contralateral triad consisting of hemianesthesia, hemianopsia, and hemihypacusis.

VISUAL PATHWAY

Retina

The rods and cones of the retina are visual receptors that react specifically to physical light (Fig. 9.26). The cones have a higher threshold of excitability and are stimulated by light of relatively high intensity. They are responsible for sharp vision and for color discrimination in adequate illumination. The rods react to low intensities of illumination and subserve twilight and night vision. Close to the posterior pole of the eye, the retina shows a small, circular, yellowish area, the macula lutea. The macula represents the retinal area for central vision, and the eyes are fixed in such a manner that the retinal image of any object is always focused on the macula. The rest of the retina is concerned with paracentral and peripheral vision. In the macular region the inner layers of the retina are pushed apart, forming a small central pit, the *fovea centralis*, which constitutes the point of sharpest vision and most acute color discrimination. Here the retina is composed entirely of closely packed slender cones.

The rods and cones are composed of an outer segment, a narrow neck, an inner segment, a cell body, and a synaptic base (Fig. 9.26). Photopigments are present in the outer segments, where the photochemical reactions to light take place that give rise to the generator potential. The outer segment is composed of a series of laminated discs derived from infoldings of the plasma membrane. The photopigments, bound to the membranes of the discs, are constantly renewed. Rhodopsin is the photopigment of the rods in primates, and three pigments with maximum absorptions for blue, green, and red are present in the cones. The synaptic base of the cone is called a *pedicle*, while that of the rod is referred to as a *spherule*. Each cone pedicle has several invaginations which contain terminals of horizontal, midget bipolar, and flat bipolar cells in a specific arrangement. Rod spherules have a single invagination containing multiple processes of horizontal and rod bipolar cells (Fig. 9.26). Each midget ganglion cell makes several synaptic contacts with a single bipolar cell. Diffuse ganglion cells establish synaptic contacts with all types of bipolar cells. Horizontal cells and amacrine cells constitute retinal interneurons. It is difficult to determine whether processes of horizontal cells are axons or dendrites, and it is possible that each process may be capable of both receiving and transmitting signals. Amacrine cells in the inner plexiform layer have no axon but make synaptic contacts with all types of bipolar cells, other amacrine cells, and the dendrites and somata of ganglion cells. The axons of ganglion cells, at first unmyelinated, are arranged in fine radiating bundles which run parallel to the retinal surface and converge at the optic disc to form the optic nerve. On emerging from the eyeball, the fibers at once acquire a myelin sheath.

Retinal ganglion cells are of different sizes, project to different sites and form at least three functional classes. Distinct classes of ganglion cells are referred to X, Y, and W cells. The X class cells have slower conduction velocities than Y cells, exhibit sustained or tonic responses and project to the dorsal nucleus of the LGB and the pretectum. The Y cells have rapid conduction, exhibit transient or phasic responses and project to the dorsal nucleus of the LGB and the superior colliculus. The W ganglion cells have either tonic or phasic responses, very slow axonal conduct velocities, and project to the superior colliculus and the pretectum. It has been suggested that (1) the largest ganglion cells correspond to the Y cells, (2) medium-sized cells with narrow dendritic arborizations correspond to the X cells, and (3) the smallest ganglion cells with the widest dendritic arborizations correspond to the W cells. Because the central projections of these classes of retinal ganglion cells differ, it is presumed that their functional roles also differ. Both X and Y cells possess properties that contribute to the highly discriminative aspects of vision. Both cell types have high resolving properties. The smaller receptive field centers of the X cells permit resolving higher spatial frequencies than Y cells, but Y cells are more sensitive to moving stimuli. X cells tend to be concentrated near the central retina, whereas Y cells occur in all parts of the retina. The Y cells are present in much smaller numbers than either X or W cells. Since W cells do not project to the dorsal nucleus of the LGB, it is presumed that X-type ganglion cells must be concerned with central vision.

Optic Nerves

These nerves enter the cranial cavity through the optic foramina and unite to form the optic chiasm, beyond which they are continued as the optic tracts (Figs. 2.7, 2.8, 9.5, and 9.27). Within the chiasm a partial decussation occurs, the fibers from the nasal halves of the retina cross to the opposite side, and those from the temporal halves of the retina remain uncrossed (Figs. 9.23 and 9.27). In binocular vision each visual field, right and left, is projected on portions of both retinae. Thus the images of objects in the right field of vision (*red* in Fig. 9.27) are projected on the right nasal and the left temporal halves of the retina. The right monocular crescent of the visual field (not shown in Fig. 9.27) projects upon retinal

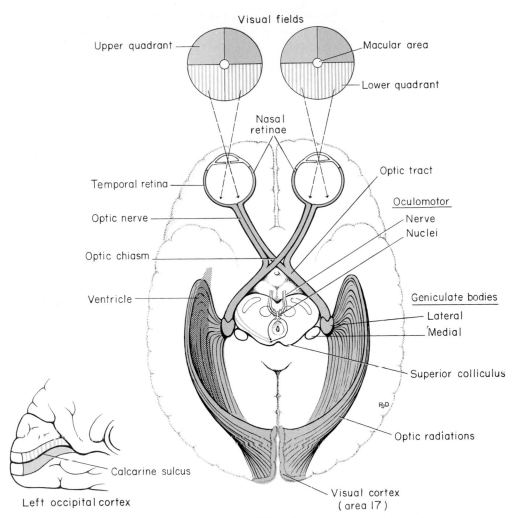

Figure 9.27. Diagram of the visual pathways viewed from the ventral surface of the brain. Light from the upper half of the visual field falls on the inferior half of the retina. Light from the temporal half of the visual field falls on the nasal half of the retina; light from the nasal half of the visual field falls on the temporal half of the retina. The visual pathways from the retina to the striate cortex are shown. The plane of the visual fields has been rotated 90 degrees toward the reader. The insert (*lower left*) shows the projection of the quadrants of the visual field on the left calcarine (striate) cortex. The macular area of the retina (*white*) is represented nearest the occipital pole. Fibers (*blue*) mediating the pupillary light reflex leave the optic tract and project to the pretectal region; fibers from the pretectal olivary nucleus relay signals bilaterally to the visceral nuclei of the oculomotor complex. (From Carpenter and Sutin, *Human Neuroanatomy,* 1983; courtesy of Williams and Wilkins.)

receptors only in the most medial part of the right nasal retina (Fig. 9.23). In the chiasm the fibers from these two retinal portions are combined to form the left optic tract. By this arrangement the whole right field of vision is projected upon the left hemisphere, and the left visual field upon the right hemisphere.

Optic Tract

Each optic tract partially encircles the hypothalamus and the rostral portions of the crus cerebri (Fig. 2.8). Most of its fibers terminate in the lateral geniculate body, though small portions continue as the brachium of the superior colliculus to the superior colliculus and pretectal area (Fig. 9.27). The lateral geniculate body gives rise to the geniculocalcarine tract, which forms the last relay of the visual path. The pretectal area (Figs.

7.12, 7.13, and 9.3) is concerned with the light reflex, and the superior colliculi with reflex movement of the eyes and head and tracking of visual stimuli. Retinohypothalamic fibers terminate bilaterally in the suprachiasmatic nucleus of the hypothalamus (Figs. 10.1 and 10.6). This direct retinal projection is functionally relevant to neuroendocrine regulation.

Geniculocalcarine Tract

This tract arises from cells in the dorsal nucleus of the LGB, passes through the retrolenticular portion of the internal capsule, and forms the optic radiation (Fig. 9.24). These fibers terminate on both sides of the calcarine sulcus in the striate cortex (Figs. 9.27 and 9.28). All fibers of the radiation do not reach the cortex by the shortest route. The most dorsal fibers pass almost directly backward to the striate cortex. More ventral fibers first turn forward and downward into the temporal lobe, spread out over the rostral part of the inferior horn of the lateral ventricle and then loop backward. These fibers pass close to the outer wall of the lateral ventricle (external sagittal stratum) to reach the occipital cortex (Fig. 2.19). The most ventral fibers make the longest loop (Figs. 9.27 and 9.28).

The retinal areas have a precise point-to-point relationship with the lateral geniculate body, each portion of the retina projecting on a specific and topographically limited portion of the layers of the lateral geniculate. The fibers from the upper retinal quadrants (representing the lower visual field) terminate in the medial half, those from the lower quadrants terminate in the lateral half of the geniculate body. The macula is represented by a wedge-shaped sector in the caudal part of the LGB on both sides of the plane representing the horizontal meridian. The peripheral field, including the monocular crescent, is represented rostrally and laterally in the LGB and is continuous across the horizontal meridian (Fig. 9.23). A similar point-to-point relation exists between the geniculate body and the striate cortex. The medial half of the lateral geniculate body, representing the upper quadrants (lower visual field) projects to the superior lip of the calcarine sulcus, and the fibers form the superior portion of the optic radiation (Fig. 9.27). The lateral half of the lateral geniculate body, representing the lower retinal quadrants (upper visual field) projects to the inferior lip of the calcarine sulcus. These fibers form the inferior portion of the optic radiation. The macular fibers, which constitute the intermediate part of the optic radiation, terminate in the caudal third of the calcarine cortex. Those from the paracentral and peripheral retinal areas end in respectively more rostral portions.

Experimental studies with stationary spots of light indicate that the receptive fields of ganglion cells in the retina are organized into two concentric zones. In the retina the receptive field is related to those receptors, rods and cones, and other retinal neurons which influence the excitability of a single ganglion cell. The retina is a composite of as many receptive fields as there are ganglion cells. Each receptive field is organized into two zones: (1) a small circular central zone, and (2) a surrounding concentric zone referred to as the periphery, or surround. These two zones are functionally antagonistic. Two general types of receptive fields have been described: (1) those with an "on" center and an "off" surround and (2) those with an "off" center and an "on" surround. If a light stimulus illuminates an "on" center, or an "on" surround, the ganglion cell will fire vigorously (Fig. 13.15). If the light stimulus illuminates both "on" and "off" zones, mutual inhibition cancels the stimulus. Retinal

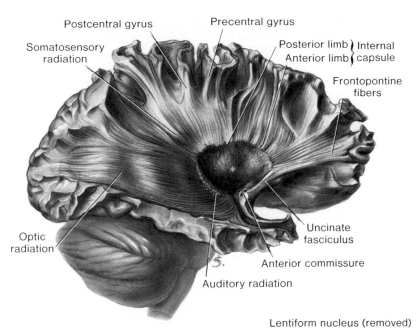

Postcentral gyrus

Precentral gyrus

Somatosensory
radiation

Posterior limb ⎫ Internal
Anterior limb ⎰ capsule

Frontopontine
fibers

Optic
radiation

Uncinate
fasciculus

Anterior commissure

Auditory radiation

Lentiform nucleus (removed)

Figure 9.28.   Drawing of a lateral brain dissection of the corona radiata showing the visual, auditory, and somatosensory radiations. The lentiform nucleus has been removed and its position is marked by an *asterisk* (*). (From Mettler's *Neuroanatomy*, 1948.)

connections account for the concentric circular receptive fields at the ganglion cell level. Impulses from the central zone are said to be mediated by direct connections between receptor cells, bipolar cells, and ganglion cells, while the antagonistic surround zone has interposed connections with amacrine cells (i.e., between bipolar and ganglion cells). The receptive fields of neurons in the lateral geniculate body appear similar to those in the retina with stationary spots of light, but LBG neurons show a greater suppression of the receptive field periphery. Cells in different laminae of the lateral geniculate body are driven from receptive fields in one eye, either ipsilaterally or contralaterally. No cells in the LGB are influenced binocularly. An important transformation of the receptive field properties occurs between the LGB and cells in the striate cortex. Cells in the striate cortex respond to "slits" of light, or moving visual patterns oriented in specific directions (Figs. 13.15 and 13.16). The transformation that occurs in the striate cortex is based upon columns of cortical cells of different functional types that encode a variety of variables in vertical and horizontal systems.

Clinical Considerations

Injury to any part of the optic pathway produces visual defects whose nature depends on the location and extent of the injury. During examination each eye is covered in turn as the retinal quadrants of the opposite eye are tested. Visual defects are said to be *homonymous* when restricted to a single visual field, right or left, and *heteronymous* when parts of both fields are involved. It is evident that homonymous defects are caused by lesions on one side anywhere behind the chiasm (i.e., optic tract, lateral geniculate body, optic radiations, and visual cortex). Complete destruction of any of these structures results in a loss of the whole opposite field of vision (*homonymous hemianopsia*, Fig. 9.29); partial injury may produce *quadrantic homonymous* defects. Lesions of the temporal lobe, de-

Figure 9.29. Schematic diagram of common lesions of the visual pathways. On the *left, black lines A through D* indicate the locations of the lesions. Corresponding visual field defects are shown on the *right*. (Modified from Haymaker, 1956.)

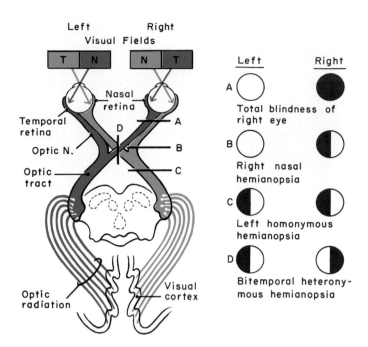

stroying the looping fibers in lower portions of the optic radiation, are likely to produce homonymous quadrantic defects in the upper visual field. Injury to the parietal lobe may involve the more superiorly placed fibers of the radiation and cause similar defects in the lower field of vision.

Lesions of the chiasm may cause several kinds of heteronymous defects. Most commonly, crossing fibers from the nasal portions of the retina are involved, with consequent loss of both temporal fields of vision (*bitemporal hemianopsia*; Fig. 9.29). Visual field defects of this type result from pituitary adenomas that break out of the sella turcica. Rarely, both lateral angles of the chiasm may be compressed; in such cases the non-decussating fibers from the temporal retinae are affected, and results in loss of the nasal visual fields (*binasal hemianopsia*). Injury of one optic nerve naturally produces blindness in the corresponding eye with loss of the pupillary light reflex (Fig. 9.29). The pupil will, however, contract consensually to light entering the other eye, since the pretectal reflex center is related to both Edinger–Westphal nuclei. The pupillary reflex will not be affected by lesions of the visual pathway above the brachium of the superior colliculus (Fig. 9.29).

FUNCTIONAL CONSIDERATIONS OF THE THALAMUS

All sensory impulses, with the sole exception of the olfactory ones, terminate in the gray masses of the thalamus, from which they are projected to specific cortical areas by the thalamocortical radiations. While portions of the dorsal thalamus serve as primary relay nuclei in various sensory pathways in which impulses are projected to specific regions of the cerebral cortex, the structure and organization of the thalamus indicate that its function is more complex and elaborate than that of a simple relay station. It seems certain that the thalamus is the chief sensory integrating mechanism of the neuraxis, but its functions are not limited to this. There is abundant evidence that specific parts of the thalamus play a dominant role in the maintenance and regulation of the state of consciousness, alertness, and attention. The thalamus is concerned not only with general and specific types of awareness, but also with the emotional correlates that accompany most sensory experiences. Other data suggest that some thalamic nuclei serve as integrative centers for motor functions, since they receive the principal efferent projections from the deep cerebellar nuclei and the corpus striatum.

Physiologically the thalamus and related neuronal subsystems are concerned with high-fidelity transmission of sensory information, input selection, output tuning, synchronization and desynchronization of cortical activity, parallel processing of information, signal storing, and signal modification.

Specific Sensory Relay Nuclei

These thalamic nuclei are in the ventral tier of the lateral nuclear group. They include the medial and lateral geniculate bodies and the two major divisions of the ventral posterior nucleus, known as the ventrobasal complex. The medial geniculate body receives fibers from the inferior colliculus. The laminated, tonotopically organized parvicellular part of this nucleus projects fibers via the geniculotemporal radiation to the transverse temporal gyrus of Heschl, the *primary auditory area* (Figs. 6.9 and 9.13). The lateral geniculate body, receiving both crossed and uncrossed fibers of the optic tract, gives rise to the geniculocalcarine fibers, which project in a specific way to the cortex surrounding the calcarine sulcus; cortex surrounding the calcarine sulcus represents the *primary visual area* (Figs. 9.13 and 9.27).

The divisions of the ventral posterior nucleus (VPLc, VPM, and VPMpc) project to the cortex of the postcentral gyrus. In the postcentral gyrus all parts of the body are represented in a somatotopical sequence; this cortical region is referred to as the *primary somesthetic area* (somatic sensory area I) (Figs. 9.13 and 9.16). The sensory representation of the body in somatic sensory area I (S I) is duplicated in a different sequence in the second somatic area (SS II) which lies buried along the superior bank of the lateral sulcus (Fig. 13.11). Somatic sensory area II receives fibers ipsilaterally from VPI and bilaterally from S I and responds mainly to cutaneous stimuli.

Signals from peripheral receptors do not pass through the thalamus without modification. Many of the impulses are modified and integrated at a thalamic level before being projected to specific cortical areas. In certain lesions of the thalamus, or of the thalamocortical connections, after a brief initial stage of complete contralateral anesthesia, pain, crude touch, and some thermal sense return. However, tactile localization, two-point discrimination, and the sense of position and movement remain severely impaired. The sensations recovered are poorly localized and are accompanied by a great increase in "feeling tone," most commonly of an unpleasant character (i.e., thalamic syndrome). Though the threshold of excitability is raised on the affected side, tactile and thermal stimuli, previously not unpleasant, evoke disagreeable sensations.

There are two aspects to sensation: the discriminative and the affective. In the former, stimuli are compared with respect to intensity, locality, and relative position in space and time. These impulses are integrated into perceptions of form, size and texture; movements are judged as to direction, amplitude, and sequence. These aspects of somatic sensation are related to VPLc and VPM and their cortical projection areas. VPLc and VPM represent a complete though distorted image of the body, and the relationship between the periphery and portions of this complex is precise. These neurons are modality specific, being concerned mainly with tactile and position sense, and respond to either superficial mechanical stimulation of the skin, mechanical distortion of deep tissues, or joint rotation, but not to more than one of these. Some impulses arising from primary endings in muscle spindles (group Ia fibers), conveyed to the outer shell of the ventrobasal complex, are relayed to the depths of the central sulcus (area 3a). These responses from muscle spindles reach the thalamus via the posterior column nuclei and VPLc.

The visual and auditory thalamic nuclei likewise are organized in a very specific manner in which point-for-point relationships exist between the receptor organ, thalamic nuclei, and the projections of thalamic nuclei to cortex. Columns of cells in all layers of the LGB receive inputs from corresponding points in the retina of each eye related to the contralateral binocular visual field. Cell columns in the dorsal nucleus of the LGB project to the striate cortex in a precise retinotopic fashion. No binocular fusion occurs in the LGB. This visual input to the striatal cortex is transformed in a manner that gives individual cortical neurons properties different from geniculate neurons, but better suited to detect shapes and patterns, and to provide binocular vision. The auditory thalamic relay nuclei are organized in a similar specific manner. The cellular laminae of the ventral nucleus of the medial geniculate body (MGB), evident only in Golgi preparation, forms the basis for the tonotopic organization. Neurons in the ventral division of the MGB project to the primary auditory cortex, while those in other cytological subdivisions of the MGB project to a belt of secondary auditory cortex surrounding the primary auditory area (Figs. 13.22 and 13.23).

The "affective" side of sensation is concerned with pain, agreeableness, and disagreeableness. Pain is a subjective sensation with considerable affective quality that often is difficult to describe and almost impossible to measure. The localization of different types of pain is often inexact and clinical judgment of its intensity must take into account the personality of the patient. Temperature and many tactile sensations likewise have a marked affective tone. This is especially true for visceral sensation, in which the discriminative element is practically absent.

Cortical Relay Nuclei

These thalamic nuclei receive impulses from specific subcortical structures and project to well-defined cortical regions. These include (1) the anterior nuclei, (2) the ventral posterolateral nucleus, pars oralis (VPLo) and the ventral lateral nucleus (VLc); and (3) the ventral lateral nucleus (VLo) and the ventral anterior nucleus (VApc). The anterior nuclei of the thalamus receive the largest efferent fiber bundle from the hypothalamus—the mammillothalamic tract (Figs. 9.7, 9.8, 10.9, and 10.10) and direct projections from the hippocampal formation via the fornix (Figs. 9.7, 10.9, 10.10, and 12.9). These nuclei in turn project to the cingulate gyrus, a cortical area demonstrated to be concerned with visceral functions (Fig. 9.13).

The contralateral deep cerebellar nuclei project most of their ascending fibers to nuclei in the "cell sparse" thalamic region (VPLo, VLc, "area x"). These afferents come from all deep cerebellar nuclei with the largest number arising from the dentate nucleus. The "cell sparse" zone in the ventral lateral thalamic region projects somatotopically on the primary motor cortex, area 4 MI. The medial segment of the globus pallidus projects topographically on the ipsilateral VLo, and VApc and none of its terminations overlap fiber systems arising from the deep cerebellar nuclei or pars reticulata of the substantia nigra. The cortical projection zone of VLo is to the supplementary motor area (M II), on the medial surface of the hemisphere. The pars reticulata of the substantia nigra projects ipsilaterally to VAmc and the paralaminar parts of MD (MDpl). The cortical projection zones for these thalamic nuclei are largely to the prefrontal cortex (Fig. 9.13). MDpl and VAmc have reciprocal connections with the frontal eye field. The distinctive subdivisions of the ventral lateral thalamic region that receive separate inputs from the deep cerebellar nuclei, the medial segment of the globus pallidus, and the pars reticulata of the substantia nigra project to cortical areas concerned with unique and different aspects of motor function. Thalamic projections from the medial pallidal segment and substantia nigra are GABAergic.

As a group the cortical relay nuclei of the thalamus possess common features, although the ventral anterior nucleus presents certain exceptions: (1) all receive substantial projections from specific parts of the neuraxis; (2) all, except for parts of VA, project to well-defined cortical areas; and (3) all, except VA, undergo extensive cell change following ablation of their cortical projection areas. These nuclei, with the exception of parts of VA, constitute the *specific thalamic nuclei*. Low frequency electrical stimulation of individual specific sensory relay nuclei, and certain cortical relay nuclei (e.g., the ventral lateral nucleus) evokes a primary surface potential followed by an augmenting sequence which is limited to the cortical projection area. This response is called the augmenting response. Characteristically, *augmenting responses* (1) have a short latency; (2) are diphasic and increase in magnitude during the initial four or five stimuli of a repetitive train; and (3) are localized to the primary cortical projection area of the specific thalamic nucleus stimulated.

Association Nuclei

The association nuclei of the thalamus receive no direct ascending systems but have abundant connections with other diencephalic nuclei. They project largely to association areas of the cerebral cortex in the frontal and parietal lobes and, to a lesser extent, in the occipital and temporal lobes. The principal association nuclei include the mediodorsal nucleus MD, the lateral dorsal nucleus (LD), the lateral posterior nucleus (LP), and the pulvinar (P). The mediodorsal nucleus, the most prominent gray mass of the medial thalamus, is highly developed in primates, especially humans (Figs. 9.9 and 9.10). It is connected with the lateral thalamic nuclei, the amygdaloid nuclear complex, and the temporal neocortex and has reciprocal connections with the frontal granular cortex (Fig. 9.13). Large bilateral injuries to the frontal lobes cause defects in complex associations, as well as changes in behavior, expressed by loss of acquired inhibitions and more direct emotional responses. These alterations in emotional behavior are produced when the pathways between the mediodorsal nucleus and the frontal cortex are severed (e.g., in frontal lobotomy).

The lateral dorsal nucleus projects upon portions of the limbic and precuneal cortex (Fig. 9.13). The larger lateral posterior nucleus has extensive connections with the association cortex of the superior and inferior parietal lobules, concerned with cognitive and symbolic functions. The pulvinar develops into a huge nuclear mass concerned with the integration of general and special somatic senses, particularly vision and audition. The inferior and parts of the lateral nuclei of the pulvinar are involved in extrageniculate projections to the secondary visual area.

Intralaminar and Midline Nuclei

Phylogenetically these nuclei are older than the specific relay nuclei that develop *pari passu* with the cerebral cortex. Afferent projections to parts of the intralaminar nuclei are derived from the spinal cord, the reticular formation, the cerebellum, the globus pallidus, and broad cortical areas.

Stimulation of the ascending reticular activating system and various kinds of sensory stimuli result in a generalized desynchronization and activation of the electroencephalogram, and behavioral arousal. The electroencephalographic (EEG) arousal response, which produces dramatic effects upon cortical activity, is mediated, in large part, by the intralaminar nuclei. Physiological studies suggest that impulses producing these changes in cortical activity reach the cortex via a diffuse, nonspecific thalamic projection system. The more rostral intralaminar thalamic nuclei (CL and PCN), which receive fibers from the midbrain reticular formation, project directly to widespread cortical regions.

Stimulation of the so-called nonspecific thalamic nuclei, produces widespread and pronounced effects on electrocortical activity. The *nonspecific*, or *diffuse*, thalamic nuclei include the intralaminar and midline nuclei and, in part, the ventral anterior nucleus. Repetitive stimulation of these thalamic nuclei alters spontaneous electrocortical activity over large areas and, under certain conditions, resets the frequency of brain waves by eliciting responses that are time-locked to the thalamic stimulus. The most characteristic effect of stimulating the nonspecific thalamic nuclei is the *recruiting response*. When the frequency of stimulation is in the range of 6–12 cycles per second, predominantly surface negative cortical responses rapidly increase to a maximum (by the fourth to sixth stimulus of the train) and then decrease over a broad area; continued stimulation causes the evoked responses to wax and wane. Stimulation of one of the nonspecific thalamic nuclei causes all others to be activated in a mass excitation.

The observation that cortical recruiting responses induced by low frequency stimulation of the nonspecific thalamic nuclei could be reduced, or blocked, by stimulation of the bulbar reticular formation provided experimental evidence that the nonspecific thalamic nuclei are within the sphere of influence of the ascending reticular formation.

The largest component of the intralaminar nuclei, the centromedian-parafascicular nuclear complex (CM-PF) receives its input mainly from forebrain derivatives. The precentral and premotor cortex project profusely upon these nuclei. The centromedian nucleus (CM) also receives collaterals of pallidofugal fibers arising from the medial pallidal segment. The principal projection of CM-PF is to the striatum, with cells in PF projecting to the caudate nucleus and CM projecting to the putamen. These connections suggest that CM-PF plays an important role in motor integration.

The thalamus is played upon by two great streams of afferent fibers one the peripheral and one central. Signals generated in receptors in all parts of the body convey information concerning changes in the external and internal environment. In addition, the thalamus receives significant subcortical inputs from the deep cerebellar nuclei, the medial segment of the globus pallidus, and the pars reticulata of the substantia nigra concerned with different aspects of motor function. Massive cortical projections bring thalamic nuclei under the influence of sensory, motor, and association areas of the cortical mantle. Most of the major sensory and motor systems converge on thalamic nuclei in a very specific manner without overlap. The thalamus integrates these systems and distributes projections to specific areas of the cerebral cortex. The thalamus is not only the key to understanding the cerebral cortex, it is the key to understanding the integration of neural systems.

SUGGESTED READINGS

AKERT, K., AND HARTMANN-VON MONAKOW, K. 1980. Relationships of precentral, premotor and prefrontal cortex to the mediodorsal and intralaminar nuclei of the monkey thalamus. Acta Neurobiol. Exp. (Warsz,), **40**: 7–25.

ASANUMA, C., THACH, W. T., AND JONES, E. G. 1983. Cytoarchitectonic delineation of the ventral lateral thalamic region in the monkey. Brain Res. Rev., **5**: 219–235.

ASANUMA, C., THACH, W. T., AND JONES, E. G. 1983a. Distribution of cerebellar terminations and their relation to other afferent terminations in the ventral lateral thalamic region of the monkey. Brain Res. Rev., **5**: 237–265.

ASANUMA, C., THACH, W. T., AND JONES, E. G. 1983b. Anatomical evidence for segregated focal groupings of efferent cells and their terminal ramifications in the cerebellothalamic pathway of the monkey. Brain Res. Rev., **5**: 267–297.

BECKSTEAD, R. M., MORSE, J. R., AND NORGREN, R. 1980. The nucleus of the solitary tract in the monkey: Projections to the thalamus and brain stem nuclei. J. Comp. Neurol., **190**: 259–282.

BENEVENTO, L. A., AND FALLON, J. H. 1975. The ascending projections of the superior colliculus in the rhesus monkey (*Macaca mulatta*). J. Comp. Neurol., **160**: 339–362.

BENEVENTO, L. A., AND REZAK, M. 1976. The cortical projections of the inferior and adjacent lateral pulvinar in the rhesus monkey (*Macaca mulatta*): An autoradiographic study. Brain Res., **108**: 1–24.

BENTIVOGLIO, M., MINCIACCHI, D., MOLINARI, M., GRANTO, A., SPREAFICO, R., AND MACCHI, G. 1988. The intrinsic and extrinsic organization of the thalamic intralaminar nuclei. In M. BENTIVOGLIO AND R. SPREAFICO (Editors), *Cerebellar Thalamic Mechanisms*. Excerpta Medica, Amsterdam, pp. 221–237.

BERKLEY, K. J. 1980. Spatial relationships between the terminations of somatic sensory and motor pathways in the rostral brainstem of cats and monkeys. I. Ascending somatic sensory inputs to lateral diencephalon. J. Comp. Neurol., **193**: 283–317.

BLOMQUIST, A. J., BENJAMIN, R. M., AND EMMERS, R. 1962. Thalamic localization of afferents from the tongue in squirrel monkey (*Saimiri sciureus*). J. Comp. Neurol., **118**: 77–87.

BLOOM, F. E., BATTENBERG, E., ROSSIER, J., LING, N., AND GUILLEMIN, R. 1978. Neurons contain β endorphin in rat brain exist separately from those containing enkephalin: Immunocytochemical studies. Proc. Natl. Acad. Sci. USA, **75**: 1591–1595.

BOIVIE, J. 1978. Anatomical observations on the dorsal column nuclei, their thalamic projection and the cytoarchitecture of some somatosensory thalamic nuclei in the monkey. J. Comp. Neurol., **178**: 17–48.

BOIVIE, J. 1979. An anatomical reinvestigation of the termination of the spinothalamic tract in the monkey. J. Comp. Neurol., **186**: 343–370.

BOYCOTT, B. B., AND WÄSSLE, H. 1974. The morphological types of ganglion cells of the domestic cat's retina. J. Physiol. (Lond.), **240**: 397–419.

BUNT, A. H., HENDRICKSON, A. E., LUND, J. S., LUND, R. D., AND FUCHS, A. F. 1975. Monkey retinal ganglion cells: Morphometric analysis and tracing of axonal projections with a consideration of the peroxidase technique. J. Comp. Neurol., **164**: 265–286.

BURTON, H., AND JONES, E. G. 1976. The posterior thalamic region and its cortical projection in new world and old world monkeys. J. Comp. Neurol., **168**: 249–302.

CARMEL, P. W. 1970. Efferent projections of the ventral anterior nucleus of the thalamus in the monkey. Am. J. Anat., **128**: 159–184.

CARPENTER, M. B. 1989. Connectivity patterns of thalamic nuclei implicated in dyskinesia. Stereotact. Funct. Neurosurg., **58**: 79–119.

CARPENTER, M. B., NAKANO, K., AND KIM, R. 1976. Nigrothalamic projections in the monkey demonstrated by autoradiographic technics. J. Comp. Neurol., **144**: 93–116.

DOWLING, J. E., AND BOYCOTT, B. B. 1966. Organization of the primate retina: Electron microscopy. Proc. R. Soc. Lond (Biol.), **166**: 80–111.

FONNUM, F., STORM-MATHISON, J., AND DIVAC, I. 1981. Biochemical evidence for glutamate as neurotransmitter in corticostriate and corticothalamic fibers in rat brain. Neuroscience, **6**: 863–873.

FRIEDMAN, D. P., AND MURRAY, E. A. 1986. Thalamic connectivity of the second somatosensory area and neighboring somatosensory fields of the lateral sulcus of the macaque. J. Comp. Neurol., **252**: 348–373.

FUKUDA, Y., AND STONE, J. 1974. Retinal distribution and central projections of Y, X and W cells of the cat's retina. J. Neurophysiol., **37**: 749–772.

GLENN, L. L., AND STERIADE, M. 1982. Discharge rate and excitability of cortically projecting intralaminar thalamic neurons during waking and sleeping states. J. Neurosci., **2**: 1387–1404.

GRAYBIEL, A. M. 1972. Some extrageniculate visual pathways in the cat. Invest. Ophthalmol., **11**: 322–332.

GIUFFRIDA, R., AND RUSTIONI, A. 1988. Glutamate and aspartate immunoreactivity in corticothalamic neurons of rats. In M. BENTIVOGLIO AND R. SPREAFICO (Editors), *Cerebellar Thalamic Mechanisms*. Excerpta Medica, Amsterdam, pp. 311–320.

HALLANGER, A. E., AND WAINER, B. H. 1988. Ultrastructure of ChAT-immunoreactive synaptic terminals in the thalamic reticular nucleus of the rat. J. Comp. Neurol., **278**: 486–497.

HAYHOW, W. R. 1958. The cytoarchitecture of the lateral geniculate body in the cat in relation to the distribution of crossed and uncrossed optic fibers. J. Comp. Neurol., **110**: 1–64.

HENDRICKSON, A. M., WILSON, M. E., AND TOYNE, M. J. 1970. The distribution of optic nerve fibers in *Macaca mulatta*. Brain Res., **23**: 425–427.

HERKENHAM, M., AND NAUTA, W. J. H. 1977. Afferent connections of the habenular nuclei in the rat: A horseradish peroxidase study, with a note on the fiber-of-passage problem. J. Comp. Neurol., **173**: 123–145.

HICKEY, T. L., AND GUILLERY, R. W. 1979. Variability of laminar patterns in the human lateral geniculate nucleus. J. Comp. Neurol., **183**: 221–246.

HIRAI, T., AND JONES, E. G. 1989. Distribution of tachykinin- and enkephalin-immunoreactive fibers in the human thalamus. Brain Res. Rev., **14**: 35–52.

HIRAI, T., AND JONES, E. G. 1989a. A new parcellation of the human thalamus on the basis of histochemical staining. Brain Res. Rev., **14**: 1–34.

ILINSKY, I. A., JOUANDET, M. L., AND GOLDMAN-RAKIC, P. S. 1985. Organization of the nigrothalamocortical system in the rhesus monkey. J. Comp. Neurol., **236**: 315–330.

ILINSKY, I. A., AND KULTAS-ILINSKY, K. 1987. Sagittal cytoarchitectonic maps of the *Macaca mulatta* thalamus with a revised nomenclature of the motor-related nuclei validated by observations on their connectivity. J. Comp. Neurol., **262**: 331–364.

JAYARAMAN, A., AND UPDYKE, B. V. 1979. Organization of visual cortical projections of the claustrum in the cat. Brain Res., **178**: 107–115.

JONES, E. G. 1975. Some aspects of the organization of the thalamic reticular complex. J. Comp. Neurol., **162**: 285–308.

JONES, E. G. 1983. Distribution patterns of individual medial lemniscus axons in the ventrobasal complex of the monkey thalamus. J. Comp. Neurol., **215**: 1–16.

JONES, E. G. 1985. *The Thalamus*. Plenum Press, New York, 935 pp.

JONES, E. G., AND BURTON, H. 1974. Cytoarchitecture and somatic sensory connectivity of thalamic nuclei other than the ventrobasal complex in the cat. J. Comp. Neurol., **154**: 395–432.

JONES, E. G., AND FRIEDMAN, D. P. 1982. Projection pattern of functional components of thalamic ventrobasal complex on monkey somatosensory cortex. J. Neurophysiol., **48**: 521–544.

JONES, E. G., AND POWELL, T. P. S. 1971. An analysis of the posterior group of thalamic nuclei on the basis of its afferent connections. J. Comp. Neurol., **143**: 185–216.

KAAS, J. H. 1988. How the somatosensory thalamus is subdivided and interconnected with areas of the somatosensory cortex in monkeys. In M. BENTIVOGLIO AND R. SPREAFICO (Editors), *Cerebellar Thalamic Mechanisms*. Excerpta Medica, Amsterdam, pp. 143–150.

KAAS, J. H., GUILLERY, R. W., AND ALLMAN, J. M. 1972. Some principles of organization in the dorsal lateral geniculate nucleus. Brain Behav. Evol., **6**: 253–299.

KAAS, J. H., HUERTA, M. F., WEBER, J. T., AND HARTING, J. K. 1977. Patterns of retinal terminations and laminar organization of the lateral geniculate nucleus of primates. J. Comp. Neurol., **182**: 517–554.

KELLY, J. P., AND GILBERT, C. D. 1975. The projection of different morphological types of ganglion cells in the cat's retina. J. Comp. Neurol., **163**: 65–80.

KIEVIT, J., AND KUYPERS, H. G. J. M. 1977. Organization of the thalamocortical connexions to the frontal lobe in the rhesus monkey. Exp. Brain Res., **29**: 299–322.

KIM, R., NAKANO, K., JAYARAMAN, A., AND CARPENTER, M. B. 1976. Projections of the globus pallidus and adjacent structures: An autoradiographic study in the monkey. J. Comp. Neurol., **169**: 263–289.

KLEIN, D. C., AND MOORE, R. Y. 1979. N-acetyltransferase and hydroxyindole-o-methyltransferase: Control by the retinohypothalamic tract and the supra–chiasmatic nucleus. Brain Res., **174**: 245–262.

KLEIN, D. C., WELLER, J. L., AND MOORE, R. Y. 1971. Melatonin metabolism: Neural regulation of the pineal serotonin N-acetyltransferase. Proc. Natl. Acad. Sci. USA, **68**: 3107–3110.

KRETTEK, J. E., AND PRICE, J. L. 1974. A direct input from the amygdala to the thalamus and the cerebral cortex. Brain Res., **67**: 169–174.

KUFFLER, S. W. 1953. Discharge patterns and functional organization of mammalian retina. J. Neurophysiol., **16**: 37–68.

KÜNZLE, H. 1976. Thalamic projections from the precentral motor cortex in *Macaca fascicularis*. Brain Res., **105**: 253–267.

KÜNZLE, H., AND AKERT, K. 1977. Efferent connections of cortical Area 8 (frontal eye field) in *Macaca fascicularis*: A reinvestigation using the autoradiographic technique. J. Comp. Neurol., **173**: 147–164.

KUO, J.-S., AND CARPENTER, M. B. 1973. Organization of pallidothalamic projections in the rhesus monkey. J. Comp. Neurol., **151**: 201–236.

LEE, H. J., RYE, D. B., HALLANGER, A. E., LEVEY, A. I., AND WAINER, B. H. 1988. Cholinergic vs. noncholinergic efferents from the mesopontine tegmentum to the extrapyramidal motor system nuclei. J. Comp. Neurol., **275**: 469–492.

LEVAY, S., AND SHERK, H. 1981. The visual claustrum of the cat. I. Structure and connections. J. Neurosci., **1**: 956–980.

LEVAY, S., AND SHERK, H. 1981a. The visual claustrum of the cat. II. The visual field map. J. Neurosci., **1**: 981–992.

MACCHI, G., AND BENTIVOGLIO, M. 1986. The thalamic intralaminar nuclei and the cerebral cortex. In E. G. Jones and A. Peters (Editors), *Cerebral Cortex*. Plenum Press, New York, **5**: 355–401.

MALONE, E. F. 1910. Über die Kerne des menschlichen Diencephalon. Aus dem Anhang zu den Abhandlungen der königl. preuss. Akademie der Wissenschaften, p. 92.

MALPELI, J. C., AND BAKER, F. H. 1975. The representation of the visual field in the lateral geniculate nucleus of the *Macaca mulatta*. J. Comp. Neurol., **161**: 569–594.

MEHLER, W. R. 1966. The posterior thalamic region. Confin. Neurol., **27**: 18–29.

MEHLER, W. R. 1966a. Further notes on the center median nucleus of Luys. In D. P. PURPURA AND M. D. YAHR (Editors), *The Thalamus*. Columbia University Press, New York, pp. 109–127.

MEHLER, W. R. 1980. Subcortical afferent connections of the amygdala in the monkey. J. Comp. Neurol., **190**: 733–762.

MOLINARI, M., HENDRY, S. H. C., AND JONES, E. G. 1987. Distribution of certain neuropeptides in the primate thalamus. Brain Res., **426**: 270–289.

MOREST, D. K. 1964. The neuronal architecture of the medial geniculate body of the cat. J. Anat., **98**: 611–638.

MOREST, D. K. 1965. The laminar structure of the medial geniculate body of the cat. J. Anat., **99**: 143–159.

MOREST, D. K. 1965a. The lateral tegmental system of the midbrain and medial geniculate body: Study with Golgi and Nauta methods in the cat. J. Anat., **99**: 611–634.

NIIMI, K., NIIMI, M., AND OKADO, Y. 1978. Thalamic afferents to the limbic cortex in the cat studied with the method of retrograde transport of horseradish peroxidase. Brain Res., **145**: 225–238.

OLIVER, D. L., AND HALL, W. C. 1978. The medial geniculate body of the tree shrew, *Tupaia glis*. I. Cytoarchitecture and midbrain connections. J. Comp. Neurol., **182**: 423–458.

OLSZEWSKI, J. 1952. *The Thalamus of the Macaca Mulatta*. S. Karger, Basel, 93 pp.

PARENT, A., AND DE BELLEFEUILLE, L. 1982. Organization of efferent projections from the internal segment of the globus pallidus in primate as revealed by fluorescence retrograde labeling method. Brain Res., **245**: 201–213.

PARENT, A., MACKEY, A., AND DE BELLEFEUILLE, L. 1983. The subcortical afferents to caudate nucleus and putamen in primate: A fluorescence retrograde double labeling study. Neuroscience, **10**: 1137–1150.

PEARSON, R. C., BRODAL, P., AND POWELL, T. P. S. 1978. The projection of the thalamus upon the parietal lobe in the monkey. Brain Res., **144**: 143–148.

PERCHERON, G. 1977. The thalamic territory of cerebellar afferents and the lateral region of the thalamus of the macaque in sterotaxic ventricular coordinates. J. Hirnforsch., **18**: 375–400.

POGGIO, G. F., AND MOUNTCASTLE, V. B. 1963. The functional properties of ventrobasal thalamic neurons studied in unanesthetized monkeys. J. Neurophysiol., **26**: 775–806.

PURPURA, D. P. 1970. Operations and processes in thalamic and synaptically related neural subsystems. In F. O. SCHMITT (Editor), *The Neurosciences, Second Study Program*. Rockefeller University Press, New York, Ch 42, pp. 458–470.

REZAK, M., AND BENEVENTO, L. A. 1979. A comparison of the organization of the projections of the dorsal lateral geniculate nucleus, the inferior pulvinar and adjacent lateral pulvinar to primary visual cortex (Area 17) in the macaque monkey. Brain Res., **167**: 19–40.

RINVIK, E., OTTERSEN, O. P., STORM-MATHISEN, J. 1987. Gamma-aminobutyrate-like immunoreactivity in the thalamus of the cat. Neuroscience, **23**: 781–805.

SCHEIBEL, M. E., AND SCHEIBEL, A. B. 1966. The organization of the nucleus reticularis thalami: A Golgi study. Brain Res., **1**: 43–62.

SCHEIBEL, M. E., AND SCHEIBEL, A. B. 1966a. The organization of the ventral anterior nucleus of the thalamus: A Golgi study. Brain Res., **1**: 250–268.

SCHELL, G. R., AND STRICK, P. L. 1984. The origin of thalamic inputs to the arcuate premotor and supplementary motor areas. J. Neurosci., **4**: 539–560.

SMITH, Y., SÉQUELA, P., AND PARENT, A. 1987. Distribution of GABA-immunoreactive neurons in the thalamus of the squirrel monkey (*Saimiri sciureus*). Neuroscience, **22**: 579–591.

STERIADE, M., AND GLENN, L. L. 1982. Neocortical and caudate projections of intralaminar thalamic neurons and their synaptic excitation from midbrain reticular core. J. Neurophysiol., **48**: 352–371.

STONE, J., AND FUKUDA, Y. 1974. Properties of cat retinal ganglion cells: A comparison of

W cells with X and Y cells. J. Neurophysiol., **37**: 722–748.

SUGIMOTO, T., HATTORI, T., MIZUNO, N., ITOH, K., AND SATO, M. 1983. Direct projections from the centre median-parafascicular complex to the subthalamic nucleus in the cat and rat. J. Comp. Neurol., **214**: 209–216.

THACH, W. T., AND JONES, E. G. 1979. The cerebellar dentatothalamic connection: terminal field, lamellae, rods and somatotopy. Brain Res., **169**: 168–172.

TRACEY, D. J., ASANUMA, C., JONES, E. G., AND PORTER, R. 1980. Thalamic relay to motor cortex: Afferent pathways from brain stem, cerebellum and spinal cord in monkeys. J. Neurophysiol., **44**: 532–554.

WALKER, A. E. 1966. Internal structure and afferent-efferent relations of the thalamus. In D. P. PURPURA AND M. D. YAHR (Editors), *The Thalamus*. Columbia University Press, New York, pp. 1–12.

WILLIS, W. D. JR. 1988. Nociception neurons in the primate ventral posterior lateral (VPL) nucleus. In M. BENTIVOGLIO AND R. SPREAFICO (Editors), *Cerebellar Thalamic Mechanisms*. Excerpta Medica, Amsterdam, pp. 77–92.

WONG-RILEY, M. T. T. 1976. Projections from the dorsal lateral geniculate nucleus to prestriate cortex in the squirrel monkey as demonstrated by retrograde transport of horseradish peroxidase. Brain Res., **109**: 595–600.

10

The Hypothalamus

The hypothalamus is the division of the diencephalon concerned with visceral, autonomic, and endocrine functions. All of these functions are intimately related to affective and emotional behavior. This structure lies in the walls of the third ventricle below the hypothalamic sulci and is continuous across the floor of this ventricle (Figs. 10.1, 10.2, and 10.3). On the ventral surface of the brain the *infundibulum*, to which the hypophysis is attached, emerges posterior to the optic chiasm (Figs. 9.4, 10.1, and 10.13). A slightly bulging region posterior to the infundibulum is the *tuber cinereum* (Fig. 10.9). The *mammillary bodies* lie posteriorly near the interpeduncular fossa.

Externally the hypothalamus is bounded rostrally by the optic chiasm, laterally by the optic tracts, and posteriorly by the mammillary bodies (Figs. 1.8, 2.7, and 2.8). This region is roughly diamond-shaped, and its surface contains several small eminences. The zone forming the floor of the third ventricle is called the *median eminence* of the tuber cinereum. The portion rostral to the infundibular stem contains the *anterior median eminence*; the portion posterior to the infundibular stem forms the posterior median eminence, which is better developed in humans (Figs. 2.7 and 2.8). Paired lateral eminences form well-defined landmarks. The ventral protrusion of the hypothalamus and the third ventricular recess form the infundibulum (Fig. 9.4). The most distal portion of the infundibular process is the neurohypophysis; tissue joining the infundibular process to the median eminence is called the infundibular stem (Fig. 10.15). The median eminence represents the final point of convergence of pathways from the central nervous system on the peripheral endocrine system (Fig. 10.8). The median eminence is the anatomical interface between brain and the anterior pituitary. Primary capillaries of the hypophysial portal vessels vascularize the median eminence. Ependymal cells lining the floor of the third ventricle have processes that traverse the width of the median eminence and terminate near the portal perivascular space. These cells, called tanycytes, provide a structural and functional link between the cerebrospinal fluid (CSF) and the perivascular space of the pituitary portal vessels.

The hypothalamus can be described as extending from the region of the optic chiasm to the caudal border of the mammillary bodies. Anteriorly it passes without sharp demarcation into the basal olfactory area (diagonal gyrus of the anterior perforated substance) (Fig. 12.2). The region immediately in front of the optic chiasm, extending to the lamina terminalis is known as the preoptic area (Fig. 10.1). The preoptic area, classically regarded as a forebrain derivative, arises from a rostral hypothalamic anlage and appears structurally and functionally a part of the hypothalamus. Caudally the hypothalamus merges imperceptibly with the periaqueductal gray of the midbrain. The thalamus lies dorsal and caudal

Figure 10.1. Schematic diagram of the medial hypothalamic nuclei. Nuclei in the supraoptic region arc in *blue*. The paraventricular and supraoptic nuclei are *dark blue*; the suprachiasmatic and anterior hypothalamic nuclei are *light blue*. Nuclei of the middle or tuberal region of the hypothalamus are *yellow*. Nuclei of the caudal or mammillary region are shades of *red*. The preoptic area lies rostral to the anterior hypothalamic region and classically is regarded as a forebrain derivative functionally related to the hypothalamus. (From Carpenter and Sutin, *Human Neuroanatomy*, 1983; courtesy of Williams & Wilkins.)

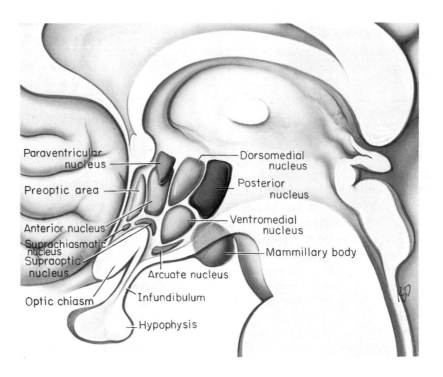

to the hypothalamus; the subthalamic region is lateral and caudal (Figs. 9.4 and 9.5).

HYPOTHALAMIC NUCLEI

Pervading the whole area is a diffuse matrix of cells constituting the central gray substance, in which are found a number of more or less distinct nuclear masses. A sagittal plane passing through the anterior pillar of the fornix roughly divides the hypothalamus into medial and lateral areas (Figs. 10.2, 10.7, and 10.9).

Preoptic Region

This region constitutes the periventricular gray of the most rostral part of the third ventricle (Figs. 10.1, 10.2, and 10.3). The *preoptic periventricular nucleus* surrounds the walls of the third ventricle in the region of the preoptic recess. The diffusely arranged small cells are poorly differentiated from the ependymal lining. The *medial preoptic nucleus*, composed of predominantly small cells, lies lateral to the preoptic periventricular nucleus and extends ventrally to the optic chiasm (Fig. 10.2). The *lateral preoptic nucleus*, rostral to the lateral hypothalamic area, is composed of diffusely dispersed medium-sized cells (Figs. 10.2 and 10.3) and is regarded as the interstitial nucleus of the median forebrain bundle.

Lateral Hypothalamic Area

This area is bounded medially by the mammillothalamic tract and the anterior column of the fornix (Figs. 10.2 and 10.3); the lateral boundary is the medial margin of the internal capsule and the subthalamic region (Fig. 10.2). Rostrally this area is continuous with the lateral preoptic nucleus, while caudally it merges with the midbrain tegmentum (Fig. 10.3). This area contains scattered groups of large, dark-staining cells—the *lateral hypothalamic nucleus*—and two or three sharply delimited circular cell groups known as the tuberal nuclei (nuclei tuberales), which often produce small visible eminences on the basal surface of the hypothalamus. They consist of small, pale, multipolar cells surrounded by a delicate fiber capsule about which are found the large cells of the lateral hypothalamic nucleus (Figs. 10.2 and 10.3).

Medial Hypothalamic Area

This part of the hypothalamus lies medial to the fibers of the fornix and the mammillothalamic tract and caudal to the preoptic region. Its medial boundary is the ependyma of the third ventricle. The medial hypothalamic area can be divided rostrocaudally into three distinct regions: (1) a rostral *supraoptic region*, lying above the optic chiasm; (2) a middle, or *tuberal region*; and (3) a *mammillary region* continuous caudally with the periaqueductal gray (Fig. 10.1).

Supraoptic Region

This region contains two of the most striking and sharply defined hypothalamic nuclei, the *paraventricular nucleus* and the *supraoptic nucleus* (Figs. 10.2, 10.3, and 10.4). Cells of the paraventricular nucleus form a vertical plate of densely packed cells immediately beneath the ependyma of the third ventricle, the dorsal part of which extends laterally toward the fornix (Fig. 10.5). The paraventricular nucleus consists of several distinct cell groups, among which are a medial predominantly parvicellular group and a prominent lateral magnocellular group. The supraoptic nucleus caps the optic chiasm and straddles the optic tract laterally; this nucleus is composed mainly of uniformly large cells. Large cells in both the paraventricular and supraoptic nucleus appear similar with peripherally distributed Nissl substance and colloidal cytoplasmic inclusions, regarded as neurosecretory products. Immunocytochemically large cells in both nuclei contain either vasopressin or oxytocin, each of which is associated with a distinctive neurophysin (Figs. 10.5 and 10.8). It is generally accepted that one large cell contains only one hormone, either oxytocin or vasopressin. Magnocellular components of both the supraoptic and paraventricular nuclei project fibers into the neural lobe of the hypophysis and transmit either oxytocin or vasopressin by distinctive fibers. A small projection from these nuclei reaches the external zone of the median eminence. Regions of the paraventricular nucleus containing parvicellular elements give rise to descending axons projecting to the brain stem and all levels of the spinal cord (Fig. 4.15).

The less differentiated central gray in the supraoptic region constitutes the *anterior hypothalamic nucleus* (Fig. 10.1). This nucleus merges imperceptibly with the preoptic area.

The *suprachiasmatic nucleus* forms a group of small round cells immediately dorsal to the optic chiasm and close to the third ventricle (Fig. 10.6). These small nuclei receive direct bilateral projections from the retina. The well-defined physiological role of the suprachiasmatic nucleus is that of a biological clock. Retinohypothalamic projections to the suprachiasmatic nucleus provide the anatomical link between a cyclical environment and the internal clock.

Tuberal Region

In this region, the hypothalamus reaches its widest extent; the fornix separates the medial and the lateral hypothalamic areas (Figs. 10.2, 10.3,

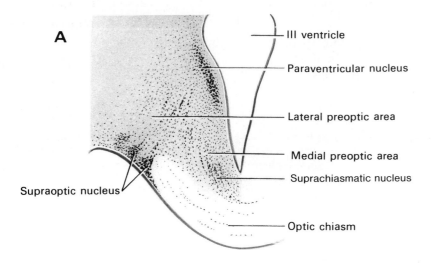

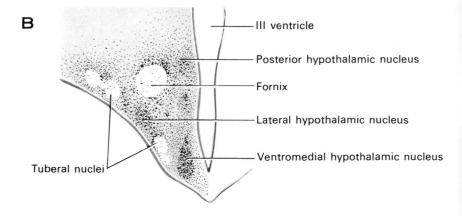

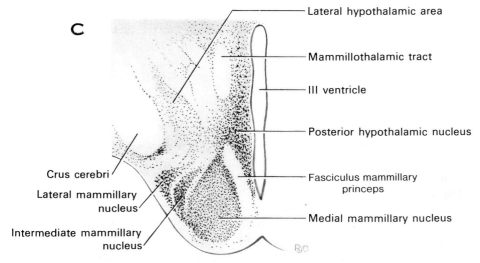

Figure 10.2. Drawings of transverse sections through portions of the human hypothalamus: *A*, Supraoptic region; *B*, infundibular region; *C*, mammillary region. (After Clark et al., 1938.) (From Carpenter and Sutin, *Human Neuroanatomy*, 1983; courtesy of Williams & Wilkins.)

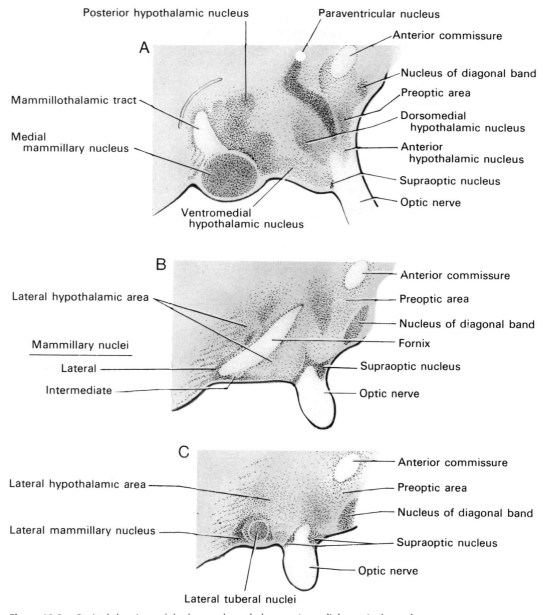

Figure 10.3. Sagittal drawings of the human hypothalamus. *A*, medial ventricular surface; *B*, through the anterior column of the fornix; *C*, near lateral border of hypothalamus. (After Clark et al., 1938.) (From Carpenter and Sutin, *Human Neuroanatomy*, 1983; courtesy of Williams & Wilkins.)

10.7, and 10.9). The medial portion forms the central gray substance of the ventricular wall, in which there may be distinguished a ventromedial and a dorsomedial nucleus.

The *ventromedial nucleus*, the largest cell group in the tuberal region, has a round or oval shape and is surrounded by a cell-poor zone that helps to delineate its boundaries (Figs. 10.1, 10.2, 10.3, and 10.7). Neurons of the ventromedial nucleus typically have dendrites that extend beyond the borders of the nucleus. The cell-free capsular zone around the nucleus is formed by a dense ring of axons and terminals (Fig. 10.7). The *dorsomedial nucleus* is a less distinct aggregation of cells that borders the third ventricle (Fig. 10.3).

The *arcuate nucleus* (infundibular nucleus) is located in the most ventral part of the third ventricle near the entrance to the infundibular

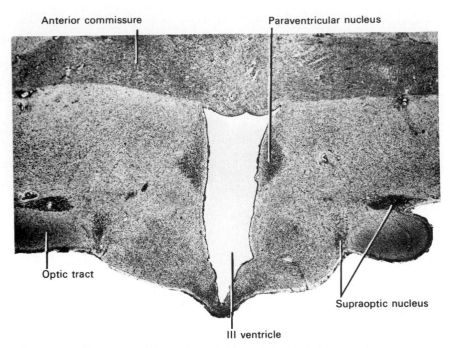

Figure 10.4. Photograph of human hypothalamus at the level of the anterior commissure demonstrating the paraventricular and supraoptic nuclei. Nissl stain. (From Carpenter and Sutin, *Human Neuroanatomy*, 1983; courtesy of Williams & Wilkins.)

recess and extends into the median eminence (Figs. 10.1 and 10.18). The small cells of this nucleus are in close contact with the ependyma lining the ventricle. In coronal sections the nucleus has an arcuate shape. The efferent projections of the arcuate nucleus have been traced to the external layer of the median eminence (Figs. 10.8 and 10.18). This connection is of great importance to adenohypophysial function. Cells of the arcuate nucleus contain dopamine, which is released into the hypophysial portal system. In addition, neurons of the arcuate nucleus are immunocytochemically reactive for the adrenocorticotrophic hormone (ACTH), β-lipotrophic hormone (β-LPH), and β-endorphin (β-END). Chemical substances from the arcuate nucleus play a major role in the regulation of hormonal output from the anterior pituitary.

Mammillary Region

This region consists of the mammillary bodies and the dorsally located posterior hypothalamic nucleus (Fig. 10.2, 10.3, 10.9, and 10.10). In humans the mammillary body consists almost entirely of the large, spherical medial *mammillary nucleus*, composed of relatively small cells invested by a capsule of myelinated fibers. Lateral to this is the small *intermediate* (*intercalated*) *mammillary nucleus* composed of smaller cells (Fig. 10.2). Even further lateral is a well-defined group of large cells, the *lateral mammillary nucleus* (Fig. 10.2).

The posterior hypothalamic nucleus lies dorsal to the mammillary body and caudal portions of the ventromedial nucleus (Fig. 10.1). This nucleus consists of a matrix of small cells in which large round or oval cells are scattered. The large cells are especially numerous in humans and extend caudally into the periaqueductal gray.

Synthetic descriptions may suggest that all hypothalamic nuclei are

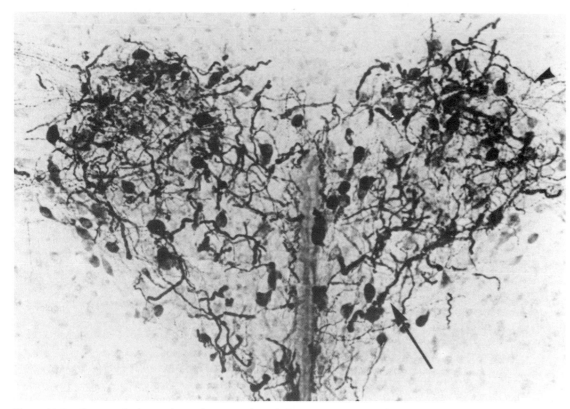

Figure 10.5. Paraventricular nuclei in the mouse hypothalamus immunoreacted with antiserum to bovine neurophysin 1 demonstrating cells and their processes. (From Silverman and Pickard, 1983, *Chemical Neuroanatomy*, Raven Press, with permission.)

sharply circumscribed, but the cellular matrix of the hypothalamus is broadly continuous with the surrounding gray matter. Tissue continuities with the surrounding gray matter contain the major afferent and efferent hypothalamic pathways. Rostrally and laterally the hypothalamus is continuous with the *basal olfactory region*, a large gray mass beneath the rostral part of the lentiform nucleus and the head of the caudate nucleus (Figs. 10.2, 10.3, 12.2, 12.16, and 12.17). Near the median plane this region extends dorsally, rostral to the anterior commissure, where it becomes the *septal region*. Beneath the lentiform nucleus is a gray mass extending toward the amygdaloid complex, referred to as the substantia innominata (Figs. 12.15 and 12.16). The *substantia innominata* contains clusters of large cholinergic neurons, which constitute the basal nucleus of Meynert. These large cholinergic neurons have widespread projections to the cortex and the amygdala. Neurons in the basal nucleus constitute the major source of cholinergic innervation of the entire neocortex. The base of the septal region is continuous with the substantia innominata laterally and with the preoptic region caudally. The septal region contains the *medial septal nucleus*, the *lateral septal nucleus*, and the *nucleus accumbens septi* (Figs. 12.6, 12.15 and 12.16).

CONNECTIONS OF THE HYPOTHALAMUS

The hypothalamus has extensive and complex connections. Some fibers are organized into definite and conspicuous bundles, while others are diffuse and difficult to trace.

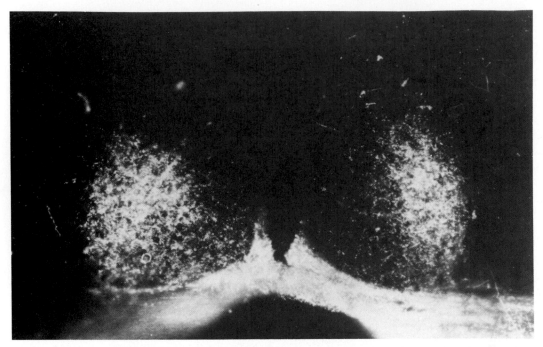

Figure 10.6. Dark-field photomicrograph of retinal fibers and terminals in the suprachiasmatic nuclei of the hamster demonstrated by transport of horseradish peroxidase (HRP). (From Pickard and Silverman, 1981, J. Comp. Neurol., with permission.)

Afferent Connections of the Hypothalamus

The afferent connections of the hypothalamus which have been established are:

The *medial forebrain bundle* is a complex group of fibers arising from the basal olfactory regions, the septal nuclei, the periamygdaloid region, and the subiculum, that passes to, and through, the lateral preoptic and lateral hypothalamic regions (Figs. 10.11 and 10.12). The bundle is formed, at levels rostral to the anterior commissure, mainly of fibers from the septal region. In its parasagittal course it receives contributions from the substantia innominata and the amygdaloid complex. This tract is well developed in lower vertebrates, but is small in humans.

Hippocampo-hypothalamic fibers originating from the hippocampal formation form the fornix (Figs. 10.2, 10.3, 10.9 and 12.9). Cells in the subiculum at the lip of the hippocampal fissure also give rise to fibers in the fornix bundle (Fig. 10.12). The hippocampal formation projects fibers to the septal nuclei (Fig. 10.12). Fibers arising from the subiculum project via the fornix to the septum and the medial and lateral mammillary nuclei (Fig. 10.12).

In the septal region fibers of the fornix form two distinct bundles: (1) a compact fornix column, or postcommissural fornix, which arches caudal to the anterior commissure, and (2) a more diffuse precommissural fornix.

Precommissural fibers of the fornix are distributed to the septal nuclei, the lateral preoptic region, the nucleus of the diagonal band, and the dorsal hypothalamic area. *Postcommissural fibers* of the fornix project to the medial mammillary nucleus, except for those that leave this bundle and terminate in the anterior thalamic nuclei.

Amygdalo-hypothalamic fibers follow two pathways to the hypothalamus: (1) the stria terminalis (Figs. 9.1 and 12.6) and (2) a course ventral to the lentiform nucleus. The stria terminalis arises mainly from

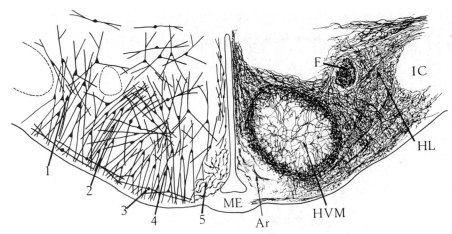

Figure 10.7. Drawings of the tuberal region of rodent hypothalamus based upon Golgi preparations. The general arrangement of dendrites and axons is shown on the *left*: (1) dendrites of HL radiate in mediolateral and dorsoventral directions; (2) there is a compression of dendritic fields of neurons located between F and HVM; (3) the dendritic fields of neurons along the hypothalamic surface are parallel with the pia; (4) the long dendrites of HVM extend in all directions from the nucleus; and (5) small bipolar neurons of the Ar nestle against the ventricle, adjacent to ME. *Abbreviations*: Ar, arcuate nucleus; F, fornix; HL, lateral hypothalamic area; HVM, hypothalamic ventromedial nucleus; IC, internal capsule; ME, median eminence. (Reproduced with permission from O. E. Millhouse: *Handbook of the Hypothalamus*, Vol. 1. *Anatomy of the Hypothalamus*, edited by P. Morgane and J. Panksepp, Marcel Dekker, New York, 1979.) (From Carpenter and Sutin, *Human Neuroanatomy*, 1983; courtesy of Williams & Wilkins.)

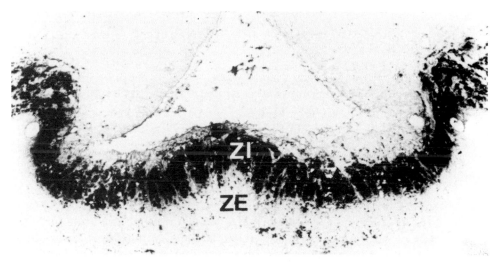

Figure 10.8. Transverse section through the rat median eminence immunoreacted with antiserum to neurophysin demonstrating the *zona interna* (ZI) and the *zona externa* (ZE). Fibers of the hypothalamo-neurohypophysial tract are abundant in ZI and a few positive fibers are evident in ZE. (From Silverman and Pickard, 1983, *Chemical Neuroanatomy*, Raven Press, with permission.)

the corticomedial part of the amygdaloid complex and distributes fibers to the medial preoptic nucleus, the anterior hypothalamic nucleus, and the ventromedial and arcuate nuclei (Fig. 12.6). Ventral amygdalofugal fibers arise from the basolateral amygdaloid nuclei and the pyriform cortex and spread medially and rostrally under the lentiform nucleus to reach the lateral hypothalamic nucleus and the medial forebrain bundle.

Brain stem reticular afferents ascend to the hypothalamus via the mammillary peduncle and the dorsal longitudinal fasciculus. The *mammillary peduncle* arises from the dorsal and ventral tegmental nuclei of

Figure 10.9. Sagittal section of the brain stem through the pillar of fornix, the mammillothalamic tract, and the stria medullaris. Weigert's myelin stain. Photograph. (From Carpenter and Sutin, *Human Neuroanatomy*, 1983; courtesy of Williams & Wilkins.)

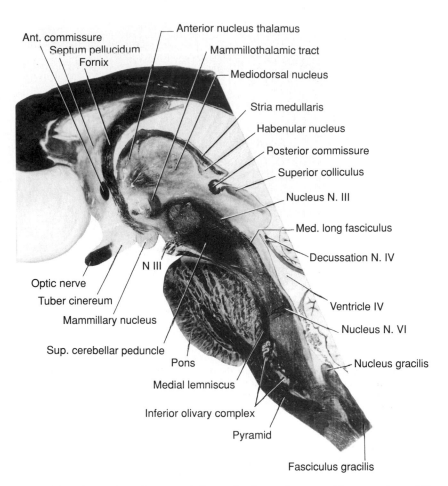

the midbrain and projects mainly to the lateral mammillary nucleus (Fig. 10.11). The ascending component of the *dorsal longitudinal fasciculus* is formed from cells in the central gray of the midbrain (Fig. 10.11). Fibers in this bundle spread out over caudal and dorsal regions of the hypothalamus where they become part of the periventricular system.

Brain stem afferents to the hypothalamus also arise from neurons in the raphe nuclei of the midbrain (Fig. 5.13), the lateral parabrachial nuclei in the pons (Fig. 5.24), and from the locus ceruleus (Figs. 6.28 and 6.29). Serotonergic fibers arising mainly from the median nucleus of the raphe (superior central nucleus), ascend in the medial forebrain bundle to, and through the lateral hypothalamus; terminals are distributed to the preoptic region, the suprachiasmatic nucleus, and the mammillary bodies. Afferents from different parts of the nucleus solitarius project to the medial and lateral parabrachial nuclei (Figs. 5.24 and 6.27). Portions of the nucleus solitarius that receive general visceral afferents (located caudally) project primarily to the lateral parabrachial nuclei (Fig. 5.24). The lateral parabrachial nuclei innervate the medial preoptic region, the paraventricular and dorsomedial hypothalamic nuclei, and the lateral hypothalamic area. Rostral portions of the nucleus solitarius that receive special visceral afferents (taste) project to the medial parabrachial nuclei. The medial parabrachial nuclei project to the substantia innominata, the amygdala, and posterolateral regions of the hypothalamus. Noradrenergic fibers originating in the locus ceruleus ascend in a dorsal tegmental bundle, which distributes terminals in the dorsomedial, supraoptic, and paraventricular hypothalamic nuclei. Afferent fibers to the hypothalamus from the brain stem and other sources are shown in Figures 10.12 and 10.14.

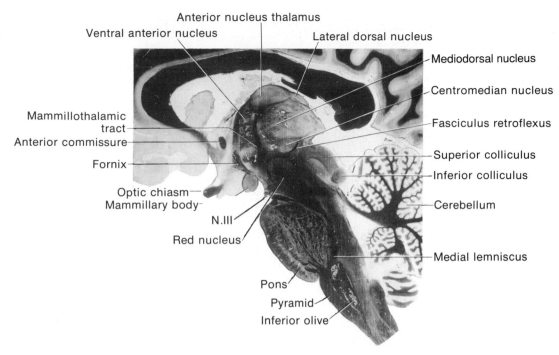

Figure 10.10. Sagittal section of the brain stem demonstrating the mammillothalamic tract, the anterior thalamic nucleus, and thalamic nuclei lateral to those shown in Figure 10.9. Weigert's myelin stain. Photograph. (From Carpenter and Sutin, *Human Neuroanatomy*, 1983; courtesy of Williams & Wilkins.)

Retinohypothalamic fibers arise from ganglion cells of the retina and project bilaterally to the suprachiasmatic nuclei via the optic nerve and chiasm (Fig. 10.6). The suprachiasmatic nuclei also receive inputs from extrahypothalamic sources, such as the ventral lateral geniculate nucleus and the paraventricular nuclei of the thalamus. This nucleus is the pacemaker for circadian rhythms.

Opinions vary concerning corticohypothalamic fibers, which are usually described as arising from the posterior orbital cortex (Fig. 12.2). Direct thalamohypothalamic pathways are sparse.

Broadly stated, the principal forebrain afferents to the hypothalamus arise from the two phylogenetically oldest cortical areas, the pyriform cortex and the hippocampal formation (Fig. 10.14). In each instance the cortical projection is reinforced by a corresponding subcortical projection, the amygdala in the case of the pyriform cortex, and the septum in the case of the hippocampal formation. Each of these subcortical nuclei is reciprocally connected with the overlying cortical area. Of the phylogenetically newer cortical areas the cingulate gyrus appears particularly favored to influence the hypothalamus indirectly through the entorhinal cortex and the hippocampal formation. The cingulate cortex can in turn be influenced by hypothalamic projections to the anterior nuclear group of the thalamus. Both the sense of taste and olfaction are directly involved in arousal mechanisms and phases of consumatory behavior. Gustatory pathways to the hypothalamus are multisynaptic, while olfactory projections to the hypothalamus are relatively direct.

Efferent Connections of the Hypothalamus

The efferent connections of the hypothalamus appear, in part, reciprocal to afferent systems. There are reciprocal connections in the me-

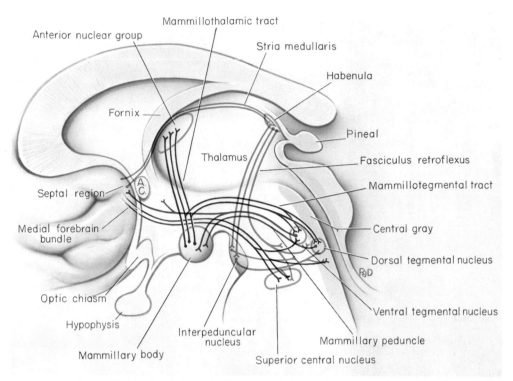

Figure 10.11. Semischematic diagram of limbic pathways interrelating the telencephalon and diencephalon with medial midbrain structures. The medial forebrain bundle and efferent fibers of the mammillary body are shown in *black*. The *medial forebrain bundle* originates from the septal and lateral preoptic regions, traverses the lateral hypothalamic area, and projects into the midbrain tegmentum. The *mammillary princeps* (*black*) divides into two bundles, the *mammillothalamic tract* and the *mammillotegmental tract*. Ascending fibers of the *mammillary peduncle*, arising from the dorsal and ventral tegmental nuclei, are shown in *red*; most of these fibers pass to the mammillary body but some continue rostrally to the lateral hypothalamus, the preoptic region, and the medial septal nucleus. Fibers arising from the septal nuclei project caudally in the medial part of the *stria medullaris* (*blue*) to terminate in the medial habenular nucleus. Impulses conveyed to the habenular nucleus are distributed to midbrain tegmental nuclei via the *fasciculus retroflexus* (*blue*). (Based on Nauta, 1958.) (From Carpenter and Sutin, *Human Neuroanatomy*, 1983; courtesy of Williams & Wilkins.)

dial forebrain bundle which provide indirect connections between the lateral hypothalamus and the hippocampal formation. In addition, there are hypothalamic projections to the amygdaloid nuclear complex via both the stria terminalis and the ventral pathway (Fig. 10.14). Reciprocal connections with the midbrain tegmentum and central gray are conducted by the dorsal longitudinal fasciculus and via pathways projecting to and from the mammillary bodies (Figs. 10.11 and 10.13). In addition, there are several efferent hypothalamic pathways which have no counterpart among afferent systems.

The *medial forebrain bundle* (Fig. 10.11) conveys impulses from the lateral hypothalamus rostrally to the nuclei of the diagonal band (Figs. 10.3 and 12.2) and to the medial septal nuclei, which in turn send fibers to the hippocampal formation via the fimbria of the fornix (Fig. 10.12). Descending hypothalamic efferents in the medial forebrain bundle project through the ventral tegmental region to the superior central nucleus, the ventral tegmental nucleus, and to the periaqueductal gray (Fig. 10.11). Hypothalamic efferents to the amygdaloid nuclear complex pass via both the stria terminalis and the ventral pathway (Fig. 12.6). Fibers from the lateral hypothalamic region follow the ventral pathway through the substantia innominata to the amygdala.

The *dorsal longitudinal fasciculus* contains descending fibers from medial and periventricular portions of the hypothalamus distributed to

Limbic brain stem connections

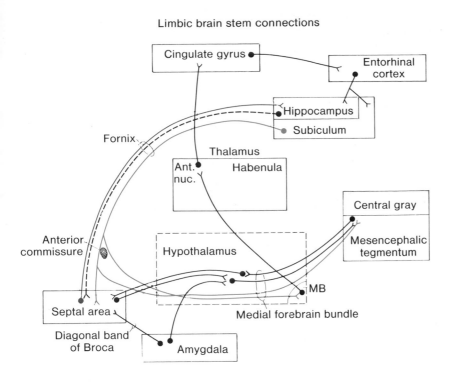

Figure 10.12. Schematic block diagram of major interconnections of structures comprising the "limbic system." Projections arising from the subiculum (*blue*) pass via the fornix to the septal area, mammillary body, and the mesencephalic tegmentum. Fibers projecting in the fornix from the hippocampal formation are shown in *black-dashed lines*. Projections from the septal area to the hippocampal formation are shown in *red*. MB indicates the mammillary body. (From Carpenter and Sutin, *Human Neuroanatomy*, 1983; courtesy of Williams & Wilkins.)

the periaqueductal gray of the midbrain and the tectum (Fig. 10.13). Some descending fibers in this system may extend to the dorsal tegmental nucleus (Fig. 10.11).

Mammillary efferent fibers, arising from the medial mammillary nucleus, and to a lesser extent from the lateral and intermediate mammillary nuclei, form a well-defined bundle, the *fasciculus mammillaris princeps* (Figs. 10.9, 10.10, and 10.11). This bundle passes dorsally for a short distance and divides into two components: the *mammillothalamic tract* and the *mammillotegmental tract* (Figs. 10.9, 10.10, and 10.11). The mammillothalamic tract contains fibers from the medial mammillary nucleus that project to the anterior thalamic nuclei. Superimposed upon this hypothalamic relay to the thalamus are projections from the hippocampal formation via the fornix to the anterior nuclei of the thalamus. The anterior thalamic nuclei project to subdivisions of the cingulate cortex (Figs. 2.6, 9.13, and 12.17). The cingulate cortex projects back to the hippocampal formation via the entorhinal cortex (Fig. 10.14).

The *mammillotegmental tract* arches caudally into the midbrain tegmentum where fibers terminate in the dorsal and ventral tegmental nuclei (Fig. 10.11).

Efferent projections of the suprachiasmatic nucleus are regarded as incomplete, even though they have been traced to multiple hypothalamic sites. Thus, it is not clear how the suprachiasmatic nucleus effects circadian rhythms, since it does not appear to innervate cell groups responsible for the motor, autonomic, or endocrine responses.

Descending hypothalamic projections to the lower brain stem and spinal cord constitute pathways by which cells of the hypothalamus exert regulatory influences on central autonomic neurons (Fig. 4.15). Parvicellular elements of the paraventricular nucleus, cells in the lateral hypothalamic area, and cells in the posterior hypothalamus project fibers directly to the dorsal motor nucleus of the vagus, the medial nucleus solitarius, portions of the nucleus ambiguus and into ventrolateral regions of the medulla. Fibers from these same hypothalamic nuclei enter the

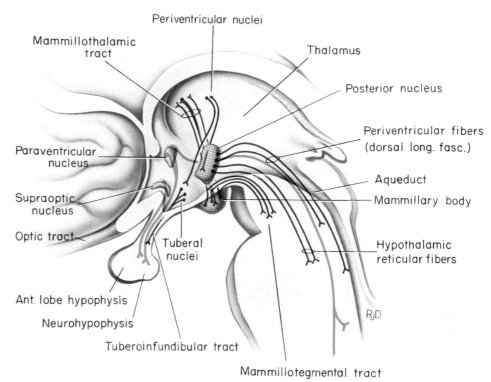

Mammillothalamic tract

Periventricular nuclei

Thalamus

Posterior nucleus

Periventricular fibers (dorsal long. fasc.)

Aqueduct

Mammillary body

Hypothalamic reticular fibers

Paraventricular nucleus

Supraoptic nucleus

Optic tract

Tuberal nuclei

Ant. lobe hypophysis

Neurohypophysis

Tuberoinfundibular tract

Mammillotegmental tract

Figure 10.13. Diagram of some efferent hypothalamic pathways. Color code is the same as in Figure 10.1. Terminations of the mammillotegmental tract are shown in Figure 10.11. (From Carpenter and Sutin, *Human Neuroanatomy*, 1983; courtesy of Williams & Wilkins.)

spinal cord, descend in the lateral funiculus, and terminate in the intermediolateral cell column at all levels.

These direct descending hypothalamic fibers influence autonomic functions in the lower brain stem and at all spinal levels. Descending fibers from the parvicellular paraventricular nucleus, which form a part of this system, appear to contain both oxytocin and vasopressin.

Supraoptic Hypophysial Tract

This tract consists of fibers arising from magnocellular elements of the supraoptic and paraventricular nuclei that project to the posterior lobe of the hypophysis (Figs. 10.13 and 10.15). The peptides specific for these large neurons, oxytocin and vasopressin, were the first brain peptides isolated and characterized. These peptides are always present in conjunction with a class of larger peptides, known as neurophysins. The neurophysins are part of a precursor molecule. Neurophysin I is related to oxytocin and neurophysin II with vasopressin (Figs. 10.5 and 10.8). Both neurophysins are present in the supraoptic and paraventricular nuclei, but oxytocin and vasopressin are present in different neurons. Secretory products are synthesized within the cell bodies and transported down axons to terminals. The neurosecretory material consists of granules 120 to 200 nm in diameter. Oxytocin and vasopressin are present in different axonal profiles. Hormones in the hypothalamic-hypophysial tract are stored in terminal axonal varicosities in dense core vesicles. The contents of the dense core vesicles are released into perivascular spaces containing fenestrated capillaries.

A second efferent projection from the magnocellular elements of the paraventricular nucleus has been described to the external zone of

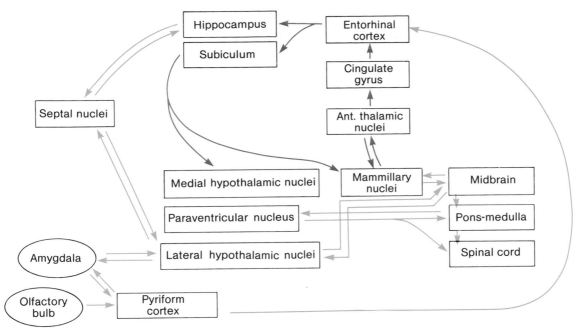

Figure 10.14. A schematic diagram of the principal fiber connections of the hypothalamus. The principal afferents to the hypothalamus from the forebrain arise from two phylogenetically older cortical areas, the *pyriform cortex* and the *hippocampal formation*. Each of these projections is reinforced by a second projection from a related subcortical nuclear mass; this secondary projection arises from the *amygdaloid complex* in the case of the pyriform cortex, and from the *septal nuclei* in the case of the hippocampal formation. Reciprocal connections exist between the hypothalamus and these subcortical nuclei. The cingulate gyrus and the pyriform cortex can exert influences upon the hypothalamus via the entorhinal area and the hippocampal formation. The mammillary nuclei and the hippocampal formation project to the anterior thalamic nuclei, which in turn influence activities in the cingulate gyrus. Pathways from the mammillary nuclei to the cortex and from the hippocampal formation and subiculum to the hypothalamus are indicated in *red*. All other connections are shown in *blue*. (Modified from Raisman, 1966.) (From Carpenter and Sutin, *Human Neuroanatomy*, 1983; courtesy of Williams & Wilkins.)

the median eminence. In addition, high levels of vasopressin have been demonstrated in the hypophysial portal system. The role of vasopressin in the zona externa of the median eminence is unresolved, but it may act as a regulator for adrenocorticotropic hormone (ACTH) release. Cells of the supraoptic and paraventricular nuclei also contain other biologically active substances, such as enkephalin, cholecystokinin, glucagon, dynorphin, and angiotensin.

Neurosecretory cells in the hypothalamus retain their capacity to conduct electrical impulses. Stimulation of the cell bodies in the hypothalamus gives rise to action potentials conducted in axons that trigger the release of the hormones.

Tuberohypophysial Tract

The tuberohypophysial or tuberoinfundibular tract arises from the tuberal region, mainly from the arcuate nucleus (Figs. 10.1 and 10.18), and can be traced only to the median eminence and the infundibular stem (Figs. 10.8, 10.13, and 10.15). Cells of the arcuate nucleus are situated in the uppermost part of the infundibulum (i.e., the median eminence) and lie directly upon the ependymal lining. Axons of these cells form the tuberoinfundibular tract, which projects to the internal and external zones of the median eminence, where they collateralize (Figs. 10.8 and 10.18). Some cells in the arcuate nucleus have projections, or collaterals, that

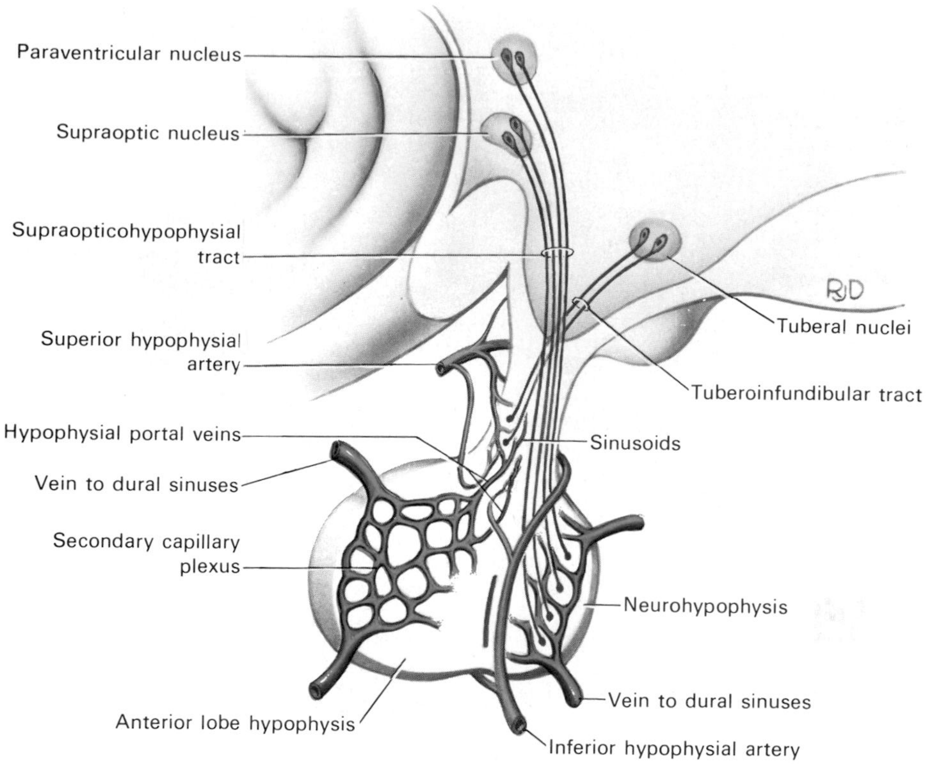

Figure 10.15. Diagram of the hypophysial portal system, the tuberoinfundibular tract, and the supraopticohypophysial tract. The hypophysis is supplied by the *superior* and *inferior hypophysial arteries*. Branches of these arteries form sinusoids about the infundibulum. Blood from the sinusoids flows to the anterior lobe of the hypophysis via the portal vessels that give rise to a second capillary plexus in the anterior lobe (Figure 10.16). The *tuberoinfundibular tract* ends in the sinusoids of the infundibular stem and transports *releasing hormones*, which enter the sinusoids. The *supraopticohypophysial tract* contains fibers from the *supraoptic* and magnocellular elements of the *paraventricular nuclei* that project to the neurohypophysis. Neurosecretory products of these cells are conveyed directly to terminals in the neurohypophysis. Separate cells in the supraoptic and paraventricular nuclei contain and produce either vasopressin (antidiuretic hormone) or oxytocin.

extend to other parts of the hypothalamus, the thalamus, and the amygdala. Although these fibers accompany those of the supraoptic hypophysial tract in part of their course, they end on capillary loops near the sinusoids of the hypophysial portal system (Figs. 10.15 and 10.16). These are fine fibers, but secretory granules can be demonstrated in their axons. Fibers of the tuberoinfundibular tract convey "releasing" hormones, which are transported via the hypophysial portal vessels to the anterior lobe of the hypophysis where they modulate the synthesis and release of adenohypophysial hormones. Functionally, the tuberoinfundibular tract and the hypophysial portal system establish the neurohumoral link between the hypothalamus and the anterior pituitary.

Dopamine was the first of many substances identified in the arcuate nucleus (Fig. 10.18). Dopaminergic neurons innervate the external zone of the median eminence and dopamine is released into the portal capillaries. Dopamine in the hypophysial portal system inhibits the release of prolactin from the anterior pituitary. A short feedback loop suggests that pituitary prolactin inhibits dopamine release from the median eminence. Increases in dopamine occur in the arcuate nucleus in pregnancy, pseudopregnancy, and lactation, suggesting there is little release of the inhibiting factor in these conditions. Physiological stimuli of major importance in the release of prolactin from the anterior lobe are estrogens and suckling. The arcuate nucleus also contains a number of peptides similar to

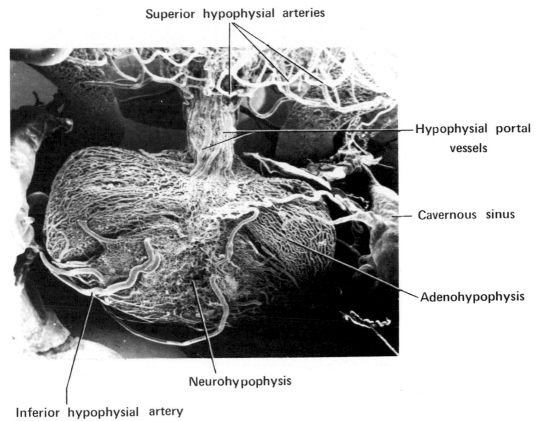

Superior hypophysial arteries

Hypophysial portal vessels

Cavernous sinus

Adenohypophysis

Neurohypophysis

Inferior hypophysial artery

Figure 10.16. Scanning electron micrograph of vascular casts of the pituitary gland, infundibular stem, and median eminence in the monkey. The pituitary is viewed from its posterior aspect. The hypophysial arteries and the portal system shown here should be compared with the schematic diagram shown in Figure 10.15. (From Page and Bergland, 1977, Am. J. Anat., with permission.) (From Carpenter and Sutin, *Human Neuroanatomy*, 1983; courtesy of Williams & Wilkins.)

hormones in the anterior pituitary, such as ACTH, β-lipotrophin (β-LPH), and β-endorphin (β-END). ACTH and β-LPH in the arcuate nucleus do not appear to coexist in neurons with dopamine. The heterogeneity of the substances found in the arcuate nucleus and the presence of releasing factors beyond the limits of this nucleus suggest it is not the sole hypophysiotrophic center in the hypothalamus.

Hypothalamic efferent projections fall into five main categories: (1) fibers that emerge via the medial forebrain bundle, (2) neurosecretory neurons that convey hormones to the neurohypophysis, (3) fibers concerned with releasing hormones into the hypophysial portal system, (4) fibers that arise from the mammillary nuclei that project to the anterior nuclear group of the thalamus and to nuclei in the midbrain tegmentum, and (5) fibers that project to the lower brain stem and spinal cord.

HYPOPHYSIAL PORTAL SYSTEM

The hypophysis is supplied by two sets of arteries, both of which arise from the internal carotid artery (Figs. 10.15 and 10.16). The superior hypophysial artery forms an arterial ring around the upper part of the hypophysial stalk; the inferior hypophysial artery forms a ring about the posterior lobe and gives branches to the lower infundibulum. Both of these arteries enter the hypophysial stalk and break up into a number of sinusoids. Both arteries are innervated by postganglionic sympathetic fibers. Blood from these sinusoids collects into vessels that pass into the anterior lobe of the hypophysis, which receives almost all of its blood supply via these vessels. These vessels are referred to as the hypophysial portal vessels. Anatomical and physiological evidence indicates that hypothalamic influences on the anterior lobe of the hypophysis are conveyed by humoral substances transported via the tuberoinfundibular tract to the sinusoids and the anterior lobe via the portal system. The pattern of blood flow in living animals is not easily deduced from anatomical studies of blood vessels. Observations in living animals leave no doubt that blood in the portal system flows from the median eminence to the anterior lobe. Hypophysiotrophic releasing factors in neuronal terminals in the median eminence are carried to the adenohypophysis via this restricted vascular route.

The hypothalamus is intimately concerned with the synthesis and transmission of factors that stimulate and inhibit the secretion of hormones by the anterior pituitary. Electrical stimulation of the hypothalamus can increase the discharges of gonadotrophic hormone and ACTH. Stimulation of the tuberal region in the rabbit has produced ovulation. Direct stimulation of the anterior lobe does not elicit these responses, because the humoral part of this pathway is not electrically excitable. The neurosecretory substances acting on cells of the anterior lobe are called *hypophysiotrophic agents* or *releasing hormones* and are named according to the hormone they release.

HYPOPHYSIOTROPHIC AGENTS

These releasing factors have most of the attributes of hormones and most appear to be neuropeptides (Fig. 10.17). Hypophysiotrophic agents include corticotrophin-releasing factor (CRF), growth hormone–releasing factor (GHRF), gonadotrophin hormone–releasing factor [or luteinizing hormone–releasing factor (LRH)], thyrotrophin-releasing factor (TRF), prolactin-inhibiting factor (PIF), somatostatin [somatic inhibiting-releasing factor (SIRF)], melanocyte-releasing hormone (MSH), as well as β-lipotrophin (β-LPH) and β-endorphin (β-END). Neurons of the arcuate nucleus are immunocytochemically positive for ACTH, β-LPH, and β-END; these peptides are derived from a common precursor. Under stressful conditions CRF is present in the plasma of the portal vessels, but it is suspected that all of these peptides are released.

Although the naturally occurring growth hormone-releasing factor has not been identified, semipurified extracts of the hypothalamus are effective in stimulating release of the growth hormone. Secretion of growth hormone (GH) is regulated by neural influences both stimulatory and inhibitory. This is achieved by two hypothalamic releasing factors, growth hormone–releasing factor (GHRF) and growth hormone–inhibiting factor (SIRF), or somatostatin. Secretion of these hormones is regulated by monoamines, dopamine (DA), norepinephrine (NE), and serotonin (5-HT), all of which appear to have stimulating effects. Growth hormone measured in the plasma is age-dependent and occurs in surges from early puberty to adolescence. Somatostatin, which also inhibits secretion of thyrotropin, has been recognized in many locations other than the hypothalamus from which it was originally isolated. Clinical studies confirm the powerful inhibitory effects of somatostatin on growth hormone, as well as on insulin and glucagon.

Thyrotropin-releasing factor (TRF) has been isolated and synthesized; the synthetic compound has an action greater than the natural

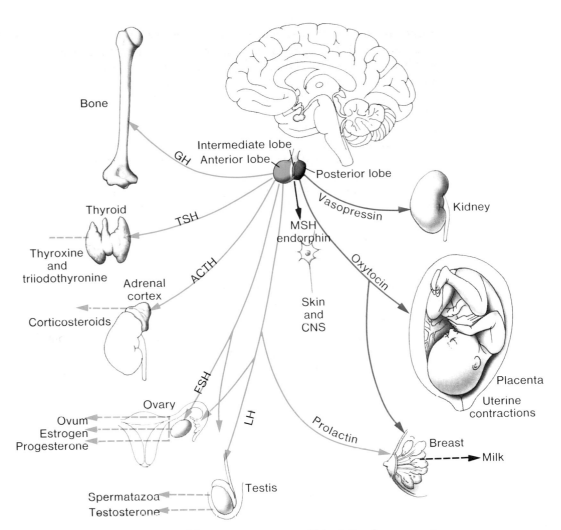

Figure 10.17. Schematic diagram of the target organs upon which pituitary hormones act. Hormones secreted by cells of the anterior (*blue*) and intermediate (*black*) lobes of the pituitary are regulated by hypothalamic hypophysiotrophic agents conveyed by the hypophysial portal system. Hormones of the anterior lobe include (1) growth hormone (GH), (2) thyrotropin (TSH), (3) corticotrophin (ACTH), (4) follicle-stimulating hormone (FSH), (5) luteinizing hormone (LH), and (6) prolactin. Melanocyte-stimulating hormone (MSH) is derived from cells in the intermediate lobe (*black*) of the pituitary. The neurohypophysis (posterior lobe, *red*) contains vasopressin and oxytocin secreted by separate populations of cells in the supraoptic and paraventricular nuclei of the hypothalamus. These hormones act on the kidney tubules (vasopressin) and the smooth muscle of the uterus and glandular tissue of the breast (oxytocin). (Modified from Schally et al., 1977.)

secretion on the thyroid-stimulating hormone (TSH). No true antagonist of TRF has been reported, but thyroxin is known to inhibit TSH. The luteinizing hormone-releasing factor (LRF) and the follicle-stimulating–releasing factor (FRH) appear to be parts of the same molecule. FRH causes the release of the follicle-stimulating hormone (FSH) from the anterior pituitary, which initiates cyclical changes in the ovaries and the production of estrogens. The discharge of LRH liberates the luteinizing hormone, which produces ovulation and the development of the corpus luteum. Ovulation appears to require both FSH and LH. The medial preoptic area is considered responsible for the cyclical nature of the female reproductive system.

The prolactin-inhibiting factor (PIF) appears to be dopamine, which has been identified in the arcuate nucleus, the portal vessels, and in

Figure 10.18. Frontal section through the hypothalamus and part of the subthalamic region showing the immunofluorescent localization of tyrosine hydroxylase (TH), the enzyme that synthesizes dopamine. Section is oblique so that the ventral region is most rostral. Fluorescent cell bodies are present in the arcuate nucleus (Ar) and in the zona incerta (ZI). The median eminence (Me) contains a dense plexus of TH-positive fibers in the external part (Figure 10.8). V indicates the third ventricle (from Hökfelt et al., 1976).

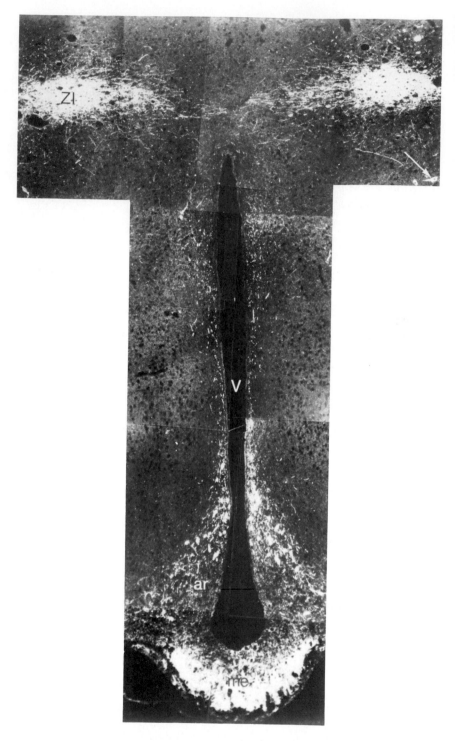

pituitary receptors (Fig. 10.18). Thyrotropin-releasing factor (TRF) also appears to potentiate the release of prolactin. Prolactin secretion increases as the effective dopamine concentrations at receptor site in the anterior pituitary are reduced.

The naturally occurring opioid peptide β-endorphin is found in rat anterior and intermediate lobes of the pituitary. Cells in the arcuate nucleus of the hypothalamus contain a common 31,000-Dalton precursor of ACTH, β-lipotrophin (β-LPH), and β-endorphin (β-END), which is cleaved in the anterior and intermediate lobes. β-LPH has no opioid activity but may be a prohormone for opioid-like peptides. β-Endorphin has 5 to 10 times the analgesic potency of morphine, but its effects are seen mainly after intracerebral administration. β-Endorphin–labeled axons are distributed along the ventricular wall to the supraoptic, periventricular, paraventricular, and suprachiasmatic nuclei, and some fibers may reach the thalamus. In severe stress, there is a coordinated release of ACTH, β-LPH, and β-END from the anterior pituitary. In syndromes characterized by hypersecretion of ACTH, the peptides that form part of the precursor molecule also are increased. There is as yet no well-defined physiological role for β-END, but it would appear to be involved in maintaining homeostasis. The enkephalins are not derived from β-lipotrophin or β-endorphin and the cells and fibers labeled for β-endorphin are distinct from those labeled by antisera specific for enkephalins.

FUNCTIONAL CONSIDERATIONS

The hypothalamus and immediately adjoining regions are related to all kinds of visceral activities. The most diverse disturbances of autonomic functions, involving water balance, internal secretion, sugar and fat metabolism, and temperature regulation, all can be produced by stimulation or destruction of hypothalamic areas. Even the mechanism for normal sleep may be altered profoundly by such lesions. The hypothalamus is the chief subcortical center for the regulation of both sympathetic and parasympathetic activities. These dual activities are integrated into coordinated responses that maintain adequate internal conditions in the body. It is improbable that each of the autonomic activities has its own discrete center in the hypothalamus. However, a specific function has been established for the supraoptic and paraventricular nuclei. There is also a fairly definite topographical organization with regard to the two main divisions of the autonomic system. Control of parasympathetic activities is related to the anterior and medial hypothalamic regions (supraoptic and preoptic areas) and the ventricular portion of the tuber cinereum. Stimulation of this region results in increased vagal and sacral autonomic responses, characterized by reduced heart rate, peripheral vasodilation, and increased tonus and motility of the alimentary and vesical walls.

The lateral and posterior hypothalamic regions are concerned with the control of sympathetic responses. Stimulation of this region, especially the posterior portion from which many descending efferents arise, activates the thoracolumbar outflow. This results in increased metabolic and somatic activities characteristic of emotional stress, combat or flight. These responses are expressed by dilatation of the pupil, piloerection, acceleration of the heart rate, elevation of blood pressure, increase in the rate and amplitude of respiration, somatic struggling movements, and inhibition of the gut and bladder. All these physiological correlates of emotional excitement can be elicited when the hypothalamus is released from cortical control. Removal of the cortex, or interruption of the cortical connections with the hypothalamus, induces many of the above visceral symptoms collectively designated as "sham rage." On the other hand, destruction of the posterior hypothalamus produces emotional lethargy, abnormal sleepiness, and a fall in temperature due to general reduction of visceral and somatic activities.

The coordination of sympathetic and parasympathetic responses is strikingly shown in the regulation of body temperature. This complex function, involving widespread physical and chemical processes, is mediated by two hypothalamic mechanisms, one concerned with the dissipation of heat and the other with its production and conservation. Experimental evidence indicates that the anterior hypothalamus is sensitive to increases in blood temperature and sets in motion the mechanisms for dissipating excess heat. In humans this consists mainly of profuse sweating and vasodilatation of the cutaneous blood vessels. These actions permit the rapid elimination of heat by convection and radiation from the surface of the engorged blood vessels, and by the evaporation of sweat. In animals heat loss is effected mainly by the rapid warming of successive streams of inspired air (panting). Lesions involving the anterior part of the hypothalamus abolish the neural mechanisms concerned with the dissipation of heat and result in hyperthermia. Thus, hyperthermia (hyperpyrexia) may result from tumors in, or near, the anterior hypothalamus.

The posterior hypothalamus, on the other hand, is sensitive to conditions of decreasing body temperature and controls mechanisms for the conservation and increased production of heat. The cutaneous blood vessels are constricted and sweat secretion ceases, so that heat loss is reduced. Simultaneously there is augmentation of visceral activities, and the somatic muscles exhibit shivering. All these activities tremendously increase the process of oxidation, with a consequent production and conservation of heat. Bilateral lesions in posterior regions of the hypothalamus usually produce a condition in which body temperature varies with the environment (poikilothermia), since such lesions effectively destroy descending pathways concerned with both heat conservation and dissipation.

These two intrinsically antagonistic mechanisms do not function independently but are continually interrelated and balanced against each other to meet changing needs of the body; the coordinated responses always are directed to the maintenance of a constant optimum temperature.

The supraoptic and paraventricular nuclei are specifically concerned with the maintenance of body water balance (Figs. 10.2, 10.3, 10.4, 10.5, 10.13, and 10.15). Destruction of these nuclei, or their hypophysial connections, invariably is followed by the condition known as *diabetes insipidus*, in which there is increased secretion of urine (polyuria) without an increase in the sugar content. The antidiuretic hormone, vasopressin, is secreted directly by the cells of the supraoptic and paraventricular nuclei. Vasopressin is transported by the unmyclinated axons of the supraopticohypophysial tract and is stored in terminals in the posterior lobe of the pituitary. The production of antidiuretic hormone varies in accordance with changes in the osmotic pressure of the blood. An increase in the osmotic pressure of the blood that supplies the magnocellular hypothalamic nuclei increases the activity of these neurons and the release of antidiuretic hormone. In states of dehydration there is a depletion of the hormone in the posterior lobe and increased secretory activity in the supraoptic nuclei. After reestablishment of water balance, there is a reaccumulation of the hormone in the posterior lobe. The antidiuretic hormone is considered to act specifically on the kidneys, although the exact mechanism by which vasopressin brings about the reabsorption of renal water is not clear (Fig. 10.17). Reabsorption of sodium chloride and bicarbonate ions is followed by passive reabsorption of water. This hormone also appears to alter the osmotic permeability of water in the distal and collecting tubules of the kidney.

There is evidence that a region of the hypothalamus is responsible for the regulation of water intake. Electrical stimulation of anterior regions on the hypothalamus in goats creates fantastic "thirst" and results in consumption of large volumes of water. This is probably part of a more extensive system which regulates the consumption of both food and water.

An increase in the osmotic pressure of body fluids may be an effective stimulus for water intake. Osmoreceptors probably are situated close to the cells of the supraoptic nucleus which have an abundant blood supply. Localized lesions in the lateral hypothalamus at the level of the ventromedial nucleus in rats cause a reduction in water intake without affecting food intake; larger lesions in the lateral hypothalamus may cause adipsia as well as aphagia. The lateral hypothalamic area can excite cells of the supraoptic nucleus, which in turn inhibit the lateral hypothalamic area in a negative feedback circuit.

The paraventricular and supraoptic nuclei also produce oxytocin, which causes contractions of uterine muscle and myoepithelial cells surrounding the alveoli of the mammary gland (Fig. 10.17).

The important role of the hypothalamus in maintaining and regulating the activity of the anterior lobe of the hypophysis has been described in relation to the hypophysial portal system (Figs. 10.15 and 10.17). This is a humoral control mechanism in which releasing hormones are transmitted via the portal system. There are no hypothalamic efferent fibers that reach the anterior lobe of the pituitary. The anterior pituitary stands in marked contrast to other endocrine organs, such as the ovary, testis, thyroid, and adrenal cortex, which may be transplanted to distant sites and still retain their endocrine functions. The anterior lobe of the pituitary cannot be transplanted to distant locations and retain its function, because it is dependent upon its close relationships with the hypothalamus. The essential hypothalamic features are the tuberoinfundibular tract and the hypophysial portal system (Figs. 10.15 and 10.16).

The hypothalamus is considered the site of elaboration of releasing hormones (peptides) related to gonadotrophic, adrenocorticotrophic (ACTH), thyrotrophic (TSH), and growth hormones. Attempts to determine the loci within the hypothalamus concerned with particular releasing factors suggest that the neural area related to TSH appears to lie on either side of the midline between the paraventricular nucleus and the median eminence. Electrical stimulation of the anterior median eminence appears to be the most effective site for increasing thyroid activity. Similarly, electrical stimulation of the hypothalamus in the rabbit can cause the discharge of gonadotrophic hormone and ACTH. While bilateral lesions in almost any region near the base of the hypothalamus reduce ACTH release, the median eminence-tuberal region has the most important controlling influence.

The brain plays an important role in the initiation and coordination of reproductive functions, and these functions are different in the two sexes. The tuberal region of the hypothalamus appears essential for the maintenance of basal levels of gonadotrophic hormone, but the integrity of the preoptic area is necessary for the cyclic surge of gonadotropin which precedes ovulation (Fig. 10.17). Electrical stimulation of the preoptic area, or the corticomedial nuclear group of the amygdaloid complex, produces ovulation in rabbits and cats. The effects of preoptic stimulation are abolished by lesions separating this area from the tuberal region of the hypothalamus; the effects of amygdaloid stimulation are blocked by a section of the stria terminalis. These observations suggest a functional linkage between the amygdala and the medial preoptic area via the stria terminalis, and fiber systems from the medial preoptic area to the tuberal region of the hypothalamus. However, the amygdaloid input to the preoptic area is not essential for ovulation, for bilateral destruction of the stria terminalis does not prevent ovulation.

Tumors and other pathological processes involving the hypothalamus frequently modify sexual development. Such lesions may be associated with precocious puberty or hypogonadism associated with underdevelopment of secondary sex characteristics. Although hypergonadism has been attributed to tumors of the pineal, most tumors of the brain associated with precocious puberty actually involve, or impinge on, the hypothalamus. These lesions frequently destroy the posterior hypothalamus and leave the anterior hypothalamus intact; the intact hypothalamic regions functioning in the absence of inhibitory influences from posterior regions leads to increased pituitary function.

The preoptic region plays an important role in regulating the release of gonadotrophic hormones from the anterior lobe of the hypophysis (Fig. 10.17). In the female, pituitary gonadotropins are released in a cyclic manner, the duration of the cycle corresponding to the menstrual period. In the male, the gonadotropins are released topically without regularly occurring fluctuations. Therefore it is not surprising that there are differences in the functional organization of the preoptic region in the male and female. A morphological expression of this difference has been observed in the preoptic region of the rat, where a nucleus of densely stained cells is larger in the male. This nucleus has been termed the "sexually dimorphic nucleus of the preoptic area." The full ontogenetic development of this nucleus, as well as the male pattern of tonic gonadotrophic release, depends on the presence in the circulation of testosterone during the first week of life. If the testes are removed from the newborn animal, the genetic male will fail to develop the sexually dimorphic nucleus of the preoptic region. Conversely, a newborn female given exogenous testosterone will, as an adult, show the male pattern of gonadotropin release. In the male the equivalent of luteinizing hormone promotes the growth and development of interstitial testicular cells (Leydig cells), which convert steroid precursors to testosterone. The role of gonadotrophins in spermatogenesis is complex and unclear, but a high level of testosterone appears essential (Fig. 10.17).

Growth hormone–releasing factor acts on acidophilic cells of the anterior pituitary that produce the growth hormone. Growth hormone functions synergistically with thyroxin, and blood levels fluctuate widely. A large part of the daily output of growth hormone is secreted in bursts following the onset of sleep. Strenuous exercise, hypoglycemia, and testosterone also appear to stimulate growth hormone secretion. Somatostatin, which inhibits the release of growth hormone, is present in the hypothalamus and in a variety of other tissues. Chronic hypersecretion of growth hormone leads to an overgrowth of bones and soft tissues, which produce a highly characteristic syndrome (acromegaly).

Tumors of the adenohypophysis may produce symptoms due to their increasing size or because they result in alterations of pituitary functions. Expanding tumors cause a ballooning of the sella turcica, may compress fibers in the optic chiasm or optic tract, and frequently produce headaches due to traction on the meninges. The most typical visual field defect is a bitemporal hemianopsia due to involvement of the decussating fibers in the optic chiasm (Fig. 9.29) but visual field defects take many forms dependent on the growth pattern of the tumor. Endocrinopathy may take the form of hypersecretion or hyposecretion depending on the type of tumor. The pituitary syndrome may be associated with excess prolactin (amenorrhea-galactorrhea), growth hormones (acromegaly), adrenocorticotrophic hormone (Cushing's syndrome). Patients with prolactin-secreting tumors have been successfully treated with dopamine agonists, particularly bromocriptine. Dopamine synthesized in the arcuate and periventricular nuclei of the hypothalamus and transported via the portal system inhibits prolactin release.

It has been known for a long time that certain lesions near the base of the brain are associated with obesity. Localized bilateral lesions in the hypothalamus involving primarily, or exclusively, the ventromedial nucleus in the tuberal region produce *hyperphagia*. Such animals eat voraciously, consuming two or three times the usual amount of food. Obesity appears to be the direct result of increased food intake. Bilateral lesions destroying portions of the lateral hypothalamic nucleus impair, or abolish, the desire to feed in hyperphagic and normal animals. These data suggest that the ventromedial nucleus of the hypothalamus is concerned with *satiety*, while the lateral hypothalamic nucleus may be regarded as a feeding center. Most animals with hyperphagia due to hypothalamic lesions exhibit savage behavior and rage reactions.

The hypothalamus is regarded as one of the principal centers concerned with emotional expression. It is acknowledged that the physiological expression of emotion is dependent on both sympathetic and parasympathetic components of the autonomic nervous system. The hypothalamus, intimately relating both of these, probably is involved directly or indirectly in most emotional reactions. Stimulation of the hypothalamus in unanesthetized cats with implanted electrodes provokes responses resembling rage and fear, which can be increased by graded stimuli of different intensities. These reactions, referred to as "pseudo-affective," are "stimulus-bound" in that they are present only during the period of stimulation. Different types of responses are elicited from different parts of the hypothalamus; flight responses are most readily evoked from lateral regions of the anterior hypothalamus, while aggressive responses characterized by hissing, snarling, baring of teeth, and biting are seen with stimulation of the region of the ventromedial nucleus. Because the emotional reactions provoked by electrical stimulation of the hypothalamus are directed, it seems likely that the cerebral cortex and thalamus play important roles in these responses. In these reactions the hypothalamus cannot be regarded as a simple efferent mechanism influencing only lower levels of the neuraxis.

Observations that selective stimulation and lesions of the ventromedial nucleus of the hypothalamus both produce aggressive behavior raise questions concerning the mechanism. Savage behavior after bilateral lesions of the ventromedial nucleus cannot be assumed to result from release of inhibitory influences. Because animals with such lesions never show spontaneous outburst of aggressive behavior and this hyperirritable state develops slowly, it has been postulated that destruction of these nuclei leads to a state of supersensitivity. Further secondary lesions involving the periaqueductal gray and the reticular formation may have a "taming" effect on this savage behavior. Hypothalamic-induced rage reactions may be blocked by midbrain lesions, indicating that structures at this level play a role in the expression of savage and aggressive behavior.

It is generally accepted that morphophysiologic substrates of abnormal and aggressive behavior involve, in some differential and selective fashion, predominantly "forebrain" brain structures. This part of the central nervous system contains the neural structures concerned with goal-directed behavior, and the motivational and emotional concomitants that make such behavior possible. Impulses generated in sensory systems, the cerebral cortex, and still undetermined neural structures may trigger mechanisms that excite visceral and somatic systems whose activities in concert provide the physiological expression of aggressive behavior.

SUGGESTED READINGS

ANTUNES, J. L., CARMEL, P. W., AND ZIMMERMAN, E. A. 1977. Projections from the paraventricular nucleus to the zona externa of the median eminence of the rhesus monkey: An immunohistochemical study. Brain Res., **137**: 1–10.

BERK, M. L., AND FINKELSTEIN, J. A. 1981. An autoradiographic determination of the efferent projections of the suprachiasmatic nucleus of the hypothalamus. Brain Res., **226**: 1–13.

BERK, M. L., AND FINKELSTEIN, J. A. 1981. Afferent projections to the preoptic area and hypothalamic regions in the rat brain. Neuroscience, **6**: 1601–1624.

CLARK, W. E. L., BEATTIE, J., RIDDOCH, G., AND DOTT, N. M. 1938. *The Hypothalamus.* Oliver & Boyd, Edinburgh.

DIFIGLIA, M., AND ARONIN, N. 1984. Immunoreactive leu-enkephalin in the monkey hypothalamus including observations on its ultrastructural localization in the paraventricular nucleus. J. Comp. Neurol., **225**: 313–326.

FAGG, G. E., AND FOSTER, A. C. 1983. Amino acid neurotransmitters and their pathways in the mammalian central nervous system. Neuroscience, **9**: 701–749.

FROHMAN, L. A. 1980. Neurotransmitters as regulators of endocrine function. In D. T. KRIEGER AND J. C. HUGHES (Editors), *Neuroendocrinology.* Sinauer Associates, Sunderland, MA, pp. 44–57.

FULWILER, C. E., AND SAPER, C. B. 1984. Subnuclear organization of the efferent connections of the parabrachial nucleus in the rat. Brain Res. Rev., **7**: 239–259.

FUXE, K., AND HÖKFELT, T. 1970. Central monoaminergic systems and hypothalamic function. In L. MARTINI, M. MOLTA, AND F. FRASCHINI (Editors), *The Hypothalamus.* Academic Press, New York, pp. 123–138.

GAINER, H. 1981. The biology of neurosecretory neurons. In J. B. MARTIN, S. REICHLIN, AND K. L. BICK (Editors), *Neurosecretion and Brain Peptides*, Raven Press, New York, pp. 5–20.

GLUSMAN, M. 1974. The hypothalamic "savage" syndrome. Proc. Assoc. Res. Nerv. Ment. Dis., **52**: 52–92.

GORSKI, R. A. 1980. Sexual differentiation of the brain. In D. T. KRIEGER AND J. C. HUGHES (Editors), *Neuroendocrinology.* Sinauer, Sunderland, MA, pp. 215–222.

GORSKI, R. A., HARLAN, R. E., JACOBSON, C. D., SHRYNE, J. E., AND SOUTHAM, A. M. 1980. Evidence for the existence of a sexually dimorphic nucleus in the preoptic area of the rat. J. Comp. Neurol., **193**: 529–539.

GUILLEMIN, R. 1978. Biochemical and physiological correlates of hypothalamic peptides. The new endocrinology of the neuron. In S. REICHLIN, R. J. BALDESSARINI AND J. B. MARTIN (Editors), *The Hypothalamus.* Raven Press, New York, pp. 155–194.

GUILLEMIN, R. 1980. Beta-lipotrophin and endorphins: Implications of current knowledge. In D. T. KRIEGER AND J. C. HUGHES (Editors), *Neuroendocrinology.* Sinauer Associates, Sunderland, MA, pp. 67–74.

HARRIS, G. W. 1948. Electrical stimulation of the hypothalamus and the mechanism of neural control of the adenohypophysis. J. Physiol., **107**: 418–429.

HARRIS, G. W., AND GEORGE, R. 1969. Neurohumoral control of the adenohypophysis and regulation of the secretion of TSH, ACTH and growth hormone. In W. HAYMAKER et al. (Editors), *The Hypothalamus.* Charles C Thomas, Springfield, IL, Ch. 10, pp. 326–388.

HARRIS, G. W., AND WOODS, J. W. 1958. The effects of electrical stimulation of the hypothalamus or pituitary gland on thyroid activity. J. Physiol., **143**: 246–274.

HAYMAKER, W. 1969. Hypothalamo-pituitary neural pathways and the circulatory system of the pituitary. In W. HAYMAKER ET AL. (Editors), *The Hypothalamus.* Charles C Thomas, Springfield, IL, Ch. 6, pp. 219–250.

HEIMER, L., AND NAUTA, W. J. H. 1969. The hypothalamic distribution of the stria terminalis in the rat. Brain Res., **13**: 284–297.

HÖKELT, T. 1967. The possible ultrastructural identification of tuberoinfundibular dopamine-containing nerve endings in the median eminence of the rat. Brain Res., **5**: 121–123.

HÖKFELT, T., JOHANSSON, O., FUXE, K., GOLDSTEIN, M., AND PARK, D. 1976. Immunohistochemical studies on the localization and distribution of monoamine neuron systems in the rat brain. I. Tyrosine hydroxylase in the mesencephalon and diencephalon. Med. Biol., **54**: 427–453.

KAWATA, N., McCABE, J. T., HARRINGTON, C., CHIKARAISHI, D., AND PFAFF, D. W. 1988. *In situ* hybridization analysis of osmotic stimulus-induced changes in ribosomal RNA in rat supraoptic nucleus. J. Comp. Neurol., **270**: 528–536.

KNIGGE, K. M., AND SILVERMAN, A.-J. 1974. The anatomy of the endocrine hypothalamus. In R. O. GREEP AND E. P. ASTWOOD (Editors), *Handbook of Physiology*, Sect. 7, Vol. IV. American Physiological Society, Washington, DC, Ch. 1, pp. 1–32.

KUHLENBECK, H. 1969. Derivation and boundaries of the hypothalamus, with atlas of hypothalamic grisea. In W. HAYMAKER ET AL. (Editors), *The Hypothalamus.* Charles C Thomas, Springfield, IL, Ch. 2, pp. 13–60.

KUYPERS, H. G. J. M., AND MAISKY, V. A. 1975. Retrograde axonal transport of horseradish peroxidase from spinal cord to brain stem cell groups in the cat. Neurosci, Lett., **1**: 9–14.

McNeill, T. H., and Sladek, J. R., Jr. 1980. Simultaneous monoamine histofluorescence and neuropeptide immunocytochemistry. II. Correlative distribution of catecholamine varicosities and supraoptic and paraventricular nuclei. J. Comp. Neurol., **193**: 1023–1033.

Mains, R. E., and Eipper, B. A. 1976. Biosynthesis of adrenocorticotrophic hormone in mouse pituitary tumor cells. J. Biol. Chem., **251**: 4115–4120.

Martin, J. B., Brazeau, P., Tannenbaum, G. S., Willoughby, J. O., Epelbaum, J., Terry, L. C., and Durand, D. 1978. Neuroendocrine organization of growth hormone regulation. In S. Reichlin, R. J. Baldessarini, and J. B. Martin (Editors), *The Hypothalamus*. Raven Press, New York, pp. 329–355.

Martin, J. B., Reichlin, S., and Brown, G. M. 1977. *Clinical Neuroendocrinology*. F. A. Davis, Philadelphia, pp. 229–246.

Meibach, R. C., and Siegel, A. 1977. Efferent connections of the hippocampal formation in the rat. Brain Res., **124**: 197–224.

Mesulam, M.-M., Mufson, E. J., Levey, A. I., and Wainer, B. H. 1983. Cholinergic innervation of cortex of the basal forebrain: Cytochemistry and cortical connections of the septal area, diagonal band nuclei, nucleus basalis (substantia innominata) and hypothalamus in the rhesus monkey. J. Comp. Neurol., **214**: 170–197.

Millhouse, O. E., 1979. A Golgi anatomy of the rodent hypothalamus. In P. J. Morgane and J. Panksepp (Editors), *Handbook of the Hypothalamus; Vol. I. Anatomy of the Hypothalamus*. Marcel Dekker, New York, pp. 221–265.

Nauta, W. J. H. 1958. Hippocampal projections and related pathways to the midbrain in the cat. Brain, **81**: 319–340.

Nauta, W. J. H., and Haymaker, W. 1969. Hypothalamic nuclei and fiber connections. In W. Haymaker et al. (Editors), *The Hypothalamus*. Charles C Thomas, Springfield, IL, Ch. 4, pp. 136–209.

Page, R. B. 1988. The anatomy of the hypothalamo-hypophyseal complex. In E. Knobil et al. (Editors), *The Physiology of Reproduction*. Raven Press, New York, pp. 1161–1233.

Page, R. B., and Bergland, R. M. 1977. The neurohypophyseal capillary bed. I. Anatomy and arterial supply. Am. J. Anat., **148**: 345–357.

Palkovits, M. 1981. Catecholamines in the hypothalamus: An anatomical review. Neuroendocrinology, **33**: 123–128.

Palkovits, M., and Zaborsky, L. 1979. Neural connections of the hypothalamus. In P. J. Morgane and J. Panksepp (Editors), *Anatomy of the Hypothalamus*. Marcel Dekker, New York.

Pickard, G. E., and Silverman, A. J. 1981. Direct retinal projections to the hypothalamus, piriform cortex, and accessory optic nuclei in the golden hamster as demonstrated by a sensitive anterograde horseradish peroxidase technique. J. Comp. Neurol., **196**: 155–172.

Porter, J. C., Ondon, J. G., and Cramer, O. M. 1974. Nervous and vascular supply of the pituitary gland. In R. O. Greep and E. P. Astwood (Editors), *Handbook of Physiology*, Sect. 7, Vol. IV. Endocrinology. American Physiological Society, Washington, DC, Ch. 2, pp. 33–43.

Rafols, J. A., Aronin, N., and DiFiglia, M. 1987. A Golgi study of the monkey paraventricular nucleus: Neuronal types, afferent and efferent fibers. J. Comp. Neurol., **257**: 595–613.

Raisman, G. 1966. Neural connexions of hypothalamus. Br. Med. Bull., **22**: 197–201.

Reichlin, S, Baldessarini, R. J., and Martin, J. B. (Editors). 1978. *The Hypothalamus*. Raven Press, New York.

Renaud, L. P. 1979. Neurophysiology and neuropharmacology of medial hypothalamic neurons and their extrahypothalamic connections. In P. J. Morgane and J. Panksepp (Editors), *Anatomy of the Hypothalamus*. Marcel Dekker, New York, pp. 593–694.

Saffran, M. 1974. Chemistry of hypothalamic and hypophysiotropic factors. In R. O. Greep and E. P. Astwood (Editors), *Handbook of Physiology*, Sect. 7, Vol. IV. Endocrinology, Part 2. American Physiological Society, Washington, DC, Ch. 43, pp. 563–586.

Saper, C. B., Loewy, A. D., Swanson, L. W., and Cowan, W. M. 1976. Direct hypothalamo-autonomic connections. Brain Res., **117**: 305–312.

Schally, A. V., Kastin, A. J., and Arimura, A. 1977. Hypothalamic hormones: The link between brain and body. Am. Sci., **65**: 712–719.

Silverman, A. J., and Pickard, G. E. 1983. The hypothalamus. In P. C. Emson (Editor), *Chemical Neuroanatomy*. Raven Press, New York, pp. 295–336.

Steinberger, E., and Steinberger, A. 1974. Hormonal control of testicular function in mammals. In R. O. Greep and E. P. Astwood (Editors), *Handbook of Physiology*: Sect. 7, Vol. IV. Endocrinology., Part 2. American Physiological Society, Washington, DC, pp. 325–345.

Swanson, L. W., and Cowan, W. M. 1977. An autoradiographic study of the organization of the efferent connections of the hippocampal formation in the rat. J. Comp. Neurol., **172**: 49–84.

Swanson, L. W., and Kuypers, H. G. J. M. 1980. The paraventricular nucleus of the hypothalamus: Cytoarchitectonic subdivisions and organization of projections to the pituitary, dorsal vagal complex, and spinal cord as demonstrated by retrograde fluorescence double-labeling methods. J. Comp. Neurol., **194**: 555–570.

Swanson, L. W., Sawchenko, P. E., Wiegand, S. J., and Price, J. L. 1980. Separate neurons in the paraventricular nucleus project to the median eminence and to the medulla or spinal cord. Brain Res., **198**: 190–195.

WATTS, A. G., AND SWANSON, L. W. 1987. Efferent projections of the suprachiasmatic nucleus. II. Studies using retrograde transport of fluorescent dyes and simultaneous immunohistochemistry in the rat. J. Comp. Neurol., **258**: 230–252.

WATTS, A. G., SWANSON, L. W., AND SANCHEZ-WATTS, G. 1987. Efferent projections of the suprachiasmatic nucleus: I. Studies using anterograde transport of *Phaseolus vulgaris* leucoagglutinin in the rat. J. Comp. Neurol., **258**: 204–229.

VAN WYK, J. J., AND UNDERWOOD, L. E. 1978. Growth hormone, somatomedins and growth failure. In D. T. KRIEGER AND J. C. HUGHES (Editors), *Neuroendocrinology*. Sinauer Associates, Sunderland, MA, pp. 299–309.

ZIMMERMAN, E. A. 1981. Organization of oxytocin and vasopressin pathways. In J. B. MARTIN, S. REICHLIN AND K. L. BICK (Editors), *Neurosecretion and Brain Peptides*. Raven Press, New York, pp. 63–75.

ZIMMERMAN, E. A., CARMEL, P. W., HUSAIN, M. K., FERIN, M., TANNENBAUM, M., FRANTZ, A. G., AND ROBINSON, A. G. 1973. Vasopressin and neurophysin: High concentrations in monkey hypophyseal portal blood. Science, **182**: 925–927.

11

Corpus Striatum and Related Nuclei

The basal ganglia are large subcortical nuclei classically considered to be derived largely, but not exclusively, from the telencephalon. The major divisions of the basal ganglia are (1) the corpus striatum, considered to be concerned primarily with somatic motor functions, and (2) the amygdaloid nuclear complex, functionally related to the hypothalamus and regarded as an integral part of the limbic system. The corpus striatum consists of the putamen, the caudate nucleus, and the globus pallidus (Figs. 11.1 and 11.2). The putamen and caudate nucleus, derived from the telencephalon, form the *neostriatum*, the largest part of the corpus striatum (Fig. 11.3). The globus pallidus consists of two parallel, cytologically similar segments medial to the putamen. Segments of the globus pallidus constitute the *paleostriatum* (Figs. 11.2, 11.4, and 11.5). The amygdaloid nuclear complex, a telencephalic derivative, is referred to as the *archistriatum*. The amygdala is located in the temporal lobe, deep to the uncus and rostral to the inferior horn of the lateral ventricle (Figs. 2.8, 11.2, and 11.3). Some functions of the basal ganglia are not easily segregated and the neostriatum appears to consist of limbic and nonlimbic subdivisions.

CORPUS STRIATUM

The *corpus striatum* consists of two distinctive parts, the *neostriatum* (caudate nucleus and putamen) and the *paleostriatum* (globus pallidus). The putamen lies deep to the external capsule in the insular region. The caudate nucleus is disposed in a C-shaped configuration and bears a constant relationship to the lateral ventricle (Figs. 11.3 and 11.4). The two parallel segments of the globus pallidus lie medial to the putamen and are separated from each other, and from the putamen, by medullary laminae, which in places contain large cholinergic neurons (Figs. 11.5 and 11.15). Both segments of the globus pallidus and the subthalamic nucleus are diencephalic derivatives. The putamen plus the globus pallidus together are referred to as the lentiform nucleus.

The neostriatum, considered the receptive component, receives massive inputs which originate from (1) broad regions of the cerebral cortex, (2) the centromedian-parafascicular (CM-PF) nuclear complex, (3) the substantia nigra, (4) several smaller mesencephalic nuclei, and (5) portions of the lateral amygdala. Most of the striatal afferent systems are associated with distinctive neurotransmitters. The neural activities of the neostriatum involve the largest number of distinctive cell types and a large number of different neurotransmitters, which include acetylcholine, monamines, peptides, and amino acids. The striatum has a form of reciprocal connections with the distinctive cytological subdivisions of the substantia nigra in which fibers arise from and terminate on different cell populations (Fig. 11.12). Impaired synthesis and transmission of neuro-

Figure 11.1. Photograph of a frontal section of the brain passing through the columns of the fornix and the anterior commissure. At this level the putamen and the lateral pallidal segment lie beneath the insular cortex. (From Carpenter and Sutin, *Human Neuroanatomy*, 1983; courtesy of Williams & Wilkins.)

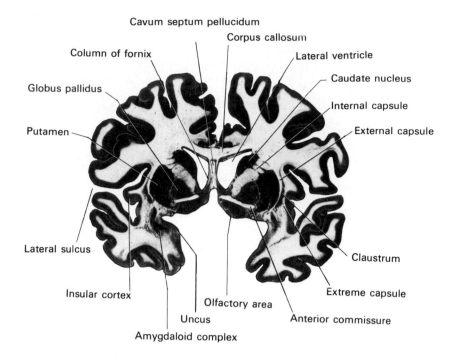

Figure 11.2. Photograph of a frontal section of the brain at the level of the mammillary bodies. In this section the main nuclear groups of the thalamus are identified and portions of all components of the basal ganglia are present. The amygdaloid nuclear complex lies in the temporal lobe internal to the uncus and ventral to the lentiform nucleus. (From Carpenter and Sutin, *Human Neuroanatomy*, 1983; courtesy of Williams & Wilkins.)

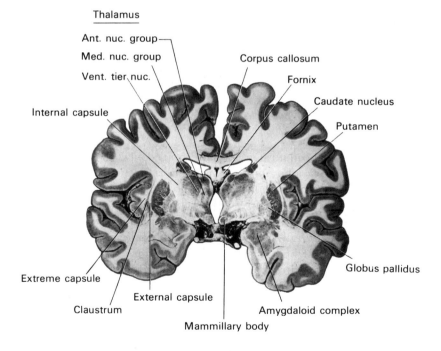

transmitters involved in striatal functions constitute one important feature of metabolic disturbances associated with two relatively common forms of dyskinesia (disturbances of movement), namely, parkinsonism and Huntington's disease.

The globus pallidus forming the smaller, most medial part of the lentiform nucleus consists of two cytologically similar segments that have input systems with both common and distinctive neurotransmitters (Figs. 11.4, 11.5, and 11.13). Each pallidal segment gives rise to different projections. Projections of the medial pallidal segment are to ipsilateral thalamic nuclei, which in turn have access to motor regions of the cerebral cortex. The lateral pallidal segment projects primarily to portions of the

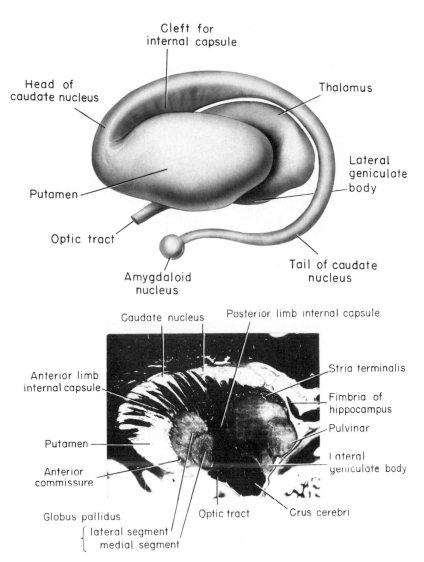

Cleft for
internal capsule

Head of
caudate nucleus

Thalamus

Putamen

Lateral
geniculate
body

Optic tract

Amygdaloid
nucleus

Tail of caudate
nucleus

Figure 11.3. Semischematic drawing of the isolated striatum, thalamus, and amygdaloid nucleus showing (1) the continuity of the putamen and head of the caudate nucleus rostroventrally, and (2) the relationships between the tail of the caudate nucleus and the amygdaloid nucleus. The cleft occupied by fibers of the internal capsule is indicated. The anterior limb of the internal capsule is situated between the caudate nucleus and the putamen (Figs. 9.25, 11.4, and 11.5), while the posterior limb of the internal capsule lies between the lentiform nucleus and the thalamus. (From Carpenter and Sutin, *Human Neuroanatomy*, 1983; courtesy of Williams & Wilkins.)

Caudate nucleus

Posterior limb internal capsule

Anterior limb
internal capsule

Stria terminalis

Fimbria of
hippocampus

Pulvinar

Putamen

Anterior
commissure

Lateral
geniculate body

Globus pallidus
  lateral segment
  medial segment

Optic tract

Crus cerebri

Figure 11.4. Sagittal section through the basal ganglia, internal capsule, and thalamus. Note the relationships of the caudate nucleus to the fibers of the anterior limb of the internal capsule. Weigert's myelin stain. Photograph. (From Carpenter and Sutin, *Human Neuroanatomy*, 1983; courtesy of Williams & Wilkins.)

subthalamic nucleus. Reciprocal connections interrelate portions of the lateral pallidal segment and the subthalamic nucleus. The output systems of the corpus striatum arise from the medial pallidal segment and from the pars reticulata of the substantia nigra.

STRIATUM

Caudate Nucleus

The caudate nucleus is an elongated, arched gray mass related throughout its extent to the surface of the lateral ventricle (Figs. 9.6, 11.1, 11.2, 11.3, 11.4, and 11.5). Its enlarged anterior portion, or *head*, lies rostral to the thalamus and bulges into the anterior horn of the lateral ventricle (Figs. 2.11, 2.12, and 11.5). The head of the caudate nucleus and the putamen are separated by fibers of the anterior limb of the internal capsule, except rostroventrally where continuity is maintained. The *body* of the caudate nucleus extends along the dorsolateral border of the thalamus, from which it is separated by the stria terminalis and the terminal vein (Fig. 9.6). This part of the caudate nucleus is regarded as suprathalamic. The *tail* of the caudate nucleus is the attenuated caudal portion that sweeps into the temporal lobe in the roof of the inferior horn of the

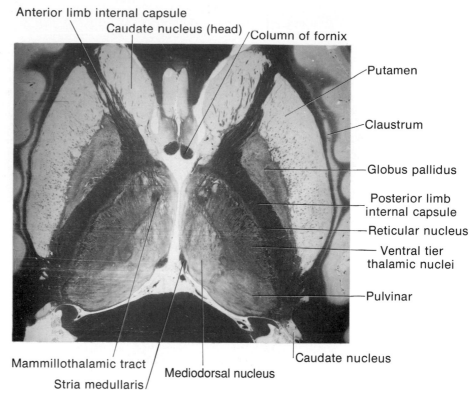

Anterior limb internal capsule
Caudate nucleus (head) / Column of fornix
Putamen
Claustrum
Globus pallidus
Posterior limb internal capsule
Reticular nucleus
Ventral tier thalamic nuclei
Pulvinar
Caudate nucleus
Mammillothalamic tract / Mediodorsal nucleus
Stria medullaris

Figure 11.5. Horizontal section of the thalamus, internal capsule, and corpus striatum. Weigert's myelin stain. Photograph. (From Carpenter and Sutin, *Human Neuroanatomy*, 1983; courtesy of Williams & Wilkins.)

lateral ventricle and comes into relationship with the central nucleus of the amygdaloid complex (Figs. 2.11, 9.6, 11.2, 11.3, and 12.13).

Putamen

The putamen, the largest and most lateral part of the basal ganglia, lies between the external capsule and the lateral medullary lamina of the globus pallidus (Figs. 11.1, 11.2, 11.3, 11.4, and 11.5). Most of the putamen is situated deep to the insular cortex and is separated from it by the extreme capsule, the claustrum, and the external capsule. In transverse sections it appears lightly stained and is traversed by numerous fascicles of myelinated fibers directed ventromedially toward the globus pallidus. The caudate nucleus and putamen are continuous rostroventrally, beneath the anterior limb of the internal capsule, and in dorsal regions where slender gray cellular bridges pass across the posterior limb of the internal capsule (Figs. 11.3 and 11.4). At levels through the septum pellucidum the nucleus accumbens lies adjacent to ventromedial portions of the striatum (Fig. 12.15). The nucleus accumbens is ontogenetically more closely related to the caudate nucleus and putamen than to the septal nuclei and has projections to both the globus pallidus and the substantia nigra.

Cytologically the caudate nucleus and the putamen appear identical and are composed of enormous numbers of cells that exhibit no lamination or special arrangements. The striatum may not be as uniform as it appears because in its development cells of different types migrate in clusters, histochemical activity has a patchy distribution (Fig. 11.9), and efferent

SI

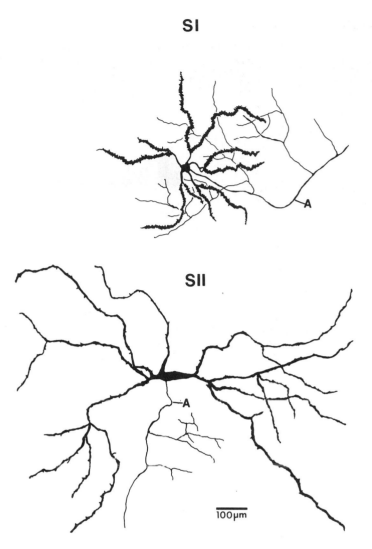

SII

100μm

Figure 11.6. Drawings of spiny striatal neurons. Spiny type I (SI) neurons have dendrites that radiate into a spheroid domain of about 200 μm, but the first 20 μm of the stem dendrites are free of spines. Spiny type II (SII) neurons are larger, vary in size and shape, and have dendrites that extend 600 μm from the somata. Axons (A) of these cells project to either the medial pallidal segment, the lateral pallidal segment, or the pars reticulata of the substantia nigra. These neurons receive most inputs to the striatum and collectively are the efferent neurons of the striatum. GABA, enkephalin, and substance P in various combinations are the neurotransmitters of these cells. (Redrawn from Groves, 1983, Brain Res. Rev.)

neurons show some segregation. Striatal neurons fall into two categories: (1) those with spiny dendrites and (2) those with smooth dendrites.

Spiny neurons, considered the most numerous striatal neuron, are round or oval medium-sized cells, emit multiple primary dendrites covered with spines, and have long axons (Fig. 11.6). Two types of spiny striatal neurons are recognized. Type I spiny neurons, present in enormous numbers, have smooth somata and proximal dendrites that distally become laden with spines; dendrites radiate into spherical space of about 200 μm. Long axons of these cells give rise to both proximal and distal collaterals. Spiny type II striatal neurons commonly are larger neurons with spiny dendrites that extend 600 μm from the somata (Figs. 11.6 and 11.13). Axons of spiny II neurons are long and give off collaterals near the somata (Fig. 11.6). Spiny striatal neurons serve as both receptive and projection neurons. Most afferents from various sources terminate on spiny processes of these neurons. All fibers projecting beyond the striatum arise from spiny striatal neurons. Immunocytochemically, spiny striatal neurons are heterogeneous, containing γ-aminobutyric acid (GABA), substance P (SP), enkephalin (ENK), and perhaps neurotensin (NT). Many spiny striatal neurons contain more than one neurotransmitter and transmitter substances occur in various combinations. In spite of this

Figure 11.7. Drawings of aspiny striatal neurons whose processes are contained within the striatum. Aspiny type I (ASI) neurons are the most frequently impregnated striatal neuron in Golgi preparations. These intrinsic striatal neurons appear to have GABA, neuropeptide Y (NPY), and somatostatin (SRIF) as neurotransmitters. Aspiny type II (ASII) neurons are giant cholinergic neurons evenly distributed within the striatum (Fig. 11.8). Axons (A) of ASII neurons contact all parts of spiny neurons. The neurotransmitter of aspiny type II (ASIII) neurons has not been identified. (Redrawn from Groves, 1983, Brain Res. Rev.)

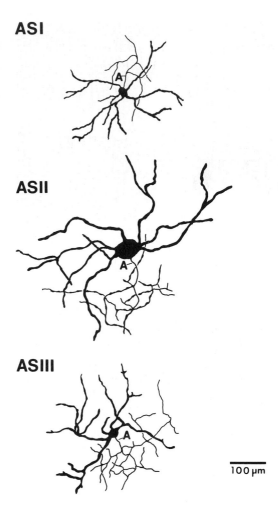

ASI

ASII

ASIII

100 µm

chemical heterogeneity, GABA is the dominant neurotransmitter (Fig. 11.13).

Aspiny neurons are intrinsic striatal neurons with short axons. Three short-axoned Golgi type II striatal neurons have been described. The aspiny type I neuron is distinguished by its small size, varicose and recurring dendrites, and a short, highly arborized axon (Figs. 11.7 and 11.13). Large numbers of aspiny type I neurons are GABAergic, but many neurons of this type are immunoreactive to neuropeptide Y (NPY) and somatostatin (SRIF). The majority of striatal neurons immunoreactive for SRIF also are immunoreactive for NPY. Aspiny type II neurons have large cell bodies, eccentric nuclei, and dendrites extending more than 250 µm. These cells correspond to a subpopulation of giant neurons distributed uniformly throughout the striatum. Immunohistochemically aspiny II neurons (Figs. 11.7, 11.8 and 11.13) stain for choline acetyltransferase (ChAT) and acetylcholinesterase (AChE). Aspiny striatal giant cholinergic neurons have been shown to establish symmetrical synapses with medium-sized spiny neurons, which are the major target of nigral dopaminergic terminals. These cholinergic neurons are considered to play a crucial role in maintaining the striatal balance of dopamine and GABA. The neurotransmitter of aspiny type III striatal neurons has not been identified (Figs. 11.7 and 11.13).

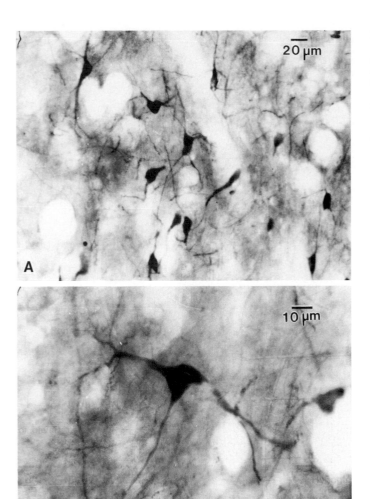

Figure 11.8. Aspiny type II striatal neurons in the monkey immunoreactive to choline acetyltransferase (ChAT). *A*, These neurons are uniformly distributed throughout the caudate nucleus and putamen. *B*, Higher magnification of a cholinergic striatal neuron. Short axons of these neurons establish symmetrical synaptic contacts with medium-sized spiny striatal neurons and play a role in maintaining the balance between dopamine and GABA.

STRIATAL COMPARTMENTS

There is considerable evidence that the striatal neuropil is organized into a mosaic of chemically distinct compartments related to the organization of afferent and efferent connections and to particular transmitter substances (Fig. 11.9). Every major striatal afferent system studied by autoradiography has been shown to terminate in a patchy fashion. A histochemical compartmentalization of the striatum has been demonstrated for a variety of neuropeptides and transmitter-related enzymes. Acetylcholinesterase (AChE) staining has been particularly useful in dramatically demonstrating these compartments (Fig. 11.9). The two major compartments of the striatum are referred to as "patches" (striosomes) and "matrix." Patches in the striatum are characterized by high levels of opiate receptors, substance P (SP), neurotensin (NT) and tyrosine hydroxylase (TH). The matrix is identified with high levels of AChE, somatostatin (SRIF), neurotensin receptors, and terminals of thalamic projections. Prefrontal, cingulate, and motor cortical areas project to both patches and matrix.

Striking changes occur in organization of striatal compartments during early development. In the fetus AChE and dopamine are in register in the patches, but postnatally AChE is largely in the matrix (Fig. 11.9).

Figure 11.9. Dark-field photograph of muscarinic cholinergic receptor binding sites in the caudate nucleus and putamen of a 22-week-old human fetus. Areas rich in binding sites appear as light patches (striosomes). GE indicates the ganglionic eminence. Scale bar = 1.0 mm. (Courtesy of Professor Ann M. Graybiel, Massachusetts Institute of Technology; Nastuk and Graybiel, 1985. J. Comp. Neurol.).

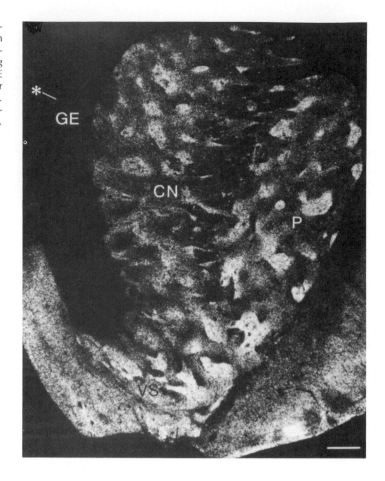

Opiate receptors, diffusely distributed prenatally, are found postnatally in the patches. Chemical compartmentalization of the striatum appears to be a mammalian evolutionary phenomenon that expresses functional differences in groups of striatal neurons.

STRIATAL CONNECTIONS

Striatal Afferents

The caudate nucleus and the putamen receive the principal afferent systems projecting to the corpus striatum. Major afferent fibers arise from the cerebral cortex, parts of the amygdala, the intralaminar thalamic nuclei, the substantia nigra, and the dorsal nucleus of the raphe (Figs. 6.30, 11.10, and 11.11).

CORTICOSTRIATE FIBERS

Virtually all regions of the neocortex project fibers to the striatum and all parts of the striatum receive fibers from the cortex. No part of the striatum is under the sole influence of one neocortex area.

Degeneration studies suggested that different regions of cortex projected to specific parts of the striatum with degrees of overlap. Autoradiographic studies revealed that (1) corticostriate terminals form mosaic-like patterns in the striatum, (2) many cortical areas have widespread projections in several parts of the striatum, and (3) widely separated cortical areas give rise to overlapping terminal fields. The terminal distribution of corticostriate fibers is extensive and characterized by a mosaic

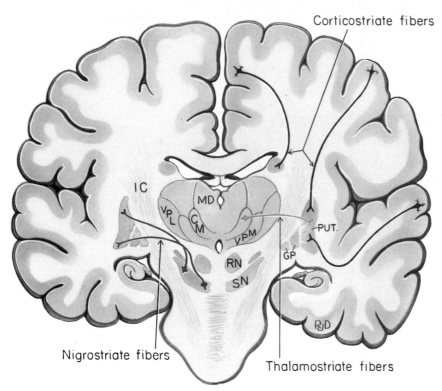

Figure 11.10.   Semischematic diagram of some major striatal afferent systems. *Corticostriate projections (black)* arise from broad regions of the cerebral cortex, are distributed to parts of both the caudate nucleus and putamen, and terminate in a mosaic pattern. These projections have glutamate as their neurotransmitter. *Nigrostriatal fibers (red)* arise from intermingled clusters of cells in the pars compacta of the substantia nigra (SNC) and convey dopamine to terminals in either the caudate nucleus or the putamen (Fig. 11.12). *Thalamostriate fibers (blue)* arise largely from cells in the centromedian-parafascicular (CM-PF) nuclear complex. Cells in CM project to the putamen and cells in PF project to the caudate nucleus. Serotonergic projections from the dorsal nucleus of the raphe are not shown here. *Abbreviations:* CM, centromedian nucleus; GP, globus pallidus; IC, internal capsule; MD, mediodorsal nucleus; PUT, putamen; RN, red nucleus; SN, substantia nigra; VPL and VPM, ventral posterolateral and ventral posteromedial thalamic nuclei.

pattern of patches or clusters. The patches of striatal terminals arising from different cortical areas not only overlap each other but also may overlap terminal projection zones of other striatal afferents.

Corticostriate fibers arising in the primary motor area (area 4) project bilaterally and somatotopically on the putamen (Fig. 11.11) where patchlike terminations are greatest in lateral regions of the putamen. The premotor area projects ipsilaterally to both the caudate nucleus and the putamen; the prefrontal cortex projects via an intranuclear trajectory to all parts of the caudate nucleus.

The laminar origin of the corticostriate system, the most massive projection system to the striatum, is mainly from smaller pyramidal cells in superficial parts of lamina V (Fig. 13.5). The implication is that these fibers constitute a distinct projection, rather than collaterals of other systems. Striatal afferents from the cerebral cortex end principally on the dendritic spines of spiny striatal neurons, are excitatory, and probably have glutamate as their neurotransmitter.

AMYGDALOSTRIATE FIBERS

Although the amygdala and the neostriatum have for many years been considered as anatomically and functionally distinct components of

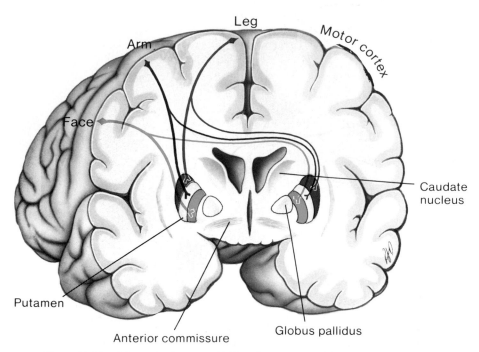

Figure 11.11.   Schematic diagram of bilateral somatotopically arranged corticostriate projections from the primary motor area (area 4) to the putamen in the monkey. The ipsilateral projection is much greater than the contralateral projection. Projections from the leg area of the motor cortex are in *red*, while those from the arm and face areas are *white* and *blue*, respectively. The premotor cortex projects ipsilateral to both the caudate nucleus and the putamen; the prefrontal cortex projects fibers to all parts of the caudate nucleus. (Based on Künzle, 1975, Brain Res.).

the basal ganglia, data now suggest a close functional relationship between parts of these structures. Projections from the basolateral amygdala to ventromedial region of the caudate nucleus and to ventrocaudal parts of the putamen suggest that the striatum may be divided into "limbic" and "nonlimbic" portions.

The smaller "nonlimbic" striatum occupies an anterodorsolateral region. In addition, the head of the caudate nucleus in the monkey receives direct projections from cells in the substantia innominata, which has inputs from the amygdala. This parcellation of the striatum into distinctive regions on the basis of amygdaloid projections suggests that large portions of the "limbic" striatum may be concerned with behavioral phenomenon.

THALAMOSTRIATE FIBERS

It has long been recognized that the largest intralaminar thalamic nuclei, the centromedian-parafascicular (CM-PF) nuclear complex, have subcortical projections to the neostriatum. In the monkey, cells in the centromedian nucleus (CM) project only to the putamen; cells in the parafascicular nucleus project only to the caudate nucleus (Figs. 9.14 and 11.10).

Cells in the central lateral (CL) and paracentral (PCN) thalamic nuclei contain two populations of neurons, one projecting to cortex and one projecting to the caudate nucleus. Monosynaptic relays in CL and PCN from the midbrain reticular formation conduct impulses separately to cortical areas and the caudate nucleus. Autoradiographic studies in

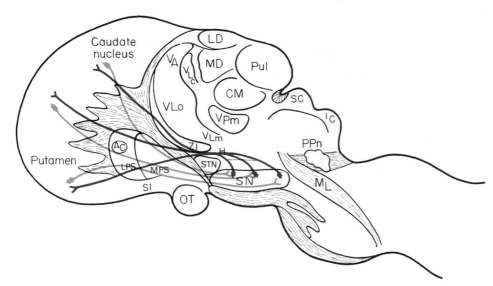

Figure 11.12. Schematic diagram of the striatonigral feedback system in a sagittal plane. *Striatonigral fibers (blue)* projecting on cells of the pars reticulata (SNR) have GABA, enkephalin (ENK), and substance P (SP) as neurotransmitters, but GABA is dominant. Intermingled clusters of cells in the pars compacta (SNC) give rise to *nigrostriatal fibers (red)*, which convey dopamine to terminals in either the caudate nucleus or the putamen that terminate in a mosaic pattern. *Abbreviations:* AC, anterior commissure; CM, centromedian nucleus; H, Forel's field; IC, inferior colliculus; LD, lateral dorsal nucleus; LPS, lateral pallidal segment; MD, mediodorsal nucleus; ML, medial lemniscus; MPS, medial pallidal segment; OT, optic tract; PPn, pedunculopontine nucleus; Pul, pulvinar; SC, superior colliculus; SI, substantia innominata; SN, substantia nigra; STN, subthalamic nucleus; VA, ventral anterior nucleus; VLc, VLo, and VLm, ventral lateral nucleus, pars caudalis, pars oralis, and pars medialis, respectively; VPM, ventral posteromedial nucleus; ZI, zona incerta.

monkey and cat show that thalamostriate fibers terminate, like corticostriate fibers, in mosaic disc-shaped aggregates or hollow rings in the caudate nucleus and putamen. Thalamostriate fibers terminate on spiny striatal neurons and are thought to be excitatory. The neurotransmitter utilized by thalamostriate fibers is not known.

NIGROSTRIATAL FIBERS

Fluorescent histochemical studies not only provided evidence that cells of the pars compacta of the substantia nigra (SNC) projected to the striatum but indicated that these cells conveyed dopamine to their terminals. The organization of ascending striatal afferents based on retrograde enzyme transport suggests cells in the rostral two-thirds of the pars compacta of the substantia nigra are related to the head of the caudate nucleus (Figs. 11.10 and 11.12), while those projecting to the putamen are in more posterior regions. One of the impressive features of the nigrostriatal project is that intermingled clusters of cells in the pars compacta project to either the caudate nucleus or the putamen, but not to both. The intermingled clusters of cells in the pars compacta of the substantia nigra projecting to different parts of the striatum may be in part responsible for the mosaic-like pattern of fiber terminations. Dendritic spines of spiny striatal neurons have been identified as the synaptic site of the majority of terminals immunoreactive of tyrosine hydroxylase, the synthesizing enzyme for dopamine.

It is generally accepted that dopamine has an inhibitory action on striatal neurons. Two different dopamine receptors have been identified pharmacologically in the mammalian striatum, designated as D_1 and D_2

receptors. The pattern of binding for both D_1 and D_2 receptors in the striatum does not match the patchy heterogeneity seen with AChE staining, but areas of greatest receptor density are found in the matrix. Activation of D_1 receptors reduces membrane excitability, while activation of D_2 receptors causes a decrease in the release of transmitter substance at synaptic terminals. Although D_1 and D_2 receptors can be distinguished, these receptors appear to function synergistically to modulate neuronal activities. Not all nigrostriatal fibers are considered dopaminergic. Some 20% of nigrostriatal fibers are said to be nondopaminergic, but their cells of origin are uncertain.

AFFERENTS FROM THE RAPHE NUCLEI

Histofluorescent technics have demonstrated several ascending pathways originating from mesencephalic indolamine cell groups in the median raphe. The dorsal and median raphe nuclei provide two distinct, but partially overlapping, ascending serotonergic (5-hydroxytryptamine, 5-HT) systems. Serotonergic projections arising from the dorsal nucleus of the raphe terminate in ventrocaudal regions of the striatum (Figs. 6.30 and 11.13). Double-labeling technics demonstrate that the majority of neurons in the dorsal nucleus of the raphe project collaterals to both the striatum and the substantia nigra. Stimulation of the dorsal nucleus of the raphe produces a long-lasting inhibition of striatal neurons.

Striatal Efferents

Different populations of spiny striatal neurons containing the same neurotransmitters (GABA, SP, and ENK) project to both the globus pallidus and the pars reticulata of the substantia nigra (SNR). Striatonigral projections that establish synaptic relationships with cells of the SNR and the GABAergic neurons of the SNR together constitute part of the output system from the corpus striatum. Striatopallidal fibers terminating in the medial pallidal segment (MPS) and the GABAergic pallidal neurons that project to the thalamus form the largest output system from the corpus striatum. Major projections from the SNR and the MPS are to different rostral ventral tier thalamic nuclei, which have projections to different regions of the cortex concerned with motor function. Striatopallidal fibers are described as pallidal afferents on page 337.

STRIATONIGRAL FIBERS

These fibers originate from spiny striatal neurons and project topographically, mainly on cells of the pars reticulata of the substantia nigra (SNR). Fibers from the head of the caudate nucleus project to rostral parts of the nigra. Putaminonigral fibers passing to more caudal parts of the nigra are arranged so that dorsal parts of the putamen project to lateral parts of the nigra and ventral parts of the putamen are related to medial parts of the nigra (Fig. 11.12). Striatonigral fibers arise from a different population of spiny neurons than striatopallidal fibers but have the same neurotransmitters, namely, GABA, SP, and ENK (Fig. 11.13). Almost all striatonigral fibers terminate in the SNR, but fibers immunoreactive for SP have been identified in both the SNR and the SNC. Neurons in the pars reticulata have smooth dendrites radiating rostrocaudally. In the rat, virtually all cells of the SNR are GABAergic, but in the monkey, neurons immunoreactive to GABA are most numerous in lateral regions of the SNR. GABAergic fibers and terminals are present in all parts of the SNR, and striatonigral synapses are of the symmetrical type. Electrical stimulation of the caudate nucleus leads to a marked increase in the release of [³H]GABA in the ipsilateral substantia nigra.

The GABAergic neurons of the pars reticulata (SNR) give rise to nigrothalamic projections that have large numbers of collaterals terminating in middle layers of the superior colliculus and in the midbrain tegmentum. Nigrothalamic fibers terminate in the ventral anterior nucleus (VAmc), parts of the ventral lateral nucleus (VLm), and in parts of the mediodorsal nucleus (MDpl). These thalamic nuclei do not receive afferents from any other part of the corpus striatum.

GLOBUS PALLIDUS

This nucleus forms the smaller and most medial part of the lentiform nucleus. Throughout its extent the pallidum lies medial to the putamen and lateral to the internal capsule (Figs. 2.11, 11.1, 11.2, 11.4, 11.5, and 11.14). A thin *lateral medullary lamina* lies on the external surface of the pallidum at its junction with the putamen. A *medial medullary lamina* divides the globus pallidus into medial and lateral segments (Figs. 11.5, 11.14, 11.16, and 11.17). A less distinct *accessory medullary lamina* divides the medial pallidal segment into outer and inner portions, which give rise to distinctive efferent fibers (Figs. 11.14 and 11.16). The globus pallidus, phylogenetically older than the striatum, is well developed in lower vertebrates. Bundles of myelinated fibers traversing the globus pallidus give it a paler appearance than the putamen or caudate nucleus in the fresh brain. Cells of the globus pallidus are predominantly large fusiform neurons with long, smooth dendrites that arborize in discoid-shaped formations parallel to the medullary laminae. Quantitative analysis of large pallidal neurons indicates they belong to a single neuronal population. No morphological or chemical differences are evident in the large neurons of the medial (MPS) and lateral (LPS) pallidal segments. In humans the LPS constitutes about 70% of the total pallidum and has the highest cell density. All large neurons within both segments of the globus pallidus are GABAergic (Fig. 11.15D). Axons of the pallidal neurons have few collaterals. Large cholinergic neurons in portions of the medial and lateral medullary laminae constitute extensions of the substantia innominata, which lies ventral to the globus pallidus (Fig. 11.15C).

PALLIDAL CONNECTIONS

Pallidal Afferents

Major afferent fibers to the globus pallidus arise from the striatum and the subthalamic nucleus. Unlike the striatum, the globus pallidus does not receive afferents from the cerebral cortex or the thalamus.

STRIATOPALLIDAL FIBERS

Massive striatal projections radiate into both segments of the globus pallidus where they traverse the discoid arbors of pallidal dendrites in a convergent fashion. In both segments of the pallidum, striatopallidal fibers arborize in elongated bands aligned parallel with the medullary laminae. Pallidal dendrites are covered with synaptic boutons, suggesting that one dendrite must receive input from multiple striatal axons. Striatofugal fibers are not a homogeneous entity. Spiny striatal neurons project to either the globus pallidus or the substantia nigra. Distinct populations of striatal neurons project to either the medial (MPS) or the lateral (LPS) pallidal segment. Oblique bands of cells in the caudate nucleus and the

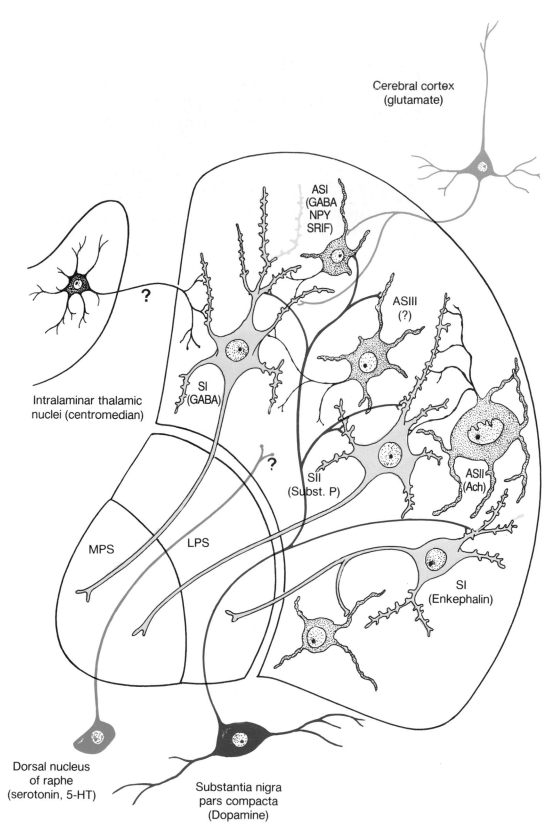

Cerebral cortex
(glutamate)

ASI
(GABA
NPY
SRIF)

ASIII
(?)

?

Intralaminar thalamic
nuclei (centromedian)

SI
(GABA)

?

SII
(Subst. P)

ASII
(Ach)

MPS

LPS

SI
(Enkephalin)

Dorsal nucleus
of raphe
(serotonin, 5-HT)

Substantia nigra
pars compacta
(Dopamine)

Figure 11.13. Schematic diagram of spiny (*yellow*) and aspiny (*gray*) striatal neurons with inputs, outputs, and suspected neurotransmitters. *Corticostriate fibers* (*blue*) arise from virtually all areas of the cerebral cortex and probably have glutamate (excitatory) as their neurotransmitter. *Thalamostriate fibers* (*black*) arise largely from the centromedian-parafascicular nuclear complex; their neurotransmitter is unidentified. *Nigrostriatal fibers* (*red*) arise from the pars compacta (SNC) and convey dopamine (inhibitory) to terminals on spiny striatal neurons. Fibers from the dorsal nucleus of the raphe (*green*) convey serotonin (5-HT) to both the striatum and the substantia nigra (SNR). Spiny striatal neurons (*yellow*) contain GABA,

338

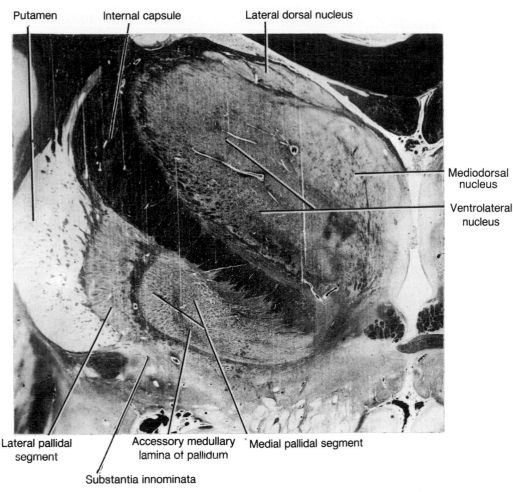

Putamen Internal capsule Lateral dorsal nucleus

Mediodorsal nucleus

Ventrolateral nucleus

Lateral pallidal segment Accessory medullary lamina of pallidum Medial pallidal segment

Substantia innominata

Figure 11.14. Photomicrograph of a transverse section of the human brain through the corpus striatum, internal capsule, and thalamus. Segments of the globus pallidus are separated by the medial medullary lamina and the accessory medullary lamina divides the medial pallidal segment into inner and outer parts. The substantia innominata lies ventral to the globus pallidus and extends rostrally. Weigert's myelin stain.

putamen project differentially to the pallidal segments, with the largest number terminating in the MPS. Large numbers of striatopallidal fibers considered to have GABA as their neurotransmitter are distributed to both pallidal segments (Fig. 11.13). GABA is conveyed to the globus pallidus via axons of spiny striatal neurons. Immunohistochemical studies indicate that striatopallidal fibers, also immunoreactive for enkephalin and substance P, are distributed in a specific pattern within the globus pallidus (Fig. 11.13). Striatopallidal fibers immunoreactive for enkephalin are dense in the lateral pallidal segment, while fibers immunoreactive for

enkephalin (ENK), and substance P (SP) in various combinations, but GABA is the dominant neurotransmitter of both spiny type I (SI) and spiny type II (SII) neurons. Fibers and terminals of different GABAergic spiny neurons project to each pallidal segment, although only projections to the medial pallidal segment (MPS) are shown here. Fibers of spiny neurons containing ENK project to the lateral pallidal segment (LPS) whereas fibers containing SP project to the MPS. A separate population of spiny striatal neurons containing these same neurotransmitters projects to the pars reticulata of the substantia nigra (not shown). Aspiny neurons (*gray*) are intrinsic striatal neurons. Aspiny type I (ASI) neurons appear to contain GABA, neuropeptide Y (NPY), and somatostatin (SRIF). Terminals of giant cholinergic neurons (AS II) contact all parts of spiny striatal neurons that receive nigrostriatal projections and these intrinsic neurons regulate striatal balance of dopamine and GABA. The neurotransmitter of aspiny type III (AS III) neurons has not been identified.

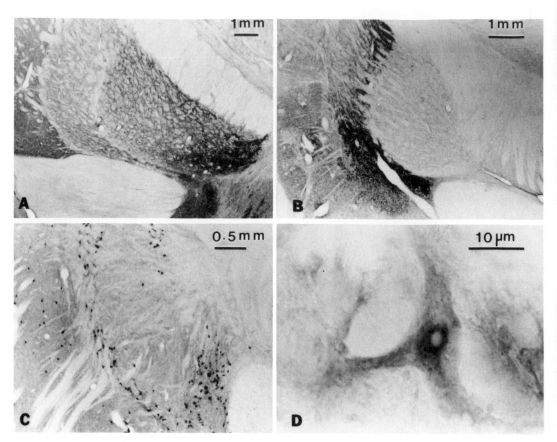

Figure 11.15. Immunocytochemical features of the globus pallidus in the monkey. *A*, Substance P immunoreactive fibers confined to the medial pallidal segment are most intense in the apical region; *B*, L-enkephalin immunoreactive fibers and terminals are limited to the lateral pallidal segment; in the middle third of the LPS immunoreactive fibers are most intense ventrally and near the medial medullary lamina. *C*, Large cholinergic neurons (choline acetyltransferase, ChAT) are abundant in the medullary laminae of the pallidum caudally; ChAT-positive aspiny type II are evenly distributed in the striatum. *D*, A large GABA immunoreactive neuron characteristic of virtually all pallidal neurons in both segments.

substance P are dense throughout the medial pallidal segment (Fig. 11.15). Regional differences in the distribution and concentration of these two peptides are evident in both pallidal segments. Substance P immunoreactivity in fibers is particularly dense in the apical region of the MPS, and enkephalin (ENK) immunoreactive fibers appear most numerous in ventral regions of the LPS caudally (Fig. 11.15). In the cat, neurotensin (NT) fibers are distributed only to the equivalent of the LPS. It is postulated the SP, ENK, and NT fibers distributed differentially in the two segments of the globus pallidus play different roles in modifying the distinctive efferent systems of these segments, which arise from intrinsic GABAergic neurons. Enkephalin-like and substance P-like immunoreactive striatopallidal fibers arise from both "limbic" and "nonlimbic" regions of the striatum. Comparisons of normal human brains with those from patients with Huntington's disease indicate substantial reductions of substance P and enkephalin in the globus pallidus and substantia nigra.

SUBTHALAMOPALLIDAL FIBERS

Subthalamopallidal fibers are topographically organized and project to both segments of the pallidum in arrays parallel to the medullary laminae (Fig. 11.26). The largest number of fibers arise from cells in the lateral two-thirds of the subthalamic nucleus (STN) and project to well-defined laminae in dorsal regions of the LPS (Fig. 11.26). Terminals in the LPS closely surround arrays of neurons that project back to the STN. Reciprocal relationships appear to exist between rostral and central portions of the LPS and the lateral two-thirds of the STN. A much smaller number of cells in medial regions of the STN project to the medial pallidal segment. Subthalamopallidal fibers are considered to have excitatory effects on pallidal neurons. Cells of the STN contain glutamate, but no specific neuropeptide has been colocalized with glutamate.

Retrograde fluorescent double-labeling technics in the rat suggested that virtually all neurons of the subthalamic nucleus project to both the globus pallidus and the SNR (Fig. 11.23). Similar studies in the primate indicate that only about 10% of the cells in the STN project to both the globus pallidus and the substantia nigra.

OTHER PALLIDAL AFFERENTS

The globus pallidus of the monkey receives a dense innervation of dopaminergic fibers that arborize mainly in the MPS. These dopaminergic fibers appear to originate from cells throughout the substantia nigra (SNC). This projection to the MPS is considered distinct from that of dopaminergic neurons projecting to the striatum. The MPS also receives a serotonergic projection derived from ascending 5-HT fiber bundles. Although cells of the two pallidal segments are morphologically and chemically similar, the activities of GABAergic neurons in each segment appear subject to modulations by different chemospecific afferents.

Pallidofugal Fibers

Each pallidal segment projects fibers to different brain stem nuclei. Fibers arising from cells of the medial pallidal segment project to thalamic nuclei, the lateral habenular nucleus, and via a descending tegmental bundle to a cell group in midbrain reticular formation (Fig. 11.21). Cells in the lateral pallidal segment project primarily to the subthalamic nucleus, although some fibers from this pallidal segment end in parts of the substantia nigra (Fig. 11.24). Pallidal efferent fibers can be divided into four main bundles: (1) the *ansa lenticularis*, (2) the *lenticular fasciculus*, (3) the *pallidotegmental fibers*, and (4) the *pallidosubthalamic fibers*. The first three of these arise exclusively from the medial pallidal segment.

ANSA LENTICULARIS

Fibers of this bundle arise from lateral portions of the medial segment of the globus pallidus and become well defined on the ventral surface of the pallidum (Figs. 11.16, 11.17, and 11.18). This bundle sweeps ventromedially and rostrally around the posterior limb of the internal capsule and then courses posteriorly to enter Forel's field H.

LENTICULAR FASCICULUS

These fibers arise from inner portions of the medial pallidal segment, issue from the dorsomedial margin of the pallidum and traverse the ventral parts of the internal capsule (Figs. 11.16, 11.17, and 11.19). Fibers cross through the internal capsule immediately rostral to the subthalamic nucleus and form a discrete bundle ventral to the zona incerta. Although most of the lenticular fasciculus lies rostral to the subthalamic nucleus, some fibers of this bundle course along its dorsal border. Fibers of the lenticular fasciculus are referred to as Forel's field H_2. While fibers of the lenticular fasciculus pursue a distinctive course through the internal

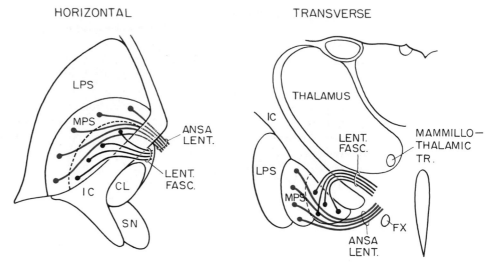

Figure 11.16. Diagrammatic representation of origin and course of pallidal efferent fibers forming the *ansa lenticularis* and *lenticular fasciculus*. Fibers of the ansa lenticularis (*red*) arise from the outer portion of the medial pallidal segment (lateral to the accessory medullary lamina, *dashed line*) and course rostrally, ventrally and medially. Fibers of the lenticular fasciculus (*black*) arise from the inner portion of the medial pallidal segment (medial to the accessory medullary lamina, *dashed line*) and course dorsally and medially through the fibers of the internal capsule. (Kuo and Carpenter, 1973.) (From Carpenter and Sutin, *Human Neuroanatomy*, 1983; courtesy of Williams & Wilkins.)

capsule, they pass medially and caudally to join fibers of the ansa lenticularis in Forel's field H (prerubral field). Fibers of the lenticular fasciculus (H_2) and the ansa lenticularis, which merge in Forel's field H, ultimately enter the thalamic fasciculus (H_1) (Fig. 11.19).

THALAMIC FASCICULUS

Pallidofugal fibers from Forel's field H pass rostrally and laterally along the dorsal surface of the zona incerta where they form part of the thalamic fasciculus (Figs. 11.17, 11.19, and 11.23). Some of the fibers of the lenticular fasciculus merely make a C-shaped loop around the medial part of the zona incerta and enter the thalamic fasciculus. The thalamic fasciculus contains pallidothalamic fibers, as well as ascending fibers from the contralateral deep cerebellar nuclei (Figs. 8.15 and 8.16). This composite bundle projects dorsolaterally over the zona incerta to terminate in specific nuclear subdivisions of the rostral ventral tier thalamic nuclei. In the region dorsal to the zona incerta, where fibers of this bundle are distinct and separate from those of the lenticular fasciculus (Figs. 11.17 and 11.19), the thalamic fasciculus is designated as bundle H_1 of forel.

PALLIDOTHALAMIC PROJECTIONS

Pallidothalamic fibers project to the ventral anterior (VApc, pars principalis) and ventral lateral (VLo, pars oralis) thalamic nuclei and give off collaterals to the centromedian (CM) nucleus (Figs. 11.20 and 11.21). Pallidal projections to the rostral ventral tier thalamic nuclei are topographically organized. Pallidothalamic terminations do not overlap the crossed projections from the deep cerebellar nuclei or the ascending projections from the substantia nigra. Each of these ascending systems terminates in separate divisions of thalamic nuclei. The ventral lateral thalamic nucleus, the pars oralis (VLo), projects to the supplementary motor area on the medial aspect of the hemisphere and to the lateral premotor area (Area 6).

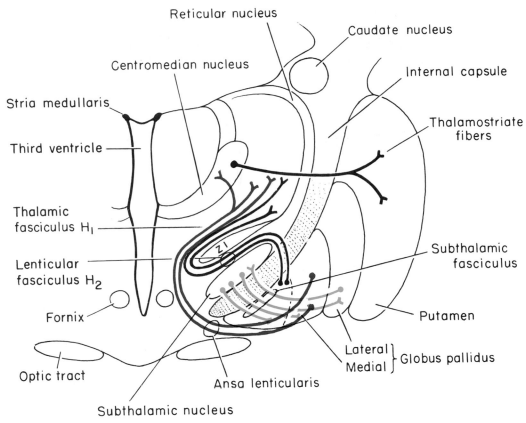

Figure 11.17. Schematic diagram of pallidofugal fiber systems in a transverse plane. Fibers of the ansa lenticularis (*red*) arise from the outer portion of the medial pallidal segment, pass ventrally, medially, and rostrally around the internal capsule and enter the prerubral field. Fibers of the lenticular fasciculus (H₂, *black*) issue from the dorsal surface of inner part of the medial pallidal segment, traverse the posterior limb of the internal capsule, and pass medially, dorsal to the subthalamic nucleus to enter the prerubral field. The ansa lenticularis and the lenticular fasciculus merge in the prerubral field (Field H of Forel, not labeled here), and project dorsolaterally as components of the thalamic fasciculus (H₁). Fibers of the thalamic fasciculus pass dorsal to the zona incerta (ZI). The subthalamic fasciculus (*blue*) consists of pallidosubthalamic fibers arising from the lateral pallidal segment, and subthalamopallidal fibers that terminate in arrays parallel to the medullary lamina in both pallidal segments. The largest number of subthalamopallidal fibers end in the lateral pallidal segment. Both components of the subthalamic fasciculus traverse the internal capsule. Thalamostriate fibers from the centromedian nucleus (*black*) project to the putamen. Compare with Figures 11.16, 11.18, and 11.19. (From Carpenter and Sutin, *Human Neuroanatomy*, 1983; courtesy of Williams & Wilkins.)

PALLIDOHABENULAR FIBERS

Fibers from the medial pallidal segment projecting to the lateral habenular nucleus separate from the ansa lenticularis and the lenticular fasciculus in Forel's field H and course through and around the medial part of the internal capsule to enter the stria medullaris. Pallidohabenular fibers arise from a different cell population than pallidothalamic fibers; most of these cells are located in a peripallidal zone.

PALLIDOTEGMENTAL FIBERS

These fibers descend from field H of Forel and terminate in the compact portion of the pedunculopontine nucleus (PPN) (Fig. 11.21). This nucleus is partially embedded in fibers of the superior cerebellar peduncle. Studies in the monkey indicate that cells in the medial pallidal segment have dichotomizing axons that project the same signal to thalamic nuclei and to the PPN.

Figure 11.18. Photograph demonstrating the ansa lenticularis in a decorticate monkey. All fibers of the internal capsule have degenerated so that pallidofugal fibers sweeping medially around the internal capsule are especially prominent. Weigert's myelin stain. (Reproduced with permission from F. A. Mettler: *Neuroanatomy*, 1948 and C. V. Mosby Company, St. Louis.)

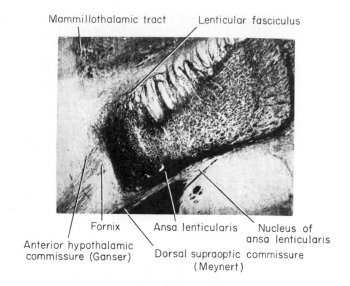

Mammillothalamic tract   Lenticular fasciculus

Fornix   Ansa lenticularis   Nucleus of ansa lenticularis

Anterior hypothalamic commissure (Ganser)   Dorsal supraoptic commissure (Meynert)

Figure 11.19. Autoradiograph of isotope transport from the medial pallidal segment (MPS) through the internal capsule and into the lenticular fasciculus. Continuity between the lenticular fasciculus and the thalamic fasciculus is seen in Forel's field H (H), medial to the zona incerta (ZI). Dark-field photomicrograph from a rhesus monkey Cresyl violet, (×16).

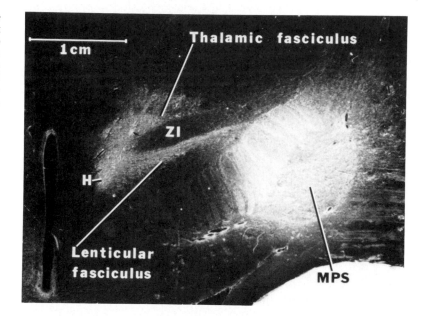

The projections of PPN are distributed to the medial pallidal segment, the subthalamic nucleus, the substantia nigra, and to thalamic nuclei (Fig. 11.24). Large cells in the PPN are strongly cholinergic. In the rat, cholinergic cells of PPN are considered to project mainly to the ventrolateral thalamic nuclei. Noncholinergic neurons in and around this nucleus are described as projecting to the corpus striatum and related nuclei. In the monkey, the major projection of PPN is to the ipsilateral substantia nigra. Special interest in this region centers around locomotor activity produced by electrical stimulation.

PALLIDOSUBTHALAMIC PROJECTIONS

Arrays of cells in the lateral pallidal segment projects mainly to the subthalamic nucleus and projections are topographically organized. Rostral parts of the lateral pallidal segment (LPS) project to medial and rostral parts of the subthalamic nucleus (STN). Cells in the central division of the LPS (flanking the medial pallidal segment) project to the lateral third of the STN throughout most of its rostrocaudal extent (Figs. 11.25

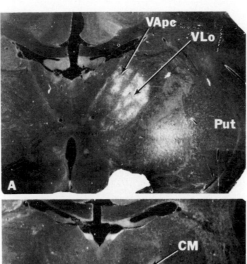

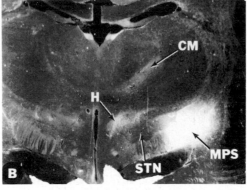

Figure 11.20. Dark-field photomicrographs of sections through the diencephalon in a monkey demonstrating transport of [³H] amino acids from the medial pallidal segment (MPS) to thalamic nuclei. *A,* Radioactive label is distributed in a patchy fashion to the pars oralis of the ventral lateral (VLo) and to the principal part of the ventral anterior nuclei (VApc) of the thalamus. *B,* The central region of the injection in the medial pallidal segment (MPS) and modest transport to the centromedian nucleus (CM) of the thalamus are shown. Radioactive label also is seen in Forel's field H and in lateral parts of the subthalamic nucleus (STN). Cresyl violet, (× 3.5). (From Carpenter and Sutin, *Human Neuroanatomy,* 1983; courtesy of Williams & Wilkins.)

and 11.26). Pallidal neurons projecting to the STN are GABAergic. Sensitive anterograde tracing technics (Phaseolus vulgaris) indicate that neurons in the LPS projecting to the STN emit collaterals that arborize in lateral parts of the SNR.

SUBTHALAMIC REGION

The subthalamic region lies ventral to the thalamus, medial to the internal capsule, and lateral and caudal to the hypothalamus (Figs. 9.5, 11.22, and 11.23). Nuclei found within the subthalamic region include the subthalamic nucleus, the zona incerta, and the nuclei of the tegmental fields of Forel. Fiber bundles passing through this region include the ansa lenticularis, the lenticular fasciculus (Forel's field H₂), the thalamic fasciculus (Forel's field H₁), and the subthalamic fasciculus (Fig. 11.17).

Subthalamic Nucleus

This nucleus, located on the inner surface of the peduncular portion of the internal capsule, has the shape of a thick biconvex lens (Figs. 9.5, 11.17, 11.22, and 11.23). Caudally the medial part of the nucleus (STN) overlies rostral portions of the substantia nigra. Cells of the subthalamic nucleus are spindle-shaped, pyramidal, or round with branching processes, but form a single population of neurons. Each STN neuron gives rise to six or seven stem dendrites that branch successively in an ellipsoidal domain parallel with the rostrocaudal axis of the nucleus. While subthalamic nucleus neurons in rat and primate are similar, their relationships to the nucleus as a whole have evolved to confer upon the primate the potential for a much more specific organization.

Cells of the STN have been shown to contain glutamate and to exert excitatory effects on pallidal and nigral neurons. Glutamate immunoreactivity in cells of the STN does not necessarily indicate that glutamate

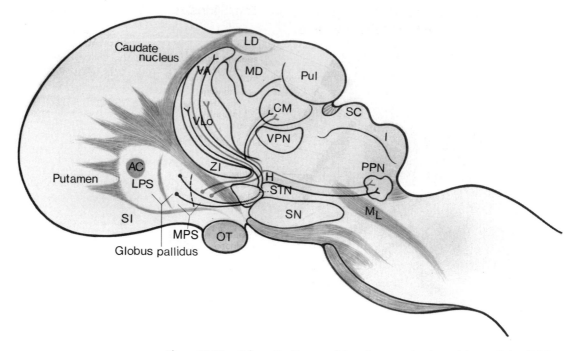

Figure 11.21.   Schematic diagram of the efferent projections of the medial pallidal segment (MPS) in a sagittal plane. Fibers of the *ansa lenticularis* (*red*) loop ventrally around the internal capsule, while fibers of the *lenticular fasciculus* (*blue*) traverse the internal capsule rostral to the subthalamic nucleus (STN). These fiber bundles merge in Forel's field H (H). Descending collaterals from field H project to the pedunculopontine nucleus (PPN) as the *pallidotegmental bundle*. *Pallidothalamic fibers* (*red* and *blue*) project mainly to the ventral lateral (VLo) and the ventral anterior (VApc) nuclei but provide collaterals to the centromedian nucleus. Abbreviations are the same as in Figure 11.12.

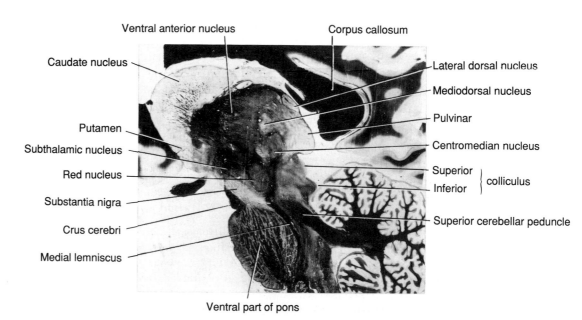

Figure 11.22.   Sagittal section through medial regions of the corpus striatum, thalamus, and upper brain stem, showing the relationships of caudate nucleus and putamen, as well as those of the subthalamic nucleus, the red nucleus, and the substantia nigra. Weigert's myelin stain. Photograph. (From Carpenter and Sutin, *Human Neuroanatomy*, 1983; courtesy of Williams & Wilkins.)

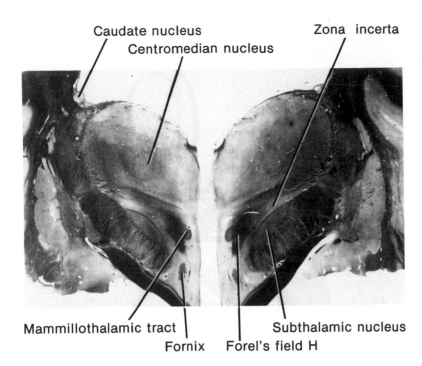

Caudate nucleus
Centromedian nucleus
Zona incerta

Mammillothalamic tract
Fornix   Forel's field H   Subthalamic nucleus

Figure 11.23. Photograph of a transverse section of the diencephalon through the subthalamic nucleus showing its relationships with the internal capsule, the zona incerta, Forel's field H, and the thalamic fasciculus. Weigert's myelin stain.

is the neurotransmitter used by these neurons, because glutamate also is involved in basic cellular metabolism.

The subthalamic nucleus is derived from the most posterior part of a lateral hypothalamic cell column. Rostral portions of this same cell column form the anlage of both segments of the globus pallidus.

Afferents to the Subthalamic Nucleus

The dominant input to the subthalamic nucleus (STN) arises from the lateral pallidal segment (Figs. 11.24, 11.25, and 11.26). Afferents to the subthalamic nucleus from the motor, premotor, and prefrontal cortex appear to be mainly collaterals of fibers destined for other loci. Relatively small numbers of afferents are derived from the thalamus (CM-PF) and from the pedunculopontine nucleus (Fig. 11.24).

PALLIDOSUBTHALAMIC PROJECTIONS

GABAergic cells in parallel arrays in the LPS project massively to the STN (Figs. 11.25 and 11.26). These fibers traverse the medial pallidal segment, the peduncular part of the internal capsule, and form one of the components of the subthalamic fasciculus (Fig. 11.17). Pallidosubthalamic fibers are topographically arranged. Cells in regions of the LPS projecting to the STN are closely surrounded by terminals of reciprocal subthalamopallidal fibers.

CORTICOSUBTHALAMIC FIBERS

Cortical projections have been regarded as the second largest group of afferents to the STN. Autoradiographic studies have identified ipsilateral somatotopic projections from motor cortex to lateral parts of the STN. Attempts to confirm the origin of this cortical projection by retrograde transport methods in monkey and cat have been repeatedly unsuccessful. Failure to confirm this projection tends to support the thesis that corticosubthalamic fibers may be collaterals of corticofugal fibers destined for other loci (Fig. 11.24).

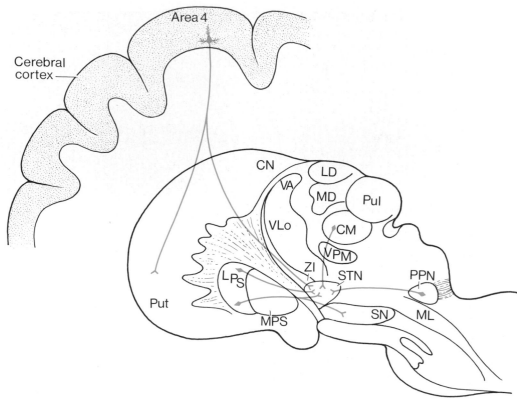

Figure 11.24. Schematic diagram of the afferent projections (*blue*) of the subthalamic nucleus (STN). *Corticosubthalamic fibers* appear to be collaterals of corticofugal projections, probably projecting to the putamen. The most massive input to the STN, *pallidosubthalamic fibers*, arises from parallel cellular arrays in the lateral pallidal segment (LPS). A few collaterals of pallidosubthalamic fibers terminate in the pars reticulata of the substantia nigra (SNR). Small numbers of cells in the centromedian (CM), parafascicular, and the pedunculopontine nucleus (PPN) project to the STN. See Figure 11.12 for abbreviations.

Figure 11.25. Dark-field photomicrographs of the subthalamic nucleus (STN) in the monkey showing regions of terminations of fibers from the lateral pallidal segment (LPS). These autoradiographs show isotope transport from rostral parts of the LPS (*A*) and from central portions of the LPS (*B*), which end in different regions of the nucleus. Terminations in *A* are in medial parts of the STN; those in *B* are in lateral parts of the nucleus. Cresyl violet.

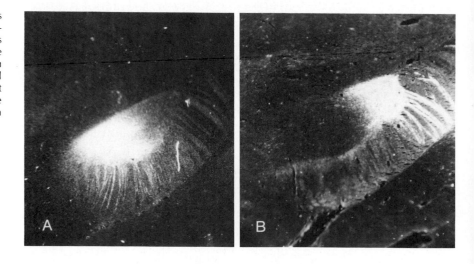

THALAMOSUBTHALAMIC FIBERS

A relatively small, but definite, projection from the centromedian-parafascicular nuclear complex (CM-PF) has been established in the monkey, cat, and rat.

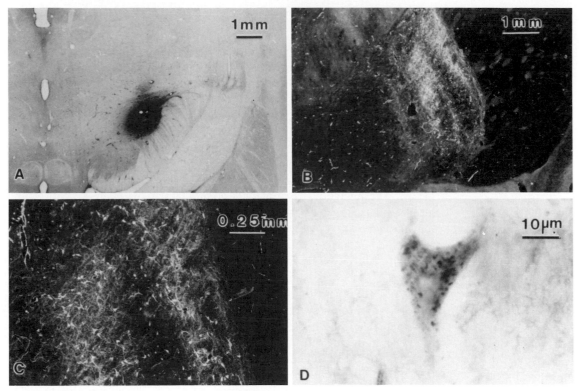

Figure 11.26.   Afferent and efferent connections of the subthalamic nucleus (STN) with the lateral pallidal segment (LPS) in the monkey demonstrated by transport of wheat germ agglutinin conjugated to horseradish peroxidase (WGA-HRP). *A*, WGA-HRP injection in the STN. *B* and *C*, Anterograde and retrograde transport of WGA-HRP to parallel arrays of terminals and cells in the LPS. *D*, Neuron in the LPS immunoreactive for GABA and retrogradely labeled with black WGA-HRP granules. (Carpenter and Jayaraman, 1990, J. Hirnforsch.)

TEGMENTOSUBTHALAMIC FIBERS

The pedunculopontine nucleus (PPN), which receives inputs from the cerebral cortex, the medial pallidal segment, and the pars reticulata of the substantia nigra (SNR), is considered to project directly to the subthalamic nucleus. This very small projection does not appear to originate from cholinergic neurons of PPN (Fig. 11.24).

Subthalamic Efferents

The efferents from the subthalamic nucleus (STN) project to both segments of the globus pallidus and to the substantia nigra (Fig. 11.26). The largest number of STN neurons project fibers to terminal arrays in the LPS. Cells in medial parts of the STN project to the MPS; few cells of the STN project to both pallidal segments. This massive projection has been described on page 340. In the primate about 10% of the cells in the STN project to both the globus pallidus and the pars reticulata of the substantia nigra.

Subthalamic Fasciculus

This bundle consists of fibers from the lateral pallidal segment that project to the STN and fibers from the STN that project to both pallidal segments. These fibers project through peduncular portions of the internal capsule caudal to the lenticular fasciculus (Fig. 11.17).

Zona Incerta

This structure is a strip of gray matter situated between the thalamic and lenticular fasciculi (Figs. 9.5, 11.17, and 11.19). It is composed of diffuse cell groups that laterally are continuous with the thalamic reticular nucleus. This zone receives corticofugal fibers from the precentral cortex.

Prerubral Field (Forel's Field H)

This field contains pallidofugal fibers and scattered cells that constitute the nucleus of the prerubral field (Figs. 9.5, 11.17, 11.21, and 11.23). The nuclei of the prerubral field, together with similar cells scattered along pallidofugal pathways, have been referred to collectively as the *subthalamic reticular nucleus*.

FUNCTIONAL CONSIDERATIONS

Nearly 80 years ago Wilson introduced the term "extrapyramidal" motor system (without definition) in his classic description of hepatolenticular degeneration. This syndrome is a familial disorder of copper metabolism characterized by degeneration of the striatum, cirrhosis of the liver, flapping tremor, muscular rigidity, and a golden-brown pigmentation of the cornea (i.e., the Kayser–Fleischer ring). There seems to be no question that the corpus striatum forms the centerpiece of this so-called system. This term has been defined, and interpreted in innumerable ways. It now appears accepted that the corpus striatum has meaningful connections with a limited array of brain stem nuclei, chief among which are the substantia nigra, the subthalamic nucleus, and portions of the ventral tier thalamic nuclei. It is difficult to conceive of the corpus striatum and this limited array of brain stem nuclei forming an independent motor system. The corpus striatum and related nuclei exert their influences on motor activities by way of thalamic neurons that project on regions of the frontal cortex that influence motor function. Motor cortical neurons, whose activities are modulated by thalamic neurons, project fibers to, and exert motor control at all levels of the neuraxis, mainly contralaterally. Neither the corpus striatum nor anatomically related brain stem nuclei project directly to spinal levels.

The corpus striatum, subthalamic nucleus, substantia nigra, and pedunculopontine nucleus are interrelated with each other by an orderly linkage and with specific parts of the neuraxis that can modulate somatic motor activities. The striatum, representing the receptive component of the corpus striatum, receives inputs from broad regions of the cerebral cortex, the intralaminar thalamic nuclei, the substantia nigra, and the midbrain raphe nuclei, mediated by a variety of neurotransmitters. Striatal output originates from different populations of spiny neurons that project selectively to the two segments of the globus pallidus and the pars reticulata of the substantia nigra. GABA is the principal neurotransmitter in striatopallidal and striatonigral fiber systems, but fibers in both projections contain enkephalin and substance P.

The output systems of the corpus striatum arise from morphologically similar cells in the medial pallidal segment (MPS) and the pars reticulata of the substantia nigra. Thalamic projections of the medial pallidal segment and the pars reticulata of the substantia nigra (SNR) are distinctive without overlap; nuclear subdivisions of the thalamus receiving these outputs do not exert their major effects on the primary motor cortex. The output of the MPS appears to project to the premotor and supplementary motor areas. Most physiological data suggest that pallidothalamic and nigrothalamic projections exert primarily inhibitory effects on thalamic neurons. The inhibitory influences of neurons in the MPS and SNR projecting to the thalamus may result in disinhibition of thalamic neurons that act on the cortical neurons.

The substantia nigra receives inputs from both components of the corpus striatum (i.e., striatum and pallidum) and from all closely related subcortical nuclei (i.e., the subthalamic nucleus, the pedunculopontine nucleus, and the dorsal nucleus of the raphe). Dopaminergic neurons in the pars compacta (SNC) provide a major feedback to the striatum and also have a small projection to the medial pallidal segment. The output system of the substantia nigra arises from GABAergic neurons in the pars reticulata (SNR), which projects to thalamic nuclei and via collaterals to the tectum and the pedunculopontine nucleus.

The subthalamic nucleus in contrast to the substantia nigra receives major inputs from only two sources, the lateral pallidal segment and the motor cortex. Cortical projections to the subthalamic nucleus probably represent collaterals of corticofugal fibers destined for other structures. A single type of STN neuron projects fibers mainly to the LPS, but a small number of these cells project collaterals to the SNR. The number of STN neurons projecting to the medial pallidal segment is modest. The neurotransmitter of cells in the STN is unknown, although these cells contain glutamate and are regarding as exerting excitatory influences on their projection targets.

Clinically two basic types of disturbances are associated with diseases of the corpus striatum. These disturbances are (1) various types of abnormal involuntary movements, referred to as *dyskinesia*, and (2) disturbances of muscle tone. Types of dyskinesia occurring in association with these diseases include *tremor*, *athetosis*, *chorea*, and *ballism*. These and other forms of dyskinesia occur with a constellation of related somatic, visceral, and behavioral disturbances resulting from progressive degenerative disease, genetic defects, and vascular lesions. The metabolic disturbances associated with these disease processes often result in deficiencies in one or more neurotransmitters essential for normal function.

Types of Dyskinesia

TREMORS

This, the most common form of dyskinesia, is a rhythmical, alternating, abnormal involuntary activity having a relatively regular frequency and amplitude. A major clinical criterion used to describe and classify different tremors is whether the tremor occurs "at rest" or during voluntary movement. The type of tremor commonly seen in paralysis agitans (parkinsonism), involves primarily the digits, the head, and the lips, and occurs during the absence of voluntary movement. During voluntary movement the tremor ceases. Tremor classically associated with cerebellar lesions becomes evident during voluntary and associated movements and ceases when the patient is "at rest." Tremor also is seen in association with weakness (paresis), emotional excitement, and as a side effect of a variety of drugs. In general tremor is exaggerated when the patient is anxious, self-conscious, or exposed to cold. Tremor disappears during sleep and under general anesthesia.

ATHETOSIS

This term is used to designate slow, writhing, vermicular involuntary movements, involving particularly the extremities. It may involve also the axial muscle groups and the muscles of the face and neck. The movements blend with each other to give the appearance of a continuous mobile spasm. Athetoid movements involving primarily the axial musculature produce severe torsion of the neck, shoulder girdle, and pelvic girdle. This form of the disturbance, referred to as *torsion spasm* or *torsion dystonia*, is considered as a variant of athetosis; differences between torsion dystonia and athetosis are considered to be due largely to inherent mechanical differences between axial and appendicular musculature.

CHOREA

Chorea is a brisk, graceful series of successive involuntary movements of considerable complexity that resemble fragments of purposeful voluntary movements. These movements involve primarily the distal portions of the extremities, the muscles of facial expression, the tongue, and the deglutitional musculature. Most forms of choreoid activity are associated with hypotonus. *Sydenham's chorea* occurs in childhood in association with rheumatic heart disease, and most patients make a complete recovery. *Huntington's disease* (chorea) is inherited through an autosomal-dominant gene localized on chromosome 4. The symptoms usually do not begin until adult life, are progressive, and are characterized by choreiform activity in the face and hands and severe behavioral disturbances with dementia. Not every family member carries the defective gene.

BALLISM

Ballism, a violent, forceful, flinging movement, involves primarily the proximal appendicular musculature, and muscles about the shoulder and pelvic girdles. It represents the most violent form of dyskinesia known. Ballism is almost invariably associated with discrete lesions in the subthalamic nucleus or its connections. The dyskinesia occurs contralateral to the lesion and is associated with marked hypotonus.

Although athetosis, chorea, and ballism each present distinguishing features, basic resemblances among these forms of dyskinesia are greater than their differences. Characteristics common to these dyskinesias include (1) variable amplitude and frequency, (2) occurrence of movements in immediate and delayed sequence, (3) variations in the duration of single movements, and (4) a highly integrated, complex activity pattern. While each of these types of involuntary motor activity is specialized to a degree, there are indications that athetosis, chorea, and ballism may form a spectrum of choreoid activity in which athetosis and ballism represent extreme forms. Although it is customary to associate increased muscle tonus with most syndromes of the corpus striatum, this is not always found. The initial symptom of paralysis agitans is frequently a *rigidity* of the muscles, which gradually increases over a period of years. The increase in muscle tone is present to a nearly equal degree in antagonistic muscle groups (i.e., in both flexor and extensor muscles). Rigidity in the early stages can be demonstrated by passively flexing or extending the muscles of the extremities, or by attempting to rotate the hand in a circular fashion at the wrist. These movements are interrupted by a series of jerks, referred to as the cogwheel phenomenon. In later stages of the disease rigidity is often the most incapacitating feature.

Athetosis usually is associated with variable degrees of paresis and spasticity. It is suggested that the slow, writing character of this dyskinesia may be due in part to the associated spasticity. Although muscle tone is increased greatly during athetoid movements and persists after the completion of the movement, muscle tone may thereafter gradually diminish. Athetosis and dystonia accompany a group of motor disorders that form important elements of the cerebral palsy syndrome. Chorea and ballism usually are associated with variable degrees of hypotonus.

NEURAL MECHANISMS INVOLVED IN DYSKINESIA

The various types of dyskinesia and excesses of muscle tone associated with diseases of the corpus striatum and related nuclei are regarded as positive disturbances. Such disturbances cannot arise directly from destruction of specific neural structures but must represent the functional capacity of surviving intact structures. Accordingly positive disturbances such as tremor, athetosis, chorea, and ballism are believed to be the result of release phenomena. This theory implies that a lesion in one structure removes the controlling and regulating influences which that structure previously exerted on another neural mechanism. This concept forms the basis for neurosurgical attempts to alleviate dyskinesia. However, not all disturbances associated with diseases of the corpus striatum can be regarded as positive phenomena. Patients with paralysis agitans also exhibit a mask-like face, infrequent blinking of the eyes, a slow dysarthric speech, a stooped posture, a slow shuffling gait, loss of associated movements (e.g., swinging of the arms while walking), slowness of voluntary movements (bradykinesia), and general poverty of movements. These disturbances can be regarded as negative symptoms. The negative symptoms of parkinsonism largely concern disorders of postural fixation, equilibrium, locomotion, phonation, and articulation and are considered to be deficits due to destroyed neural structures.

In most forms of dyskinesia, categorized as extrapyramidal, the corpora striata suffer severe pathological alterations, but specific brain stem nuclei and parts of the cerebral cortex may be affected also.

In parkinsonism (paralysis agitans) pathological changes most consistently affect the substantia nigra. In this syndrome the synthesis and transmission of dopamine from cells of the pars compacta of the nigra to the striatum is greatly impaired. Dopamine is regarded as an inhibitory neurotransmitter. Terminals containing dopamine synapse mainly on dendrites and dendritic spines of spiny striatal neurons. Two types of dopamine receptors have been identified. Spiny striatal neurons also receive extrinsic excitatory inputs from the cortex and thalamus. Intrinsic cholinergic striatal neurons form symmetrical synaptic endings on all parts of spiny striatal neurons. The special importance of intrinsic cholinergic neurons concerns their modulating influences on spiny striatal neurons known to project to the substantia nigra. Dopamine tonically inhibits the release of acetylcholine (ACh) in the striatum, whereas ACh, or cholinomimetic drugs, enhance the release of GABA. In Parkinson's disease there is an imbalance between ACh and dopamine that favors ACh. This imbalance can be modified by elevating dopamine levels by giving L-dihydroxyphenylalanine (L-dopa), a precursor of dopamine that passes the blood-brain barrier, or by reducing the action of ACh with receptor antagonists. This rationale forms the basis for giving L-dopa in Parkinson's disease. The effectiveness of L-dopa can be enhanced by the use of a peripheral decarboxylase inhibitor, which prevents systemic decarboxylation of L-dopa to dopamine.

It has been discovered that a meperidine-analogue (1-methyl-4-phenyl-4-1,2,56-tetrahydropyridine, MPTP) appearing in illicit drugs (cocaine, meperidine) in concentrations of 2.5 to 3% was sufficient when given intravenously to produce a chronic form of parkinsonism. This compound was the product of a clandestine laboratory attempting to synthesize 1-methyl-4-phenyl-4-propionoxypiperdine (MPPP). Individuals taking this drug presented with a classic picture of Parkinson's disease. In a patient who died of a drug overdose, destruction within the substantia nigra was comparable in severity with that seen in idiopathic parkinsonism. All patients exhibiting this syndrome responded to L-dopa and carbidopa. Using this meperidine analogue, it has been possible to produce in the monkey a model of Parkinson's disease with many of its major clinical features. This meperidine analogue selectively destroys cells of the substantia nigra that synthesize dopamine.

With respect to chorea, there is relatively little information available, except concerning chronic progressive chorea, or Huntington's chorea. This hereditary disease, due to a gene defect on the fourth chromosome, is characterized by an insidious onset in adult life. Pathological changes are widespread but have a special predilection for the cerebral cortex and striatum. In brains of patients dying with Huntington's chorea it has been demonstrated that striatal neurons have reduced concentrations of glutamic acid decarboxylase (GAD), γ-aminobutyric acid (GABA), and choline acetyltransferase (ChAT). GAD is the enzyme responsible for the biosynthesis of GABA and is localized mainly in inhibitory neurons that release GABA as their transmitter. In these same patients concentrations of tyrosine hydroxylase (TH) and dopamine were normal in the striatum. The most consistent neurotransmitter disturbance in Huntington's chorea appears to be a loss of GABA-containing neurons in the striatum, which causes an imbalance in striatal levels of GABA and dopamine in favor of dopamine. The large cholinergic striatal neurons are involved in this imbalance because dopamine inhibits ACh and ACh enhances the release of GABA. It is well known that L-dopa given in large doses to patients with Parkinson's disease may cause choreiform movements to appear. L-Dopa also tends to exacerbate choreiform activity in patients with Huntington's chorea. The most effective drugs for ameliorating choreiform dyskinesia are those which deplete catecholamines, such as reserpine and dopamine receptor antagonists. The presence of normal dopaminergic systems in association with reduced availability of GABA and acetylcholine may be the key neuropharmacological feature of Huntington's disease. Clinical attempts to overcome deficiencies of GABA and acetylcholine by administering GABA-mimetic drugs or inhibitors of acetylcholine hydrolysis have so far met with limited success. This has been explained by the inability of GABA or the GABA agonists to cross the blood-brain barrier in sufficient concentrations.

The biochemical changes that characterize Huntington's (chorea) disease in humans can be mimicked in the rat by striatal injections of kainic acid, an analogue of glutamate. After injections of kainic acid, the GAD and ChAT activities were reduced whereas the activity of TH was increased. The striatal content of dopamine was unchanged. The neurotoxic effects of kainic acid appear related to the excessive stimulation of glutamate receptors that result in degeneration. The long-term effects of striatal kainic acid lesions and the reduction in activities of GABAergic and cholinergic neurons are not as severe as those in Huntington's disease.

Athetosis most frequently is associated with pathological processes involving the striatum and cerebral cortex, though lesions are sometimes found in the globus pallidus and thalamus. Hemiathetosis may develop after a hemiparesis, or in association with it, as a consequence of a necrotizing cerebrovascular lesion destroying portions of the internal capsule and striatum (Figs. 14.9 and 14.10). Athetoid activity occurs contralateral to the lesion.

Ballism appears to be the only form of dyskinesia resulting from a discrete, destructive lesion. Small lesions confined to the subthalamic nucleus, or its immediate connections, usually are vascular in nature and occur mainly in elderly hypertensive individuals. The dyskinesia has a sudden onset, occurs contralateral to the lesion, usually involves both upper and lower extremities, and displays a forceful, flinging repetitive pattern. Affected limbs exhibit a marked hypotonus.

Attempts to produce dyskinesia in experimental animals by creating lesions in parts of the basal ganglia have been notoriously unsuccessful. For reasons not understood, large electrolytic lesions destroying large parts of the substantia nigra do not produce any of the disturbances associated with parkinsonism. The only form of dyskinesia, aside from cerebellar tremor, produced in an experimental animal is that resulting from discrete lesions in the subthalamic nucleus. This dyskinesia closely resembles that which occurs in humans with lesions in the same nucleus. In the monkey, violent choreoid and ballistic activity occurs contralateral to localized lesions in the subthalamic nucleus that (1) destroy approximately 20% of the nucleus, and (2) preserve the integrity of surrounding pallidofugal fiber systems. This abnormal involuntary activity has been called subthalamic dyskinesia and becomes apparent immediately upon recovery from anesthesia. Subthalamic dyskinesia in the monkey is enduring, associated with distinct hypotonus, and can be ameliorated or abolished contralaterally by subsequent stereotaxic lesions in the medial pallidal segment, the ventral lateral nucleus of the thalamic and the motor cortex. Similar subthalamic dyskinesia has been produced in the monkey by kainic acid lesions involving the STN, but its onset usually is delayed. A transitory form of similar dyskinesia has been produced in the awake primate by injections of GABA antagonists (picrotoxin and bicuculline methiodide) into the subthalamic region. The site of action of these antagonists remains unclear. Original studies of subthalamic dyskinesia in the monkey suggested that lesions of the STN resulted in a removal of inhibitory influences acting on cells of the medial pallidal segment. Physiological observations indicating that STN efferents are excitatory suggest more complex neural mechanisms. There is general agreement that the cells of the STN do not contain GABA but that GABAergic terminals of pallidal projections closely surround individual cells.

Surgical attempts to ameliorate and abolish various forms of dyskinesia and excesses of muscle tone are based on the thesis that these disturbances are the physiological expression of release phenomena. This implies that disease or pathological alterations of certain neural structures have removed inhibitory influences normally acting on other intact neural structures, and that this overactivity, or excessive function, is responsible for the dyskinesia. Attention has been focused mainly upon the globus pallidus and the ventral lateral nucleus of the thalamus, since these structures appear to be of greatest importance in the subcortical integration of nonpyramidal motor function. In some instances localized lesions produced by different technics in these structures have abolished, or significantly reduced, various forms of dyskinesia. Sterotaxic surgery in humans is often unpredictable, unless carefully controlled by physiological studies and sophisticated imaging technics.

The cerebral cortex is acknowledged to play an important role in the neural mechanisms of all forms of dyskinesia. Almost all forms of abnormal involuntary movement cease during sleep and are abolished by general anesthesia. Most forms of dyskinesia are exaggerated in situations where the patient becomes self-conscious, overly anxious, or excited. The fact that ablations of the motor cortex or interruption of the corticospinal tract at various locations abolish dyskinesia suggests that impulses responsible for the dyskinesia probably are transmitted to segmental levels via the corticospinal tract.

SUGGESTED READINGS

ANDÉN, N.-E., FUXE, K., HAMBERGER, B., AND HÖKFELT, T. 1966. A quantitative study on the nigro-neostriatal dopamine neuron system in the rat. Acta Physiol. Scand., **67**: 306–312.

ARIKUNI, T., AND KUBOTA, K. 1984. Substantia innominata projection to caudate nucleus in macaque monkeys. Brain Res., **302**: 184–189.

ARSENAULT, M.-Y., PARENT, A., SÉQUÉLA, P., AND DESCARRIES, L. 1988. Distribution and morphological characteristics of dopamine-immunoreactive neurons in the midbrain of the squirrel monkey (*Saimiri sciureus*). J. Comp. Neurol., **267**: 489–506.

ANDERSON, M. E., AND YOSHIDA, M. 1980. Axonal branching patterns and location of nigrothalamic and nigrocollicular neurons in the cat. J. Neurophysiol., **43**: 883–895.

BECKSTEAD, R. M., AND KERSEY, K. S. 1985. Immunohistochemical demonstration of differential substance P-, met-enkephalin-, and glutamic-acid-decarboxylase-containing cell body and axon distribution in the corpus striatum of the cat. J. Comp. Neurol., **232**: 481–498.

BOLAM, J. P., CLARKE, D. J., SMITH, A. D., AND SOMOGYI, P. 1983. A type of aspiny neurons in the rat neostriatum accumulate [³H] γ-aminobutyric acid: combination of Golgi-staining, autoradiography and electron microscopy. J. Comp. Neurol., **213**: 121–134.

BOLAM, J. P., POWELL, J. F., WU, J.-Y., AND SMITH, A. D. 1985. Glutamate decarboxylase-immunoreactive structures in rat neostriatum: A correlated light and electron microscopic study including a combination of Golgi-impregnation with immunocytochemistry. J. Comp. Neurol., **237**: 1–20.

BOLAM, J. P., WAINER, B. H., AND SMITH, A. D. 1984. Characterization of cholinergic neurons in the rat neostriatum. A combination of choline acetyltransferase immunocytochemistry, Golgi-impregnation and electron microscopy. Neuroscience, **12**: 711–718.

BIRD, E. D., AND IVERSON, L. L. 1974. Huntington's chorea: Postmortem measurement of glutamic acid decarboxylase, choline acetyltransferase and dopamine in basal ganglia. Brain, **97**: 457–472.

CARPENTER, M. B. 1981. Anatomy of the corpus striatum and brain stem integrating systems. In V. BROOKS (Editor), *Handbook of Physiology*, Sect. 1, Vol. II. Motor Control. American Physiological Society, Washington, DC, Ch. 19, pp. 947–995.

CARPENTER, M. B. 1987. Anatomy of the basal ganglia. In P. J. VINKEN, G. W. BRUYN, and H. L. KLAWANS (Editors), *Handbook of Clinical Neurology*. Elsevier Science Publ., New York, pp. 1–18.

CARPENTER, M. B. 1989. Connectivity patterns of thalamic nuclei implicated in dyskinesia. Stereotact. Funct. Neurosurg., **52**: 79–119.

CARPENTER, M. B., BATTON, R. R., CARLETON, S. C., AND KELLER, J. T. 1981. Interconnections and organization of pallidal and subthalamic nucleus neurons in the monkey. J. Comp. Neurol., **197**: 579–603.

CARPENTER, M. B., CARLETON, S. C., KELLER, J. T., AND CONTE, P. 1981. Connections of the subthalamic nucleus in the monkey. Brain Res., **224**: 1–29.

CARPENTER, M. B., AND JAYARAMAN, A. 1990. Subthalamic nucleus of the monkey: Connections and immunocytochemical features of afferents. J. Hirnforsch., **31**: 653–668.

CARPENTER, M. B., NAKANO, K., AND KIM, R. 1976. Nigrothalamic projections in the monkey demonstrated by autoradiographic technics. J. Comp. Neuro., **144**: 93–116.

CARPENTER, M. B., WHITTIER, J. R., AND METTLER, F. A. 1950. Analysis of choreoid hyperkinesia in the rhesus monkey: Surgical and pharmacological analysis of hyperkinesia resulting from lesions of the subthalamic nucleus of Luys. J. Comp. Neurol., **92**: 293–331.

CHANG, H. T., KITA, H., AND KITAI, S. T. 1984. The ultrastructural morphology of the subthalamic-nigral axon terminals intracellularly labeled with horseradish peroxidase. Brain Res., **299**: 182–185.

CHESSELET, M. F., AND GRAYBIEL, A. M. 1986. Striatal neurons expressing somatostatin-like immunoreactivity: Evidence for a peptidergic interneuronal system in the cat. Neuroscience, **17**: 547–571.

CROSSMAN, A. R., SAMBROOK, M. A., AND JACKSON, A. 1984. Experimental hemichorea/

hemiballismus in the monkey: Studies on the intracerebral site of action in a drug-induced dyskinesia. Brain, **107**: 579–596.

DAHLSTRÖM, A., AND FUXE, K. 1964. Evidence for the existence of monoamine-containing neurons in the central nervous system. I. Demonstration of monoamines in the cell bodies of brain stem neurons. Acta. Physiol. Scand., **62** (Suppl. 232): 1–55.

DENIAU, J. M., HAMMOND, C., RIZK, A., AND FÉGER, J. 1978. Electrophysiological properties of identified output neurons of the rat substantia nigra (pars compacta and pars reticulata): Evidences for the existence of branched neurons. Exp. Brain Res., **32**: 409–422.

DIFIGLIA, M. 1987. Synaptic organization of cholinergic neurons in the monkey neostriatum. J. Comp. Neurol., **255**: 245–258.

DIFIGLIA, M., AND ARONIN, N. 1982. Ultrastructural features of immunoreactive somatostatin neurons in the rat caudate nucleus. J. Neurosci., **2**: 1267–1274.

DIFIGLIA, M., ARONIN, N., AND LEEMAN, S. E. 1981. Immunoreactive substance P in the substantia nigra of the monkey: Light and electron microscopic localization. Brain Res., **233**: 381–388.

DIFIGLIA, M., AND CAREY, J. 1986. Large neurons in the primate neostriatum examined with the combined Golgi-electron microscopic method. J. Comp. Neurol., **244**: 36–52.

DIFIGLIA, M., PASIK, P., AND PASIK, T. 1976. A Golgi study of neuronal types in the neostriatum of monkeys. Brain Res., **114**: 245–256.

DIFIGLIA, M., PASIK, P., AND PASIK, T. 1982. A Golgi and ultrastructural study of the monkey globus pallidus. J. Comp. Neurol., **212**: 53–75.

DRAY, A. 1980. The physiology and pharmacology of mammalian basal ganglia. Progress in Neurology, **14**: 221–335.

EMSON, P. C., ARREGUI, A., CLEMENT-JONES, V., SANDBERG, B. E. B., AND ROSSOR, M. 1980. Regional distribution of methionine-enkephalin and substance P-like immunoreactivity in normal human brain and in Huntington's disease. Brain Res., **199**: 147–160.

FONNUM, F., GOTTESFELD, Z., AND GROFOVA, I. 1978. Distribution of glutamate decarboxylase, choline acetyltransferase and aromatic amino acid decarboxylase in the basal ganglia of normal and operated rats. Evidence for striatopallidal, striatoentopeduncular and striatonigral GABAergic fibers. Brain Res., **143**: 125–138.

FRANÇOIS, C., PERCHERON, G., YELNIK, J., AND HEYNER, S. 1984. A Golgi analysis of the primate globus pallidus. I. Inconstant processes of large neurons, other neuronal types and afferent axons. J. Comp. Neurol., **227**: 182–199.

FREUND, T. F., POWELL, J. F., AND SMITH, A. D. 1984. Tyrosine hydroxylase-immunoreactive synaptic boutons in contact with identified striatonigral neurons, with particular reference to dendritic spines. Neuroscience, **13**: 1189–1215.

GALE, K., HONG, J.-S., AND GUIDOTTI, A. 1977. Presence of substance P and GABA in separate strionigral neurons. Brain Res., **36**: 371–375.

GARCIA-RILL, E. 1986. The basal ganglia and the locomotor regions. Brain Res. Rev., **11**: 46–63.

GERFEN, C. R. 1989. The neostriatal mosaic: Striatal patch–matrix organization is related to cortical lamination. Science, **246**: 358–388.

GOEDERT, M., MANTYH, P. W., EMSON, P. C., AND HUNT, S. P. 1984. Inverse relationship between neurotensin receptors and neurotensin-like immunoreactivity in cat striatum. Nature, **307**: 543–546.

GOLDMAN, P. S., AND NAUTA, W. J. H. 1977. An intricately patterned prefrontocaudate projection in the rhesus monkey. J. Comp. Neurol., **171**: 369–386.

GRAYBIEL, A. M. 1984. Correspondence between the dopamine islands and the striosomes of the mammalian striatum. Neuroscience, **13**: 1157–1187.

GRAYBIEL, A. M., PICKEL, V. M., JOH, T. H., REIS, D. J., AND RAGSDALE, C. W. 1981. Direct demonstration of a correspondence between the dopamine islands and acetylcholinesterase patches in the developing striatum. Proc. Natl. Acad. Sci. USA, **78**: 5871–5875.

GRAYBIEL, A. M., AND RAGSDALE, C. W. 1983. Biochemical anatomy of the striatum, In P. C. Emson (Editor), *Chemical Neuroanatomy.* Raven Press, New York, pp. 427–504.

GRAYBIEL, A. M., RAGSDALE, C. W., YONEOKA, E. S., AND ELDE, R. P. 1981. An immunohistochemical study of enkephalins and other neuropeptides in the striatum of the cat with evidence that the opiate peptides are arranged to form mosaic patterns in register with the striosomal compartments visible by acetylcholinesterase staining. Neuroscience, **6**: 377–397.

GREENAMYRE, J. T., YOUNG, A. B., AND PENNY, J. B. 1984. Quantitative autoradiographic distribution of L-[^{3}H]glutamate-binding sites in rat central nervous system. J. Neurosci., **4**: 2133–2144.

GROVES, P. M. 1983. A theory of the functional organization of the neostriatum and the neostriatal control of voluntary movement. Brain Res. Rev., **5**: 109–132.

GUSELLA, J. F., WEXLER, N. S., CONNEALLY, P.-M., NAYLOR, S. L., ANDERSON, M. A., TANZI, R. E., WATKINS, P. C., OTTINA, K., WALLACE, M. R., SAKAGUCHI, A. Y., YOUNG, A. B., SHOULSON, I., BONILLA, E., AND MARTIN, J. B. 1983. A polymorphic DNA marker genetically linked to Huntington's disease. Nature, **306**: 234–238.

HABER, S., AND ELDE, R. 1981. Correlation between met-enkephalin and substance P immunoreactivity in the primate globus pallidus. Neuroscience, **6**: 1291–1297.

HAMMOND, C., AND YELNIK, J. 1983. Intracellular labeling of rat subthalamic neurones with horseradish peroxidase: Computer analysis of dentrites and characterization of axon arborization. Neuroscience, **8**: 781–790.

HAMMOND, C., DENIAU, J. M., RIZK, A., AND FÉGER, J. 1978. Electrophysiological demonstration of an excitatory subthalamo-nigral pathway in the rat. Brain Res., **151**: 235–244.

HAMMOND, C., FÉGER, J., BIOULAC, B., AND SOUTEYRAND, J. P. 1979. Experimental hemiballism in the monkey produced by unilateral kainic acid lesion in corpus Luysii. Brain Res., **171**: 577–580.

HAMMOND, C., SHIBAZAKI, T., AND ROUZAIRE-DUBOIS, B. 1983. Branched output neurons of the rat subthalamic nucleus: Electrophysiological study of the synaptic effects on identified cells in the two main target nuclei, the entopeduncular nucleus and the substantia nigra. Neuroscience, **9**: 511–520.

HARNOIS, C., AND FILION, M. 1980. Pallidal neurons branching to the thalamus and to the midbrain in the monkey. Brain Res., **186**: 222–225.

HARTMANN-VON MONAKOW, K., AKERT, K., AND KÜNZLE, H. 1978. Projections of the precentral motor cortex and other cortical areas of the frontal lobe to the subthalamic nucleus in the monkey. Exp. Brain Res., **33**: 395–403.

HENDERSON, Z. 1981. Ultrastructure and acetylcholinesterase content of neurones forming connections between the striatum and substantia nigra of rat. J. Comp. Neurol., **197**: 185–196.

HERKENHAM, M., AND PERT, C. B. 1981. Mosaic distribution of opiate receptors, parafascicular projections and acetylcholinesterase in the rat striatum. Nature, **291**: 415–418.

HORNYKIEWICZ, O. 1966. Metabolism of brain dopamine in human parkinsonism: Neurochemical and clinical aspects. In E. COSTA et al. (Editors), *Biochemistry and Pharmacology*, Raven Press, Hewlett, New York, pp. 171–185.

ILINSKY, I. A., JOUANDET, M. L., AND GOLDMAN-RAKIC, P. S. 1985. Organization of the nigrothalamocortical system in the rhesus monkey. J. Comp. Neurol., **236**: 315–330.

INAGAKI, S., AND PARENT, A. 1984. Distribution of substance P and enkephalin-like immunoreactivity in the substantia nigra of the rat, cat and monkey. Brain Res. Bull, **13**: 319–329.

IZZO, P. N., AND BOLAM, J. P. 1988. Cholinergic synaptic input to different parts of spiny striatonigral neurons in the rat. J. Comp. Neurol., **269**: 219–234.

IZZO, P. N., GRAYBIEL, A. M., AND BOLAM, J. P. 1987. Characterization of substance P- and [met] enkephalin-immunoreactive neurons in the caudate nucleus of cat and ferret by a single section Golgi procedure. Neuroscience, **20**: 577–587.

JAYARAMAN, A., BATTON, R. R., AND CARPENTER, M. B. 1977. Nigrotectal projections in the monkey: An autoradiographic study. Brain Res., **135**: 147–152.

JESSELL, T. M., EMSON, P. C., PAXINOS, G., AND CUELLO, A. C. 1978. Topographical projections of substance P and GABA pathways in the striato- and pallido-nigral system: A biochemical and immunohistochemical study. Brain Res., **152**: 487–498.

KALIL, K. 1978. Patch-like termination of thalamic fibers in the putamen of the rhesus monkey: An autoradiographic study. Brain Res., **140**: 333–339.

KANAZAWA, I., MARSHALL, G. R., AND KELLY, J. S. 1976. Afferents to the rat substantia nigra studied with horseradish peroxidase, with special reference to fibers from the subthalamic nucleus. Brain Res., **115**: 485–491.

KELLEY, A. E., DOMESICK, V. B., AND NAUTA, W. J. H. 1982. The amygdalostriate projection in the rat: An anatomical study by anterograde and retrograde tracing methods. Neuroscience, **7**: 615–630.

KEMEL, M. L., GAUCHY, C., ROMO, R., GLOWINSKI, J., AND BESSON, M. J. 1983. *In vivo* release of [³H] GABA in cat caudate nucleus and substantia nigra. I. Bilateral changes induced by a unilateral nigral application of muscimol. Brain Res., **272**: 331–340.

KEMP, J. M., AND POWELL, T. P. S. 1971. The structure of the caudate nucleus of the cat: Light and electron microscopy. Philos. Trans. R. Soc. Lond. (Biol.), **262**: 383–401.

KEMP, J. M., AND POWELL, T. P. S. 1971. The site of termination of afferent fibers in the caudate nucleus. Philos. Trans. R. Soc. Lond. (Biol.), **262**: 413–427.

KEMP, J. M., AND POWELL, T. P. S. 1971. The connexions of the striatum and globus pallidus: Synthesis and speculation. Philos. Trans. R. Soc. Lond. (Biol.), **262**: 441–457.

KIM, R., NAKANO, K., JAYARAMAN, A., AND CARPENTER, M. B. 1976. Projections of the globus pallidus and adjacent structures: An autoradiographic study in the monkey. J. Comp. Neurol., **169**: 263–289.

KITA, H., CHANG, H. T., AND KITAI, S. T. 1983. Pallidal inputs to subthalamus: Intracellular analysis. Brain Res., **264**: 255–265.

KITA, H., CHANG, H. T., AND KITAI, S. T. 1983. The morphology of intracellularly labeled rat subthalamic neurons: A light microscopic analysis. J. Comp. Neurol., **215**: 245–257.

KITAI, S. T. 1981. Anatomy and physiology of the neostriatum. In G. DICHIARA and G. L. GESSA (Editors), *GABA and the Basal Ganglia*. Raven Press, New York, pp. 1–21.

KITAI, S. T., AND DENIAU, J. M. 1981. Cortical inputs to the subthalamus: Intracellular analysis. Brain Res., **214**: 411–415.

VAN DER KOOY, D., FISHELL, G., KRUSCHEL, L. A., AND JOHNSTON, J. 1987. The development of striatal compartments: from proliferation to patches. In M. B. CARPENTER AND A. JAYARAMAN (Editors), *The Basal Ganglia II, Structure and Function—Current Concepts*. Plenum Press, New York, pp. 81–98.

VAN DER KOOY, D., AND HATTORI, T. 1980. Dorsal raphe cells with collateral projections to the caudate-putamen and substantia nigra: A fluorescent retrograde double labeling study in the rat. Brain Res., **186**: 1–7.

VAN DER KOOY, D., AND HATTORI, T. 1980a. Single subthalamic nucleus neurons project to both the globus pallidus and substantia nigra in rat. J. Comp. Neurol., **192**: 751–768.

KUO, J.-S., AND CARPENTER, M. B. 1973. Organization of pallidothalamic projections in the rhesus monkey. J. Comp. Neurol., **151**: 201–236.

KÜNZLE, H. 1975. Bilateral projections from precentral motor cortex to the putamen and other parts of the basal ganglia. Brain Res., **88**: 195–210.

LANGSTON, J. W., BALLARD, P., TETRUD, J. W., AND IRWIN, I. 1983. Chronic parkinsonism in humans due to a product of meperidine-analog synthesis. Science, **249**: 979–980.

LAVOIE, B., SMITH, Y., AND PARENT, A. 1989. Dopaminergic innervation of the basal ganglia in the squirrel monkey revealed by tyrosine hydroxylase immunohistochemistry. J. Comp. Neurol., **289**: 36–52.

LEE, H. J., RYE, D. B., HALLANGER, A. E., LEVEY, A. I., AND WAINER, B. H. 1988. Cholinergic vs noncholinergic efferents from the mesopontine tegmentum to the extrapyramidal motor system nuclei. J. Comp. Neurol., **275**: 469–492.

LEHMAN, J., AND LANGER, S. Z. 1983. The striatal cholinergic interneuron: Synaptic target of dopaminergic terminals. Neuroscience **10**: 1105–1120.

MARTIN, J. P. 1967. *The Basal Ganglia and Posture*. Pitman, London, 152 pp.

MOON EDLEY, S., AND GRAYBIEL, A. M. 1983. The afferent and efferent connections of the feline nucleus tegmenti pedunculopontinus, pars compacta. J. Comp. Neurol., **217**: 187–215.

MORIIZUMI, T., NAKAMURA, Y., KITAO, Y., AND KUDO, M. 1987. Ultrastructural analysis of afferent terminals in the subthalamic nucleus of cat with a combined degeneration and horseradish peroxidase tracing method. J. Comp. Neurol., **265**: 159–174.

MUGNAINI, E., AND OERTEL, W. H. 1985. An atlas of the distribution of GABAergic neurons and terminals in the rat CNS as revealed by GAD immunohistochemistry. In A. BJÖRKLUND AND T. HÖKFELT (Editors), *Handbook of Chemical Neuroanatomy, GABA and Neuropeptides in the CNS*. Elsevier, Amsterdam, 4 (Part I). pp. 436–595.

NASTUK, M. A., AND GRAYBIEL, A. M. 1985. Patterns of muscarinic cholinergic binding in the striatum and their relation to dopamine islands and striosomes. J. Comp. Neurol., **237**: 176–194.

NAUTA, H. J. W., AND COLE, M. 1978. Efferent projections of the subthalamic nucleus: An autoradiographic study in monkey and cat. J. Comp. Neurol., **180**: 1–16.

NAUTA, W. J. H., AND MEHLER, W. R. 1966. Projections of the lentiform nucleus in the monkey. Brain Res., **1**: 3–42.

PARENT, A., BOUCHARD, C., AND SMITH, Y. 1984. The striatopallidal and striatonigral projections: Two distinct systems in primate. Brain Res., **303**: 385–390.

PARENT, A., AND DE BELLEFEUILLE, L. 1982. Organization of efferent projections from the internal segment of the globus pallidus in primate as revealed by fluorescence retrograde labeling method. Brain Res., **245**: 201–213.

PARENT, A., HAZRATI, L.-N., AND LAVOIE, B. 1991. The pallidum as a dual structure in primates. In G BERNARDI, M. B. CARPENTER, G. DI CHIARA, M. MORELLI, AND P. STANZIONE (Editors), *Basal Ganglia III*. Plenum Press, New York, pp. 81–88.

PARENT, A., MACKEY, A., AND DE BELLEFEUILLE, L. 1983. The subcortical afferents to caudate nucleus and putamen in primate: A fluorescence retrograde double labeling study. Neuroscience, **10**: 1137–1150.

PARENT, A., MACKEY, A., SMITH, Y., AND BOUCHER, R. 1983. The output organization of the substantia nigra in primate as revealed by a retrograde double labeling method. Brain Res. Bull., **10**: 529–537.

PARENT, A., AND SMITH, Y. 1987. Differential dopaminergic innervation of the two pallidal segments in the squirrel monkey (*Saimiri sciureus*). Brain Res., **426**: 397–400.

PARENT, A. AND SMITH, Y. 1987. Organization of efferent projections of the subthalamic nucleus in the squirrel monkey as revealed by retrograde labeling methods. Brain Res., **436**: 296–310.

PARK, M. R., FALLS, W. M., AND KITAI, S. T. 1982. An intracellular HRP study of the rat globus pallidus. I. Responses and light microscopic analysis. J. Comp. Neurol., **211**: 284–294.

PASIK, P., PASIK, T., AND DIFIGLIA, M. 1979. The internal organization of the neostriatum in mammals. In I. DIVAC (Editor), *The Neostriatum*, Pergamon Press, Oxford, pp. 5–36.

PASIK, P., PASIK, T., HOSTEIN, G. R., AND HÁMORI, J. 1988. GABAergic elements in the neuronal circuits of the monkey neostriatum: A light and electron microscopic immunocytochemical study. J. Comp. Neurol., **270**: 157–170.

PENNY, G. R., AFSHARPOUR, S., AND KITAI, S. T. 1986. The glutamic acid decarboxylase-, leucine-enkephalin- methionine-enkephalin- and substance P-immunoreactive neurons in the neostriatum of the rat and cat: Evidence for partial population overlap. Neuroscience, **17**: 1011–1045.

PENNY, G. R., WILSON, C. J., AND KITAI, S. T. 1988. Relationships of the axonal and dentritic geometry of spiny projection neurons to the compartmental organization of the neostriatum. J. Comp. Neurol., **269**: 275–289.

RADKE, J. M., MARTIN-IVERSON, M. T., AND VINCENT, S. R. 1987. Somatostatin-dopamine interactions in the rat striatum. In M. B. CARPENTER AND A. JAYARAMAN (Editors), *The Basal Ganglia II*, Structure and Function—Current Concepts. Plenum Press, New York, pp. 99 113.

RIBAK, C. E. 1979. The GABA neurons and their axons terminals in rat corpus striatum as demonstrated by GAD immunocytochemistry. J. Comp. Neurol., **187**: 261–284.

RIBAK, C. E. 1981. The GABAergic neurons of the extrapyramidal system as revealed by immunocytochemistry. In DI CHIARA AND G. L. GESSA (Editors), *GABA and the Basal Ganglia*. Raven Press, pp. 23–36.

RIBAK, C. E., VAUGHN, J. E., AND ROBERTS, E. 1980. GABAergic nerve terminals decrease in the substantia nigra following hemitransections of the striatonigral and pallidonigral pathways. Brain Res., **192**: 413–420.

RICHFIELD, E. K., YOUNG, A., AND PENNY, J. B. 1987. Comparative distribution of dopamine D_1 and D_2 receptors in the basal ganglia of turtles, pigeons, rats, cats and monkeys. J. Comp. Neurol., **262**: 446–463.

RICHTER, E. 1965. *Die Entwichlung des Globus Pallidus und des Corpus Subthalamicum*. Springer-Verlag, Berlin, pp. 131.

RUSSCHEN, F. T., AND PRICE, J. L. 1984. Amygdalostriatal projections in rat. Topographical organization and fiber morphology shown using lectin PHA-L as an anterograde tracer. Neurosci. Lett., **47**: 15–22.

SCHELL, G. R., AND STRICK, P. L. 1984. The origin of thalamic inputs to the arcuate premotor and supplementary motor areas. J. Neurosci., **4**: 539–560.

SEROOGY, K., AND FALLON, J. H. 1989. Forebrain projections from cholecystokinin-like immunoreactive neurons in the rat midbrain. J. Comp. Neurol., **279**: 415–435.

SEROOGY, K. B., DANGARAN, K., LIM, S., HAYCOCK, J. W., AND FALLON, J. 1989. Ventral mesoencephalic neurons containing both cholecystokinin- and tyrosin hydroxylase-like immunoreactivities project to forebrain regions. J. Comp. Neurol., **279**: 397–414.

SIGGINS, G. R., HOFFER, B. J., BLOOM, F. E., AND UGERSTEDT, U. 1976. Cytochemical and electrophysiological studies of dopamine in the caudate nucleus. Res. Publ. Assoc. Res. Nerv. Ment. Dis., **55**: 227–248.

SMITH, Y., AND PARENT, A. 1986. Differential connections of the caudate nucleus and putamen in the squirrel monkey (*Saimiri sciureus*). Neuroscience, **18**: 347–371.

SMITH, Y., AND PARENT, A. 1987. Neuropeptide Y-immunoreactive neurons in the striatum of cat and monkey. Morphological characteristics, intrinsic organization and co-localization with somatostatin. Brain Res., **372**: 241–252.

SMITH, Y., AND PARENT, A. 1988. Neurons of the subthalamic nucleus in primates display glutamate but not GABA immunoreactivity. Brain Res., **453**: 353–356.

SMITH, Y., PARENT, A., SÉQUELA, P., AND DESCARRIES, L. 1987. Distribution of GABA-immunoreactive neurons in the basal ganglia of the squirrel monkey (*Saimiri sciureus*). J. Comp. Neurol., **259**: 50–64.

SOMOGYI, P., BOLAM, J. P., AND SMITH, A. D. 1981. Monosynaptic cortical input and local axon collaterals of identified striatonigral neurons: A light and electron microscopic study using the Golgi-peroxidase transport-degeneration procedure. J. Comp. Neurol., **185**: 567–584.

STRICK, P. L., AND STERLING, P. 1974. Synaptic terminations of afferents from the ventro-lateral nucleus of the thalamus in the cat motor cortex: A light and electron microscope study. J. Comp. Neurol., **153**: 77–106.

SUGIMOTO, T., AND HATTORI, T. 1983. Confirmation of thalamosubthalamic projections by electron microscopic autoradiography. Brain Res., **267**: 335–339.

SUGIMOTO, T., AND MIZUNO, N. 1987. Neurotensin in projection neurons of the striatum and nucleus accumbens, with reference to coexistence with enkephalin and GABA: An immunohistochemical study in the cat. J. Comp. Neurol., **257**: 383–395.

TOKUNO, H., MORIIZUNI, T., KUDO, M., KITAO, Y., AND NAKAMURA, Y. 1989. Monosynaptic striatal inputs to the nigrotegmental neurons: An electron microscopic study in cat. Brain Res., **485**: 189–192.

WHITTIER, J. R. 1947. Ballism and the subthalamic nucleus (nucleus hypothalamicus: corpus luysi). Arch. Neurol. and Psychiat., **58**: 672–692.

WHITTIER, J. R., AND METTLER, F. A. 1949. Studies on the subthalamus of the rhesus monkey. II. Hyperkinesia and other physiologic effects of subthalamic lesions with special reference to the subthalamic nucleus of Luys. J. Comp. Neurol., **90**: 319–372.

WILSON, S. A. K. 1912. Progressive lenticular degeneration: A familial nervous disease associated with cirrhosis of the liver. Brain, **34**: 295–509.

YELNIK, J., AND PERCHERON, G. 1979. Subthalamic neurons in primates: A quantitative and comparative analysis. Neuroscience, **4**: 1717–1743.

12

Olfactory Pathways, Hippocampal Formation, and the Amygdala

Olfactory sense plays a crucial role in the survival of many animals in that this sense monitors the chemical environment for molecules that reveal food sources, detect predators, and influence social and sexual behavior. Olfaction is well developed in vertebrates, although the importance of this sense is diminished in humans. Clinically the olfactory system can provide important diagnostic information. The term "rhinencephalon" refers to the olfactory brain. The rhinencephalon includes the olfactory bulb, tract, tubercle and striae, the anterior olfactory nucleus, parts of the amygdaloid complex, and parts of the pyriform cortex. In this restricted sense the term rhinencephalon is equivalent to the *paleopallium* or primitive olfactory lobe.

The *archipallium*, the oldest cortical derivative, is represented by the hippocampal formation, the dentate gyrus, the fasciolar gyrus, and the indusium griseum (supracallosal gyrus). The hippocampal formation reaches its greatest development in microsomatic humans and is well formed in anosomatic cetaceans, some of which lack olfactory bulbs. The hippocampal formation has little, if any, relationship to the sense of smell.

OLFACTORY PATHWAYS

Olfactory Receptors

The olfactory membrane is a yellowish-brown patch of specialized epithelium in the upper, posterior part of the nasal cavity. Olfactory receptors are bipolar neurons that possess unique dendrites that extend among supporting cells in the olfactory epithelium to the mucosal surface, where they end in enlargements known as olfactory vesicles (Fig. 12.1). Several hair-like kinocilia extend from the olfactory vesicle into the overlying mucus. The membranes of the cilia contain receptors capable of detecting odoriferous molecules. The delicate unmyelinated central processes of bipolar cells which constitute the *olfactoria fila*, pass from nasal cavity via foramina in the cribriform plate of the ethmoid bone. (Figs. 12.1 and 12.3). These exceedingly small fibers, with a very slow conduction rate, enter the ventral surface of the olfactory bulb. The olfactory fila, originating from bipolar cells in the olfactory epithelium, collectively constitute the *olfactory nerve* (N.I.). Morphologically the olfactory epithelium represents a primitive type of sensory cell, which supports the concept that olfaction is the oldest and most primitive of the special senses. The olfactory receptor has a life span measured in days; new axons are continually growing into the olfactory bulb and form new synapses.

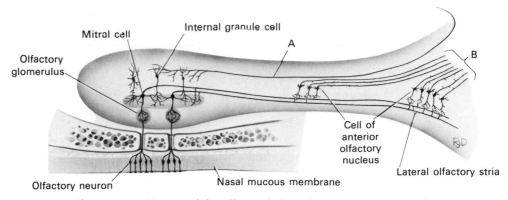

Figure 12.1. Diagram of the olfactory bulb and tract showing relationships of primary olfactory neurons and receptors in the nasal mucosa. Cells of the anterior olfactory nucleus form scattered groups caudal to the olfactory bulb. *A,* Peripherally projecting fibers from the anterior olfactory nucleus. *B,* Centrally projecting fibers from the anterior olfactory nucleus. (After Cajal, 1911.)

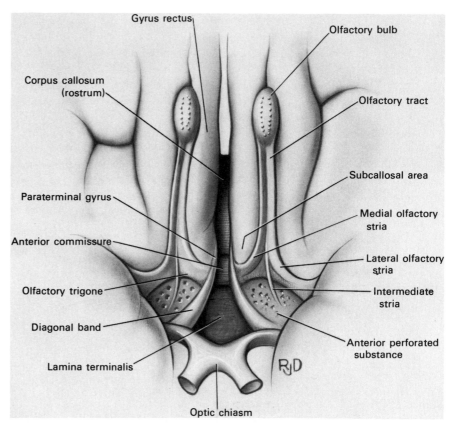

Figure 12.2. Drawing of olfactory structures on the inferior surface of the frontal lobe. The optic nerves and chiasm have been retracted to expose the olfactory striae and the anterior perforated substance.

Olfactory Bulb

This flattened ovoid body resting on the cribriform plate of the ethmoid bone is the terminal "nucleus" of the olfactory nerve (Figs. 12.1 and 12.2). The olfactory bulb is the first processing station in the olfactory pathway. Most of the fibers of the olfactory nerve enter the anterior tip of the olfactory bulb. Structurally the olfactory bulb has a laminar organization arranged in both radial and tangential fashion. Within the gray matter of the olfactory bulb are several types of nerve cells, the most striking of which are the large, triangular *mitral cells*, so named because of their resemblance to a bishop's mitre (Figs. 12.1 and 12.3). Primary olfactory fibers synapse with the brush-like terminals of vertically descending dendrites of the mitral cells to form the *olfactory glomeruli*. Smaller cells of the olfactory bulb, known as *tufted cells*, have a number of dendrites, one of which participates in the formation of the glomerulus.

The olfactory glomeruli consist of rows of spherical acellular islands where olfactory nerve fibers establish synaptic contact with the apical dendrites of mitral and tufted neurons. Numerous interneurons surround the glomeruli. Axons of mitral and tufted cells project to deeper layers of the olfactory bulb where they merge to form the lateral olfactory tract. Glutamate and aspartate are considered the excitatory transmitters of both mitral and tufted neurons.

Granule cells of various sizes are found throughout the olfactory bulb but are most dense toward the center of the bulb, forming the granular cell layer (Fig. 12.3). Dendritic processes of granule cells extend radially from the somata toward both the surface of the olfactory bulb and its central region (Fig. 12.3). Granule cells have no axons, and their dendrites have spines, or gemmules, which form dendrodendritic synapses with mitral cells. The morphological features of these junctions suggest reciprocal synapses; one from granule cell to mitral cell, and one from mitral cell to granule cell (Fig. 12.3). Granule cells inhibit mitral cells, and the mitral cells appear to excite the granule cells. Although afferent fibers in the olfactory bulb do not appear to be localized in any patterned way, a regional organization of olfactory nerve projections to the olfactory bulb has been demonstrated in mammals. Localized lesions in different regions of the olfactory epithelium produce degeneration in specific regions of the glomerular layer. Axons of the mitral and tufted cells entering the lateral olfactory tract are *secondary olfactory fibers* (Fig. 12.1).

Caudal to the olfactory bulb are scattered groups of neurons, intermediate in size between mitral and granule cells, that form the *anterior olfactory nucleus* (Fig. 12.4). Some cells of this loosely organized nucleus are found along the olfactory tracts near the base of the hemisphere. Dendrites of these cells pass among the fibers of the olfactory tract, from which they receive impulses. Axons of the cells of the anterior olfactory nucleus cross in the anterior part of the anterior commissure and enter the contralateral anterior olfactory nucleus and olfactory bulb (Fig. 12.4).

Excitation of mitral and tufted cells via their primary dendrites is controlled by synaptic contacts with a heterogeneous population of periglomerular cells. Periglomerular cells and some external tufted cells are considered to contain dopamine, γ-aminobutyric acid (GABA), and substance P (SP). The inner elements of the olfactory bulb include tufted and mitral cells (output neurons) and the internal granule cells. Internal granule cells and intrinsic short axon cells receive central projections conveying acetylcholine (ACh), serotonin (5-HT), noradrenalin, enkephalin (ENK), and SP.

Olfactory Tract

This tract passes toward the anterior perforated substance and divides into well-defined *lateral* and *medial olfactory striae*. A thin covering of gray substance over the olfactory striae composes the *lateral* and *medial olfactory gyri* (Figs. 12.2 and 12.4). The lateral olfactory stria and gyrus pass along the lateral margin of the anterior perforated substance to reach the pyriform region (Figs. 12.5 and 12.6). These fibers terminate in the

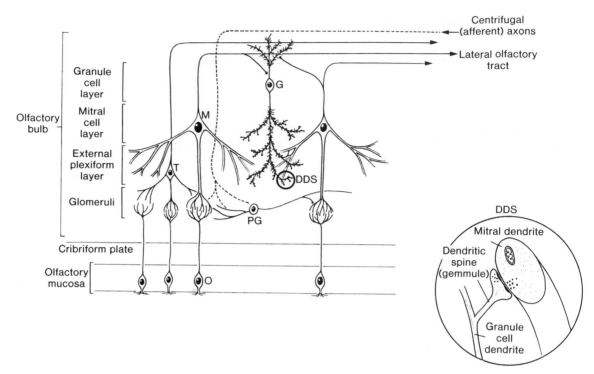

Figure 12.3. Schematic diagram of the major cells in the olfactory bulb and their relationships. Sensory neurons and receptor elements (*O*) are in the olfactory mucosa. Central processes of primary sensory neurons enter the olfactory bulb and synapse upon dendrites of mitral cells (*M*), forming a complex known as olfactory glomeruli. Axons of mitral cells projecting centrally form the lateral olfactory tract. Granule cells (*G*) have no axons, but dendritic spines on external dendrites form dendrodendritic synapses (*DDS* in insert) with mitral cell dendrites. Periglomerular cells (*PG*), representing several morphological cell types, provide a linkage bewteen glomeruli. Tufted cells (*T*) are similar to mitral cells, but their cell bodies are dispersed throughout the external plexiform layer.

pyriform cortex and in the corticomedial part of the amygdaloid nuclear complex.

Olfactory Lobe

This lobe develops as a longitudinal bulge on the basal surface of the hemisphere, where it is separated from the neopallium by the rhinal sulcus (Fig. 2.8). The posterior portion of this lobe differentiates into the olfactory area (anterior perforated substance) and other olfactory structures on the anteromedial part of the temporal lobe, collectively known as the pyriform lobe.

The *pyriform lobe*, so named because of its pear shape in certain species, is divided into several regions (Fig. 12.5). These include the *pyriform*, the *periamygdaloid*, and the *entorhinal areas*. The pyriform area, often referred to as the lateral olfactory gyrus, extends along the lateral olfactory stria to the rostral amygdaloid region (Fig. 12.6). Since its afferent fibers are derived from the lateral olfactory stria, it is regarded as an olfactory relay center. The periamygdaloid area is a small region dorsal and rostral to the amygdaloid nuclear complex. The entorhinal area, the most posterior part of the pyriform lobe, corresponds to area 28 of Brodmann and constitutes a major portion of the anterior parahippocampal gyrus in humans (Figs. 12.6 and 13.9). Fibers of the lateral olfactory stria, arising in the olfactory bulb, give collaterals to the anterior olfactory nucleus and the olfactory tubercle and terminate in the pyriform cortex and in parts of the amygdaloid nuclear complex.

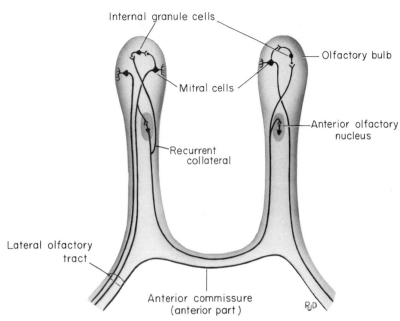

Figure 12.4. Schematic diagram of the interconnections of the olfactory bulbs. Collaterals of mitral cell axons synapse upon the apical dendrites of pyramidal-shaped cells of the anterior olfactory nucleus. These cells give rise to fibers that project centrally, cross in the anterior part of the anterior commissure (Fig. 12.9), and synapse upon cells of the anterior olfactory nucleus and internal granule cells in the contralateral olfactory bulb. Recurrent collaterals of cells of the anterior olfactory terminate upon internal granules in the ipsilateral olfactory bulb. The principal axons of mitral cells enter the lateral olfactory tract. (Based upon Valverde, 1965.)

The pyriform cortex and the periamygdaloid area, which receive fibers from the lateral olfactory stria, constitute the *primary olfactory cortex*. Olfaction appears to be unique among the sensory systems, in that impulses in this system project to the cortex without being relayed by thalamic nuclei.

The pyriform cortex projects fibers to the entorhinal cortex (area 28), the basal and lateral amygdaloid nuclei, the lateral preoptic area, the nucleus of the diagonal band, and parts of the mediodorsal nucleus of the thalamus. The entorhinal cortex is the *secondary olfactory cortical area* (Figs. 12.5 and 13.9). Efferent fibers from the entorhinal cortex are projected to the hippocampal formation, and to the anterior insular and frontal cortex via the uncinate fasciculus (Fig. 2.13). No fibers from the pyriform cortex pass to the hippocampal formation.

The lateroposterior quadrant of the orbitofrontal cortex receives olfactory information via relays in the pyriform and entorhinal cortex (Fig. 12.5). In addition, the pyriform cortex projects to the mediodorsal nucleus (MDmc) of the thalamus, which in turn projects to the orbitofrontal cortex.

Different parts of the amygdaloid nuclear complex receive olfactory inputs. Direct projections from the olfactory bulb pass to the cortical and medial amygdaloid nuclei, while indirect olfactory impulses pass to the basal and lateral amygdaloid nuclei, via relays in the pyriform cortex. Direct and indirect olfactory pathways to the amygdaloid complex terminate in different components that probably influence almost the entire complex.

Fibers originating from the cells of the anterior olfactory nucleus project (1) peripherally to internal granule cells of the ipsilateral olfactory bulb, and (2) via the anterior part of the anterior commissure to the

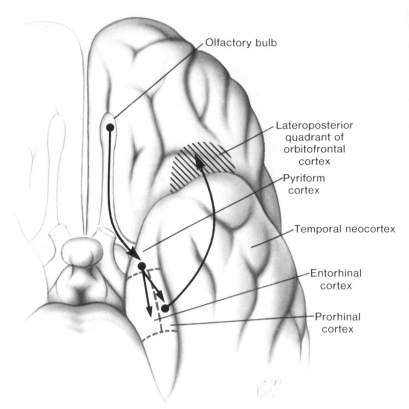

Figure 12.5. Diagram of the inferior surface of the frontal and temporal lobes of the primate brain showing olfactory connections. The lateroposterior quadrant of the orbitofrontal cortex receives olfactory information from the lateral entorhinal area (prorhinal cortex). The lateral entorhinal area also receives an olfactory input indirectly from the pyriform cortex. (Based upon Potter and Nauta, 1979.)

contralateral anterior olfactory nucleus and olfactory bulb. Projections from the anterior olfactory nucleus on one side thus reach internal granule cells of the olfactory bulb on both sides and the contralateral anterior olfactory nucleus (Fig. 12.4).

The medial olfactory stria becomes continuous with the subcallosal area and the paraterminal gyrus (Figs. 12.2 and 12.6). Some of the fibers in this stria may reach the olfactory tubercle.

The *anterior perforated substance* is a rhomboid-shaped region bounded by the medial and lateral olfactory striae and the optic tract (Figs. 2.8, 12.2, and 12.8). This region is studded with perforations made by penetrating blood vessels (Fig. 14.8). The posterior border of this region is formed by the *diagonal band of Broca* (Fig. 12.2).

The *subcallosal area* and the *paraterminal gyrus* together constitute the septal area. The term *septal area* refers to the cortical part of this region, beneath which are the septal nuclei. The *medial* and *lateral septal nuclei* lie rostral to the anterior commissure and the preoptic area near the base of the septum pellucidum (Figs. 12.6 and 12.7). The medial septal nucleus becomes continuous with the nucleus and tract of the diagonal band and has connections with the amygdaloid nuclear complex. Cells of the medial septal nuclei and the nuclei of the diagonal band are strongly cholinergic (Fig. 12.16*A* and *B*). The septal nuclei receive afferents from the hippocampal formation via the fornix; afferents to the medial septal nucleus ascend in the medial forebrain bundle and mammillary peduncle (Figs. 12.7 and 12.14). Efferent fibers from the septal nuclei project via (1) the stria medullaris to the medial habenular nucleus, (2) the medial forebrain bundle to the lateral hypothalamus and midbrain

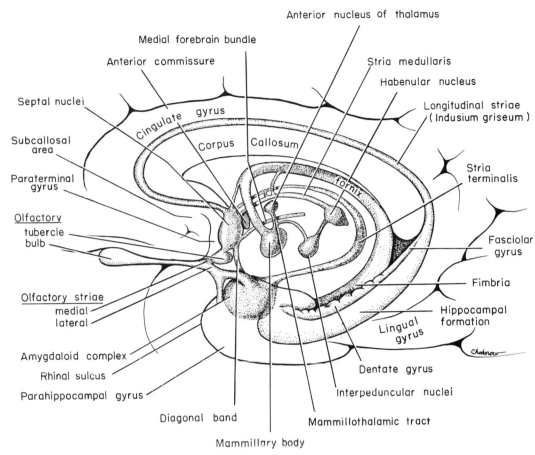

Figure 12.6. Schematic drawing of rhinencephalic and limbic structures and their connections as seen in medial view of the right hemisphere. Both deep and superficial structures are shown. (Modified from Kreig, 1953.)

tegmentum, and (3) the fornix to the hippocampal formation (Figs. 10.14 and 12.14).

Clinical Considerations

The ability of the human nose, in concert with the brain, to discriminate thousands of different odors is well known, but the physiological and psychological bases for such discriminations are unknown. Olfactory discrimination is not based on morphologically distinct types of receptors, but there is some evidence that certain odors may be distinguished by their effectiveness in stimulating particular regions of the olfactory epithelium. Current theories suggest that spatial and temporal factors probably play important roles in coding of olfactory responses.

Other evidence indicates that the sense of smell is based on molecular geometry. Molecules identical in every respect, except that one is the mirror image of the other, may have different odors. Seven primary odors (i.e., camphoraceous, musky, floral, pepperminty, ethereal [ether-like], pungent, and putrid) are considered to be equivalent to the three primary colors, because every known odor can be produced by appropriate mixtures of primary odors. Molecules with the same primary odor appear to have particular configurations, and these configurations are thought to fit appropriately shaped receptors. Molecules that may fit more than one receptor are considered to signal complex odors.

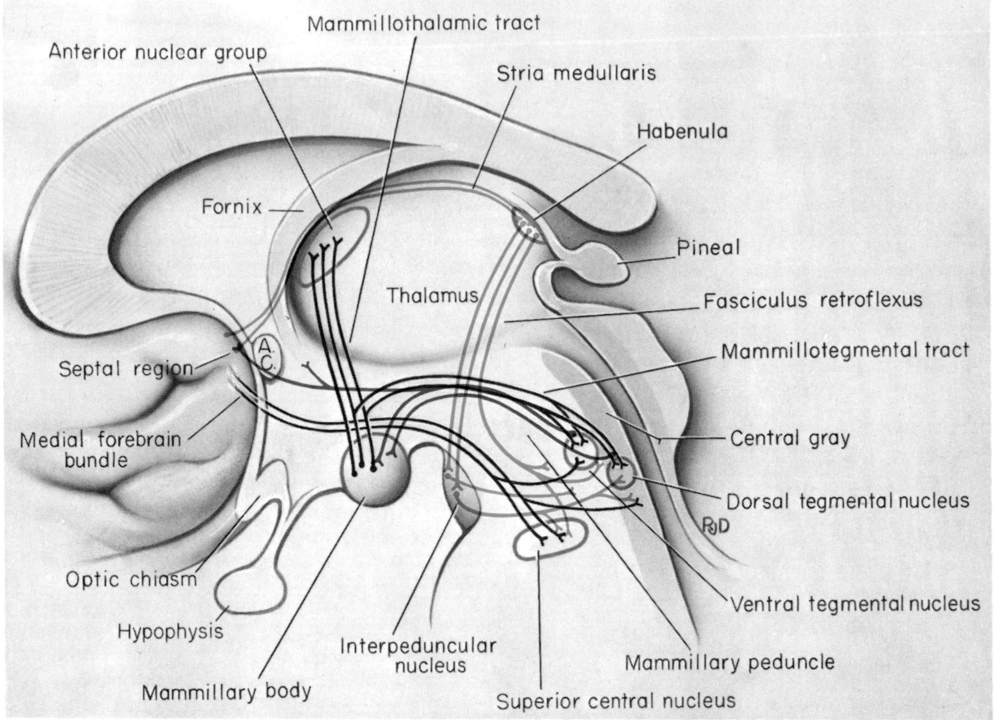

Figure 12.7. Semischematic diagram of limbic pathways interrelating the telencephalon and diencephalon with medial midbrain structures. The medial forebrain bundle and efferent fibers of the mammillary body are shown in *black*. The *medial forebrain bundle* originates from the septal and lateral preoptic regions, traverses the lateral hypothalamic area, and projects into the midbrain tegmentum. The mammillary princeps (*black*) divides into two bundles, the *mammillothalamic tract* and the *mammillotegmental tract*. Ascending fibers of the *mammillary peduncle*, arising from the dorsal and ventral tegmental nuclei, are shown in *red*; most of these fibers pass to the mammillary body, but some continue rostrally to the lateral hypothalamus, the preoptic regions, and the medial septal nucleus. Fibers arising from the septal nuclei project caudally in the medial part of the *stria medullaris* (*blue*) to terminate in the medial habenular nucleus. Impulses conveyed by this bundle are distributed to midbrain tegmental nuclei via the fasciculus retroflexus. (Based on Nauta, 1958.) (From Carpenter and Sutin, *Human Neuroanatomy*, 1983; Williams & Wilkins.)

From a clinical viewpoint the importance of the olfactory system in humans is slight, since this special sense plays a less essential role than in lower vertebrates. In certain instances valuable clinical information can be obtained by testing olfactory sense by appropriate methods. Olfaction is tested in each nostril separately by having the patient inhale or sniff nonirritating volatile oils or liquids with characteristic odors. Substances that stimulate gustatory end organs or peripheral endings of the trigeminal nerve in the nasal mucosa are not appropriate for testing olfaction. Comparisons between the two sides are of great importance. Fractures of the cribriform plate of the ethmoid bone or hemorrhage at the base of the frontal lobes may cause tearing of the olfactory filaments. The olfactory nerves may be involved as a consequence of meningitis or abscess of the frontal lobe.

Unilateral anosmia may be of diagnostic significance in localizing intracranial neoplasms, especially meningiomas of the sphenoidal ridge or olfactory groove. Hypophysial tumors affect the olfactory bulb and tract only when they extend above the sella turcica. Olfactory "hallucinations" frequently are a consequence of lesions involving or irritating the parahippocampal gyrus, the uncus, or adjoining areas. The olfactory sensations which these patients experience usually are described as disagreeable in character and may precede a generalized convulsion. Such seizures are referred to as "uncinate fits."

ANTERIOR COMMISSURE

The anterior commissure crosses the median plane as a compact fiber bundle immediately in front of the anterior columns of the fornix (Figs. 2.6, 2.23, 9.8, 12.8, and 12.9). Proceeding laterally it splits into two portions. The small anterior, or olfactory, portion, greatly reduced in humans, loops rostrally and connects the gray substance of the olfactory tract on one side with the olfactory bulb of the opposite side. Fibers in this part of the anterior commissure arise from the anterior olfactory nucleus (Fig. 12.4).

The larger posterior portion forms the bulk of the anterior commissure. From its central region fibers of the anterior commissure pass laterally and backward through the most inferior parts of the lateral segments of the globus pallidus and putamen (Figs. 9.8, 9.9, and 11.1). Further laterally the fibers of the anterior commissure enter the external capsule and come into apposition with the inferior part of the claustrum. Fibers of the posterior portion of the anterior commissure mainly interconnect the middle temporal gyri, although some fibers pass into the inferior temporal gyrus (Fig. 12.9).

HIPPOCAMPAL FORMATION

The hippocampal formation is laid down in the embryo on the medial wall of the hemisphere along the hippocampal fissure. This fissure lies immediately above and parallel to the choroidal fissure, which marks the invagination of the choroid plexus into the ventricle (Fig. 12.10). With the formation of the temporal lobe, both these fissures are carried downward and forward, each forming an arch extending from the region of the interventricular foramen to the tip of the inferior horn of the lateral ventricle. The various parts of the hippocampal arch do not develop to the same extent. The dorsal portion of the hippocampal fissure is invaded by commissural fibers of the corpus callosum and ultimately becomes the callosal sulcus (Fig. 2.6). The part of the hippocampal formation that remains above the corpus callosum forms a thin vestigial convolution, the indusium griseum (Fig. 12.8).

The temporal part of the arch, not affected by the corpus callosum, differentiates into the hippocampal formation. As the hippocampal fissure deepens, the invaginated portion bulges into the inferior horn and becomes the *hippocampal formation* (Fig. 12.9). The lips of the fissure gives rise to the *dentate* and *parahippocampal gyri*. These relationships can be seen in transverse sections (Fig. 12.10). Proceeding from the collateral sulcus, the *parahippocampal gyrus* extends to the hippocampal fissure, where it dips into the ventricle to form the *hippocampal formation*. The latter curves dorsally and medially and, on reaching the medial surface, curves inward again to form a semilunar convolution, the *dentate gyrus* or *fascia dentata* (Figs. 12.6, 12.8, and 12.11). The whole ventricular surface of the hippocampal formation is covered by a white fibrous layer, the *alveus*, composed of axons from cells of the hippocampus (Fig. 12.10). These fibers converge on the medial surface of the hippocampus to form the *fimbria*. Fibers from the alveus entering the fimbria constitute the beginning of the fornix system (Figs. 12.8, 12.9, and 12.11). The choroid plexus, invaginated into the ventricle along this fissure, partly covers the hippocampus (Fig. 12.10).

The superior portion of the parahippocampal gyrus adjoining the hippocampal fissure is known as the *subiculum*, and the area of transition

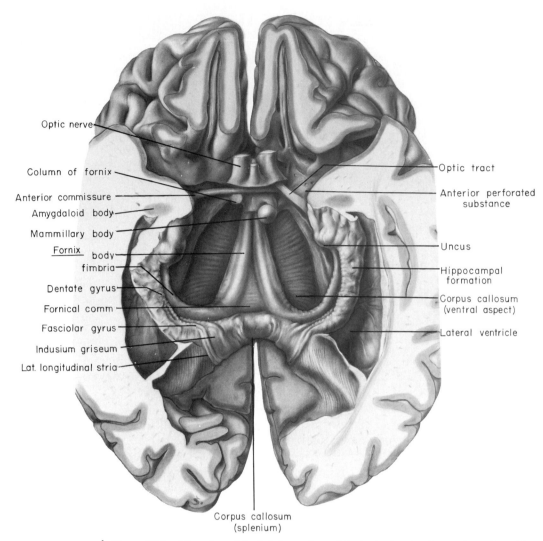

Optic nerve

Column of fornix

Anterior commissure

Amygdaloid body

Mammillary body

Fornix { body

fimbria

Dentate gyrus

Fornical comm

Fasciolar gyrus

Indusium griseum

Lat. longitudinal stria

Optic tract

Anterior perforated
substance

Uncus

Hippocampal
formation

Corpus callosum
(ventral aspect)

Lateral ventricle

Corpus callosum
(splenium)

Figure 12.8.   Dissection of the inferior surface of the brain showing the configuration of the fornix, the hippocampal formation, the dentate gyrus, and related structures. (From Mettler, _Neuroanatomy_, Ed. 2; The C. V. Mosby Company, St. Louis, 1948.) (From Carpenter and Sutin, _Human Neuroanatomy_, 1983; Williams & Wilkins.)

between it and the parahippocampal gyrus, as the _presubiculum_ (Fig. 12.10). The presubiculum, subiculum, prosubiculum, hippocampal formation, and dentate gyrus all belong to the archipallium. The larger inferior portion of the parahippocampal gyrus near the collateral sulcus has a six-layered transitional lamination resembling isocortex.

When the hippocampal fissure is opened up, the _dentate gyrus_ is seen as a narrow, notched band of cortex between the hippocampal fissure below and the fimbria above (Figs. 12.8 and 12.10). In sagittal sections (Fig. 12.11) the relationships between the hippocampal formation, the dentate gyrus, the amygdaloid nucleus, and the inferior horn of the lateral ventricle can be appreciated. Traced backward, the gyrus accompanies the fimbria almost to the splenium of the corpus callosum. There it separates from the fimbria, loses its notched appearance, and, as the delicate _fasciolar gyrus_, passes on to the superior surface of the corpus callosum (Fig. 12.8). It spreads out into a thin gray sheet representing a vestigial convolution, the _indusium griseum_ or supracallosal gyrus (Fig. 12.8). Imbedded in the indusium are two slender bands of myelinated fibers, which appear as longitudinal ridges on the superior surface of the corpus

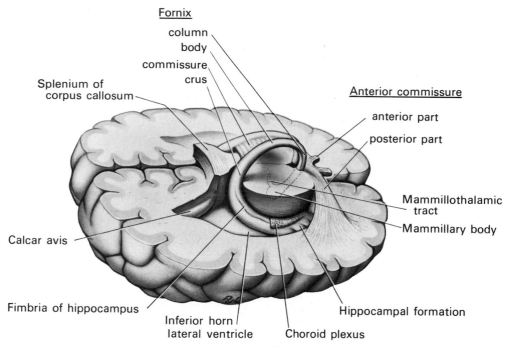

Fornix
column
body
commissure
crus
Splenium of
corpus callosum
Anterior commissure
anterior part
posterior part
Mammillothalamic
tract
Mammillary body
Calcar avis
Fimbria of hippocampus
Hippocampal formation
Inferior horn
lateral ventricle
Choroid plexus

Figure 12.9. Drawing of the brain dissection showing the hippocampal formation, the fornix system, and the anterior and posterior parts of the anterior commissure. Only postcommissural fibers of the fornix project to the mammillary body.

callosum. These are the *medial* and *lateral longitudinal striae* (Lancisii), which constitute the white matter of these vestigial convolutions (Fig. 2.9). The indusium griseum and the longitudinal striae extend the length of the corpus callosum, pass over the genu, and become continuous with the paraterminal gyrus and the diagonal band (Fig. 12.2).

The cortical zones from the parahippocampal gyrus through the presubiculum, the subiculum, and the prosubiculum to the hippocampal formation and the dentate gyrus show a gradual transition from a six- to a three-layered cellular organization (Fig. 12.11). Although the entorhinal region (area 28) is six-layered cortex, in more medial regions certain layers drop out and undergo rearrangement. The cortex of the hippocampal formation has three fundamental layers. These are the *polymorphic layer*, the *pyramidal layer*, and the *molecular layer* (Fig. 12.11). Several secondary laminae are formed by the arrangement of axons and dendrites of cells within the fundamental layers. Axons of pyramidal cells project into the alveus and the fimbria of the fornix.

The most characteristic layer of the hypocampal formation consists of large and small pyramidal cells, which exhibit many morphological differences, especially in dendritic development. Some of the cells, described as double pyramids, have rich dendritic plexuses arising from both poles. Basal and apical dendrites of pyramidal cells enter adjacent layers while their axons enter the alveus (Fig. 12.12).

Dentate Gyrus

Like the hippocampus, the dentate gyrus consists of three layers: a *molecular layer*, a *granular layer*, and a *polymorphic layer* (Fig. 12.11). Layers of the dentate gyrus are arranged in a U- or V-shaped configuration in which the open portion is directed toward the fimbria (Figs. 12.10 and 12.12). The molecular layer of the dentate gyrus is continuous with that

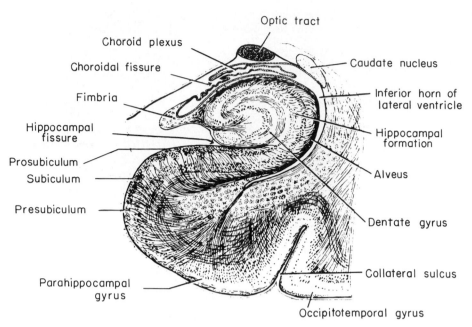

Figure 12.10. Transverse section through the human hippocampal formation and parahippocampal gyrus. The presubiculum, subiculum, and prosubiculum represent the region of transition between parahippocampal gyrus and the hippocampus and are archipallial. (From Carpenter and Sutin, *Human Neuroanatomy*; 1983; courtesy of Williams & Wilkins.)

of the hippocampus in the depths of the hippocampal fissure. The granular layer, made up of densely arranged spherical or oval neurons, gives rise to axons that pass through the polymorphic layer to terminate on dendrites of pyramidal cells in the hippocampus. Dendrites of granule cells enter mainly the molecular layer. Cells of the polymorphic layer are of several types, including modified pyramidal cells and so-called basket cells. The dentate gyrus does not give rise to fibers passing beyond the hippocampal formation.

Histochemical studies provide some clues concerning the operations of the hippocampal formation. Septohippocampal projections contain acetylcholinesterase (AChE) and fibers positive for choline acetyltransferase (ChAT). Few intrinsic hippocampal neurons are cholinergic. Noradrenergic innervation of the hippocampal formation arises from cells in the locus ceruleus that project via the septal region. Enkephalin-like immunoreactive axons emerge from the hilar region of the dentate gyrus and terminate as mossy fibers on proximal apical dendrites of hippocampal pyramidal cells. A second group of enkephalin-containing axons follow the "perforant path" from the lateral entorhinal cortex to the hippocampus (Fig. 12.12).

The anatomical connections of the hippocampal formation indicate that it does not receive an olfactory input and suggest that it is largely an effector structure. Afferent fibers to this structure arise mainly from the entorhinal area, a portion of the pyriform lobe that does not receive direct olfactory fibers (Figs. 12.5 and 12.12). Fibers from the entorhinal area (area 28) are distributed to the dentate gyrus and hippocampus in their entire posterior part. Fibers arising from the medial part of the entorhinal area follow the so-called alvear path to enter the hippocampus from its ventricular surface (Fig. 12.12). Fibers from the lateral parts of the entorhinal cortex pursue the so-called perforant path and traverse the subiculum (Fig. 12.12). These fibers are distributed to all sectors of the hippocampus except the region transitional to the dentate gyrus.

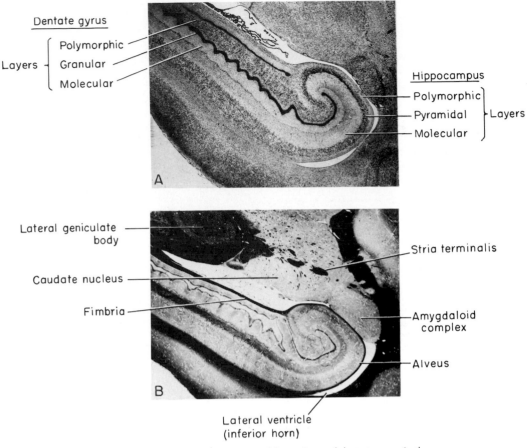

Figure 12.11. Sagittal sections through the hippocampal formation and dentate gyrus in the rhesus monkey demonstrating relationships of these structures to the inferior horn of the lateral ventricle, the tail of the caudate nucleus and the amygdaloid nuclear complex. In *A*, the cellular layers of the hippocampal formation and dentate gyrus are identified. In *B*, the alveus, fimbria, tail of the caudate nucleus, stria terminalis, amygdaloid complex, and part of the lateral geniculate body are identified. *A*, Nissl stain (×8); *B*, Weil stain (×9). (From Carpenter and Sutin, *Human Neuroanatomy*, 1983; courtesy of Williams & Wilkins.)

Other afferents to the hippocampal formation project from the medial septal nucleus via the fimbria (Figs. 12.14 and 12.16 *A*, *B*). Projections from the cingulate cortex reach the presubiculum and entorhinal cortex via the cingulum but do not enter the hippocampal formation. Because the entorhinal cortex projects to the hippocampus, impulses from the cingulate cortex can be relayed to the hippocampus (Fig. 12.14).

Fornix

This band of white fibers constitutes the main efferent fiber system of the hippocampal formation. It includes both projection and commissural fibers (Figs. 12.8 and 12.9). It is composed of axons of cells in the subicular cortex (presubiculum, subiculum, and prosubiculum) and pyramidal cells of the hippocampus, which spread over the ventricular surface as the alveus and converge to form the *fimbria*. Proceeding backward, the fimbriae of the two sides increase in thickness. On reaching the posterior end of the hippocampus, they arch under the splenium of the corpus callosum as the crura of the fornix, at the same time converging toward each other. In this region a number of fibers pass to the opposite side, forming a thin sheet of crossing fibers, the *fornical commissure* (hippocampal commissure, or psalterium) a structure rather poorly developed

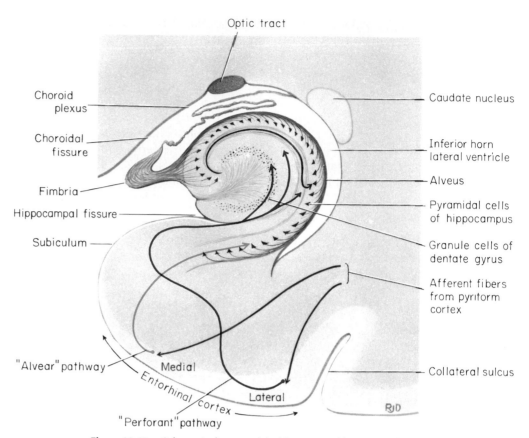

Figure 12.12. Schematic diagram of the hippocampal formation, dentate gyrus, and entorhinal cortex. In the dentate gyrus only the granular layer is indicated. In the hippocampal formation only pyramidal cells and their axons projecting into the alveus are shown. Afferent fibers from pyriform cortex projecting to the entorhinal cortex are shown in *black*. Projections of the entorhinal cortex to the hippocampal formation follow two pathways: (1) the lateral region gives rise to fibers that follow the so-called perforant pathway (*red*), and (2) the medial region gives rise to fibers that follow the so-called alvear pathway (*blue*). Axons of pyramidal cells in the hippocampal formation entering the alveus pass to the fimbria of the hippocampus. Cells of the dentate gyrus project only to the hippocampal formation. (Based on Lorente de Nó, 1934.) (From Carpenter and Sutin, *Human Neuroanatomy*, 1983; courtesy of Williams & Wilkins.)

in humans (Figs. 12.8 and 12.9). The two crura then join to form the *body of the fornix*, which runs forward under the corpus callosum to the rostral margin of the thalamus. Here the bundles separate again and, as the *anterior columns of the fornix*, arch ventrally in front of the interventricular foramina and caudal to the anterior commissure (Figs. 10.9 and 10.10). The fimbriae, thin bands of fibers situated laterally, accompany the fornices throughout most of their extent, but rostrally they become incorporated within the anterior columns of the fornix. The largest number of the fibers descend caudal to the anterior commissure as the *post-commissural fornix*. Remaining fibers of the fornix pass rostral to the anterior commissure as the *precommissural fornix*.

Postcommissural fornix fibers, originating from the subicular cortex, traverse the hypothalamus en route to the mammillary body. In their course they give off fibers to the thalamus. Fornix fibers passing directly to the mammillary body terminate mainly in the medial nucleus (Figs. 10.2, 10.9, and 12.14). Fibers leaving the postcommissural fornix in the rostral hypothalamus are distributed to the lateral septal nuclei and the anterior and lateral dorsal thalamic nuclei (Figs. 9.7 and 9.10). Other efferent fibers from the subiculum project directly to the medial frontal cortex, the caudal cingulate gyrus, and the parahippocampal gyrus. Some postcommissural fornix fibers descend caudally beyond the mammillary bodies to enter the midbrain tegmentum (Fig. 10.12).

Precommissural fornix fibers constitute a smaller, less compact group of fibers that cannot be detected grossly. These fibers originate from hippocampal pyramidal cells in all sectors and have a restricted projection via the precommissural fornix to the caudal septal nuclei.

These anatomical connections indicate the complex pathways by which signals from the hippocampal formation can be projected to different parts of the neuraxis. Both direct and indirect pathways connect the hippocampal formation and the subiculum with the septal nuclei, the hypothalamus, the thalamus, and widespread regions of the cerebral cortex and the midbrain reticular formation (Figs. 12.7 and 12.14).

Functional Considerations

Anatomical and physiological evidence indicate that the hippocampus has no significant olfactory function. The hippocampus and dentate gyrus are well developed in cetaceans that are said to be completely anosmatic and lack olfactory bulbs and nerves.

Localized lesions in the hippocampus and local stimulation of this structure in conscious cats tend to produce similar phenomena. Behavioral changes observed in these animals resemble those occurring in psychomotor epilepsy, and it seems likely that the abnormal fears, hyperesthesia, and pupillary dilatation seen may represent fragments of a seizure. The behavioral changes noted initially after lesions tend to disappear but recur at a later time. The hippocampus has an exceedingly low threshold for seizure activity.

The hippocampus appears to be concerned particularly with recent memory. Relatively large bilateral lesions of the hippocampus are associated with profound impairment of memory for recent events and with relatively mild behavioral changes. Memory for remote events usually is unaffected. Although general intellectual functions may remain at a fairly high level, these patients demonstrate an inability to learn new facts and skills. Even though the fornix contains most of the efferent fibers from the hippocampal formation, evidence that interruption of these fibers produces memory loss is meager. The mammillary bodies, like the fornix, would seem to be implicated in memory, but experimental data do not support this thesis.

The intrinsic pathways in the hippocampal formation suggest that the subiculum may be the final recipient of the extensively processed output of the dentate gyrus and the hippocampus. The subiculum is the major source of efferents in the fornix and the sole source of direct cortical projections. The functional implications of direct projections from the subiculum to the cortex are numerous. First, they provide a plausible explanation for the discrepancies between clinical and experimental observations concerning memory loss. Second, they provide a direct pathway by which seizure activity might spread to the cerebral cortex. Finally, the cortical areas that receive direct projections from the subiculum have rich connections with the association areas of the frontal and parietal lobe.

Korsakoff's syndrome (amnestic confabulatory syndrome) appears as a sequel to Wernicke's encephalopathy and probably is related to a thiamine deficiency associated with alcoholism. This syndrome is characterized by severe impairment of memory without clouding of consciousness, confusion, and confabulatory tendencies. Lesions in this syndrome almost always involve the mammillary bodies and adjacent areas. Amnesia is said to be present in this syndrome only if there is additional thalamic involvement.

Particularly prominent among concepts relating the hippocampal formation to emotion is the theory proposed by Papez. Realizing that the term "emotion" denotes both subjective feelings and the appropriate autonomic and somatic responses, Papez concluded that (1) the cortex is essential for subjective emotional experience, and (2) emotional expression must be dependent on the integrative actions of the hypothalamus. The hippocampal formation and its principal projection system, the fornix, appeared to provide the main pathway by which impulses from the cortex could reach the hypothalamus. Impulses reaching the hypothalamus could be projected caudally through the brain stem to effector structures, as well as rostrally to thalamic and cortical levels. The "central emotive process of cortical origin" was considered to be formed in the hippocampal formation and transmitted to the mammillary bodies, the anterior nuclei of the thalamus, and the cingulate gyrus. The cingulate cortex was regarded as the receptive cortical region for impulses concerned with emotion. Signals transmitted from the cingulate gyrus to other cortical regions were considered to add emotional coloring to the psychic process.

AMYGDALOID NUCLEAR COMPLEX

The amygdaloid nuclear complex is a gray mass situated in the mediodorsal portion of the temporal lobe rostral and dorsal to the tip of the inferior horn of the lateral ventricle (Figs. 2.8, 11.2, 12.6, 12.8, and 12.13). It is covered by a rudimentary cortex and caudally is continuous with the uncus of the parahippocampal gyrus.

The amygdaloid complex is divided into two main nuclear masses: (1) a corticomedial nuclear group and (2) a basolateral nuclear group. A central nucleus frequently is included as part of the corticomedial nuclear group. Nuclear subdivisions of the corticomedial group include (1) the anterior amygdaloid area, (2) the nucleus of the lateral olfactory tract, (3) the medial amygdaloid nucleus, and (4) the cortical amygdaloid nucleus. The corticomedial amygdaloid nuclear group lies closest to the putamen and tail of the caudate nucleus.

The largest and best differentiated part of the amygdaloid complex in humans is the *basolateral nuclear group*. Subdivisions of this nuclear group are (1) the lateral amygdaloid nucleus, (2) the basal amygdaloid nucleus, and (3) an accessory basal amygdaloid nucleus. Caudally the amygdaloid complex is in contact with the tail of the caudate nucleus, which sweeps anteriorly in the roof of the inferior horn of the lateral ventricle (Figs. 11.3, 12.11, and 12.13).

Among the afferent connections of the amygdaloid complex, olfactory fibers are well established (Fig. 12.6). Fibers of the lateral olfactory tract terminate in the corticomedial nuclear group. No fibers from the lateral olfactory tract appear to enter the basolateral nuclear group. The basolateral amygdaloid nuclei receive an indirect olfactory input via relays in the pyriform cortex. Thus nearly all parts of the amygdaloid nuclear complex receive either direct or indirect olfactory pathways.

Important diencephalic projections to the amygdala follow pathways which parallel efferent systems. Fibers arising in the rostral half of the hypothalamus pass to all amygdaloid nuclei except the central nucleus. Hypothalamic afferents to the amygdala arise chiefly from the ipsilateral

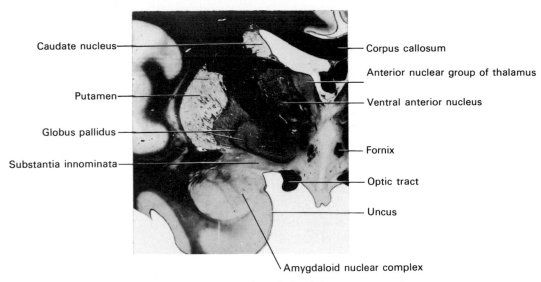

Caudate nucleus

Putamen

Globus pallidus

Substantia innominata

Corpus callosum

Anterior nuclear group of thalamus

Ventral anterior nucleus

Fornix

Optic tract

Uncus

Amygdaloid nuclear complex

Figure 12.13. Photograph of a transverse section through the thalamus, corpus striatum, and the amygdaloid nuclear complex. The substantia innominata lies ventral to the globus pallidus and dorsal to the amygdala. Weil stain. (From Carpenter and Sutin, *Human Neuroanatomy*, 1983; courtesy of Williams & Wilkins.)

lateral hypothalamic area (Fig. 10.14); the ventromedial hypothalamic nucleus projects mainly to medial regions of the amygdala. The amydgala receives small ipsilateral projections from midline paraventricular thalamic nuclei. The lateral parabrachial nuclei, which receive ipsilateral afferents from the nucleus solitarius, project ipsilaterally to the central nucleus of the amygdala.

Cytochemical Features of the Amygdala

The amygdala receives noradrenergic afferents from the locus ceruleus and dopaminergic afferents from the region of the ventral tegmental area and substantia nigra in the midbrain. Dopamine-containing terminals and noradrenergic varicosities are distributed in a similar manner with the greatest densities in the central nucleus. Axons utilizing each of these neurotransmitters reach the amygdala via both the stria terminalis and ventral pathways.

Choline acetyltransferase (ChAT) immunoreactivity in the amygdala is present only in fibers and terminals with the greatest density in the basal nuclei and in the lateral olfactory tract. These cholinergic fibers originate from the large cholinergic neurons in the substantia innominata. Serotonergic fibers in the amygdala arise from the dorsal nucleus of the raphe (Fig. 6.30) and have a high density in the basal and lateral nuclei.

Peptides found in cells and terminals within the amygdaloid nuclear complex include somatostatin (SRIF), enkephalin (ENK), substance P (SP), cholecystokinin (CCK), neurotensin (NT), and vasoactive intestinal polypeptide (VIP). SRIF-immunoreactive cells, fibers, and terminals in the monkey are distributed throughout all subdivision of the amygdala. The levels of SRIF in the amygdala are among the highest in the brain and appear to have an intrinsic origin. Cells and terminals immunoreactive for ENK, SP, and NT have an intrinsic origin and are localized mainly in the central and medial nuclei. Cells containing CCK and VIP are present in the lateral amygdaloid nuclei and in the pyriform cortex. Many of the amygdaloid neurons synthesizing these peptides project to the preoptic region and hypothalamic nuclei.

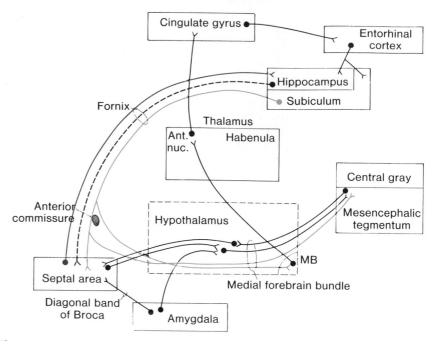

Figure 12.14. Schematic diagram of the major interconnections of structures composing the "limbic system." Fibers arising from the subiculum (*blue*) project via the fornix to the septal area, hypothalamus, and mesencephalic tegmentum. Projection fibers from the hippocampal formation in the fornix are represented by *black-dashed lines*. Fibers from the septal area passing to the hippocampus via the fornix are indicated in *red*. *MB* indicates the mammillary body. (From Carpenter and Sutin, *Human Neuroanatomy*, 1983; courtesy of Williams & Wilkins.)

Stria Terminalis

The best established amygdaloid nuclear complex is the stria terminalis (Figs. 2.21, 2.26, 9.3, 9.5, 11.4, and 12.6). Most, but not all, of the fibers in this bundle originate from the corticomedial part of the amygdaloid complex. Fibers of the stria terminalis arch along the entire medial border of the caudate nucleus near its junction with the thalamus (Fig. 9.6). Rostrally large numbers of these fibers terminate in the nuclei of the stria terminalis located lateral to the columns of the fornix and dorsal to the anterior commissure. This is the most massive termination of the stria terminalis. Postcommissural fibers of the stria terminalis end in the anterior hypothalamic nucleus, and some of the fibers may join the medial forebrain bundle. Fibers of the precommissural part of the stria terminalis terminate in the medial preoptic area and continue caudally to end in a cell-poor zone surrounding the ventromedial hypothalamic nucleus (Fig. 10.7).

Ventral Amygdalofugal Projection

This projection, considered to arise from both the basolateral amygdaloid nuclei and pyriform cortex, emerges from the dorsomedial part of the amygdala and spreads medially and rostrally beneath the lentiform nucleus. These fibers pass through the substantia innominata (Figs. 12.13, and 12.16C and D) and enter the lateral preoptic and hypothalamic areas, the septal region, and the nucleus of the diagonal band (Broca) (Figs.

12.2 and 12.14). Some fibers in the projection arise from the periamygdaloid cortex.

Amygdalofugal fibers, bypassing the preoptic region and hypothalamus, enter the inferior thalamic peduncle (Fig. 9.9). These fibers project to the midline periventricular nuclei and the magnocellular division of the mediodorsal nucleus (MDmc) of the thalamus. The amygdaloid complex also has projections to the neostriatum, the magnocellular nuclei of the substantia innominata (Figs. 12.15 and 12.16), the hippocampal formation, the subiculum, and the entorhinal cortex. In addition, the central nucleus of the amygdala projects descending fibers to the parabrachial nuclei (Fig. 6.27), the nuclei of the solitary fasciculus, and the dorsal motor nucleus of the vagus. Most of these projections to brain stem nuclei are reciprocal. Targets of descending projections from the amygdala are directly involved in the regulation of cardiovascular, respiratory, and gastric functions, all of which participate in the expression of fear and stress-related behavior.

Amygdalocortical Projections

Although it was long accepted that the amygdala was primarily associated with subcortical structures that controlled visceral and autonomic functions, many observations suggested that the functions of the complex are not restricted to this role. The widespread projections of the amygdala to multiple regions of the cerebral cortex suggest that this complex plays important roles in higher cognitive and motivational functions. Projections from the amygdala are to regions of the frontal, insular, temporal, and occipital cortex. Amygdalocortical projections include the somatosensory cortex and nearly all regions of the temporal lobe.

Amygdalostriate Projections

Axoplasmic transport studies indicate that portions of the amygdaloid complex, which project to the neostriatum, also project to what is collectively called the ventral striatum. The *ventral striatum* consists of the nucleus accumbens (Fig. 12.15) and striate-like portions of the olfactory tubercle (Fig. 12.6). Projections to the neostriatum arise from the basal lateral amygdaloid nucleus and pass via the longitudinal association bundle and the stria terminalis. Rostrally this projection is dense only in ventromedial regions of the caudate nucleus while caudal to the anterior commissure it encompasses larger parts of the putamen. No fibers project to the rostrodorsolateral region of the striatum. Most amygdalostriate fibers are ipsilateral, but a modest symmetrical contralateral distribution is conveyed by the anterior commissure. These observations suggest a division of the striatum into "limbic" and "nonlimbic" parts. Corticostriate projections from the sensorimotor cortex are mainly to rostrodorsolateral, "nonlimbic" regions. The amygdalostriate projections may integrate motor activities appropriate to emotional and motivational states.

Functional Considerations

Even though the amygdaloid complex receives an olfactory input, its importance for olfactory sense is uncertain. The amygdaloid complex cannot be closely related to olfaction since it is well developed in anosmatic aquatic mammals, and bilateral destruction of this complex does not impair olfactory discrimination.

Pronounced behavioral changes are elicited by stimulation of the amygdala in unanesthetized animals. The most common response to amygdaloid stimulation under such conditions is an "arrest" reaction in which all spontaneous ongoing activities cease as the animal assumes an attitude of aroused attention. The "arrest" reaction appears as the initial phase of flight or defense reactions. Flight (fear) and defensive (rage and aggression) reactions, termed agonistic behavior, have been elicited from different regions of the amygdaloid complex. In the amygdaloid complex the intensity of the stimulus determines the magnitude of the response, which builds gradually and outlasts the period of stimulation. Intense reactions of fear and rage are associated with pupillary dilatation, pilo-erection, growling, hissing, unmistakable signs of emotional involvement, and activity of the autonomic nervous system. Electrical stimulation of the stria terminalis, or of the ventral amygdalofugal fibers, produces components of the defense reaction, but lesions of the stria terminalis do not alter the response obtained by stimulating the amygdala. After completely interrupting the ventral amygdalofugal projections, defense reactions can no longer be obtained by stimulating the amygdaloid complex. These findings suggest that the basolateral part of the amygdaloid complex may play an important role in defense reactions.

Stimulation of the amygdaloid region in man produces feelings of fear, confusional states, disturbances of awareness, and amnesia for events taking place during the stimulation. Although rage is the most common behavioral response to amygdaloid stimulation in animals, it rarely is associated with temporal lobe seizures.

Bilateral lesions of the amygdaloid complex in animals consistently produce disturbances of emotional behavior. Animals become placid and display no reactions of fear, rage, or aggression. Previously dominant and abusive animals became tame and did not retaliate to the threats or molestations of other animals. Hypersexuality has been noted as a prominent feature in some experimental studies. Hypersexual behavior may occur only when the lesions concomitantly involve the pyriform cortex, since amygdaloid lesions sparing this region do not alter sexual behavior.

The *Klüver–Bucy syndrome* is characterized by conversion of wild intractable animals (monkeys) to docile beasts which show no evidence of fear, rage, or aggression. These animals display apparent "psychic blindness," a compulsion to examine objects visually, tactually, and orally, bizarre sexual behavior and certain changes in dietary habits. Almost all objects are examined, smelled, and mouthed; if the object is not edible, it is discarded. Hypersexuality is characterized by the indiscriminate partnerships sought with both male and female animals.

Observations in humans concerning the effects of bilateral lesions in the amygdaloid complex indicate that these lesions cause a decrease of aggressive and assaultive behavior. Stereotaxic lesions in the amygdaloid complex in human beings produce a marked reduction in emotional excitability and tend to normalize social behavior in individuals with severe behavior disturbances. Unilateral lesions in some cases proved sufficient to bring about improvement. Bilateral lesions did not produce the signs and symptoms suggestive of the Klüver–Bucy syndrome.

Visceral and autonomic responses include alterations of respiratory rate, rhythm, and amplitude, as well as inhibition of respiration. The most common response of amygdaloid stimulation in unanesthetized animals is an acceleration of the respiratory rate associated with a reduction in amplitude. Cardiovascular responses involve both increases and decreases in arterial blood pressure and alterations in heart rate. Pressor responses appear to predominate following amygdaloid stimulation in the unanesthetized animal. Gastrointestinal motility and secretion may be inhibited or activated, and both defecation and micturition may be induced. Piloerection, salivation, pupillary changes, and alterations of body temperature can occur. These responses may be either sympathetic or parasympathetic in nature.

Somatic responses obtained by stimulation of the amygdaloid complex include turning of the head and eyes to the opposite side, and complex rhythmic movements related to chewing, licking, and swallowing. The varied somatic and autonomic effects of electrical stimulation of the amygdaloid complex constitute an insignificant part of the syndrome produced by lesions in this complex.

Endocrine responses to stimulation of the amygdaloid nuclear complex include the release of ACTH and gonadotrophic hormone, and lactogenic responses. Stimulation of the amygdaloid areas that produce arousal and emotional responses also produce increased adrenocortical output. Bilateral lesions in the medial amygdaloid nuclei produce an elevation of serum levels of ACTH, presumably due to release of an inhibitory influence on the secretion of ACTH. Stimulation of the corticomedial division of the amygdala may induce ovulation, but this response is abolished by transection of the stria terminalis. The corticomedial amygdaloid nuclei in the female appear to have estrogen concentrating neurons which are part of a system of similar cells extending into hypothalamic and limbic structures. The amygdala also is concerned with the luteinizing (LH) and follicle-stimulating (FSH) hormones. It is quite clear that the amygdala participates with the hypothalamus in the control and regulation of hypophysial secretions.

The amygdaloid complex also plays a role in food and water intake. Bilateral ablations of the amygdala may result in striking hyperphagia, or in hypophagia. Lesions of the basolateral nucleus of the amygdala result in hyperphagia, while stimulation of this part of the amygdala produces an arrest of feeding behavior. It has been postulated that this part of the amygdaloid complex inhibits the lateral hypothalamic area, which is regarded as the feeding center of the hypothalamus. The corticomedial part of the amygdaloid complex is a facilitatory area concerned with food intake. Stimulation of this region produces increases in food intake. The amygdala appears to exert its influence upon feeding by modulating the activity of hypothalamic mechanisms.

The role of the amygdala as an integrator of autonomic and visceral functions through its reciprocal connections with the hypothalamus and visceral nuclei of the brain stem is widely accepted. It has become increasingly evident that the amygdala also is involved in complex cognitive functions that influence emotion and behavior in a global fashion. These functions appear to involve virtually all regions of the cerebral cortex and all sensory modalities. Cortical inputs to the amygdala derived from modality-specific association areas appear unique among central limbic structures. It has been suggested that the amygdala represents the interface between the hypothalamus and brain stem visceral centers, and regions of the cerebral cortex concerned with cognitive functions. The Klüver–Bucy syndrome provides an example of this interrelationship. In the presence of lesions in the amygdala, monkeys respond to visual stimuli in a bizarre fashion because the visual stimuli have no meaning. This may also apply to other sensory modalities whose cortical inputs to the amygdala are disconnected by destruction of the amygdalae. Broadly stated, impulses generated in sensory systems, the cerebral cortex, and probably

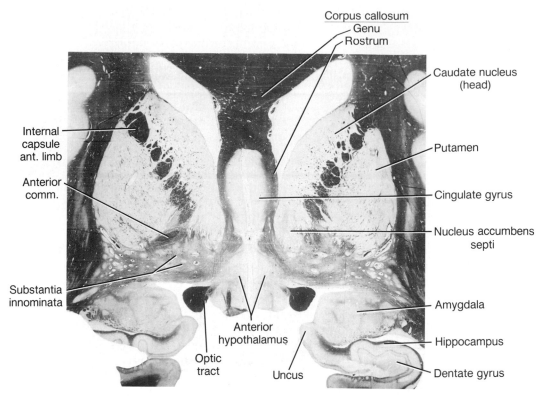

Figure 12.15. Section cut parallel to longitudinal axis of the brain stem through the genu and rostrum of the corpus callosum, the head of the caudate nucleus, the putamen, the substantia innominata, the amygdala, and the hippocampal formation. This section reveals the nucleus accumbens septi, ventromedial to the head of the caudate nucleus. The *substantia innominata* lies in the subcommissural region, ventral to the corpus striatum, and contains the large hyperchromic neurons known as the *basal nucleus of Meynert*. Cells of the basal nucleus are a major source of cholinergic innervation of the entire cerebral cortex. Human brain, Weigert's myelin stain.

still-undetermined neural structures trigger mechanisms that excite visceral and somatic systems whose activities in concert provide the physiological expression of emotion and goal-directed behavior. Reciprocal connections between areas of the cerebral cortex and the amygdala appear essential to the correlation of emotional expression and meaningful behavior.

SUBSTANTIA INNOMINATA

A heterogeneous group of telencephalic structures on the medial and ventral aspect of the cerebral hemispheres collectively are referred to as the basal forebrain. Despite the location of these structures near the surface of the brain, they lack a cortical organization. The basal forebrain extends from the olfactory tubercle rostrally to the hypothalamic region caudally and overlaps the area known as the anterior perforated substance (Fig. 12.2). Although the precise boundaries of the basal forebrain are not clearly defined, it appears generally agreed to include the septal area, the olfactory tubercle, parts of the amygdala, and the area under the anterior commissure known as the *substantia innominata* (Figs. 11.14, 12.13, and 12.15). The subcommissural region contains a number of cell groups in contact with fiber bundles traversing the region, which include the diagonal band (Broca), the anterior commissure, the medial forebrain bundle, the ansa lenticularis, the ansa peduncularis, and the

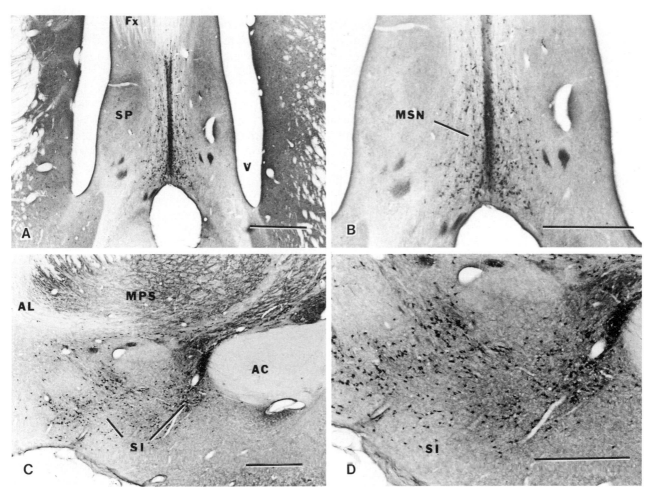

Figure 12.16. Cells in the septal nuclei and the substantia innominata immunoreactive to choline acetyltransferase (ChAT) in the monkey. *A* and *B*, Cells in the medial septal nuclei (MSN). *C* and *D* ChAT immunoreactive cells in portions of the substantia innominata (SI) ventral to the medial pallidal segment (MPS). Collections of large cholinergic neurons in this complex constitute the basal nuclei. The substantia innominata extends rostrally beneath the anterior commissure. *Abbreviations:* AC, anterior commissure; AL, ansa lenticularis; Fx, fibers of the fornix; SP, septum pellucidum; V, anterior horn of the lateral ventricle. Bar scales represent 1 mm.

inferior thalamic peduncle (Fig. 9.9). In the subcommissural region the most conspicuous cells are a group of magnocellular hyperchromic neurons, known as *nucleus basalis* (Fig. 12.16*C* and *D*). The term substantia innominata is used inconsistently and frequently as a synonym for the nucleus basalis (Figs. 11.14, 12.13, and 12.16). Large basophilic neurons with similar morphological characteristics are present in the medial septum, vertical and horizontal parts of the nucleus of the diagonal band, and in largest numbers along the ventral and lateral margins of the pallidal segments (Fig. 12.16). Similar cells are present in parts of the medullary laminae of the globus pallidus (Fig. 11.15*C*). In the nucleus basalis most neurons are cholinergic. Clusters of small GABA-immunoreactive cells are scattered among the large cholinergic neurons of the nucleus basalis. Afferents to the substantia innominata and the nucleus basalis arise mainly from the amygdala, portions of the insular and temporal cortex, and from the pyriform and entorhinal cortices. About 90% of the cholinergic neurons in the nucleus basalis project to widespread regions of the cerebral cortex. It has been suggested that the nucleus basalis may be the single major source of cholinergic innervation of the entire cerebral cortex. In this sense, the basal nucleus appears analogous to the raphe nuclei and the locus ceruleus, which constitute the major sources of serotonergic and noradrenergic innervation, respectively, to widespread regions of the cerebral cortex.

Interest in the basal nucleus (substantia innominata) is related to the discovery that neurons in this nucleus selectively degenerate in Alzheimer's disease and its variant, senile dementia of the Alzheimer's type, the most common dementia occurring in middle and late life. The loss of cholinergic input from neurons in the nucleus basalis appears to be a highly significant factor in the well-documented cortical cholinergic deficiency that occurs in these patients. Alzheimer's disease usually develops between the ages of 40 and 60 and is characterized by progressive dementia with apraxia and speech disturbances. There is loss of memory, slurred speech, and disorientation. The pathological picture is associated with diffuse degeneration of the cerebral cortex involving all layers, senile amyloid plaques in the cortex, intraneuronal fibrillary tangles, and selective degeneration of the cells in the nucleus basalis.

LIMBIC SYSTEM

On the medial surface of the cerebral hemisphere, a large arcuate convolution, formed primarily by the cingulate and parahippocampal gyri, surrounds the rostral brain stem and interhemispheric commissures. These gyri, which encircle the upper brain stem, constitute what Broca referred to as the "grand lobe limbique" (Fig. 12.17).

Limbic Lobe

The limbic lobe includes the subcallosal, cingulate, and parahippocampal gyri, as well as the underlying hippocampal formation and dentate gyrus (Fig. 12.17). The limbic lobe consists of *archicortex* (hippocampal formation and dentate gyrus), *paleocortex* (pyriform cortex of the anterior parahippocampal gyrus), and *juxtallocortex* or *mesocortex* (cingulate gyrus). The striking feature of the limbic lobe is that it appears early in phylogenesis and possesses a certain constancy in gross and microscopic structure. The extent to which these various cortical areas form a functional unit is not fully understood.

Limbic System

An even more extensive and inclusive designation is the *limbic system*. This term is used to include all of the limbic lobe (Fig. 12.17) as well as associated subcortical nuclei (Fig. 12.6), such as the amygdaloid complex, septal nuclei, hypothalamus, epithalamus, and various thalamic nuclei. The medial tegmental region of the midbrain also is regarded as a part of the limbic system since this region contains both ascending and descending pathways which directly or indirectly are related to the hippocampal formation and the amygdaloid nuclear complex (Figs. 12.7 and 12.14). Despite the heterogeneity and diffuse nature of the so-called limbic system, there are compelling observations that structures comprising this system are involved in neural circuitry that gives rise to a subcortical continuum that begins in the septal area and extends in a paramedian zone through the preoptic region and hypothalamus into the rostral mesencephalon. This longitudinal continuum has extensive reciprocal connections with the amygdala and the substantia innominata.

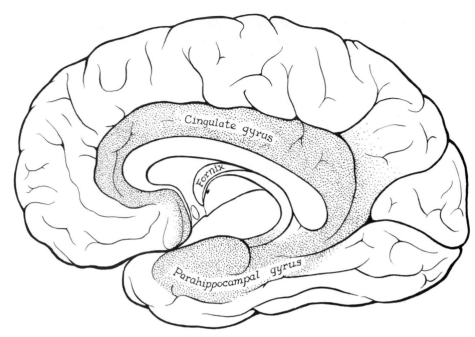

Figure 12.17.   Drawing of the medial surface of the brain with the *shaded* area indicating the limbic cortex. The limbic cortex lies at the most medial margin of the hemisphere (i.e., the limbus) and includes archicortex, paleocortex, and juxtallocortex.

The role of the cerebral cortex in the subjective aspects of emotion has been emphasized repeatedly, yet the neocortex appears to have relatively few hypothalamic connections. Both the amygdala and the substantia innominata have reciprocal connections with regions of the cerebral cortex, although projections from these structures to the cortex are most extensive. These nuclear masses appear to represent the principal interface between visceral and autonomic centers in the hypothalamus and brain stem and broad expanses of the cortical mantle. These extensive cortical connections of forebrain nuclei appear to provide part of the mechanism by which sensory stimuli and psychic phenomena influence emotional aspects of behavior. These connections may also explain the close adjustment of visceral and somatic activities in emotional expression.

Various visceral, somatic, and behavioral responses are obtained by electrical stimulation of the anterior cingulate cortex and the orbital-insular-temporal cortex. Elevation, as well as depression, of arterial blood pressure results from electrical stimulation of these regions in experimental animals. Points from which pressor and depressor effects can be obtained frequently are only a few millimeters apart. Effects on arterial pressure do not appear to be secondary to respiratory changes. Other autonomic responses obtained in experimental animals include inhibition of peristalsis, pupillary dilatation, salivation, and bladder contraction. Perhaps the most striking effect of stimulating these regions is profound inhibition of respiratory movements which involves mainly the inspiratory phase, occurs almost instantaneously, and cannot be held in abeyance for long.

Somatic effects of stimulating the anterior cingulate and the orbital-insular-temporal cortex resemble those obtained by stimulating the amygdala in awake animals. These responses include (1) inhibition of spontaneous movements; (2) chewing, licking, and swallowing movements;

and (3) the "arrest" reaction. The arrest reaction consists of an immediate cessation of other activities, an expression of attention or surprise, and movements of the head and eyes to the opposite side. Animals remain alert during stimulations and respond to external stimuli. Stimulation of posterior cingulate areas may induce enhanced grooming and seemingly pleasurable reactions. Neither unilateral nor bilateral ablations of the cingulate cortex, or of the cortex of the orbital-insular-temporal polar region, appear to disturb basic somatomotor or autonomic functions.

Electrical stimulation of certain subcortical structures via implanted electrodes in unanesthetized rats, cats, and monkeys produces a patterned self-stimulation behavior. In these studies the experimental arrangement is such that the animals can deliver an electrical stimulus to localized areas of their own brains by pressing a pedal. Self stimulations of the septal region, the anterior preoptic area, and the posterior hypothalamus by bar pressing may be at rates as high as 5000 per hour in the rat. The compulsive behavior seen in these situations, where the only reward is an electric shock to a localized region of the brain, suggests that the stimulus may provide a primary reinforcement for drives related to food or sex. Repeated self-stimulation may occur in the monkey from electrodes implanted in a variety of subcortical sites, such as the head of the caudate nucleus, the amygdaloid complex, the medial forebrain bundle, and the midbrain reticular formation. Self-stimulation of certain regions of the thalamus and hypothalamus may produce unpleasant or avoidance reactions, but these regions appear relatively small in number compared to those from which some gratification appears to result.

The limbic lobe and system occupy central positions in the neural mechanisms that govern behavior and emotion. Components of the limbic system appear to have their main afferent and efferent relationships with two great functional realms, the neocortex and the visceroendocrine periphery. The amygdala with complex connections, to and from the cerebral cortex and with subcortical autonomic centers, appears to represent the linchpin of the system.

SUGGESTED READINGS

AGGLETON, J. P., BURTON, M. J., AND PASSINGHAM, R. E. 1980. Cortical and subcortical afferents to the amygdala of the rhesus monkey (*Macaca mulatta*). Brain Res., **190**: 347–368.

ALHEID, G. F., AND HEIMER, L. 1988. New perspectives in basal forebrain organization of special relevance for neuropsychiatric disorders: The striatopallidal, amygdaloid and corticopedal components of the substantia innominata. Neuroscience, **27**: 1–39.

ALLEN, W. F. 1941. Effect of ablating the pyriform-amygdaloid areas and hippocampi on positive and negative olfactory conditioned reflexes and on conditioned olfactory differentiation. Am. J. Physiol., **132**: 81–92.

AMARAL, D. G., AVENDAÑO, C., AND BENOIT, R. 1989. Distribution of somatostatin-like immunoreactivity in the monkey amygdala. J. Comp. Neurol., **284**: 294–313.

AMARAL, D. G., AND BASSETT, J. L. 1989. Cholinergic innervation of the monkey amygdala: An immunohistochemical analysis with antisera to choline acetyltransferase. J. Comp. Neurol., **281**: 337–361.

AMOORE, J. E., JOHNSTON, J. W., JR., AND RUBIN, M. 1964. The stereochemical theory of odor. Sci. Am., **210**: 42–49.

ARIKUNI, T., AND KUBOTA, K. 1984. Substantia innominata projection to caudate nucleus in macaque monkeys. Brain Res., **302**: 184–189.

ARMSTRONG, D. M., SAPER, C. B., LEVEY, A. I., WAINER, B. H., AND TERRY, R. D. 1983. Distribution of cholinergic neurons in rat brain: Demonstration by immunocytochemical localization of choline acetyltransferase. J. Comp. Neurol., **216**: 53–68.

BOVARD, E. W., AND GLOOR, P. 1961. Effect of amygdaloid lesions on plasma corticosterone response of the albino rat to emotional stress. Experientia, **17**: 521.

BRADY, J. V. 1960. Temporal and emotional effects related to intracranial electrical self-stimulation. In S. R. RAMEY AND D. S. O'DOHERTY (Editors), *Electrical Studies on the Unanesthetized Brain*. Paul B. Hoeber, New York, Ch. 3, pp. 52–77.

BROADWELL, R. D. 1975. Olfactory relationships of the telencephalon and diencephalon in the rabbit. II. An autoradiographic and horseradish peroxidase study of the efferent connections of the anterior olfactory nucleus. J. Comp. Neurol., **164**: 389–410.

BRODAL, A. 1947. The hippocampus and the sense of smell. Brain, **70**: 179–222.

BROWN-GRANT, K., AND RAISMAN, G. 1972. Reproductive function in the rat following selective destruction of afferent fibres to the hypothalamus from the limbic system. Brain Res., **46**: 23–42.

CARPENTER, M. B. AND SUTIN, J. 1983. Human Neuroanatomy, 8th Ed. Williams & Wilkins, Baltimore, pp. 872.

CLARK, W. E. L. 1951. The projection of the olfactory epithelium on the olfactory bulb in the rabbit. J. Neurol. Neurosurg. Psychiatry, **14**: 1–10.

CLARK, W. E. L. 1957. Inquiries into the anatomical basis of olfactory discrimination. Proc. R. Soc. Lond. (Biol.), **146**: 299–319.

CLARK, W. E. L., AND WARWICK, R. T. 1946. The pattern of olfactory innervation. J. Neurol. Neurosurg. Psychiatry, **9**: 101–111.

COWAN, W. M., RAISMAN, G., AND POWELL, T. P. S. 1965. The connexions of the amygdala. J. Neurol. Neurosurg. Psychiatry, **28**: 137–151.

DAITZ, H. M., AND POWELL, T. P. S. 1954. Studies of the connections of the fornix system. J. Neurol. Neurosurg. Psychiatry, **17**: 75–82.

DANIELSEN, E. H., MAGNUSON, D. J., AND GRAY, T. S. 1989. The central amygdaloid innervation of the dorsal vagal complex in rat: A *Phaseolus vulgaris* leucogglutinin lectin anterograde tracing study. Brain Res. Bull., **22**: 705–715.

DAVIES, P., AND MALONEY, A. J. P. 1976. Selective loss of central cholinergic neurons in Alzheimer's disease. Lancet, **2**: 1403.

ELEFTHERIOU, B. E., ZOLOVICK, A. J., AND PEARSE, R. 1966. Effects of amygdaloid lesions on pituitary-adrenal axis in the deer-mouse. Proc. Soc. Exp. Biol. Med., **122**: 1259.

FEINDEL, W., AND PENFIELD, W. 1954. Localization of discharge in temporal lobe automatism. Arch. Neurol. Psychiat., **72**: 605–630.

FONBERG, E. 1968. The role of the amygdaloid nucleus in animal behavior. Prog. Brain Res., **22**: 273–281.

FULWILER, C. E., AND SAPER, C. B. 1984. Subnuclear organization of the efferent connections of the parabrachial nucleus in the rat. Brain Res. Rev., **7**: 229–259.

GETCHELL, T. V., AND SHEPHERD, G. M. 1975. Short-axon cells in the olfactory bulb: Dendrodendritic synaptic interactions. J. Physiol. (Lond.), **251**: 523–548.

GLOOR, P. 1960. Amygdala. In J. FIELD (Editor), *Handbook of Physiology*, Sect. 1, Vol. II. American Physiological Society, Washington, DC, Ch. 57, pp. 1395–1420.

GLOOR, P. 1972. Temporal lobe epilepsy: Its possible contribution to the understanding of the functional significance of the amygdala and of its interaction with neocortical-temporal mechanisms. In B. E. ELEFTHERIOU (Editor), *The Neurobiology of the Amygdala*. Plenum Press, New York, pp. 423–457.

GREEN, J. D. 1964. The hippocampus. Physiol. Rev., **44**: 561–608.

HALÁSZ, N., LJUNGDAHL, Å., AND HÖKFELT, T. 1978. Transmitter histochemistry of the rat olfactory bulb. II. Fluorescence histochemical, autoradiographic and electron microscopic localization of monoamines. Brain Res., **154**: 253–272.

HALÁSZ, N., LJUNGDAHL, Å., AND HÖKFELT, T. 1979. Transmitter histochemistry of the rat olfactory bulb. III. Autoradiographic localization of [³H] GABA. Brain Res., **167**: 221–240.

HALÁSZ, N., AND SHEPHERD, G. M. 1983. Neurochemistry of the vertebrate of olfactory bulb. Neuroscience, **10**: 579–619.

HERZOG, A. G., AND VAN HOESEN, G. W. 1976. Temporal neocortical afferent connections to the amygdala in the rhesus monkey. Brain Res., **115**: 57–70.

HILTON, S. M., AND ZBROŻYNA, A. 1963. Defense reaction from the amygdala and its afferent connections. J. Physiol., **165**: 160–173.

IWAI, E., AND YUKIE, M. 1987. Amygdalofugal and amygdalopetal connections with modality-specific visual cortical areas in macaques (*Macaca fuscata, M. mulatta,* and *M. fascicularis*). J. Comp. Neurol., **261**: 362–387.

JAYARAMAN, A. 1985. Organization of thalamic projections in the nucleus accumbens and caudate nucleus in cats and its relation with hippocampal and other subcortical afferents. J. Comp. Neurol., **231**: 396–420.

KAADA, B. R. 1972. Stimulation and regional ablation of the amygdaloid complex with reference to functional representation. In B. E. ELEFTHERIOU (Editor), *The Neurobiology of the Amygdala*. Plenum Press, New York, pp. 205–281.

KATZMAN, R. 1976. The prevalence and malignancy of Alzheimer's disease. A major killer. Arch. Neurol., **33**: 217–218.

KELLEY, A. E., DOMESICK, V. B., AND NAUTA, W. J. H. 1982. The amygdalostriate projection in the rat: An anatomical study by anterograde and retrograde tracing methods. Neuroscience, **7**: 615–630.

KLÜVER, H. 1952. Brain mechanisms and behavior with special reference to the rhinencephalon. Lancet, **72**: 567–574.

KLÜVER, H., AND BUCY, P. 1939. Preliminary analysis of functions of the temporal lobe in monkeys. Arch. Neurol. Psychiatry, **42**: 979–1000.

KOSEL, K. C., VAN HOESEN, G. W., AND WEST, J. R. 1981. Olfactory bulb projections to the parahippocampal area of the rat. J. Comp. Neurol., **198**: 467–482.

KREIG, W. J. S. 1953. *Functional Neuroanatomy*. Blakiston Company, New York.

KRETTEK, J. E., AND PRICE, J. L. 1974. Projections from the amygdala to the perirhinal and entorhinal cortices and the subiculum. Brain Res., **71**: 150–154.

KRETTEK, J. E., AND PRICE, J. L. 1978. Amygdaloid projections to subcortical structures within the forebrain and brainstem in the rat and cat. J. Comp. Neurol., **178**: 225–254.

LORENTE DE NÓ, R. 1934. Studies on the structure of the cerebral cortex. II. Continuation of the study of the ammonic system. J. Psychol. Neurol., **46**: 113–177.

MACRIDES, F., AND DAVIS, B. J. 1983. The olfactory bulb. In P. C. Emson (Editor), *Chemical Neuroanatomy*. Raven Press, New York, pp. 391–426.

MEHLER, W. R. 1980. Subcortical afferent connections of the amygdala in the monkey. J. Comp. Neurol., **190**: 733–762.

MEIBACH, R. C., AND SIEGEL, A. 1977. Efferent connections of the hippocampal formation in the rat. Brain Res., **124**: 197–224.

MESULAM, M.-M., AND GEULA, C. 1988. Nucleus basalis (Ch4) and cortical cholinergic innervation in the human brain: Observations based on the distribution of the acetylcholinesterase and choline acetyltransferase. J. Comp. Neurol., **275**: 216–240.

MESULAM, M.-M., AND MUFSON, E. J. 1984. Neural inputs into the nucleus basalis of the substantia innominata (Ch4) in the rhesus monkey. Brain, **107**: 253–274.

MESULAM, M.-M., MUFSON, E. J., LEVEY, A. I., AND WAINER, B. H. 1983. Cholinergic innervation of cortex of the basal forebrain: Cytochemistry and cortical connections of the septal area, diagonal band nuclei, nucleus basalis (substantia innominata) and hypothalamus in the rhesus monkey. J. Comp. Neurol., **214**: 170–197.

METTLER, F. A. 1948. *Neuroanatomy*, Ed. 2, C. V. Mosby Co., St. Louis.

NARABAYASHI, H., NAGAO, T., SAITO, Y., YOSHIDA, M., AND NAGAHATA, M. 1963. Sterotaxic amygdalotomy for behavior disorders. Arch. Neurol., **9**: 1–16.

NAUTA, W. J. H. 1958. Hippocampal projections and related neural pathways to the midbrain in the cat. Brain, **81**: 319–340.

NAUTA, W. J. H. 1962. Neural associations of the amygdaloid complex in the monkey. Brain, **85**: 505–520.

NAUTA, W. J. H. 1972. The central visceromotor system: A general survey. In C. H. HOCKMAN (Editor), *Limbic System Mechanisms and Automatic Function*. Charles C Thomas, Springfield, IL, Ch. 2, pp. 21–33.

OLDS, J., AND MILNER, P. 1954. Positive reinforcement produced by electrical stimulation of septal area and other regions of the rat brain. J. Comp. Physiol. Psychol., **47**: 419–427.

OOMURA, Y., ONO, T., AND OOYAMA, H. 1970. Inhibitory action of the amygdala on the lateral hypothalamic area in rats. Nature, **228**: 1108–1110.

PAPEZ, J. W. 1937. A proposed mechanism of emotion. Arch. Neurol. Psychiat., **38**: 725–743.

PARENT, A., CSONKA, C., AND ÉTIENNE, P. 1984. The occurrence of large acetylcholinesterase-containing neurons in human neostriatum as disclosed in normal and Alzheimer's disease brains. Brain Res., **291**: 154–158.

POTTER, H., AND NAUTA, W. J. H. 1979. A note on the problem of olfactory associations of the orbitofrontal cortex in the monkey. Neuroscience, **4**: 361–369.

POWELL, T. P. S., COWAN, W. M., AND RAISMAN, G. 1965. The central olfactory connexions. J. Anat., **99**: 791–813.

PRICE, J. L., AND AMARAL, D. G. 1981. An autoradiographic study of the projections of the central nucleus of the monkey amygdala. J. Neurosci., **1**: 1242–1259.

PRICE, J. L., AND POWELL, T. P. S. 1970. The mitral and short axon cells of the olfactory bulb. J. Cell Sci., **7**: 631–652.

RAISMAN, G., COWAN, W. M., AND POWELL, T. P. S. 1965. The extrinsic afferent, commissural and association fibres of the hippocampus. Brain, **88**: 963–996.

RAISMAN, G., COWAN, W. M., AND POWELL, T. P. S. 1966. An experimental analysis of the efferent projections of the hippocampus. Brain, **89**: 83–108.

ROSENE, D. L., AND VAN HOESEN, G. W. 1977. Hippocampal efferents reach widespread areas of cerebral cortex and amygdala in the rhesus monkey. Science, **198**: 315–317.

RUSSCHEN, F. T., AMARAL, D. G., AND PRICE, J. L. 1985. The afferent connections of the substantia innominata in the monkey, *Macaca fascicularis*. J. Comp. Neurol., **242**: 1–27.

RUSSCHEN, F. T., AMARAL, D. G., AND PRICE, J. L. 1987. The afferent input to the magnocellular division of the mediodorsal thalamic nucleus in the monkey, *Macaca fascicularis*. J. Comp. Neurol., **256**: 175–210.

RUSSCHEN, F. T., BAKST, I., AMARAL, D. G., AND PRICE, J. L. 1985. The amygdalostriatal projections in the monkey. An anterograde tracing study. Brain Res., **329**: 241–257.

SHEPARD, G. 1979. *The Synaptic Organization of the Brain*. Oxford University Press, New York, pp. 436.

SHIOSAKA, S., SAKANAKA, M., INAGAKI, S., SENBA, E., HARA, Y., TAKATSUKI, K. TAKAGI, H., KAWAI, Y., AND TOHYAMA, M. 1983. Putative neurotransmitters in the amygdaloid complex with special reference to peptidergic pathways. In P. C. EMSON (Editor), *Chemical Neuroanatomy*. Raven Press, New York, pp. 359–389.

SMITH, Y., PARENT, A., SÉQUELA, P., AND DESCARRIES, L. 1987. Distribution of GABA-immunoreactive neurons in the basal ganglia of the squirrel monkey (*Saimiri sciureus*). J. Comp. Neurol., **259**: 50–64.

SWANN, H. G. 1934. The function of the brain in olfaction. II. The results of destruction of olfactory and other nervous structures upon the discriminaton of odors. J. Comp. Neurol., **59**: 176–201.

SWANSON, L. W., AND COWAN, W. M. 1977. An autoradiographic study of the organization of the efferent connections of the hippocampal formation in the rat. J. Comp. Neurol., **172**: 49–84.

SWITZER, R. C., DeOLMOS, J., AND HEIMER, L. 1985. Olfactory system. In G. PAXINOS (Editor), *The Rat Nervous System*. Academic Press, Sydney, Australia, pp. 1–36.

TAKEUCHI, Y., MATSUSHIMA, S., MATSUSHIMA, R., AND HOPKINS, D. A. 1983. Direct amygdaloid projections to the dorsal motor nucleus of the vagus nerve: A light and electron microscopic study in the rat. Brain Res., **280**: 143–147.

TANABE, T., YARITA, H., IINO, M., OOSHIMA, Y., AND TAKAGI, S. F. 1975. An olfactory projection area in orbitofrontal cortex of the monkey. J. Neurophysiol., **38**: 1269–1283.

TURNER, B. H., MISHKIN, M., AND KNAPP, M. 1980. Organization of the amygdalopetal projections from modality-specific cortical association areas in the monkey. J. Comp. Neurol., **191**: 515–543.

URSIN, H., AND KAADA, B. R. 1960. Functional localization within the amygdaloid complex in the cat. Electroencephalogr. Clin. Neurophysiol., **12**: 1–20.

VALVERDE, F. 1965. *Studies on the Piriform Lobe*. Harvard University Press, Cambridge, Mass., 131 pp.

VEENING, J. G., SWANSON, L. W., AND SAWCHENKO, P. E. 1984. The organization of projections from the central nucleus of the amygdala to brainstem sites involved in central autonomic regulation: A combined retrograde transport-immunohistochemical study. Brain Res., **303**: 337–357.

VELASCO, M. E., AND TALEISNIK, S. 1969. Release of gonadotropins induced by amygdaloid stimulation in the rat. Endocrinology, **84**: 132–139.

VICTOR, M. 1964. Functions of memory and learning in man and the relationship to lesions in the temporal lobe and diencephalon. In M. A. B. BRAZIER (Editor), *Brain Function, RNA in Brain Functions: Memory and Learning*, Vol. III. American Institute of Biological Sciences, Washington, DC.

WALAAS, I. 1983. The hippocampus. In P. C. EMSON (Editor), *Chemical Neuroanatomy*, Raven Press, New York, pp. 337–358.

WANG, H. S. 1977. Dementia of old age. In W. L. SMITH AND M. KINSBORN (Editors), *Aging and Dementia*. Spectrum, New York, pp. 1–24.

WHITEHOUSE, P. J., PRICE, D. L., CLARK, A. W., COYLE, J. T., AND DeLONG, M. R. 1981. Alzheimer's disease: evidence for selective loss of cholinergic neurons in the nucleus basalis. Ann Neurol., **10**: 122–126.

WHITEHOUSE, P. J., PRICE, D. L., STRUBLE, R. G., CLARK, A. W., COYLE, J. T., AND DeLONG, M. R. 1982. Alzheimer's disease and senile dementia: loss of neurons in the basal forebrain. Science, **215**: 1237–1239.

ZBROŻYNA, A. W. 1972. The organization of the defense reaction elicited from amygdala and its connections. In B. E. ELEFTHERIOU (Editor), *The Neurobiology of the Amygdala*. Plenum Press, New York, pp. 597–606.

ZOLOVICK, A. J. 1972. Effects of lesions and electrical stimulation of the amygdala on hypothalamic-hypophyseal regulation. In B. E. ELEFTHERIOU (Editor), *The Neurobiology of the Amygdala*. Plenum Press, New York, pp. 643–683.

13

The Cerebral Cortex

The cerebral cortex has an area of approximately 2.5 square feet, but only a third of this is found on the free surface. The cortex is thickest over the crest of a convolution, thinnest in the depth of a sulcus, and contains an estimated 14 billion neurons.

The cerebral cortex develops from portions of the telencephalic vesicle. Cells originating from the germinal zone surrounding the lumen migrate peripherally to form the cortical mantle. After the sixth month of fetal life, cortical neurons begin to form six horizontal layers. Cells formed at the same time migrate to the same cortical layer; cells migrating later pass through deep layers to form more superfical laminae. A six-layer cellular arrangement is characteristic of the entire neopallium, which is referred to as the *neocortex*, isocortex, or homogenetic cortex. The *paleopallium* (olfactory cortex) and the *archipallium* (hippocampal formation and dentate gyrus) have three basic layers and collectively constitute the *allocortex* or *heterogenetic cortex*.

CORTICAL CELLS AND FIBERS

Although the cerebral cortex contains a prodigious number of cells, the number of cell types is surprisingly small. The principal types of cells in the cerebral cortex are classified as pyramidal, stellate, and fusiform (Fig. 13.1).

The *pyramidal cells* have the form of a pyramid with an *apical dendrite* extending upward toward the pial surface and numerous basal dendrites projecting horizontally from the cell body. The axon emerges from the base of the cell and enters the white matter. Pyramidal cells vary in height from 10 to 50 μm, with the giant pyramidal cells, found in the precentral gyrus, more than 100 μm in height.

Stellate, or *granule cells* have a polygonal shape, scant cytoplasm, and range in size from 4 to 8 μm. These cells have numerous dendrites and a short axon. Stellate cells are most numerous in layer IV (Figs. 13.1, 13.2, and 13.3).

The *fusiform* or *spindle cells* are found mainly in the deepest cortical layers, with their long axis vertical to the surface. Numerous dendrites arise from the poles of the cell; the axon arises from the lower part of the cell body and enters the white matter (Fig. 13.1).

Other cell types found in the cortex are the *horizontal cells of Cajal*, and the cells with ascending axons, known as the *cells of Martinotti*. Small horizontal fusiform cells are found in the most superficial cortical layer (Fig. 13.4). Axons of Martinotti cells extend toward the surface.

Fibers in the cerebral cortex are disposed both radially and tangentially. Radially arranged fiber bundles run vertically from the medullary substance toward the cortical surface (Fig. 13.1). They include axons of

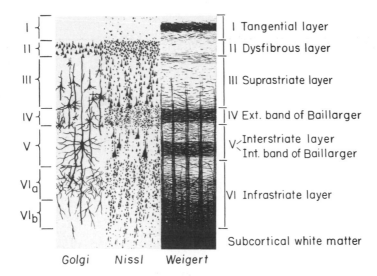

I Tangential layer

II Dysfibrous layer

III Suprastriate layer

IV Ext. band of Baillarger

V Interstriate layer
Int. band of Baillarger

VI Infrastriate layer

Subcortical white matter

Golgi   Nissl   Weigert

Figure 13.1. Cell layers and fiber arrangements in the human cerebral cortex, as revealed by Golgi, Nissl, and Weigert stains. Semischematic. (After Brodmann, 1909.)

pyramidal, fusiform, and stellate cells, which leave the cortex as projection or association fibers, and the entering afferent projection and association fibers, which terminate within the cortex. Tangential fibers run parallel to the cortical surface. These fiber bundles are composed of the terminal branches of afferent projection and association fibers, axons of horizontal and granule cells, and collateral branches of pyramidal and fusiform cells. Horizontal fibers in large part represent terminal portions of radial fibers. Tangential fibers are not distributed evenly throughout the cortex but are concentrated at varying depths into horizontal bands. The two most prominent bands are known as the *bands of Baillarger*, which form delicate white stripes in sections of the fresh cortex (Figs. 13.1 and 13.14).

CORTICAL LAYERS

In Nissl-stained sections the cell bodies are arranged in superimposed horizontal layers. Layers are distinguished by the types, density, and arrangement of their cells. The lamination seen in myelin-sheath-stained sections is determined primarily by the disposition of horizontal or tangential fibers, which vary in different layers (Figs. 13.1, 13.2, and 13.3.). The *neopallium* (neocortex or isocortex), which forms 90% of the hemispheric surface, has six fundamental layers.

The following layers are distinguished in the neocortex in passing from the pial surface to the underlying white matter (Figs. 13.1, 13.2, 13.3, and 13.4):

I. The *molecular layer* containing cells with horizontal axons and Golgi type II cells.

II. The *external granular* layer consisting of closely packed granule cells.

III. The *external pyramidal layer* composed of two sublayers of pyramidal neurons.

IV. The *internal granular layer* composed of closely packed stellate cells, many of which have short axons ramifying within the layer. Some larger stellate cells project axons to deeper layers. Myelinated fibers of the external band of Baillarger form a prominent horizontal plexus in this layer (Fig. 13.1).

Figure 13.2. Cytoarchitecture of frontal agranular (areas 6 and 4) and granular cortex (area 46). (After Campbell, 1905.)

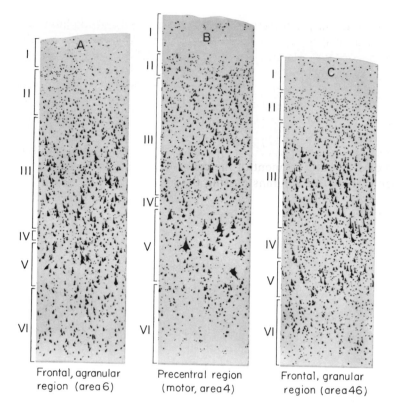

Frontal, agranular region (area 6)

Precentral region (motor, area 4)

Frontal, granular region (area 46)

Figure 13.3. Cytoarchitecture of parietal (area 39) and occipital (areas 18 and 17) cortex. Area 17 represents koniocortex, composed mainly of small granule cells. (After Campbell, 1905.)

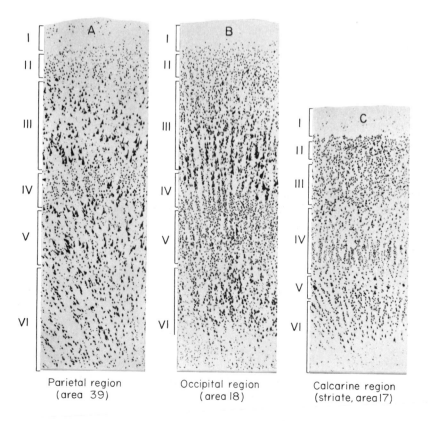

Parietal region (area 39)

Occipital region (area 18)

Calcarine region (striate, area 17)

V. The *internal pyramidal layer* consisting mainly of medium and large-size pyramidal neurons. Apical dendrites of large pyramidal cells ascend to the molecular layer (Figs. 13.1 and 13.5). Axons of pyramidal cells leave the cortex chiefly as projection fibers.

VI. The *multiform layer* containing predominantly spindle-shaped cells whose long axes are perpendicular to the cortical surface. Axons of these cells enter the white matter mainly as projection fibers. (Figs. 13.1 and 13.5).

Besides the horizontal cellular lamination, the cortex also exhibits a vertical or radial arrangement of the cells, which gives the appearance of slender vertical cell columns passing through the whole thickness of the cortex (Fig. 13.3). These vertical columns are quite distinct in the parietal, occipital, and temporal lobes but are practically absent in the frontal lobe (Fig. 13.2). The columnar arrangement of cells in the cerebral cortex is determined largely by the mode of termination of corticocortical afferents.

INTERRELATION OF CORTICAL NEURONS

The structure of the cerebral cortex as seen in Nissl or myelin sheath–stained sections is incomplete; these stains show only the type and arrangement of cell bodies, or the course and distribution of myelinated fibers. An understanding of the neuronal relationships and of the intracortical circuits can be obtained only by impregnation methods, which give a total picture of the cell body and all its processes (i.e., the Golgi method). The arrangement of the axonal and dendritic branchings within the cerebral cortex form one of its most constant features (Fig. 13.4).

The afferent fibers of the cortex include projection fibers from the thalamus, association fibers from other cortical areas, and commissural fibers from the opposite side. The thalamocortical fibers, especially the specific afferents from the ventral tier thalamic nuclei and the geniculate bodies, pass unbranched to layer IV (Figs. 4.1, 4.2, 4.3, 6.9, 9.12, 9.28, and 13.4). Fibers of the so-called nonspecific thalamocortical system project directly to the cortex from parts of the rostral intralaminar thalamic nuclei. The synaptic termination of nonspecific fibers in the cortex is chiefly axodendritic and widely distributed in all layers.

Commissural fibers arise from cells in all cortical regions and interconnect homologous cortical areas via the corpus callosum. Exceptions to this generalization are found in the regions of the primary motor (area 4) and somesthetic cortex (S I) that represent the hand and foot, in the visual cortex, area 17, and in parts of the auditory cortex. Commissural cells are large pyramidal cells in deep parts of layer III (Fig. 13.5). Cortical afferents from commissural neurons extend throughout all cortical layers and fill a column about 200 to 300 μm in diameter. Ipsilateral corticocortical association fibers arise from cells in more superficial parts of layer III and from parts of layer II (Fig. 13.4).

All the pyramidal cells of layer V give off basilar dendrites to their own layer and an apical dendrite extending toward the molecular layer (Figs. 13.4 and 13.5). The spindle cells of layer VI have similar branches. The axons of pyramidal and spindle neurons are continued as projection fibers. All of these axons send horizontal collaterals to layers V and VI (Fig. 13.5).

The horizontal laminar arrangements of the cells in the cerebral cortex has served as a major criteria to map the distinctive cytoarchitec-

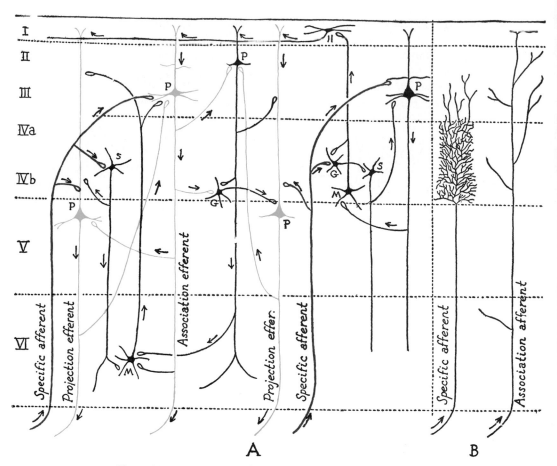

Figure 13.4. *A*, Diagram of some intracortical circuits. Synaptic terminals are represented by loops. *Red*, afferent thalamocortical fibers; *blue*, efferent cortical neurons; *black*, intracortical neurons. *G*, granule cells; *H*, horizontal cell; *M*, Martinotti cell; *P*, pyramidal cells; *S*, stellate cells. *B*, Indicates the mode of termination of afferent cortical fibers. (Based on Lorente de Nó, 1949.)

tonic areas. This lamination also serves to segregate different efferent projections from the cortex (Fig. 13.5). Each of the major efferent pathways emanating from sensory-motor cortex has a specific laminar or sublaminar origin. The somata of the majority of cells whose axons are distributed intracortically (both ipsilaterally and contralaterally) lie in the supragranular layers (layers II and III). Cortical neurons whose axons project to subcortical structures are located in the infragranular layers, particularly layer V and VI. In the infragranular layers (layers V and VI) the somata of corticostriate neurons lie in the most superficial part of layer V while somata giving rise to corticospinal and corticotectal fibers are in the deepest part of the same layer. Cells in layer VI of the cortex give rise to corticothalamic projections. Cells giving rise to particular efferent connections are of nearly the same size and do not vary in their laminar distribution. Only neurons giving rise to corticospinal fibers show great variation in cell size.

Functional Columnar Organization

Studies of the somatosensory and visual cortex provide evidence that a vertical column of cells, extending across all cellular layers, constitutes the elementary functional cortical unit. This conclusion in the somatosensory cortex is supported by the following: (1) neurons of a particular vertical column are all related to the same, or nearly the same,

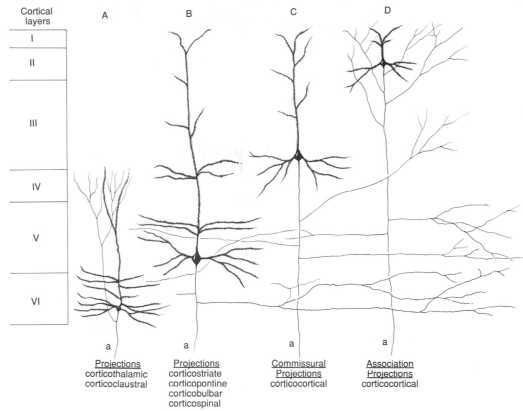

Cortical layers

I

II

III

IV

V

VI

A

B

C

D

a

a

a

a

Projections
corticothalamic
corticoclaustral

Projections
corticostriate
corticopontine
corticobulbar
corticospinal

Commissural
Projections
corticocortical

Association
Projections
corticocortical

Figure 13.5. Schematic diagram of the major projection neurons in different layers of the cerebral cortex. Cortical layers are indicated on the *left* by *Roman numerals* and *columns A, B, C,* and *D* depict individual projection neurons in different layers which have separate targets. Subcortical projections of neurons in column *B* arise from pyramidal cells located in different parts of layer V, with corticostriate neurons most superficial, and corticospinal neurons in the deepest part. Intracortical ramifications of dendrites and axonal collaterals are shown. Projection axons (a) are indicated as they enter the white matter. (Redrawn from Jones (1986) with permission of the author and Plenum Press, New York.)

peripheral receptive field; (2) neurons of the same vertical column are activated by the same kind of peripheral stimulus; and (3) all cells of a vertical column discharge at more or less the same latency following a brief peripheral stimulus. The topographic pattern present on the cortical surface extends throughout its depth. Studies of the visual (striate) cortex demonstrate similar discrete functional columns extending from the pial surface to the white matter that are responsive to specific kinds of retinal stimulation. Functional cell columns are arranged radially, perpendicular to the cortical layers and display variations in size and cross-sectional area. Complex axonal branching suggests that intracortical circuits involve cells in all parts of the column. These vertical circuits are interconnected by short neuronal links, represented primarily by the short axons of granule cells. Through these linkages, cortical excitation may spread horizontally and involve a progressively larger number of vertical units (Fig. 13.4).

The cerebral cortex has been envisaged as a mosaic of columnar units of remarkably similar internal structure. In addition to the functional columnar arrangement described in the sensory cortical areas, there are corticocortical columns delineated by the pattern of termination of association and commissural fibers. Columnar units of corticocortical projections and the functional columns of the sensory cortex are roughly the

Figure 13.6. Photomicrographs of layer V of the primary motor cortex (M I) in the rat processed immunocytochemically for glutamate (*A*) and aspartate (*B*). Colloidal gold coupled with enzymatically inactive horseradish peroxidase conjugated to wheat germ agglutinin (WGAapoHRP-Au) injected into the spinal cord retrogradely labeled corticospinal neurons (*black granules*). Three types of neurons can be seen: (a) cells immunoreactive for glutamate or aspartate only (*arrows*), (2) cells retrogradely labeled only with WGAapoHRP-Au (*arrowheads*), and (3) cells retrogradely labeled with WGAapoHRP-Au and immunoreactive for either glutamate or aspartate (*tailed arrows*). Calibration: 50 μm. (Courtesy of Drs. Giuffrida, Istituto di Fisiologia Umana, Catania, Italy, and Rustioni, University of North Carolina; from Giuffrida and Rustioni, 1989, with permission of the authors and Alan R. Liss, Inc., New York.)

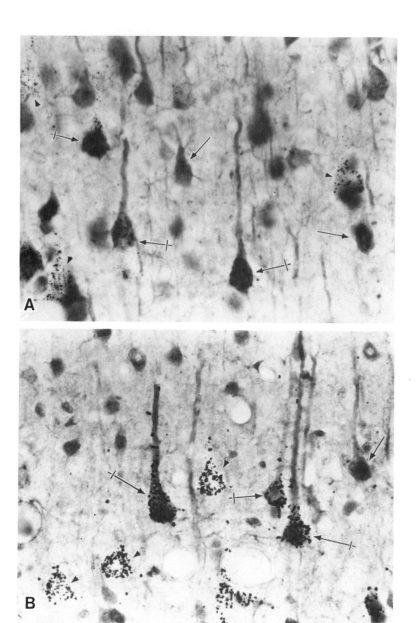

same size. Inputs from the thalamus and other cortical areas are considered to be processed through a column-oriented circuitry composed of both excitatory and inhibitory neurons. Both excitatory and inhibitory influences within the cerebral cortex are exerted upon pyramidal cells that represent the principal cortical output neurons.

CYTOCHEMISTRY OF THE CEREBRAL CORTEX

Glutamate (GLU) and aspartate (ASP) are generally accepted as the most widely distributed excitatory neurotransmitters in the CNS. Although GLU is involved in basic cellular metabolism, it satisfies the criteria for classification as a neurotransmitter. There are strong indications that GLU and ASP are the principal neurotransmitters of most cortical projection neurons, forming corticospinal, corticostriate, corticothalamic and corticopontine pathways (Fig. 13.6).

γ-Aminobutyric acid (GABA), widely accepted as the most important central nervous system inhibitory neurotransmitter, plays a partic-

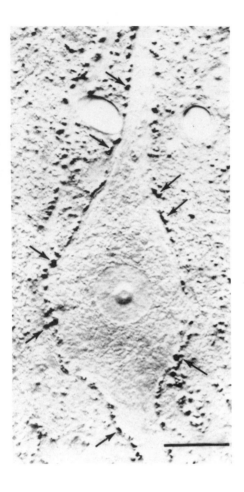

Figure 13.7. Glutamic acid decarboxylase (GAD) immunoreactive terminals (*arrows*) on the soma and proximal dendrites of a pyramidal neuron in the motor cortex of a monkey. Photographed with Nomarski optics. Calibration: 20 μm. (From Houser et al., 1984; courtesy of Dr. Carolyn R. Houser, Brain Research Institute, UCLA, with the permission of Plenum Press, New York.)

ularly important role in cortical function. GABAergic neurons are intrinsic nonpyramidal cortical neurons whose dendrites form both vertical and horizontal arborizations. The unique feature of GABAergic cortical neurons is their extensive synaptic contacts with receptive surfaces of pyramidal neurons (Fig. 13.7). These intrinsic neurons are organized to inhibit pyramidal output neurons irrespective of their sources of excitation. Cortical sites identified as the focus of chronic epileptiform activity, demonstrate significant loss of GABA in cells and terminals. Barbiturates and anticonvulsant drugs are considered to potentiate GABAergic inhibition.

Peptides identified mainly in the cerebral cortex include cholecystokinin (CCK), vasoactive intestinal polypeptide (VIP), and neuropeptide Y (NPY). These peptides are found in superficial layers close to capillaries and may control local metabolism and blood flow. VIP is a potent vasodilator and NPY is a vasoconstrictor (Fig. 13.8). Somatostatin-like immunoreactivity in the cortex is significantly reduced in Alzheimer's disease.

Although cholinergic, adrenergic, and serotonergic cells are not present in the cortex, fibers and terminals contain these neurotransmitters. Neurons projecting these fibers to the cortex via extrathalamic pathways lie in the basal forebrain and the brain stem. Cholinergic neurons in the substantia innominata (Figs. 12.15 and 12.16) project directly to widespread neocortical areas. Noradrenergic fibers in the cerebral cortex originate from the locus ceruleus (Figs. 6.28 and 6.29). Serotonergic fibers and terminals in the cortex arise from the median and dorsal nuclei of the raphe (Fig. 6.30). While the cerebral cortex does not contain dopa-

Figure 13.8. *A, B,* Neurons immunoreactive to neuropeptide Y (NPY) in layer VI of the cingulate gyrus of the monkey. NPY coexists with somatostatin (SRIF) in some cortical neurons in the rat and human. Calibration bars = 10 μm.

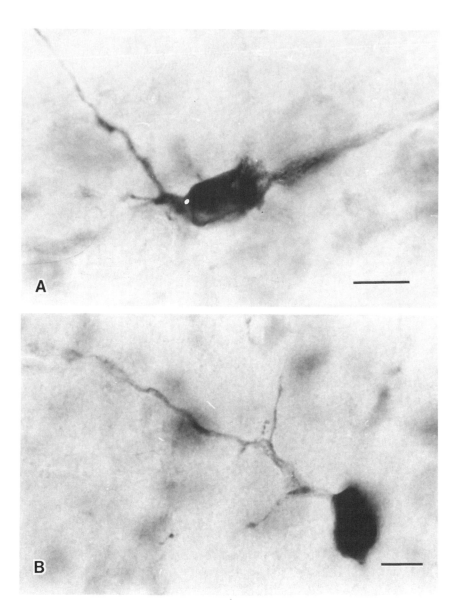

minergic neurons, it receives a rich innervation of dopamine fibers distributed preferentially in the frontal and temporal cortex. The laminar distribution of dopaminergic fibers suggests that this neurotransmitter may modulate activities of corticocortical, corticostriate, and corticobulbar projections.

CORTICAL AREAS

The cerebral cortex does not have a uniform structure. It has been mapped and divided into a number of distinctive areas that differ from each other in total thickness, in the thickness and density of individual layers, and in the arrangement and number of cells and fibers. Structural variations are so extreme in some areas that the basic six-layered pattern is practically obscured. Such areas are termed *heterotypical*, as opposed to *homotypical*, which describes cortex in which all six layers are easily distinguished.

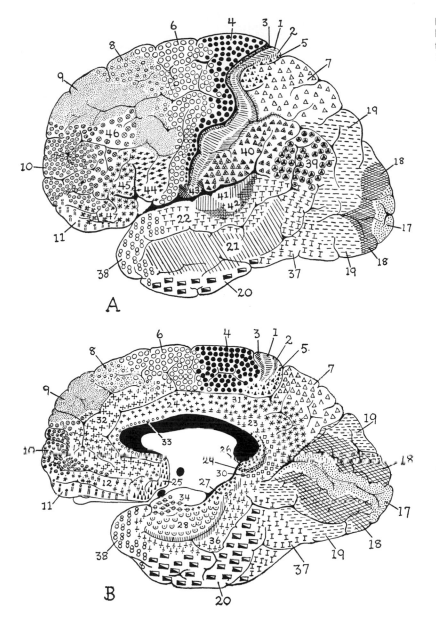

Figure 13.9. Cytoarchitectural map of the human cerebral cortex. *A*, Lateral convex surface; *B*, medial surface. (After Brodmann, 1909.)

Differences in the arrangements and types of cells, as well as the patterns of myelinated fibers, have been used to construct several fundamentally similar cytological maps of the cortex (Fig. 13.9). The Broadmann map of the cerebral cortex has been used widely for reference (Fig. 13.9).

SENSORY AREAS OF THE CEREBRAL CORTEX

Primary Sensory Areas

The localized cortical regions to which impulses concerned with specific sensory modalities are projected constitute the primary sensory areas. Although aspects of the sensation probably enter consciousness at thalamic levels, the primary sensory areas are concerned especially with integration of sensory experience and with the discriminative qualities of

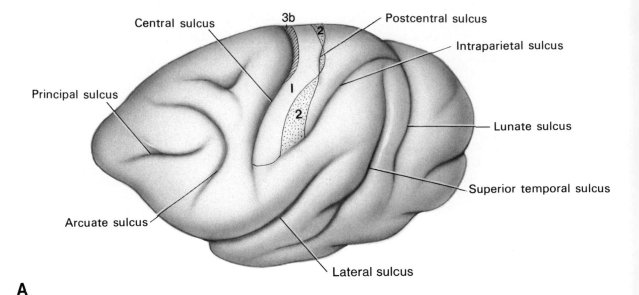

Figure 13.10. *A*, Diagram of the lateral surface of the monkey cerebrum showing the extent of the three cytoarchitectonic areas that compose the primary somesthetic cortex. Area 3b, which forms the posterior wall of the central sulcus, is hidden, except for a small dorsomedial region. Areas 1 and 2 form the crown and posterior wall of the postcentral gyrus. *B*, Bar graph indicating the prevalence in each cytoarchitectural area of the postcentral gyrus of neuronal column activated by cutaneous stimuli and joint movement. (Based on Powell and Mountcastle, 1959 and Mountcastle and Powell, 1959.)

sensation. With the exception of olfaction, impulses involved in all forms of sensation reach localized areas of the cerebral cortex via thalamo-cortical projection systems.

Established primary sensory areas in the cerebral cortex are (1) the *somesthetic area*, consisting of the postcentral gyrus and its medial ex-

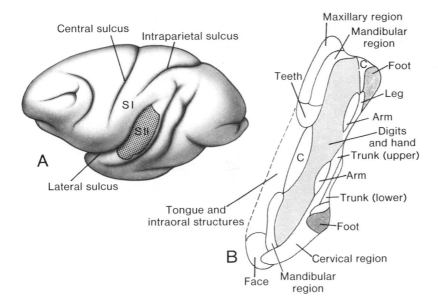

Figure 13.11. Diagram of the somatic sensory area II (SS II) in the *Macaca cynomologus* monkey. Most of SS II lies buried in the depths of the lateral sulcus. This area has been identified on the basis of its cytoarchitecture and connections with the ventrobasal complex (VPLc and VPM) and the primary somesthetic area (S I). In *A*, SS II has been flattened on the cortical surface to show its extent. In *B* the somatotopic features of SS II as determined from recordings in awake monkeys. Different regions of the body are represented by serial oblique strips parallel to the lateral sulcus, with the face and intraoral structures most rostral (*white*). The area in *blue* represents the hand and the digits, while areas in *red* represent the foot. The areas designated as *C* are poorly defined receptive fields. (Based on Robinson and Burton, 1980.)

tension in the paracentral lobule (areas 3, 1, and 2); (2) the *visual* or *striate area*, located along the lips of the calcarine sulcus (area 17); and (3) the *auditory area*, located on the two transverse gyri (Heschl; areas 41 and 42; see Figs. 2.4, 2.9, 6.9, 13.9, 13.10, 13.11, and 13.13). The *gustatory area* is localized to the most ventral part (opercular) of the postcentral gyrus (area 43). The primary olfactory area, consisting of the allocortex of the pyriform and periamygdaloid regions, has not been assigned numbers under the Brodmann parcellation.

Secondary Sensory Areas

Near each primary receptive area are cortical zones which also receive sensory inputs directly from the thalamus, from the primary sensory area, or from both. Cortical zones, adjacent to the primary sensory areas are referred to as *secondary sensory areas*. Secondary sensory areas have been defined primarily in animals by recording evoked potentials in response to sensory stimuli. Secondary sensory areas are smaller than the primary sensory areas, and the sequence of representation is the reverse or different than that found in the primary area. Ablations of the secondary sensory areas produce only minor sensory disturbances compared with those resulting from ablations of the primary sensory areas.

Primary Somesthetic Area (S I)

The cortical area subserving general somatic sensibility, superficial as well as deep, is located in the postcentral gyrus and in the posterior part of the paracentral lobule. Histologically the gyrus is composed of three narrow strips of cortex (areas 3, 1, 2) which differ in their architectural structure (Fig. 13.9). Cortical area 3 is characterized by its thinness and lies along the posterior wall of the central sulcus. Area 3 has been divided into two parts, 3b on the posterior wall of the sulcus and 3a in the depths of the central sulcus (Fig. 13.12). Areas 1 and 2 form, respectively, the crown and posterior wall of the postcentral gyrus (Fig. 13.10).

The postcentral gyrus receives the thalamic projections from the ventral posterior nuclei (VPLc and VPM), which relay impulses from the medial lemniscus, the spinothalamic tracts, and ascending trigeminothalamic pathways (Figs. 9.12 and 9.13). In the ventrobasal complex (VB) of the thalamus (VPLc and VPM) the central core region receives cutaneous input and a thinner outer shell receives input from receptors in deep tissues. The inner part of the central core project to area 3b; the outer part of the central core (cutaneous) projects to areas 3b and 1 (Fig. 13.12). The narrower outer shell concerned with input from deep receptors projects to areas 3a and 2. All thalamocortical projections from the VB complex to the primary somesthetic cortex are somatotopically organized.

Cortical area 3a in the depths of the central sulcus receives input from group Ia muscle afferents (muscle spindles). In the somatosensory cortex most of the thalamic afferents terminate in layer IV.

Studies in the monkey indicate that the majority of neurons in the postcentral gyrus are activated by mechanical stimulation and are selectively excited by stimulation of receptors within either skin or deep tissues, but not by stimulation of both (Fig. 13.10). Over 90% of the neurons in area 2 are related to receptors in deep tissues of the body (joint receptors), while the majority of neurons in area 3b are activated only by cutaneous stimuli; different columns of neurons in area 1 are related to either cutaneous or deep receptors. This differential representation of sensory modalities is closely correlated with the morphological changes that characterize these three cytoarchitectural areas. Afferent impulses from receptors in joint capsules and pericapsular tissues, stimulated by joint movement, are conveyed by the posterior columns, the medial lemnicus, and thalamic relay neurons to particular cell columns in the postcentral gyrus. Impulses conveyed by this system subserve position sense and kinesthesis. Cell columns of the postcentral gyrus responsive to cutaneous stimuli have constant unchanging receptive fields on the body surface. The majority of cortical neurons driven by cutaneous stimuli adapt quickly to steady stimuli. This is a system of great synaptic security, poised for action at high frequency levels, and possessing the neural attributes required for discriminatory functions.

Stretch receptors in muscle and tendons probably do not provide information useful in perception of joint position. Although most of the afferent impulses from stretch receptors project to the cerebellum, the rostral margin of the primary somesthetic area, designated as area 3a, receives impulses from Ia muscle afferents via the ventrobasal complex. The medullary relay centers for group I muscle afferents are in the rostral part of the nuclei gracilis and cuneatus and project only to VPLc. This region is considered as part of the somesthetic cortex.

Although fibers of the spinothalamic tract project to the ventral posterolateral nucleus (VPLc) of the thalamus, fibers of this system also project bilaterally on portions of the intralaminar and posterior thalamic nuclei. Cells of the ventral posterolateral nucleus (VPLc) project to areas 3, 1, and 2 (S I), as well as to the second somatic sensory area (SS II) (Figs. 13.10, 13.11, and 13.13). Both of these cortical projections are topographically organized. Studies in the monkey disclose that the primary somesthetic area (S I) and somatic sensory area II (SS II) are reciprocally and topographically connected with each other within the same hemisphere. The remarkable feature of these somatic sensory areas is the interlocking of topographic subdivisions.

The various regions of the body are represented somatotopically in specific portions of the postcentral gyrus, in a pattern corresponding to

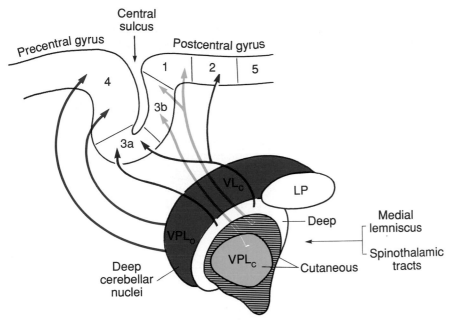

Figure 13.12. Schematic diagram in a sagittal plane showing projections of thalamic sub-divisions to the sensorimotor cortex. Neurons in the ventral posterolateral nucleus (VPLc) (and the ventral posteromedial nucleus (VPM), not shown) form a central core (*blue*) consisting of two parts (one represented in solid *blue* and one lined *blue*) responsive to cutaneous stimuli. An outer shell (*white*) of neurons in these nuclei is responsive to deep stimuli. Input to VPLc is via the medial lemniscus and the spinothalamic tracts; input to VPM is via trigeminothalamic projections (not illustrated). These thalamic afferents terminate somatotopically (Fig. 9.15). Cells in the outer shell project to cortical area 3a (muscle spindles) and to area 2 (deep receptors). Cells in the inner central core (*blue*) project to areas 3b (cutaneous). Cells in the outer central core (lined *blue*) project to areas 3b and 1 (cutaneous). Input to the ventral posterolateral nucleus, pars oralis (VPLo), and the ventral lateral nucleus, pars caudalis (VLc) (*red*), is from the contralateral deep cerebellar nuclei. Cerebellar input to these thalamic nuclei is considered to terminate somatotopically in the same fashion as sensory input in VPLc and VPM. VPLo and VLc project somatotopically upon the primary motor area (area 4) (Based upon Jones and Friedman, 1982; redrawn with permission of authors and Journal of Neurophysiology.)

that of the motor area (Fig. 13.13). Thus the face area lies in the most ventral part, while above it are the sensory areas for the hand, arm, trunk, leg, and foot in the order named; the lower extremity is represented in the paracentral lobule (Fig. 2.6). The cortical areas representing the hand, face, and mouth regions are disproportionally large. The digits of the hand, particularly the thumb and index finger, are well represented. The cortical area related to sensations from the face occupies almost the entire lower half of the postcentral gyrus; the upper part of the face is represented above, while the lips and mouth are represented below. The tongue and pharyngeal region are localized in more ventral areas. In attempts to present a readily apparent visual pattern of the sequence of sensory representation in the cerebral cortex, Penfield has drawn a "sensory homunculus" relating different parts of the body to appropriate areas of the cortex. The "sensory homunculus" corresponds to the "motor homunculus" (Fig. 13.13). The distorted representation of the body surface in the primary sensory area has been said to reflect peripheral innervation density. Those regions of the body with higher densities of receptor elements have more extensive cortical representation, while those regions with relatively few receptors have a minimal representation.

Stimulation of the postcentral gyrus in humans produces sensations described by the patient as numbness, tingling, or a feeling of electricity.

Figure 13.13. Schematic representation of the somatotopical localization of the body in the sensory and motor cortex. The resulting distorted and inverted figure is called the sensory or motor "homunculus." The distortion reflects the disproportional representation of various parts of the body in the cerebral cortex. Representations of the body in the postcentral (sensory) and precentral (motor) gyri show a close correspondence. (Based on Penfield and Rasmussen, 1950.)

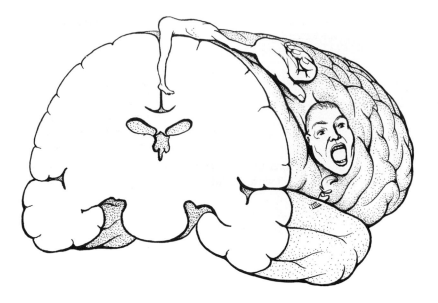

Occasionally the patient may report a sensation of movement in a particular part of the body, though no actual movement is observed. A sensation of pain is rarely produced by these stimulations. Sensations are referred to contralateral parts of the body, except in response to stimulations of the face area. The face and tongue are represented bilaterally. Position sense and kinesthetics are represented only contralaterally in the cerebral cortex. Sensory deficits caused by lesions in the postcentral gyrus are detectable only on the opposite side.

Microelectrode multi–unit mapping of the primary somatosensory cortex in the monkey suggests that the representation of the body surface may be far more complex than indicated by most earlier studies. These studies suggest two large systematic representations of the body surface, each activated by low threshold stimuli. One representation of the body surface is coextensive with area 3b and the other with area 1 (Fig. 13.10). Each of these somatotopic transformations of the skin surface has some discontinuities. While the two fields of cutaneous representation are basically similar and are approximate mirror images of each other, the sequence of representation in the trunk and parts of the limbs are reversed. The two fields differ in size and in the relative proportion of cortex devoted to the representation of various body parts. Because the proportions in each representation differ, both cannot be simple reflections of peripheral innervation density. Area 2 is considered to contain a systematic representation of deep body structures (Fig. 13.10). Studies in the monkey suggest that the somatotopical organization of area 2 only roughly parallels area 1 and some parts of the body are represented in more than one location. The three distinctive cytoarchitectonic areas that compose the postcentral gyrus may each represent different aspects of somatic sensation.

Somatic Sensory Area II (SS II)

This area lies along the superior bank of the lateral sulcus and extends posteriorly into the parietal lobe (Fig. 13.11). In the monkey the greater part of SS II lies buried in the lateral sulcus. Representation of the various parts of the body is in reverse sequence to that found in the primary somesthetic area with the two face areas adjacent. Representation of the body is bilateral in the secondary somatic sensory area, although contralateral representation predominates.

The boundaries of SS II in different animals are not easily defined physiologically. Anatomically SS II is the area on the superior bank of the lateral sulcus (or buried in it) that receives afferents from (1) the ventral posterior nuclei (VPLc and VPM) of the thalamus and (2) both the ipsilateral and contralateral primary somesthetic cortex (S I). The somatotopic organization of SS II in the monkey (Fig. 13.11) indicates that the different body regions are represented in successive, obliquely oriented cortical strips parallel with the lateral sulcus. These cortical strips representing various parts of the body in SS II do not form a topological map of the body surface as depicted in the figurines for S I. Most of the neurons in SS II respond to cutaneous stimuli in a manner similar to that reported for S I. The efferent cortical connections of SS II are with the primary somesthetic cortex (S I) and the primary motor area within the same hemisphere.

Primary Visual Area

Area 17 is located in the walls and floor of the calcarine sulcus. It occasionally extends onto the lateral surface of the hemisphere (Figs. 9.27 and 13.9). The exceedingly thin cortex of this area is the most striking example of the heterotypical granulous cortex. Layers II and III are narrow and contain numerous small pyramidal cells (Fig. 13.3). A thick layer IV is subdivided by a light band into three sublayers. The upper and lower sublayers are packed with small granule cells. In the middle, lighter layer, fewer small cells are scattered between the large stellate cells (Fig. 13.17). The middle layer contains the greatly thickened outer band of Baillarger, here known as the band of Gennari and is visible to the naked eye in sections of the fresh cortex (Fig. 13.14). The visual cortex contains GABAergic interneurons and fibers in layers II and III which exhibit a periodicity suggesting a correlation with the functional columnar subdivisions. These small neurons make symmetrical (inhibitory) synapses upon the apical and basilar dendrites of pyramidal cells.

The visual cortex receives the geniculocalcarine tract, whose course and projection have been discussed (Fig. 9.28; see p. 286). Geniculocalcarine fibers pass in the *external sagittal stratum*, separated from the wall of the inferior and posterior horns of the lateral ventricle by the *internal sagittal stratum*, and by fibers of the *tapetum* (Fig. 2.19). Fibers of the internal sagittal stratum are corticofugal fibers projecting from the occipital cortex to the superior colliculus and the lateral geniculate body (LGB). The macular fibers terminate in the caudal third of the calcarine area, and those from the paracentral and peripheral retinal areas end in respectively more rostral portions (Fig. 9.27). Parts of each macular area are represented only in the visual cortex of one hemisphere. Clinically, sparing of macular vision associated with vascular lesions involving the occipital cortex usually is attributed to collateral circulation provided by branches of the middle cerebral artery (Fig. 14.6). Following occlusion of the posterior cerebral artery, these collateral vessels may be sufficient to preserve some macular vision.

Complete unilateral destruction of the visual cortex in man produces a contralateral homonymous hemianopsia in which there is blindness in the ipsilateral nasal field and the contralateral temporal field. Thus a lesion in the right visual cortex produces a left homonymous hemianopsia

Figure 13.14. Section through the calcarine cortex (area striata) demonstrating the line of Gennari, the greatly thickened band of Baillarger in layer IV. Weigert's myelin stain. Photograph.

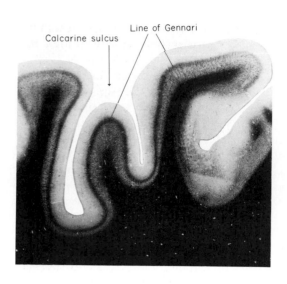

Calcarine sulcus   Line of Gennari

(Fig. 9.29). Lesions involving portions of the visual cortex, such as the inferior calcarine cortex, produce an *homonymous quadrantanopsia*, in which blindness results in the superior half of the visual field contralaterally. Homonymous hemianopsia can result from lesions involving all fibers of either the optic tract or the optic radiation (Fig. 9.29), but lesions in these locations tend to be incomplete and the visual defects in the two eyes are rarely identical. Patients frequently are unaware of an existing homonymous hemianopsia and complain of bumping into people and objects on the side of the visual field defect.

An image falling upon the retina initiates a tremendously complex process that results in vision. The transformation of a retinal image into a perceptual image occurs partly in the retina, but mostly in the brain.

The receptive field of a cell in the visual system is defined as the region of the retina (or visual field) over which one can influence the firing of that cell. In the retina the receptive field comprises those receptor sets (i.e., rods and cones) and other retinal neurons which influence the firing of one retinal ganglion cell (Fig. 9.26). Receptive fields of retinal ganglion cells are circular, vary somewhat in size, and are of two types: (1) those with an "on" (excitatory) center and an "off" (inhibitory) surround, and (2) those with an "off" (inhibitory) center and an "on" (excitatory) surround (Fig. 13.15). Retinal ganglion cells fire at a fairly steady rate even in the absence of stimulation. An "on" response is characterized by an increased firing rate of the cell to a light stimulus; in an "off" response the cell's firing rate diminishes when the light stimulus decreases. The physiological basis for the "on" and "off" retinal responses are the concentric receptive fields with either an "on" and "off" center and the reverse type of surround (Fig. 13.15). Lighting up the entire retina diffusely does not affect retinal ganglion cells as strongly as a small circular spot that just covers the excitatory region of the receptive field.

Cells of the lateral geniculate body have physiological characteristics similar to retinal ganglion cells, in that (1) each cell is driven from a circumscribed retinal region (the receptive field), and (2) each receptive field has either an "on" or "off" center with an opposing surround (Fig. 13.15). Cells in different laminae of the lateral geniculate body are driven from receptive fields in one eye, either ipsilaterally or contralaterally, depending upon the uncrossed or crossed connections. Visual processing by the brain begins in the lateral geniculate body.

The striate cortex does not have cells with concentric receptive fields. Cells of the striate cortex show a marked specificity in their responses to restricted retinal stimulation. The most effective stimulus shapes are long narrow rectangles of light ("slits"), dark bars against a light background ("dark bars"), and straight-line borders separating areas of different brightness ("edges"). A given cell responds vigorously when an appropriate stimulus is shone on its receptive field, or moves across it, provided the stimulus is presented in a specific orientation (Fig. 13.16). This orientation is referred to as the *receptive-field axis of orientation* and it is critical and constant for any particular cell, but it differs for cells in other locations. Cells with the same receptive field axis of orientation are arranged in columns extending from the pial surface to the white matter (Fig. 13.17).

The cortical columns of the striate cortex may be looked upon as the structural expression of the necessity to encode more than two variables. The two surface coordinates (eccentricity from fovea and distance above or below the horizontal meridian) encode topographical representation in the visual fields. Engrafted upon this representation are two more variables in columnar form concerned with receptive-field orientation and ocular dominance (Fig. 13.17). The topographical representation of the retinae upon the striate cortex is primary and for each position in the visual field there is neuronal machinery for each orientation and for each eye. In the striate cortex there exist two independent and overlapping systems of columns referred to as orientation columns and ocular dominance columns. Ocular dominance columns are parallel sheets or slabs arranged perpendicular to the cortical surface which are subdivided into a mosaic of alternating left eye and right eye stripes 250 to 500 μm in width (Figs. 13.17 and 13.18). Orientation columns are an order of magnitude smaller than the ocular dominance columns. The horizontal distance corresponding to a complete cycle of orientation columns, representing a rotation through 180°, is roughly equal to a set of left plus right ocular dominance columns with a thickness of 0.5 to 1 mm.

ORIENTATION COLUMNS

The visual cortex is subdivided into discrete columns extending from the pial surface to the white matter; all cells within each column have the same receptive-field axis orientation. The many varieties of cells in the striate cortex have been grouped into two main types, referred to as "*simple*" and "*complex.*"

"Simple"-type cells respond to slits of light having the proper receptive-field axis of orientation. A slit of light, oriented vertically in the visual field, may activate a given "simple" cell, whereas the same cell will not respond, though other cells will if the orientation of the slit of light is moved out of the vertical position. The retinal region over which a "simple" type cell can be influenced is, like the receptive fields of retinal and geniculate cells, divided into "on" and "off" areas (Fig. 13.15). In "simple" cells these "on" areas are narrow rectangles, adjoined on each side by larger rectangular "off" regions. The magnitude of the "on" response depends upon how much of the "on" region is covered by the stimulus light. A narrow slit of light that just fills the elongated "on" region produces a powerful "on" response; stimulation with a slit of light having a different orientation produces a weaker response, because it includes part of the adjacent antagonistic "off" regions (Fig. 13.16). A slit of light at right angles to the optimum orientation for a particular cell, usually produces no response. Thus a large spot of light covering

Figure 13.15. *A,* Receptive fields of retinal ganglion cells and lateral geniculate neurons are concentric with either an "on" (excitatory) center and an "off" (inhibitory) surround, or the reverse. In *a,* a spot of light (*red*) filling the "on" center causes the cell to fire vigorously. If the spot of light strikes the surrounding "off" zone (gray), firing of the neuron is suppressed until the light is turned off. In *b,* the responses of a cell with an "off" center and an "on" surround are the reverse. *B,* Simple cells of striate cortex receive their input from sets of lateral geniculate neurons whose "on" or "off" centers are arranged in straight lines. The receptive field axis of orientation varies for simple cells, as in *a, b,* and *c,* with excitatory areas represented by *red dots* and inhibitory areas by *black dots.* Although simple cells always have excitatory and inhibitory areas parallel and in a straight line, these areas may be asymmetrical as in *d* and *e.* (Based on Hubel and Wiesel, 1962.)

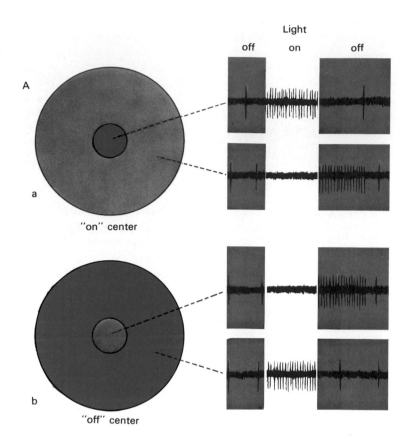

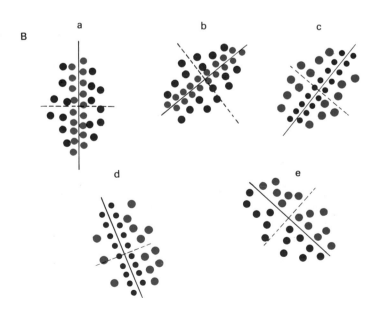

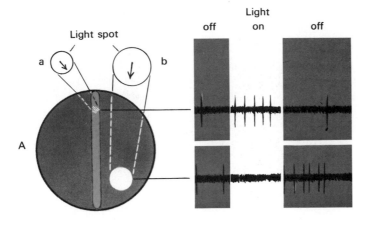

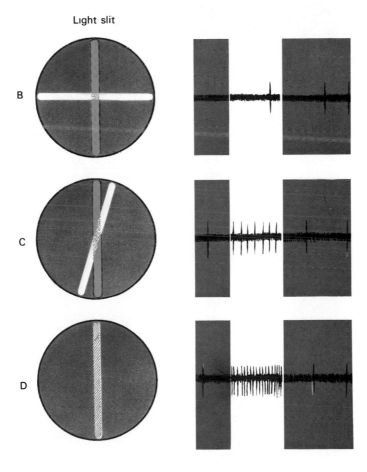

Figure 13.16. Schematic diagram of the functional characteristics of "simple" cells in the striate cortex. In *A*, a small circular spot of light (*a*) shone on the excitatory part of the receptive field (*red*) of a simple cortical cell produces a weak response. A larger spot of light (*b*) shone on the inhibitory surround produces no response. Small spots of light (*a*) produce vigorous responses in retinal ganglion cells and lateral geniculate neurons. The receptive field of the simple cell (*red*) shown above is similar to *a* in Figure 13-15*B*.

A narrow split of light perpendicular to the receptive field axis of orientation (*red*) in *B* produces virtually no response. Tilting the slit of light as in *C* produces a weak response, while a vertical slit of light, as in *D* which corresponds to the receptive field axis of the simple striate cell, produces a vigorous response. (After Hubel, 1963.)

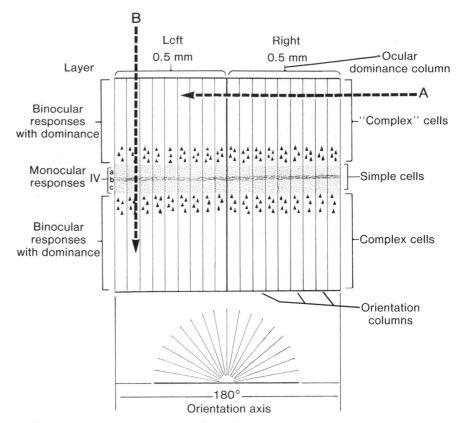

Figure 13.17. Schematic representation of the organization of ocular dominance and orientation columns in the striate cortex. Ocular dominance columns (0.25 to 0.5 mm) are an order of magnitude larger than orientation columns and a pair of left-right ocular dominance columns (0.5 to 1 mm) are roughly equal to a set of orientation columns representing a complete cycle of orientations through 180°. Input from the lateral geniculate to layer IV is strictly monocular and consists of a series of parallel and alternating stripes—one for the left eye and one for the right eye. Most of the cells in layer IV (*blue*) are "simple" cells. Binocularly influenced cells are predominantly "complex" cells in layers above and below layer IV. A recording electrode inserted tangential to the pial surface, as in *arrow A*, will detect responses to successive stimuli with different orientations, first with right eye dominance and then with left eye dominance. A recording electrode inserted vertically, as in *arrow B*, will indicate responses only to stimuli presented in one axis of orientation. About 50% of the cell above and below layer IV (*blue*) will respond to binocular stimuli, but with consistent left ocular dominance. When the electrode is in layer IV, only monocular responses will be recorded. (Based on Hubel and Wiesel, 1974; Hubel et al., 1977).

the whole retina evokes no response in "simple" cortical cells, because "on" and "off" effects apparently balance. A particular cortical cell's optimum receptive-field axis of orientation appears to be a property built into the cell by its anatomical connections. The receptive-field axis of orientation differs from one cell column to the next and may be vertical, horizontal, or oblique. No one orientation is more common than any other.

"Simple" cells, located in layer IV, receive their impulses directly from the lateral geniculate body. A typical "simple" cell receives an input from a large number of lateral geniculate neurons whose "on" centers correspond to the receptive field orientation of the simple cell (Fig. 13.15*B*). Thus, for each area of the retina stimulated, each line, and each orientation of the stimulus, there is a particular set of "simple" striate cortical cells that respond. Changing any of the stimulus arrangements will cause an entirely new and different population of "simple" striate cells to respond.

"Complex"-type cells, like "simple" cells, respond best to "slits," "bars," or "edges," provided the orientation is suitable. Unlike "simple" cells, these cells respond with sustained firing as the slits of light are moved across the retina, preserving the same receptive field axis of orientation. These cells have peculiar characteristics in that a slit of light with the appropriate receptive-field axis of orientation can cause cells to fire vigorously as it moves across the retina in one direction, but reversing the direction of movement of the light stimulus may produce a diminished, or different, response.

Although "complex" cells in the striate cortex have some characteristics similar to those of simple cells, their receptive-fields cannot be mapped into antagonistic "on" and "off" regions. A "complex" cell receives its input from a large number of "simple" cells—all of which have the same receptive-field axis of orientation. Most simple cells in the striate cortex are stellate cells located in layer IV (Fig. 13.17); the majority of complex and hypercomplex cells are pyramidal neurons lying in layers superficial or deep to layer IV. Hypercomplex cells have the properties of two or more complex cells from which they are believed to receive their input. Most cells in layer IV are driven by only one eye while cells in other layers are driven binocularly.

Orientation columns appear to have the form of narrow slabs, as do ocular dominance columns. The arrangement of the columns is highly ordered and recordings made along a tangential microelectrode penetration show that the preferred orientations of cells change in a systematic fashion, in either a clockwise or counterclockwise direction with advancement of the electrode (Fig. 13.17). There is a continuous variation in the preferred orientation with horizontal distance along the cortex. When the electrode crosses from a left-eye region to a right-eye region, there is no noticeable disturbance in the sequence of orientation columns (Fig. 13.17). The horizontal distance along the cortex corresponding to a complete cycle of orientation columns, representing rotations through 180°, is said to be equal in size to a set of left and right ocular dominance columns (0.5 to 1 mm). Orientation columns are arranged with great regularity so that a probe moving along the cortex horizontally generally can be expected to encounter all preferred orientations in a regular sequence before any one is repeated.

OCULAR DOMINANCE COLUMNS

In the lateral geniculate body, the first point at which convergence is possible, no binocularly influenced cells have been observed. No crossed and uncrossed optic tract fibers terminate in an overlapping manner in layers of the lateral geniculate body. It has long been recognized that the primary visual cortex receives projections from both eyes. The receptive fields of all binocularly influenced cortical cells occupy corresponding sites in the two retinas (Fig. 9.23). About 80% of the cells in the striate cortex are influenced independently by the two eyes. In a binocularly influenced cell of the two receptive fields have the same organization, the same axis of orientation, and a summation occurs when corresponding parts of the two retinas are stimulated simultaneously.

In the monkey, binocular convergence in area 17 is delayed beyond the first and second synaptic stages. Projections of the lateral geniculate body terminate in deep parts of layer IV where they are segregated into a series of parallel alternating stripes, one set connected with the left eye and the other to the right eye. Although input to deep parts of layer IV is essentially monocular, ocular dominance columns extend vertically

Figure 13.18. Autoradiographic montage of tangential sections of area 17 on the left in a monkey (269) whose right eye was removed as an adult. The left eye was injected 4 months later with [³H]proline. The montage shows the normal mosaic pattern of ocular dominance columns (produced by transneuronal transport of [³H]proline) with uniformly labeled bands alternating with unlabeled bands. The uniformly labeled area (*disc*) represents the monocular area which covers the blind spot (optic disc) of the enuculated right eye. (From LeVay et al., 1980, courtesy of Dr. David Hubel and Alan R. Liss, Inc., New York.) Bar equals 1 mm.

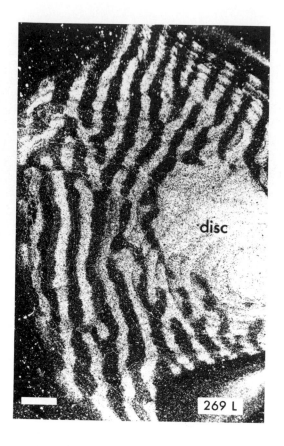

from the pial surface to the white matter, and show alternate preference for left and right eyes (Figs. 13.17, 13.18, and 13.19). This columnar arrangement is demonstrated by vertical electrode penetrations of the striate cortex in which there is no change in eye preference. In tangential penetrations of the striate cortex, the electrode moves from a region in which one eye gives the best response to an adjacent region where the other eye dominates. In layer IV the responses are monocular, while cells in other layers respond binocularly, but with definite dominance by one eye. The widths of the ocular dominance columns innervated by the ipsilateral or contralateral eye are the same (Fig. 13.17). Iontophoretic application of a GABA antagonist (bicuculline) to the visual cortex cancels the "on" and "off" subregions of simple cells and abolishes orientation selectivity. It also produces a shift in ocular dominance columns from one eye to the other. These effects are reversible and appear correlated with the loss of GABAergic inhibition.

The striate cortex is organized into both vertical and horizontal systems. The vertical or columnar system is concerned with retinal position, line orientation, ocular dominance, and perhaps detection of direction of movement; these functional features are mapped in sets of superimposed, but independent, mosaics (Figs. 13.18 and 13.19). The horizontal system segregates cells of different orders of complexity. Cells of the lowest order (simple cells), located in layer IV, are driven monocularly, while those of higher orders (complex and hypercomplex), located in the other layers, are driven by impulses from both eyes (Fig. 13.17).

Ocular dominance columns in the striate cortex have been demonstrated by a variety of neuroanatomical technics. The boundaries of

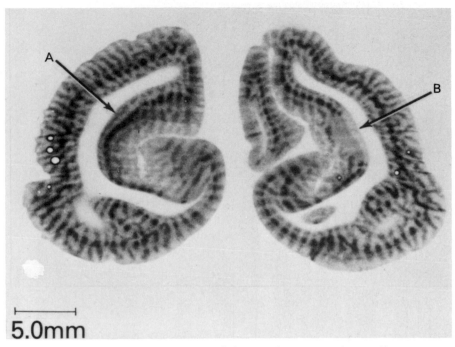

Figure 13.19. Autoradiographic mapping of the visual system in the monkey using 2–[¹⁴C]deoxyglucose. Coronal sections of the striate cortex in an animal with the right eye occluded. The alternate dark and light striations, each 0.3 to 0.4 mm in width, represent ocular dominance columns. These columns are darkest in a band which corresponds to layer IV, but they extend the entire thickness of the cortex. *Arrows A* and *B* point to regions without ocular dominance columns, these regions receive only monocular input. The region indicated by *arrow A* is contralateral to the occluded eye (Fig. 13.18). The region indicated by *arrow B* is ipsilateral to the occluded eye and shows no evidence of radioactivity. Both *arrows* indicate loci believed to be the cortical representation of the blind spots. See Figures 13.20 and 13.21. (From Kennedy et al., 1976; courtesy of Dr. Louis Sokoloff, Laboratory of Cerebral Metabolism, National Institute of Mental Health, Bethesda, Maryland.)

ocular dominance columns correspond with a mosaic pattern of dark bands seen in tangential autoradiographs of the striate cortex (Fig. 13.18). Using the principle of transneuronal transport or 2-[¹⁴C]deoxyglucose as a metabolic marker to measure glucose utilization also reveals the characteristic pattern of ocular dominance columns (Figs. 13.20 and 13.21). Two regions of the striate cortex do not contain ocular dominance columns: (1) the region representing the blind spot of the retina (Fig. 13.18) and (2) the cortical region representing the monocular temporal crescent of the visual field (Fig. 9.23). These regions of striate cortex, receiving only monocular visual inputs, have been identified (Figs. 13.18, 13.19, 13.20, and 13.21). The area of the optic disc in the nasal half of each retina transits no visual impulses to the contralateral striate cortex; this region of striate cortex receives its sole input from the temporal half of the ipsilateral retina (Figs. 13.20 and 13.21).

When an animal is deprived of vision in the right eye and the 2-[¹⁴C]deoxyglucose method is employed as a metabolic marker (1) the left striate cortex shows the striped pattern of ocular dominance columns, except in the representation of the blind spot where metabolic activity is evidenced by a continuous band of isotope uptake, and (2) the right striate cortex shows a similar pattern of striped columns but no evidence of metabolic activity or isotope in the cortical areas representing the blind spot (Figs. 13.19, 13.20, and 13.21). The cortical area representing the

Figures 13.20 and 13.21. Schematic diagrams demonstrating the ocular dominance columns and the blind spot in the striate cortex with the 2–[¹⁴C]deoxyglucose metabolic mapping technic in the monkey. In an animal with an intact visual system silver grains are distributed throughout the striate cortex with greatest concentrations in layer IV; neither the blind spot or ocular dominance columns can be demonstrated. Following removal of the right eye, or section of the right optic nerve (*Heavy black line*), silver grains are distributed evenly in the representation of the blind spot on the left (Fig. 13.20), but no isotope is evident in the blind spot on the right (Fig. 13.21). Other regions of the striate cortex demonstrated ocular dominance columns on both sides. Fibers from the ipsilateral temporal retina (left) normally cover the blind spot of the opposite (right) eye. The autoradiographs in Figure 13.19 represent the striate cortex of right and left hemispheres which are here depicted diagrammatically. (Courtesy of Dr. Louis Sokoloff, National Institute of Mental Health, Bethesda, Maryland.)

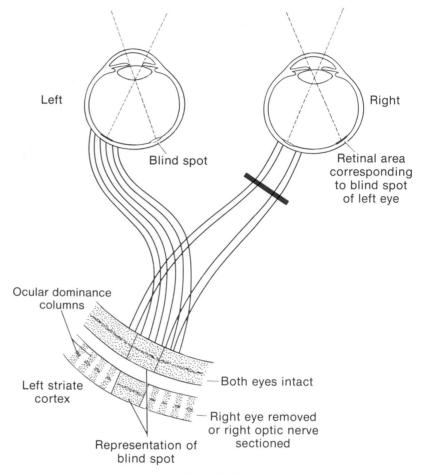

Figure 13.20.

monocular crescent of the right visual field, which lies in the left striate cortex, would not contain isotope because all of its input is crossed.

VISUAL DEPRIVATION

In very young, visually inexperienced kittens and monkeys, deprived of all vision from birth by visual occluders, responses in the striate cortex indicate that orientation columns are as highly ordered as in the adult. The connections responsible for this highly organized function of the visual cortex must be present at birth and appear to be genetically determined. The surprising finding in young monkeys deprived of binocular vision for a few weeks after birth was the marked reduction in number of cells in the striate cortex that could be influenced by both eyes. Deprivation of binocular vision for a few weeks after birth may result in deterioration of innate cortical connections subserving binocular vision.

Ocular dominance columns in the monkey are only partially formed at birth and undergo rapid development during the first 6 weeks of life. Monocular visual deprivation during the first 6 postnatal weeks causes ocular dominance columns in the deep parts of layer IV related to the open eye to be expanded, while dominance columns related to the closed eye appear to shrink. Normal binocular vision, in the first 6 weeks of life, is necessary for the development of cortical connections that subserve binocular vision.

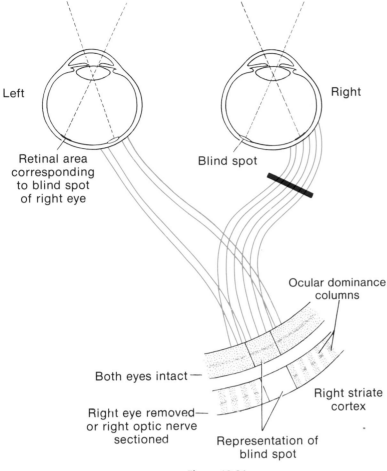

Figure 13.21.

Secondary Visual Areas

A second visual area (visual area II) has been mapped in a number of different animals. Visual area II is a smaller mirror image representation of the primary visual area and is identified as area 18 (Fig. 13.9). Lateral to visual area I and II is a third systematic projection of the contralateral visual field (visual area III) which corresponds with area 19.

Cells in visual areas II and III respond to slits of light, dark bars, and edges that have a specific receptive-field orientation. The majority of cells in visual area II are "complex"; in visual area III about half of the cells are complex. Other cells in these areas are referred to as "hypercomplex" cells because of more elaborate properties.

Area 18 is six-layered granular cortex which lacks the band of Gennari and rostrally merges with area 19. This area 18 interrelates areas 17 and 19 of the same and opposite hemispheres by association and commissural fibers. The retinotopic organization of area 18 indicates that the border between areas 17 and 18 corresponds to the vertical meridian of the contralateral visual hemifield. Thus as successive recordings are made moving from area 17 to area 18 there is a reversal of the receptive fields (i.e., from peripheral to central followed by a central to peripheral sequence) about the vertical meridian. The isoelevation lines running through both areas 17 and 18 are perpendicular to the representation of the vertical meridian. Visual area II (area 18) represents roughly the central 50° of the visual hemifield which corresponds to the binocular overlap zone.

Figure 13.22. Schematic diagram of the cortical auditory areas in the cat. The primary auditory area (A I, *dark blue*) has a tonotopic organization with high frequencies (*H*) represented rostrally and low frequencies (*L*) caudally. *Dashed vertical lines* in A I represent isofrequency bands. The primary auditory area is surrounded by a belt of secondary auditory areas, of which A II (*light blue*) is the largest. Other secondary auditory areas are SF, suprasylvian fringe; EP, posterior ectosylvian area (*stippled*); SS II, second somatic area; I, insular area; and T, temporal area. (Based on Woolsey, 1960 and Merzenich et al., 1975.)

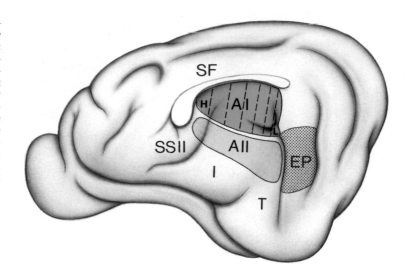

Cells of the six layers of the dorsal division of the lateral geniculate nucleus (LGB) project mainly upon area 17 but some fibers also reach areas 18 and 19. The inferior pulvinar and the adjacent part of the lateral pulvinar, each containing a representation of the contralateral visual hemifield, project retinotopically upon areas 18 and 19. Fibers projecting to areas 18 and 19 from these parts of the pulvinar constitute important links in the extragenicular visual projection. Although there are few commisural connections between area 17 in the two hemispheres, commissural fibers interconnect the junctional region near the border between areas 17 and 18. Cells near the boundary between areas 17 and 18 functionally represent the vertical meridian of the visual hemifield. Thus the vertical meridian of the visual field is bilaterally represented in the visual cortex because of commissural connections. This bilateral representation ensures a uniform visual field free of interruptions along the vertical midline.

Primary Auditory Area

In man this area (areas 41 and 42) is located on the two transverse gyri (Heschl) which lie on the dorsomedial surface of the superior temporal convolution, and are buried in the floor of the lateral sulcus (Figs. 2.9, 6.9, 9.13, and 13.9). The middle part of the anterior transverse gyrus and a portion of the posterior gyrus constitute the principal auditory receptive areas (area 41). Remaining parts of the posterior transverse gyrus and adjacent portions of the superior temporal gyrus compose area 42, largely an auditory association area (Figs. 2.4 and 2.9). Area 41 is typical koniocortex, resembling that of areas 3 and 17.

The cortical auditory area receives geniculotemporal fibers (auditory radiation) from the medial geniculate body (Fig. 2.9). The auditory radiation reaches its cortical projection site by passing through the sublenticular portion of the internal capsule (Figs. 6.9 and 9.24). The greater part of the auditory radiation projects to area 41.

The ventral laminated part of the medial geniculate body (MGB) has a tonotopic organization in which high frequencies are represented medially and low frequencies laterally. The auditory radiation arises from the ventral laminated part of the MGB (Fig. 9.19) and projects to the primary auditory cortex where there is a spatial representation of tonal frequencies. Fibers passing to the primary auditory cortex constitute the *core projection* (Figs. 13.22 and 13.23).

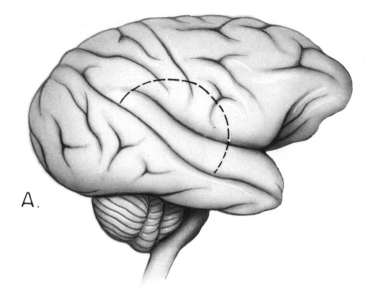

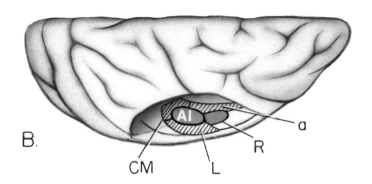

Figure 13.23. Auditory cortex in the rhesus monkey. *A,* Drawing of the lateral aspect of the brain with *dashed lines* indicating the region excised to expose the superior temporal plane. *B,* Dorsal view of the auditory cortex in the superior temporal plane. The primary auditory cortex is represented by areas A I and R (*blue*) where low frequencies are represented rostrolaterally and high frequencies caudomedially in both areas. Both areas A I and R contain orderly representations of the auditory spectrum. The primary auditory areas are surrounded by a belt of secondary auditory cortex (*shaded*) designated as *a, L,* and *CM* (Based on Merzenich and Brugge, 1973, and Imig et al., 1977).

The medial geniculate body also has two nonlaminated divisions which receive auditory inputs. These divisions of the MGB, referred to as dorsal and medial (magnocellular), project ipsilaterally via the auditory radiation to cytoarchitectonic areas forming a cortical belt around the primary auditory area (Figs. 13.22 and 13.23). Fibers arising from the nonlaminated parts of the medial geniculate body passing to the secondary auditory areas constitute the *belt projection*.

In the cat, two auditory areas were defined originally on the lateral aspect of the hemisphere below the suprasylvian sulcus, designated as auditory area I (A I) and auditory area II (A II) (Fig. 13.22).

Frequency representation in auditory area I (A I), indicate an orderly series of isofrequency strips oriented vertically in which high frequencies are represented rostrally and low frequencies caudally (Fig. 13.22). In A II no clear tonotopic representation has been established because of the broad tuning curves of its neurons. A II receives most of its fibers from the medial magnocellular nucleus of the MGB. The other secondary auditory areas receive their inputs via the belt projection from nonlaminated parts of the MGB.

The primary auditory area in the monkey lies caudally on the superior surface of the superior temporal gyrus and can be exposed by resection of the overlying parietal cortex (Fig. 13.23). Best frequencies in the full auditory range for the monkey were represented in an orderly fashion in the primary auditory area. This is a cytoarchitectonic field coextensive with the koniocortex. Lowest frequencies were represented rostrally and laterally whereas highest frequencies were found caudally and medially (Fig. 13.23). A cortical region immediately rostral to the primary auditory area (A I) has a cytoarchitecture similar to that of A I and appears to respond as vigorously to acoustic stimulation. This rostral field, smaller than A I, contains a complete and orderly representation of the audible frequency spectrum with lower frequencies represented rostral and higher frequencies represented in progressively more caudal and medial regions (Fig. 13.23). The primary auditory area (A I) and the field rostral to it, designated R, appear to constitute the central core of the auditory cortex in the monkey. The primary auditory cortex in the monkey is surrounded by a belt of auditory cortex which is not cytoarchitectonically uniform. This cortical belt represents the secondary auditory cortex in the monkey (Fig. 13.23).

The functional architecture of the auditory cortex appears similar to that of the visual and somesthetic cortex in that cells in the same cell column share the same functional properties. Functional columns in the auditory cortex appear less discrete, do not have sharp boundaries, and are considered to be smaller units than in other sensory areas. The isofrequency strips oriented across the primary auditory cortex probably represent, or are composed of, isofrequency cell columns. In these columns units throughout the depth of the cortex respond to the same frequency.

Each cochlea is represented bilaterally in the auditory cortex, with only slight differences between the two sides. The cortical effects of sound stimulating each ear separately are nearly the same, but significant differences occur when the position of the stimulus is varied with respect to both ears. When sound is presented on one side, the cortical response is greatest contralaterally. If the sound is presented in a median plane, the cortical activity in the two hemispheres is equal. Although these observations suggest that localization of sound in space is dependent upon the relative amounts of neural activity at higher levels of the auditory system, this conclusion is not correct. Localization of sound in space involves a two-stage process: (1) convergence and comparison of auditory input from the two ears and (2) a distribution of this "computer analysis" to the appropriate side of the system. The trapezoid body is the only auditory commissure essential to sound localization; above this level mechanisms for detecting sound localization are present only on one side (contralateral to the source). Attempts to physiologically identify a place map for sound direction have been elusive, but most evidence suggests it is likely to be in the deep layers of the superior colliculus, or the brain stem tegmentum. Because audition is represented bilaterally at a cortical level, unilateral lesions of the auditory cortex cause only a partial deafness. The deficits, however, are bilateral, and the greatest loss is contralateral. Lesions in Broadmann's area 22 in the dominant hemisphere produce word deafness or sensory aphasia. Although hearing is unimpaired by such lesions, patients cannot interpret the meaning of the sounds.

Gustatory Area

Taste sensibility is represented in the parietal operculum (area 43) and in the adjacent parainsular cortex. Gustatory representation in the parietal operculum is adjacent to the somesthetic area for the tongue, but separate from the nongustatory lingula area. In the cat and monkey the taste pathway ascends ipsilateral (Fig. 5.24). Rostral regions of the nucleus of the solitary fasciculus project fibers ipsilaterally to the ventral posteromedial nucleus, pars parvicellularis (VPMpc) (Figs. 9.14 and 9.17), while cells in more caudal regions project ascending fibers to both the parabrachial nuclei and VPMpc (Fig. 5.24). Thalamic cell groups subserving taste in VPMpc are distinct from neurons related to other sensory modalities of the tongue. The ventral posteromedial nucleus, pars parvicellularis (VPMpc) projects to both the insular and parietal opercular cortex. Lesions in either VPMpc or the parietal operculum cause loss of gustatory sensation.

Vestibular Representation

In the cerebral cortex vestibular sense is poorly defined. In humans, electrical stimulation of portions of the superior temporal gyrus, particularly regions rostral to the auditory area, provoke sensations of turning movements and dizziness. These sensations are mild compared with the violent vertigo produced by direct stimulation of the labyrinth. Less distinct illusions of body movement have been reported following stimulation of parietal cortex.

Two cortical areas have been identified as receiving vestibular input in the cat and monkey. These are area 3a and the posterior margin of area 2, which has been designated as area 2v. The common feature of these areas is the convergence of vestibular inputs and signals from deep somatic receptors. Area 3a also receives an input from muscle spindles and area 2v receives inputs from joint receptors (Fig. 13.12). Neurons in area 2v appear to have perceptive functions in that they are sensitive to head and visual field motion. Thalamic projections to these cortical areas originate from portions of the ventrobasal complex and are not localized to a single subdivision (i.e., VPLc, VPM, and VPI). Vestibular projections to the cortex are bilateral with contralateral dominance. Regions of the vestibular nuclear complex projecting to the thalamus are poorly understood.

MOTOR CORTICAL AREAS

Corticofugal fibers arise from all regions of the cerebral cortex. These projections convey impulses concerned with motor function, modification of muscle tone and reflex activity, modulation of sensory signals, and the alterations of awareness. Corticofugal fibers, originating mainly from the deeper cortical layers, project to spinal levels, a variety of brain stem nuclei at all levels, the thalamus and to all parts of the neostriatum.

The somata of the cells of origin of particular corticofugal fiber systems have a specific laminar or sublaminar distribution (Fig. 13.5). Corticospinal neurons lie in the deepest part of layer V, occur in clusters, and show great variation in cell size, particularly in area 4. Corticostriate fibers arise from the smallest pyramidal cells in superficial regions of layer V. Corticopontine, corticobulbar, and corticorubral neurons lie in middle regions of layer V. The majority of corticothalamic cells are found in layer VI.

Three principal motor areas are recognized in the cerebral cortex: (1) *the primary* (precentral) *motor area*, (2) *the premotor area*, and (3) *the supplementary motor area* (Figs. 13.25 and 13.26). The primary motor area is preeminently concerned with voluntary motor activity. The premotor area, rostral to the primary motor cortex, is concerned with voluntary motor function dependent upon sensory inputs. The supplementary motor area, on the medial aspect of the frontal lobe, participates in the programming and planning of motor activities, and perhaps their initiation.

Primary Motor Area (M I)

Area 4 of Brodmann, commonly designated as the primary motor area M I, is located on the anterior wall of the central sulcus and adjacent portions of the precentral gyrus (Fig. 13.9). This area is broad at the superior margin of the hemisphere, but near the inferior frontal gyrus, it is practically limited to the anterior wall of the central sulcus. On the medial surface of the hemisphere it comprises the anterior portion of the paracentral lobule (Fig. 2.6). The unusually thick cortex of the motor area is agranular in structure, and its ganglionic layer contains the giant pyramidal cells of Betz (Fig. 13.2). These cells are largest in the paracentral lobule, and smallest in the opercular region. The density of Betz cells also varies in different parts of area 4. Cytoarchitecturally area 4 represents a modification of the typical six-layered isocortex in which the pyramidal cells in layers III and V are increased in number and the internal granular layer is obscured. For this reason the cortex is called agranular.

The corticospinal tract, considered to transmit impulses for highly skilled volitional movements to lower motor neurons, arises in large part from area 4. The larger corticospinal fibers are the axons of giant pyramidal cells. Axons of the giant cells of Betz account for only a little over 3% of corticospinal fibers. Approximately 90% of the fibers of the corticospinal tract range from 1 to 4 μm in diameter. Of the total number of fibers in the tract, about 40% are poorly myelinated.

Virtually all fibers of the corticospinal tract arise from area 4, area 6, and parts of the parietal lobe. Approximate percentages of corticospinal fibers arising from these areas are (1) area 4, 31%, (2) area 6, 29%, and (3) parietal lobe, 40% (Fig. 4.7). Complete decortication, or hemispherectomy, causes all fibers of the corticospinal tract to degenerate. Cells giving rise to corticospinal projections occur in clusters aligned to form strips oriented mediolaterally across the cortex. Most of the cells contributing fibers to the corticospinal tract have glutamate or aspartate as their excitatory neurotransmitter (Fig. 13.6). Major differences exist in the pattern of terminal labeling in the spinal gray following injections of tracers into different cytoarchitectonic areas. Isotope injected into cortical areas 3, 1, 2, and 5 label terminals in parts of the posterior horn which correspond to Rexed's laminae III and IV, while injections into areas 4 and 3a label terminals largely in Rexed's lamina VII, but with extensions into regions of spinal motor neurons. No corticospinal neurons project into Rexed's laminae I and II. Some corticospinal neurons in the monkey end directly upon anterior horn cells in the brachial and lumbosacral enlargements. Branches of corticospinal fibers in the spinal cord innervate several spinal segments, but axons supplying motor neuronal pools innervating distal limb muscles have few collaterals. This arrangement is related to discrete contractions of individual distal limb muscles. Anatomically the corticospinal tract is not somatotopically organized.

Electrical stimulation of the primary motor area (M I) evokes discrete isolated movements on the opposite side of the body. Contractions usually involve functional muscle groups concerned with specific movements, but individual muscles may be contracted separately. While the general pattern of excitable foci is the same for all mammals, the number of such foci, and hence the number of discrete movements, is increased in humans. Thus flexion or extension at a single finger joint, twitchings

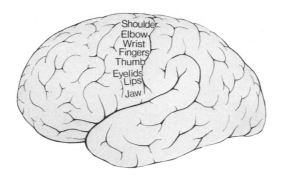

Figure 13.24. Diagrammatic representation of parts of the body in the primary motor area (M I) on the lateral aspect of the hemisphere in the human. Parts of the lower extremity are represented in sequential fashion in the anterior portion of the paracentral lobule on the medial aspect of the hemisphere.

at the corners of the mouth, elevation of the palate, protrusion of the tongue, and even vocalization, all may be evoked by careful stimulation of the proper areas. Charts of motor representation have been furnished by a number of investigators (Figs. 13.13 and 13.24). Data concerning the human brain were collected during neurosurgical procedures in patients operated on under local anesthesia. The location of centers for specific movements may vary from individual to individual, but the sequence of motor representation appears constant. Ipsilateral movements have not been observed in humans, but bilateral responses occur in the extraocular muscles and muscles of the face, tongue, jaw, larynx, and pharynx. The center for the pharynx (swallowing) lies in the most inferior opercular portion of the precentral gyrus; it is followed, from below upward, by centers for the tongue, jaw, lips, larynx, eyelid, and brow, in the order named (Figs. 13.13 and 13.24). Next come the extensive areas for finger movements, the thumb being lowest and the little finger highest; these are followed by areas for the hand, wrist, elbow, and shoulder. Finally in the most superior part are the centers for the hip, knee, ankle, and toes. The last named are situated at the medial border of the hemisphere and extend into the paracentral lobule, which also contains the centers for the anal and vesicle sphincters (Fig. 2.6).

The movements elicited by electrical stimulation of the motor cortex probably are not voluntary movements, although they are interpreted by the patient as "volitional." Responses are never skilled movements, comparable to those of complex acquired movements. Most movements consist of simple flexions or extensions at one or more joints. The threshold in different topographical parts of area 4 varies. The thumb region appears to have the lowest threshold, while the face area has the highest. Excessive stimulation of area 4 produces either a focal seizure, or one resembling a Jacksonian convulsion.

The classical view of the somatotopic organization in the motor cortex is a single continuous, distorted representation of the body within the primary motor area (Fig. 13.13). This pattern of organization, represented by the motor homunculus or its equivalent, has been extrapolated from studies in which movements have been produced by surface stimulation in a variety of animals and in man (Fig. 13.24). The summation of cortical representation depicted in a single line drawing is regarded as an oversimplification because it rarely takes into account the extent of overlap of various body regions. Studies indicating a double representation of the body surface within areas 3 and 1 in the monkey have raised questions concerning multiple representations of body parts in the primary motor cortex. The possibility of dual representation of motor function appears to have some foundation. Although there is little evidence that cells in the motor cortex are organized into discrete functional cell col-

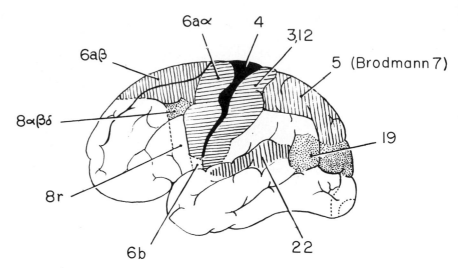

Figure 13.25. Areas of electrically excitable cortex on the lateral aspect of the human brain. The primary motor area (M I) is in *black*. Area 6aα on the lateral aspect of the hemisphere constitutes the premotor area. The part of area 6aα on the medial aspect of the hemisphere constitutes the supplementary motor area (M II, Fig. 13.26). The frontal eye field (*stippled*) lies in part of the middle frontal gyrus, but does not correspond to a single architectonic area. (Based upon Foerster, 1936.)

umns as in the somesthetic and visual cortex, microstimulation in a vertical column produces the same response in all layers.

Ablations of area 4 in the monkey produce a contralateral flaccid paralysis, marked hypotonia, and areflexia. Within a relatively short time myotatic reflexes reappear, along with withdrawal responses to nociceptive stimuli. There is recovery of some motor function in both proximal and distal musculature, but skilled movements are performed slowly with deliberation. No significant spasticity develops in these animals.

Lesions of the motor cortex in humans produce neurological deficits similar to those described in the primate. Ablations limited to the "arm" or "leg" area of the precentral gyrus result in a paralysis of a single limb. The ultimate loss of movement is always greatest in the distal muscle groups, but motor recovery in the affected limb usually is more complete than that associated with nearly total lesions of the motor area. Immediately after complete or partial lesions of the precentral gyrus, there is a flaccid paralysis of the contralateral limbs or limb, marked hypotonia, and loss of superficial and myotatic reflexes. Within a relatively short time the Babinski sign can be elicited. The myotatic reflexes generally return early in an exaggerated form.

Premotor Area

The region designated as 6aα on the lateral convexity of the hemisphere is considered the premotor area; area 6aα on the medial aspect of the hemisphere is the supplementary motor area (M II) (Fig. 13.25). The premotor area has a specific role in sensorially guided movements. Units of the premotor area are activated in response to visual, auditory, and somatosensory stimuli. Like the primary motor area (MI), units are clearly related to voluntary motor function; it differs from MI in that it

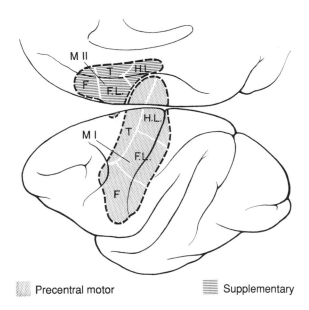

Figure 13.26. Diagram of the precentral (M I) and supplementary motor (M II) areas in the monkey. The somatotopic arrangement of different parts of the body are indicated: *F*, face; *T*, trunk; *FL*, forelimb; *HL*, hindlimb. The precentral motor area (M I) on the lateral convexity extends onto the medial aspect of the hemisphere; the *outlined area* shown posterior to the central sulcus represents cortex in the depths of the central sulcus. The supplementary motor area (M II) on the medial aspect of the hemisphere is shown *above*. (Based on Travis, 1955.)

▦ Precentral motor ▤ Supplementary

has a higher threshold and its neurons are activated by visuospatial signals. The histological structure of the premotor area resembles that of the motor area, but there are no giant cells of Betz (Fig. 13.2). The presence of pyramidal cells in layers III and V and the narrowness of layer IV make it difficult to distinguish an internal granular layer. For this reason area 6, like area 4, is referred to as agranular frontal cortex. The premotor area discharges via the corticospinal tract. Unilateral ablations of area 6, not involving the primary or supplementary motor areas, do not produce paresis, grasp reflexes or hypertonia.

Supplementary Motor Area (M II)

In man and monkey the supplementary motor area occupies the medial surface of the superior frontal gyrus rostral to area 4 and corresponds to the medial part of area 6 (area 6aα) (Fig. 13.25). Detailed descriptions of somatotopic representation within the supplementary motor area of the monkey have been provided. The sequential representation of body parts in this area is shown in Figure 13.26.

Movement-related neurons in M II (cells firing during movement) are of three types: (1) cells related to proximal movements, (2) cells related to distal movements, and (3) cells activated throughout a motor task. The majority of cortical neurons in this area (94%) exhibit movement-related activity regardless of whether the motor task is performed with the contralateral or ipsilateral limbs.

The threshold for stimulation of the supplementary motor area (M II) in the human and monkey is slightly higher than for the precentral region. Motor responses obtained by stimulating the supplementary motor area are abolished by ablations of M I. The somatotopic features of M II also are less distinct after ablations of M I.

Unilateral ablations of the supplementary motor area in man and monkey produce no permanent deficit in the maintenance of posture or the capacity for movement. In the monkey of removals of the supplementary motor area (M II) in combination with the precentral motor area

(M I) on the same side result in a contralateral spastic hemiparesis in which marked hypertonus develops in both proximal and distal flexor muscles. Combined ablations of M II and M I in monkeys with longitudinal section of the corpus callosum (i.e., split-brain preparations) result in more pronounced spasticity, suggesting that part of the bilateral influences of M II involve fibers that cross in the corpus callosum.

Cortical projections from M II are ipsilateral to areas 4, 6 (lateral part), 5, and 7, and to contralateral M II. Connections between M II and these cortical areas are almost completely reciprocal. Approximately 5% of the neurons in M II project directly to spinal cord with a bilateral disposition. Subcortical projections of M II are profuse to parts of the caudate nucleus and putamen and to thalamic nuclei [ventral anterior (VApc), ventral lateral (VLO), and mediodorsal (MD)]. Afferents to the primary motor area, the premotor area, and the supplementary motor area have distinctive features and will be discussed together in "Inputs to Motor Cortical Areas," later.

Studies in conscious, behaving monkeys indicate that neurons in the supplementary motor area are related to movements on both sides of the body and involve distal and proximal musculature equally. Most of the neurons in the supplementary motor area increase their activity before the onset of movement and large numbers of neurons in this area discharge during movement of either arm. Only a small number of cells in this area respond to peripheral stimuli and the responses are weaker than in the primary motor area.

While the supplementary motor area, as described in humans and the monkey, is recognized as a distinct and separate motor area with striking bilateral influences upon both proximal and distal musculature, it precise contribution to motor function has not been defined. M II has been considered to be involved in mechanisms that influence muscle tone and modify posture, the automatic grasp reflex response, bimanual coordination, and voluntary movement. There appears to be general agreement that neurons in M II modify the activities of cells in the primary motor area and probably are involved in the programming of learned skilled motor sequences. Some evidence suggests that M II may play a role in initiating voluntary movement. Studies in humans indicate that lesions in M II are associated with a reduction of voluntary motor activity (akinesis) and poverty of spontaneous speech.

Inputs to Motor Cortical Areas

Although impulses generated in neurons in the primary motor area (M I), the premotor area, and in the supplementary motor area (M II) are responsible for movement, motor control, changes in muscle tone, and maintenance of posture, these motor activities are initiated by inputs that arise from the thalamus, other cortical regions, and peripheral receptors. Particularly potent drives on the motor cortical areas are derived from all divisions of the ventral lateral, and the ventral posterolateral, pars oralis (VPLo) thalamic nuclei (Figs. 9.12, 9.13, and 13.12). Crossed projections from the deep cerebellar nuclei terminate somatotopically in VPLo and in the cell-sparse region of the ventral lateral thalamic nuclear complex, which includes the ventral lateral nucleus (VLc) and area x. The somatotopical cortical projection area of VPLo and the cell-sparse region of VL has been identified as projecting to area 4, the primary motor area (M I).

The uncrossed pallidothalamic fibers, originating from the medial pallidal segment, project to the ventral anterior (VApc), ventral lateral (VLo), and the centromedian (CM) thalamic nuclei (Fig. 9.12). Pallidal inputs to the rostral ventral tier thalamic nuclei do not overlap cerebellothalamic terminations. The cortical projections of VLo are to the supplementary (M II) and the lateral premotor area (area 6aα) (Figs. 9.13, 13.25, and 13.26). The thalamic terminations of projections from the substantia nigra are distinct from those arising from the deep cerebellar nuclei and the globus pallidus. The cortical projections of the magnocellular division of the ventral anterior (VAmc) and the mediodorsal (MDpl) thalamic nuclei, which receive nigral terminations, appear to exclude area 4, and probably project to frontal areas rostral to area 6 (Figs. 9.12 and 9.13).

Neurons of the ventral posterolateral nucleus (VPLo) and the cell sparse zone of the ventral lateral nucleus (VLc) show increased activity prior to any movement. This finding suggests that these neurons may play a role in initiating activity in muscles that effect discrete movements and control posture. Thalamic neurons that project to the primary motor area, the premotor cortex and the supplementary motor area are distinct and separate from those that terminate in somatic sensory areas. Electron microscopic evidence in the cat indicates that fibers from VLc and VPLo projecting to the motor cortex make synaptic terminations largely in three cortical layers: (1) layer I (18%), (2) layer III (66%), and (3) layer VI (13%). Fibers terminating directly in layer V were relatively sparse (3%). The majority of thalamocortical projections synapse on dendrite spines of cells in layer III, the apical dendrites of motor neurons (Betz cells of layer V) and on interneurons in layer III.

The primary motor area (M I) also receives inputs from the primary somesthetic area (S I) and the supplementary motor area. Area 4 has reciprocal connections with areas 1, 2, and parts of area 5. The supplementary motor area (M II) receives inputs from the same sensory areas but has reciprocal connections only with area 4 (M I). Neither M I nor M II receives inputs from any part of area 3.

It has been postulated that are 5 contains the "command apparatus" for limb and hand movements in immediate extrapersonal space. The "command" hypothesis suggests that the cortical pathway from area 5 to area 4 is involved in initiating limb and hand movements.

Physiological studies indicate that the primary motor cortex (M I) receives inputs from cutaneous and deep receptors. Impulses from joint receptors projecting to areas 1 and 2 appear to have access to M I and M II directly and via area 5. Inputs from cutaneous receptors may be involved in instinctive grasping as well as in the startle reaction.

Cortical Eye Fields

Rostral to the premotor area is a cortical region particularly concerned with voluntary eye movements. The *frontal eye field* in humans occupies principally the caudal part of the middle frontal gyrus (corresponding to parts of area 8, shown in Fig. 13.25). The entire frontal eye field does not lie within a single cytoarchitectonic area. Electrical stimulation of the frontal eye field in man causes strong conjugate deviation of the eyes, usually to the opposite side. This cortical field is believed to be a center for voluntary movements of the eyes, independent of visual stimuli. These conjugate eye movements are called "movements of command," since they can be elicited by instructing the patient to look to the right or left. The frontal eye field participates in the initiation of purposeful saccades (rapid eye movements to targets of behavioral importance) and is implicated in the coordination of eye movements necessary for accurate gaze changes.

The concept of an *occipital eye center* for conjugate eye movements is based on the fact that stimulation of occipital cortex produces conjugate eye movements to the opposite side, and lesions in this area are associated with transient deviation of the eyes to the side of the lesion. Unlike the frontal eye field, the occipital eye center is not localized to a small area. Eye responses can be obtained from a wide region of the occipital lobe in the monkey, but the lowest threshold is in area 17. The occipital eye centers subserve movements of the eyes induced by visual stimuli, such as following moving objects. These pursuit eye movements are largely involuntary, though they are not present in young infants. Parts of the occipital eye centers are interconnected by fibers passing in the splenium of the corpus callosum. The threshold for excitation in the occipital eye center is higher than in the frontal eye fields, the latency of responses is longer, and eye movements tend to be smoother.

With a lesion of the occipital eye field, the patient may have difficulty following a slow moving object, but on command can direct the eyes to a particular location. Eye movements on command are impaired by lesions in the frontal eye field, particularly in the dominant hemisphere.

The pathways by which responses from the frontal field are mediated involve multiple subcortical loci, chief among which are the rostral interstitial nucleus of the MLF (RiMLF), the interstitial nucleus of Cajal, the pontine paramedian reticular formation (PPRF), and layer IV of the superior colliculus. These structures are known to have direct and indirect influences on eye movements (see pp. 175). None of the corticofugal fibers from the frontal eye field project directly to the nuclei of the extraocular muscles. The occipital eye center appears to influence eye movements via substantial and highly organized direct projections from the visual cortex to the superior colliculus, even though this projection is to the superficial layers.

CORTICOTHALAMIC PROJECTIONS

The major corticofugal fibers systems have been discussed regionally, except for corticothalamic projections which were described briefly only as components of the internal capsule (see p. 281). In general, cortical areas receiving projections from particular thalamic nuclei give rise to reciprocal fibers which pass back to the same nuclei (Figs. 9.12 and 9.13). The granular frontal cortex has reciprocal connections with the mediodorsal nucleus (pars parvicellularis, (MDpc) of the thalamus. The frontal eye field (area 8) has reciprocal connections with the paralaminar part of the mediodorsal (MDpl) and the magnocellular part of the ventral anterior (VAmc) thalamic nuclei. Area 6 projects fibers to VA, VLc, "area x," VPLo, MDpl, and the parafascicular nucleus of the thalamus. In general, the premotor area shows projections to thalamic nuclei related to either the precentral or prefrontal cortex. Corticothalamic fibers from the precentral area are widespread and include projections to VLo, VLc, and VPLo, as well as to portions of the intralaminar thalamic nuclei. Cortical projections from area 4 to parts of VL and VPLo are reciprocal and topographically arranged. Projections from area 4 to VLc are not as impressive as those from area 6. These data indicate that corticofugal fibers from the precentral gyrus project to thalamic nuclei which receive selective inputs from the deep cerebellar nuclei, the globus pallidus, and the substantia nigra.

Efferent fibers from the parietal cortex pass via the sensory radiations to the ventral posterolateral (VPLc) and posteromedial (VPM) thalamic nuclei. Corticothalamic projections from areas 3, 1, and 2 are confined to the ventrobasal complex, except for small projections to the reticular and central lateral thalamic nuclei. No terminals from parietal areas project to VPLo.

Parts of the auditory cortex project to the medial geniculate body (MGB) via the sublenticular part of the internal capsule (Fig. 9.24). The cortical projections from the primary and secondary auditory areas are back to the subdivisions of the geniculate body (MGB) (Fig. 9.19) from which they receive inputs. The medial geniculate body (MGB) does not give rise to descending fibers that influence auditory relay nuclei at lower levels of the brain stem, but projections from the auditory cortex to the inferior colliculus (pericentral nucleus; Fig. 7.4) are involved in this activity.

The striate cortex (area 17) sends fibers to the lateral geniculate body (LGB), the superior colliculus, the pretectum, and the inferior pulvinar. Fibers from area 17, projecting retinotopically to all layers of the LGB, arise from cells in layer VI.

While reciprocal relationships exist between the principal thalamic nuclei and their cortical projection sites, a different relationship pertains to the reticular and intralaminar thalamic nuclei (Figs. 9.10, 9.11, 9.12, and 9.14). The reticular nucleus of the thalamus receives afferents from almost all cortical areas but does not project back to the cerebral cortex. However, collaterals of thalamocortical fibers terminate in particular parts of the reticular nucleus. Also corticothalamic fibers give collaterals to the same portion of the reticular nucleus as the thalamic nucleus which receives the main cortical projection. Thus, the reticular nucleus of the thalamus is strategically situated to sample activities passing in both directions between cerebral cortex and thalamic relay nuclei. The intralaminar thalamic nuclei receive corticofugal fibers; the prefrontal cortex projects on the rostral intralaminar nuclei, while the premotor and motor cortex send fibers respectively, to the parafascicular (PF) and centromedian (CM) nuclei. The parietal and occipital cortex do not project fibers to the intralaminar thalamic nuclei.

CEREBRAL DOMINANCE

Although the two cerebral hemispheres appear as mirror image duplicates, many functions are not represented equally at cortical levels. This appears true even though (1) impulses from receptors on each side of the body seem to project nearly equally, though largely contralaterally, to symmetrical cortical areas, and (2) information received in the cortex of one hemisphere can be transferred to the other via interhemispheric commissures.

In certain higher functions, believed to be cortical in nature, one hemisphere appears to be the "leading" one and, in this sense, is referred to as the *dominant hemisphere*. With respect to most of the higher functions, cerebral dominance appears to be one of degree. Cerebral dominance probably is most complete in relation to highly evolved aspects of language. Handedness also is related to cerebral dominance, though its relationship is less clear-cut than has been assumed. It seems likely that handedness is a graded characteristic. Left-handedness, in particular, is less definite than right-handedness and less regularly associated with dominance in either hemisphere. There also appears to be a group of disturbances related to language that are said to be commonly associated with imperfectly developed cerebral dominance. These include improper development of reading, writing, and drawing abilities; poor spatial judgment; and imperfect directional control. In true right-handed individuals it is nearly always the left hemisphere that is dominant and governs language and related processes. Even in left-handed individuals, the left hemisphere is most often dominant for language, but this function may be represented bilaterally. The degree of cerebral dominance appears to vary widely, not only among individuals, but with respect to different functions.

Although a degree of "cerebral ambilaterality" would appear to be a distinct advantage with respect to recovery of speech following a unilateral cerebral injury, it carries the risk, or possibility, of difficulty in learning to read, spell and draw. The relationship between handedness and speech is perhaps a more natural one than is commonly realized, since gesturing often accompanies speech and in certain situations may substitute for it. Most clinicians relate handedness and speech to the dominant hemisphere.

The dominant hemisphere, usually the left, is primarily concerned with processing language, arithmetic, and analytic functions, while the nondominant hemisphere is concerned with simple spatial concepts, recognition of faces, some elements of music, and many aspects of emotion. Ideographic (pictographic) language (i.e., Japanese Kanji) may be processed by the nondominant hemisphere because of its spatial and pictorial features, while grammatical language (i.e., Japanese Kana) using script depends on analytic functions of the dominant hemisphere. Visual sign language used by deaf persons appears to be processed primarily in the left hemisphere.

Cerebral dominance is considered to have a genetic basis, but its hereditary determination probably is not absolute. Pathological and psychological factors also influence handedness, but most determining factors remain unknown. Theoretical arguments suggest that variations in levels of testosterone, and perhaps other hormones, during pregnancy may alter the patterns of migrations of cortical neurons. Every neuron in the cerebral cortex has migrated during fetal life from the germinal zone of the neural tube to its final location. The brain of the male matures later than in the female and the left hemisphere matures later than the right. If fetal levels of testosterone are altered by maternal stress, or other factors, the right hemisphere may become more developed and assume functions for language and handedness which the left hemisphere cannot support. The effects of testosterone on brain development is most pronounced in the male, which may account for the higher incidence of left-handedness, dyslexia (reading problems), and stuttering in the male. Anomolous cerebral dominance appears to be a major factor in learning disorders, even in individuals not totally left-handed. The left dominant hemisphere is particularly concerned with ability to handle sequential information, such as language, musical rhythms, Morse code, and complex spatial tasks.

Many cortical functions are concerned only with contralateral regions of the body, and unilateral lesions affecting these functions produce contralateral disturbances, regardless of cerebral dominance. This appears particularly true of the primary motor and sensory areas. It also is the case with lesions of the parietal cortex which result in *asterognosis*, or inability to recognize form, size, texture, and identity of an object by touch alone. In lesions of the inferior parietal lobule, particular deficits occur more commonly in the nondominant hemisphere. One such syndrome is characterized by a disorder of the body image in which the patient (1) fails to recognize parts of his or her own body, (2) fails to appreciate the existence of hemiparesis, and (3) neglects the part of the body that is denied. Lesions of the angular and supramarginal gyri in the dominant hemisphere produce devastating neurological disturbances of a curious nature. Disturbances in the *Gerstmann syndrome* include (1) finger agnosis (inability to name and identify individual fingers), (2) agraphic (inability to write), (3) acalculia (impaired ability to make simple mathematical calculations) and (4) right-left disorientation. Patients with this syndrome can copy written material and write their name but cannot convert spoken words to script.

INTEGRATED CORTICAL FUNCTIONS

One of the striking and unique features of the human brain is its elaborate neural mechanisms for complex correlations, sensory discriminations and the utilization of former experiences and reactions. These mechanisms involve *associative memory* and *mnemonic reactions*. The ability to retain, modify, and reuse neuronal circuits probably provides the basis of conscious and unconscious memory.

In a general way, the central sulcus divides the cerebral cortex into a posterior receptive portion and an anterior part related to motor functions. The posterior portion contains all the primary receptive areas that receive specific sensory signals from the spinal cord and brain stem. Regions immediately adjacent to the receptive centers, known as *parasensory areas*, serve for the combination and elaboration of primary impulses into more complex sensory perceptions. In more distant *association areas* signals conveyed from various sensory regions may overlap (e.g., the inferior parietal lobule) and form the basis for multisensory perceptions. The interaction of different sensory modalities initiated by "feeling" and "seeing" an object or person excite memory constellations which lead to recognition. The arousal of associative mnemonic complexes has been termed "gnosis," and it forms the basis of understanding and knowledge. Disorders of these mechanisms caused by lesions in association areas of the cerebral cortex are known as gnostic disturbances, or *agnosias*. In these conditions tactile, visual, or auditory stimuli may no longer evoke appropriate memory constellations. When these gnostic disturbances involve the associative mechanisms underlying the comprehension of language, they form part of the complex known as the *aphasias*.

Closely related to both agnosia and aphasia is another group of disorders characterized by difficulty in performing skilled, learned movements even though no paralysis or sensory loss is present. Disorders that affect the motor side of sensory-motor integration are referred to as the *apraxias*. There are only two ways a patient can show that he or she recognizes an object: (1) by naming or describing the object, or (2) by demonstrating its use. If the patient can demonstrate the use of an object but is unable to name it, the individual has an aphasia. If the patient can name the object, or describe it, but does not know how to use it, he or she has an apraxia. The above examples demonstrate that agnosia partially underlies both aphasia and apraxia.

SUGGESTED READINGS

AIKTINS, L. M., IRVINE, D. R. F., AND WEBSTER, W. R. 1984. Central neural mechanisms of hearing. In I. DARIAN-SMITH (Editor), *Handbook of Physiology*. American Physiological Society, Washington, DC, **3**: 675–737.

ALLMAN, J. M., AND KAAS, J. H. 1974. The organization of the second visual area (VII) in the owl monkey: a second order transformation of the visual hemifield. Brain Res., **76**: 247–265.

ANGEVINE, J. B., JR., AND SIDMAN, R. L. 1961. Autoradiographic study of cell migration during histogenesis of the cerebral cortex in the mouse. Nature, **192**: 766–768.

BERTRAND, G. 1956. Spinal efferent pathways from the supplementary motor area. Brain, **79**: 461–473.

BINDMAN, L., AND LIPPOLD, O. 1981. *The Neurophysiology of the Cerebral Cortex*. University of Texas Press, Austin, pp. 495.

BRINKMAN, C., AND PORTER, R. 1983. Supplementary motor area and premotor area of monkey cerebral cortex: functional organization and activities of single neurons during performance of a learned movement. In J. C. DESMEDT (Editor), *Motor Control Mechanisms in Health and Disease*. Raven Press, New York, pp. 393–420.

BRODMANN, K. 1909. *Vergleichende Lokalisation lehre der Grosshirnrinde in ihren Prinzipien dargestellt auf Grund des Zellenbaues*. J. A. Barth, Peipzig, 324 pp.

BRUGGE, J. F., AND REALE, R. A. 1985. Auditory cortex. In A. PETERS AND E. G. JONES (Editors), *Cerebral Cortex*. Plenum Press, New York, **4**: 229–271.

BUCY, P. C. 1949. Effects of extirpation in man. In P. C. BUCY (Editor), *The Precentral Motor Cortex*, Ed. 2. University of Illinois Press, Urbana, Ch. 14, pp. 353–394.

BURTON, H. 1986. Second somatosensory cortex and related areas. In E. G. JONES AND A. PETERS (Editors), *Cerebral Cortex*. Plenum Press, New York, **5**: 31–98.

CAMPBELL, A. W. 1905. *Histological Studies on the Localization of Cerebral Function*. Cambridge University Press, New York, 360 pp.

COXE, W. S., AND LANDAU, W. M. 1965. Observations upon the effect of supplementary motor cortex ablation in the monkey. Brain, **88**: 763–772.

DENNY-BROWN, D., AND BOTTERELL, E. H. 1948. The motor functions of the agranular frontal cortex. Proc. Assoc. Res. Nerv. Ment. Dis., **27**: 235–345.

DIAMOND, I. T., JONES, E. G., AND POWELL, T. P. S. 1968. Interhemispheric fiber connections of the auditory cortex in the cat. Brain Res., **11**: 177–193.

DIVAC, I., LAVAIL, J. H., RAKIC, P., AND WINSTON, K. R. 1977. Heterogenous afferents to the inferior parietal lobule of the rhesus monkey revealed by the retrograde transport method. Brain Res., **123**: 197–207.

ECONOMO, C. F. VON. 1929. *The Cytoarchitectonics of the Human Cerebral Cortex*. Oxford Medical Publications, London.

EMSON, P. C., AND HUNT, S. P. 1984. Peptide-containing neurons of the cerebral cortex. In E. G. JONES AND A. PETERS (Editors), *Cerebral Cortex*. Plenum Press, New York, **2**: 145–169.

FELLEMAN, D. J., NELSON, R. J., AND KAAS, J. H. 1983. Representations of the body surface in areas 3b and 1 of postcentral cortex of cebus monkeys. Brain Res., **268**: 15–26.

FOERSTER, O. 1936. Symptomatologie der Erkrankungen des Grosshirns. Motorische Felder und Bahnen. In O. BUMKE AND O. FOERSTER (Editors), *Handbuch der Neurologie*, Vol. 60. Julius Springer, Berlin, pp. 1–357.

FONNUM, F. 1984. Glutamate: a neurotransmitter in mammalian brain. J. Neurochem., **42**: 1–11.

FREDERICKSON, J. M. AND RUBIN, A. M. 1986. Vestibular cortex. In E. G. JONES AND A. PETERS (Editors), *Cerebral Cortex*. Plenum Press, New York, **5**: 99–111.

FRIEDMAN, D. P., JONES, E. G., AND BURTON, H. 1980. Representation pattern in the second somatic sensory area of the monkey cerebral cortex. J. Comp. Neurol., **192**: 21–41.

GESCHWIND, J., AND GALABURDA, A. M. 1984. *Cerebral Dominance: The Biological Foundation*. Harvard University Press, Cambridge, Massachusetts, 232 pp.

GESCHWIND, N., AND GALABURDA, A. M. 1987. *Cerebral Lateralization: Biological Mechanisms, Associations and Pathology*. MIT Press, Cambridge, Massachusetts, 283 pp.

GIUFFRIDA, R., AND RUSTIONI, A. 1988. Glutamate and aspartate immunoreactivity in corticothalamic neurons of rats. In M. BENTIVOGLIO AND R. SPREAFICO (Editors), *Cellular Thalamic Mechanisms*. Elsevier, Amsterdam, pp. 311–320.

GIUFRIDA, R. AND RUSTIONI, A. 1989. Glutamate and aspartate immunoreactivity in corticospinal neurons of rat. J. Comp. Neurol., **288**: 154–164.

HENDRICKSON, A. E., HUNT, S. P., AND WU, J-Y. 1981. Immunocytochemical localization of glutamic acid decarboxylase in monkey striate cortex. Nature, **292**: 605–607.

HOUSER, C. R., VAUGHN, J. E., HENDRY, S. H. C., JONES, E. G., AND PETERS, A. 1984. GABA neurons in the cerebral cortex. In E. G. JONES AND A. PETERS (Editors), *Cerebral Cortex*. Plenum Press, New York, **2**: 63–89.

HUBEL, D. H. 1963. The visual cortex of the brain. Sci. Am., **209**: 54–62.

HUBEL, D. H., AND WIESEL, T. N. 1959. Receptive fields of single neurons in the cat's striate cortex. J. Physiol., **148**: 574–591.

HUBEL, D. H., AND WIESEL, T. N. 1962. Receptive fields, binocular interaction and functional architecture in the cat's visual cortex. J. Physiol., **160**: 106–154.

HUBEL, D. H., AND WIESEL, T. N. 1963. Receptive fields of cells in striate cortex of very young, visually inexperienced kittens. J. Neurophysiol., **26**: 994–1002.

HUBEL, D. H., AND WIESEL, T. N. 1963. Shape and arrangement of columns in the cat's striate cortex. J. Physiol., **165**: 559–568.

HUBEL, D. H., AND WIESEL, T. N. 1967. Cortical and callosal connections concerned with the vertical meridan of visual fields in the cat. J. Neurophysiol., **30**: 1561–1573.

HUBEL, D. H., AND WIESEL, T. N. 1970. Stereoscopic vision in macaque monkey. Nature, **225**: 41–42.

HUBEL, D. H., AND WIESEL, T. N. 1972. Laminar and columnar distribution of geniculo-cortical fibers in the macaque monkey. J. Comp. Neurol., **146**: 421–450.

HUBEL, D. H., AND WIESEL, T. N. 1974. Sequence regularity and geometry of orientation columns in the monkey straite cortex. J. Comp. Neurol., **158**: 267–294.

HUBEL, D. H., WIESEL, T. N., AND LeVAY, S. 1977. Plasticity of ocular dominance columns in monkey striate cortex. Philos. Trans. R. Soc. Lond. (Biol.), **278**: 377–409.

HUERTA, M. F., KRUBITZER, L. A., AND KAAS, J. H. 1986. Frontal eye field as defined by intracortical microstimulation in squirrel monkeys, owl monkeys and macaque monkeys. I. Subcortical connections. J. Comp. Neurol., **253**: 415–439.

HUERTA, M. F., KRUBITZER, L. A., AND KAAS, J. H. 1987. Frontal eye field as defined by intracortical microstimulation in squirrel monkeys, owl monkeys and macaque monkeys. II. Cortical connections. J. Comp. Neurol., **265**: 332–361.

IMIG, T. J., AND MOREL, A. 1985. Tonotopic organization of the ventral nucleus of the medial geniculate body in the cat. J. Neurophysiol., **53**: 309–340.

IMIG, T. J., RUGGERO, M. A., KITZES, L. M., JAVEL, E., AND BRUGGE, J. F. 1977. Organization of auditory cortex in the owl monkey (*Aotus Trivirgatus*). J. Comp. Neurol., **171**: 111–128.

JONES, E. G. 1981. Anatomy of cerebral cortex: columnar input-output organization. In F. O. SCHMITT, F. G. WORDEN, G. ADELMAN, AND S. G. DENNIS (Editors), *The Organization of the Cerebral Cortex*. MIT Press, Cambridge, Massachusetts, pp. 199–235.

JONES, E. G. 1986. Connectivity of primate sensory-motor cortex. In E. G. JONES AND A. PETERS (Editors), *Cerebral Cortex*. Plenum Press, New York, **5**: 113–183.

JONES, E. G. 1987. Ascending inputs to, and internal organization of, cortical motor areas. In *Motor Areas of the Cerebral Cortex*, CIBA Foundation Symposium. J. Wiley & Sons, Chichester, **132**: 21–39.

JONES, E. G., COULTER, J. D., AND HENDRY, S. H. C. 1978. Intracortical connectivity of architectonic fields in the somatic sensory, motor and parietal cortex of monkeys. J. Comp. Neurol., **181**: 291–348.

JONES, E. G., AND FRIEDMAN, D. P. 1982. Projection pattern of functional components of thalamic ventrobasal complex on monkey somatosensory cortex. J. Neurophysiol. **48**: 521–544.

JONES, E. G., AND HENDRY, S. H. C. 1980. Distribution of callosal fibers around the hand representation in monkey somatic sensory cortex. Neurosci. Lett., **19**: 167–172.

JONES, E. G., AND LEAVITT, R. Y. 1974. Retrograde axonal transport and the demonstration of non-specific projections to the cerebral cortex and striatum from thalamic intralaminar nuclei in the cat, rat and monkey. J. Comp. Neurol., **154**: 349–378.

JONES, E. G., AND POWELL, T. P. S. 1969. Connexions of the somatic sensory cortex of the rhesus monkey. I. Ipsilateral cortical connexions. Brain, **92**: 477–502.

JONES, E. G., AND POWELL, T. P. S. 1969. Connexions of the somatic sensory cortex of the rhesus monkey. II. Contralateral cortical connexions. Brain, **92**: 717–730.

JONES, E. G., AND POWELL, T. P. S. 1970. Connexions of the somatic sensory cortex of the rhesus monkey. III. Thalamic connexions. Brain, **93**: 37–56.

JONES, E. G., AND WISE, S. P. 1977. Size, laminar and columnar distribution of efferent cells in the sensory-motor cortex of monkeys. J. Comp. Neurol., **175**: 391–438.

JÜRGENS, J. 1984. The efferent and afferent connections of the supplementary motor area. Brain Res., **300**: 63–81.

KENNEDY, C., DES ROSIERS, M. H., SAKURADA, O., SHINOHARA, M., REIVICH, M., JEHLE, J. W., AND SOKOLOFF, L. 1976. Metabolic mapping of the primary visual system of the monkey by means of the autoradiographic [^{14}C] deoxyglucose technique. Proc. Natl. Acad. Sci. USA, **73**: 4230–4234.

KIEVIT J., AND KUYPERS, H. G. J. M. 1977. Organization of the thalamo-cortical connexions to the frontal lobe in the rhesus monkey. Exp. Brain Res., **29**: 299–322.

KONISHI, M., AND KNUDSEN, E. I. 1982. A theory of neural auditory space. In C. N. WOOLSEY (Editor), *Cortical Sensory Organization*. Humana Press, Clifton, New Jersey, **3**: 219–229.

KRNJEVIĆ, K. 1984. Neurotransmitters in cerebral cortex. In E. G. JONES AND A. PETERS (Editors), *Cerebral Cortex*. Plenum Press, New York, **2**: 39–61.

KUFFLER, S. W. 1953. Discharge patterns and functional organization of mammalian retina. J. Neurophysiol., **16**: 37–68.

KUYPERS, H. G. J. M., AND BRINKMAN, J. 1970. Precentral projections to different parts of the spinal intermediate zone in the rhesus monkey. Brain Res., **24**: 29–48.

LeVAY, S., WIESEL, T. N., AND HUBEL, D. H. 1980. The development of ocular dominance columns in normal and visually deprived monkeys. J. Comp. Neurol., **191**: 1–51.

LEWIS, D. A., CAMPBELL, M. J., FOOTE, S. L., GOLDSTEIN, M., AND MORRISON, J. H. 1987.

The distribution of tyrosine hydroxylase-immunoreactive fibers in primate neocortex is widespread but regionally specific. J. Neurosci., **7**: 279–290.

LORENTE DE NÓ, R. 1949. The structure of the cerebral cortex. In J. F. FULTON (Editor), *Physiology of the Nervous System*, Ed. 3. Oxford University Press, New York, pp. 288–330.

LUND, J. S., LUND, R. D., HENDRICKSON, A. E., BUNT, A. H., AND FUCHS, A. F. 1975. The origin of efferent pathways from the primary visual cortex, area 17, of the macaque monkey as shown by retrograde transport of horseradish peroxidase. J. Comp. Neurol., **164**: 287–304.

MASH, D. C., WHITE, W. F., AND MESULAM, M.-M. 1988. Distribution of muscarinic receptor subtypes within architectonic subregions of the primate cerebral cortex. J. Comp. Neurol., **278**: 265–274.

MASTERTON, R. B., AND IMIG, T. J. 1984. Neural mechanisms for sound localization. Ann. Rev. Physiol., **46**: 275–287.

MERZENICH, M. M., AND BRUGGE, J. F. 1973. Representation of the cochlear partition on the superior temporal plane of the macaque monkey. Brain Res., **50**: 275–296.

MERZENICH, M. M., KAAS, J. H., SUR, M., AND LIN, C. S. 1978. Double representation of the body surface with cytoarchitectonic areas 3b and 1 in "S 1" in the owl monkey. (*Aotus trivigatus*). J. Comp. Neurol., **181**: 41–74.

MERZENICH, M. M., KNIGHT, P. L., AND ROTH, G. L. 1975. Representation of cochlea within the primary auditory cortex in the cat. J. Neurophysiol., **38**: 231–249.

MESULAM, M.-M., AND GEULA, C. 1988. Nucleus basalis (Ch4) and cortical cholinergic innervation in the human brain: observations based on the distribution of acetylcholinesterase and choline acetyltransferase. J. Comp. Neurol., **275**: 216–240.

MESULAM, M.-M., MUFSON, E. J., LEVEY, A. I., AND WAINER, B. H. 1983. Cholinergic innervation of cortex by the basal forebrain: cytochemistry and cortical connections of the septal area, diagonal band nuclei, nucleus basalis (substantia innominata), and hypothalamus in the rhesus monkey. J. Comp. Neurol., **214**: 170–197.

MOLLIVER, M. E., GRZANNA, R., LIDOW, H. G. W., MORRISON, J. H., AND OLSCHOWKA, J. A. 1983. Monomine systems in the cerebral cortex. In J. CHAN-PALAY AND S. L. PALAY, *Cytochemical Methods in Neuroanatomy*. Alan Liss, New York, pp. 255–277.

MOUNTCASTLE, V. B., LYNCH, J. C., GEORGOPOULOS, A., SAKATA, H., AND ACUNA, C. 1975. Posterior parietal association cortex of the monkey: command functions for operation within extrapersonal space. J. Neurophysiol., **38**: 871–908.

MOUNTCASTLE, V. B., AND POWELL, T. P. S. 1959. Central nervous mechanisms subserving position sense and kinesthesis. Bull. Johns Hopkins Hosp., **105**: 173–200.

MRIGANKA SUR, NELSON, R. J., AND KAAS, J. H. 1982. Representations of the body surface in cortical areas 3b and 1 of squirrel monkeys: comparisons with other primates. J. Comp. Neurol., **211**: 177–192.

OTTERSEN, O. P., AND STORM-MATHISEN, J. 1984. Glutamate- and GABA-containing neurons in the mouse and rat brain, as demonstrated with a new immunocytochemical technique. J. Comp. Neurol., **229**: 374–392.

PARNAVELAS, J. G., AND MCDONALD, J. K. 1983. The cerebral cortex. In P. C. EMSON (Editor), *Chemical Neuroanatomy*. Raven Press, New York, pp. 505–549.

PENFIELD, W., AND BOLDREY, E. 1937. Somatic motor and sensory representation in the cerebral cortex of man as studied by electrical stimulation. Brain, **60**: 389–443.

PENFIELD, W., AND JASPER, H. H. 1954. *Epilepsy and the Functional Anatomy of the Human Brain*. Little, Brown, Boston.

PENFIELD, W., AND RASMUSSEN, T. 1950. *The Cerebral Cortex of Man: A Clinical Study of Localization of Function*. Macmillan, New York.

POOGIO, G. F., AND MOUNTCASTLE, V. B. 1960. A study of functional contributions of the lemniscal and spinothalamic systems to somatic sensibility. Bull. Johns Hopkins Hosp., **106**: 266–316.

PONS, T. P., GARRAGHTY, P. E., CUSIK, C. G., AND KAAS, J. H. 1985. The somototopic organization of area 2 in macaque monkeys. J. Comp. Neurol., **241**: 445–466.

POWELL, T. P. S. AND MOUNTCASTLE, V. B. 1959. The cytoarchitecture of the postcentral gyrus of the monkey *Macaca mulatta*. Bull. Johns Hopkins Hosp., **105**: 108–131.

ROBERTS, T. S., AND AKERT, K. 1963. Insular and opercular cortex and its thalamic projection in *Macaca mulatta*. Schweiz. Arch. Neurol. Neurochir. Psychiatr., **92**: 1–43.

ROBINSON, C. J., AND BURTON, H. 1980. Somatotopographic organization in the second somatosensory area of *M. fascicularis*. J. Comp. Neurol., **192**: 43–67.

ROBINSON, C. J., AND BURTON, H. 1980a. The organization of somatosensory receptive fields in cortical area 7b, retroinsular, postauditory and granular insular of *M. fascicularis*. J. Comp. Neurol., **192**: 69–92.

RUSSELL, J. R., AND DEMYER, W. 1961. The quantitative cortical origin of pyramidal axons of *macaca rhesus*. Neurology (Minneap.), **11**: 96–108.

SHINODA, Y., ZARZECKI, P., AND ASANUMA, H. 1979. Spinal branching of pyramidal tract neurons in the monkey. Exp. Brain Res., **34**: 59–72.

SIDMAN, R. L. 1970. Cell proliferation, migration and interaction in the developing mammalian central nervous system. In F. O. SCHMITT (Editor), *The Neurosciences*, Second Study Program. Rockefeller University Press, New York, pp. 100–116.

SILLITO, A. M. 1984. Functional consideration of the operation of GABAergic inhibitory processes in the visual cortex. In E. G. JONES AND A. PETERS (Editors), *Cerebral Cortex*. Plenum Press, New York, **2**: 91–117.

SPERRY, R. W. 1974. Lateral specialization in the surgically separated hemispheres. In F. O. SCHMITT AND F. G. WORDEN (Editors), *The Neurosciences*, Third Study Program. MIT Press, Cambridge, Massachusetts, pp. 5–19.

STERIADE, M., AND GLENN, L. L. 1982. Neocortical and caudate projections of intralaminar thalamic neurons and their synaptic excitation from midbrain reticular core. J. Neurophysiol., **48**: 342–371.

STREIT, P. 1984. Glutamate and aspartate as transmitter candidates for systems of the cerebral cortex. In E. G. JONES AND A. PETERS (Editors), *Cerebral Cortex*. Plenum Press, New York, **2**: 119–143.

STRICK, P. L. 1976. Anatomical analysis of ventrolateral thalamic input to primate motor cortex. J. Neurophysiol., **39**: 1020–1031.

STRICK, P. L., AND KIM, C. C. 1978. Input to primate motor cortex from posterior parietal cortex (area 5). I. Demonstration by retrograde transport. Brain Res., **157**: 325–330.

STRICK, P. L., AND PRESTON, J. B. 1978. Multiple representation in the primate motor cortex. Brain Res., **154**: 366–370.

SZENTÁGOTHAI, J. 1978. The neuron network of the cerebral cortex: a functional interpretation. Proc. R. Soc. Lond (Biol.), **201**: 219–248.

TANJI, J., AND WISE, S. P. 1981. Submodality distribution in sensorimotor cortex of the unanesthetized monkey. J. Neurophysiol., **45**: 467–481.

TRACEY, D. J., ASANUMA, C., JONES, E. G., AND PORTER, R. 1980. Thalamic relay to motor cortex: afferent pathways from brain stem, cerebellum, and spinal cord in monkeys. J. Neurophysiol., **44**: 532–553.

TRAVIS, A. M. 1955. Neurological deficiencies after ablation of the precentral motor area in *Macaca mulatta*. Brain, **78**: 155–173.

TRAVIS, A. M. 1955. Neurological deficiencies following supplementary motor area lesions in *Macaca mulatta*. Brain, **78**: 174–198.

TUSA, R. J., ROSENQUIST, A. C., AND PALMER, L. A. 1979. Retinotopic organization of areas 18 and 19 in the cat. J. Comp. Neurol., **185**: 657–678.

VOGT, B. A., AND PANDYA, D. N. 1978. Cortico-cortical connections of somatic sensory cortex (areas 3, 1, and 2) in the rhesus monkey. J. Comp. Neurol., **177**: 170–192.

WEINRICH, M., AND WISE, S. P. 1982. The premotor cortex in the monkey. J. Neurosci., **2**: 1329–1345.

WIESEL, T. N., HUBEL, D. H., AND LAM, D. M. K. 1974. Autoradiographic demonstration of ocular-dominance columns in the monkey striate cortex by means of transneuronal transport. Brain Res., **79**: 273–279.

WIESENDANGER, M. 1986. Recent developments in studies of the supplementary motor area of primates. Rev. Physiol. Biochem. Pharmacol., **103**: 1–57.

WIESENDANGER, M., HUMMELSHEIM, H., BIANCHETTI, M., CHEN, D. F., HYLAND, B., MAIER, V., AND WIESENDANGER, R. 1987. Input and output organization of the supplementary motor area. In *Motor Areas of the Cerebral Cortex*, CIBA Foundation Symposium. J. Wiley & Sons, Chichester, **132**: 40–62.

WISE, S. P., AND STRICK, P. L. 1984. Anatomical and physiological organization of the nonprimary motor cortex. Trends in Neuroscience, **7**: 442–446.

WISE, S. P., AND TANJI, J. 1981. Supplementary and precentral motor cortex: contrast in responsiveness to peripheral input in the hindlimb area of the unanesthetized monkey. J. Comp. Neurol., **195**: 433–451.

WONG-RILEY, M. T. T. 1979. Columnar cortico-cortical interconnections within the visual system of the squirrel and macaque monkeys. Brain Res., **162**: 201–217.

WOOLSEY, C. N. 1958. Organization of somatic sensory and motor areas of the cerebral cortex. In H. P. HARLOW AND C. N. WOOLSEY (Editors), *Biological and Biochemical Bases of Behavior*. University of Wisconsin, Madison, pp. 63–81.

WOOLSEY, C. N. 1960. Organization of cortical auditory system: A review and synthesis. In G. L. RASMUSSEN AND W. F. WINDLE (Editors), *Neural Mechanisms of the Auditory and Vestibular Systems*. Charles C Thomas, Springfield, IL, pp. 271–282.

WOOLSEY, C. N., AND WALZL, E. M. 1942. Topical projection of nerve fibers from local regions of the cochlea to the cerebral cortex of the cat. Bull. Johns Hopkins Hosp., **71**: 315–344.

WOOLSEY, C. N., AND WALZL, E. M. 1982. Cortical auditory area of *Macaca mulatta* and its relation to the second somatic sensory area (Sm II): determination by electrical excitation of auditory nerve fibers in the spiral osseous lamina and by click stimulation. In C. N. WOOLSEY (Editor), *Cortical Sensory Organization*. Humana Press, Clifton, New Jersey, **3**: 231–256.

ZANGWILL, O. L. 1960. *Cerebral Dominance and Its Relation to Psychological Function*. Charles C Thomas, Springfield, IL.

ZARZECKI, P., STRICK, P. L., AND ASANUMA, H. 1978. Input to primate motor cortex from posterior parietal cortex (area 5). II. Identification by antidromic activation. Brain Res., **157**: 331–335.

14

Blood Supply of the Central Nervous System

Metabolically the central nervous system is one of the most active systems of the body. Although the brain constitutes only about 2% of the body weight, it requires 17% of the cardiac output and 20% of the oxygen utilized by the body. Estimates of cerebral blood flow based on the nitrous oxide method indicate a normal blood flow of about 50 ml/100 g of brain tissue per minute. Thus, a brain of average weight has a normal blood flow of about 750 ml per minute and a mean oxygen consumption of about 3.3 ml/100 g of brain tissue per minute (about 46 ml per minute for the entire brain). The brain is not a homogeneous organ and metabolic activity in various regions reflect the functional activity of separate neuronal systems. This differential functional activity is neuronal systems can be demonstrated autoradiographically by the 2-[^{14}C] deoxy-glucose metabolic mapping technique, which uses a glucose analogue, that passes the blood-brain barrier, is partially metabolized by functionally active neurons and is trapped in the neurons (Figs. 13.19, 13.20, and 13.21).

Even brief interference with cerebral circulation can cause neurological or mental disturbances. Neural tissue deprived of an adequate blood supply undergoes necrosis. Impairment of local or regional blood supply constitutes the most common cause of central nervous system lesions. Vascular lesions most commonly result from arteriosclerosis of cerebral and cervical (i.e., internal carotid artery) vessels which reduce blood flow and can lead to thrombosis. Vascular occlusions also may result from emboli (i.e., fragments of blood clots, fat, and tumors or air bubbles). Hemorrhage into brain tissue, the brain ventricles, or the meninges may result from vascular lesions. Probably the most common cause of spontaneous hemorrhage into the brain and subarachnoid space is rupture of cerebral aneurysms (abnormal sacculations), most of which are of congenital origin. Neural lesions resulting from interruptions of the blood supply often can be localized to specific cerebral arteries on the basis of characteristic sensory and motor deficits.

BLOOD SUPPLY OF THE SPINAL CORD

The spinal cord is supplied by (1) branches of the *vertebral arteries* that descend, and (2) multiple *radicular arteries derived from segmental vessels* (Fig. 14.1). As the vertebral arteries ascend along the anterolateral surfaces of the medulla, each gives rise to two paired descending vessels: (1) the posterior spinal artery, and (2) the anterior spinal artery.

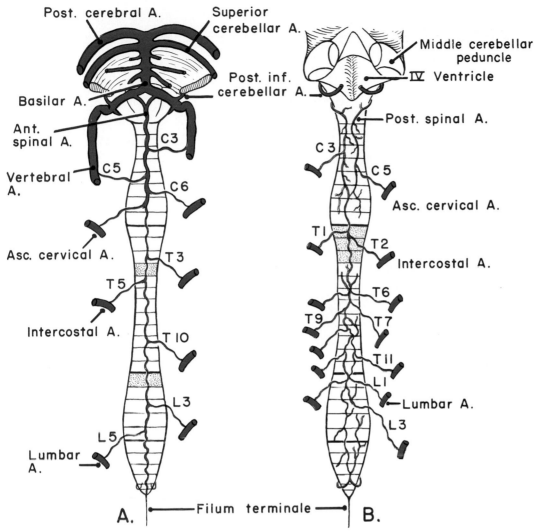

Figure 14.1.   Schematic diagrams of the arterial supply of the spinal cord. *A*, Anterior surface; *B*, posterior surface. Vulnerable segments of the spinal cord are *stippled*. *Letters* and *numbers* indicate important radicular arteries. (Based on Bolton, 1939; Suh and Alexander, 1939; Zulch, 1954.)

Posterior Spinal Arteries

Paired posterior spinal arteries descend on the posterior surface of the spinal cord, medial to the dorsal roots. These vessels receive variable contributions from the posterior radicular arteries and form two longitudinal plexiform channels near the dorsal root entry zone (Fig. 14.2). In places the posterior spinal arteries become discontinuous, or so small they appear discontinuous. These arteries are distributed to the posterior third of the spinal cord.

Anterior Spinal Arteries

The paired anterior spinal arteries unite to form a single descending midline vessel that supplies midline rami to the lower medulla and sulcal branches that enter the anterior median fissure of the spinal cord (Fig. 14.1). The continuity of the anterior spinal artery is dependent on anastomotic branches which it receives from the anterior radicular arteries. Anterior radicular arteries join the anterior spinal artery by branching

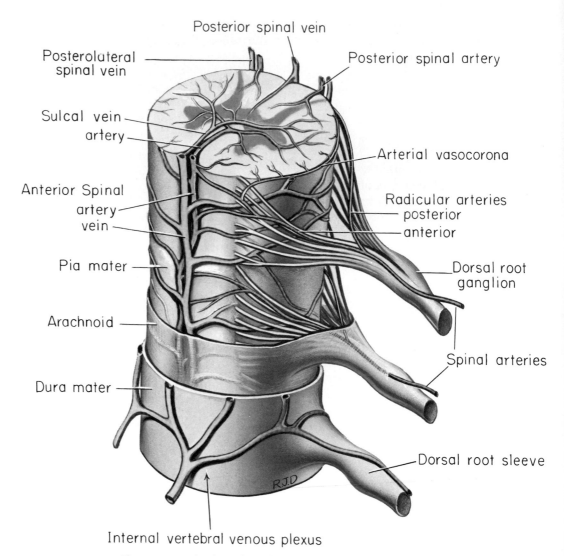

Figure 14.2. Blood supply and venous drainage of the spinal cord shown with respect to the meninges, nerve roots, and internal structure.

gently upward or sharply downward. Where two anterior radicular arteries reach the same level of the spinal cord a diamond-shaped arterial configuration results. In the thoracic region the anterior spinal artery narrows. If the anterior radicular arteries above or below it should be occluded, the anastomoses may not be adequate. An arterial ring encircling the conus medullaris communicates with the most caudal part of the anterior spinal artery.

The anterior and posterior spinal arteries are anastomotic channels extending the length of the spinal cord which receive branches from the radicular arteries. Branches of the vertebral arteries provide the principal blood supply of virtually the entire cervical spinal cord.

Radicular Arteries

These arteries are derived from segmental vessels at various levels (i.e., ascending cervical, deep cervical, intercostal, lumbar, and sacral arteries) that pass through the intervertebral foramina and divide into *anterior* and *posterior radicular arteries*. These arteries provide the principal blood supply of thoracic, lumbar, sacral, and coccygeal spinal segments (Fig. 14.2). Radicular arteries are most frequently on the left side in the thoracic and lumbar regions of the spinal cord, while cervical spinal cord segments are supplied equally on both sides. Radicular arteries course along the ventral surface of the roots they accompany. Where the epineurium blends with the dura mater, the radicular arteries enter the subarachnoid space. A single radicular artery may become either an anterior or posterior radicular artery, or divide to form both. Small twigs leave the arteries to supply the dura mater and the spinal roots they accompany.

Anterior radicular arteries contributing to the anterior spinal artery vary from 2 to 17, but commonly number between 6 and 10 arteries. The cervical spinal cord receives up to six anterior radicular arteries, while the thoracic cord receives two to four and the lumbar cord has one or two. One anterior radicular artery in the lumbar region, appreciably larger than all others, is known as the *artery of Adamkiewicz* or the artery of the lumbar enlargement. This radicular artery usually travels with a lower thoracic or upper lumbar spinal root most frequently on the left side. Thoracic spinal cord segments have the greatest length between radicular arteries, which means that occlusion of one of these vessels may seriously compromise its circulation. Certain spinal regions which receive their blood supply from more than one source are particularly vulnerable if they are suddenly deprived of blood from one of these sources (Fig. 14.1). The upper thoracic (T1–T4) and first lumbar spinal segments are among the most vulnerable regions of the spinal cord. The intercostal arteries do not interconnect with other arteries in the same extensive fashion as the extraspinal arteries in the cervical and lumbosacral regions. Thus occlusion of one intercostal artery in a vulnerable region can result in a spinal cord infarction. This clinical picture is seen with dissecting aneurysms of the aorta or as a result of surgery on the aorta where more than one intercostal artery may be occluded. Spinal cord segment L1 is another vulnerable region, where the anterior aspect of the cord is susceptible to vascular insult (Fig. 14.1).

The *posterior radicular arteries*, numbering between 10 and 23, divide on the posterolateral surface of the spinal cord and join the paired posterior spinal arteries. Although these vessels are more often on the left side, left predominance is not as evident as with the anterior radicular arteries.

The *anterior spinal artery* gives rise to a number of sulcal branches which enter the anterior median fissure of the spinal cord; these branches pass alternately to the right or left except for an occasional sulcal artery that divides into both right and left branches (Fig. 14.2). Central branches arising from the anterior spinal artery are more numerous and of larger caliber in the cervical and lumbar regions of the spinal cord. Sulcal branches of the anterior spinal artery supply the anterior horn, the lateral horn, the central gray, and the basal part of the posterior horn. In addition, these branches supply the anterior and lateral funiculi. Peripheral portions of the lateral funiculi receive branches from the *arterial vasocorona*. The *posterior spinal arteries* supply the posterior horns and the posterior funiculus (Fig. 14.2).

Spinal Veins

Veins draining the spinal cord have a distribution generally similar to that of spinal arteries. Anterior longitudinal venous trunks consist of anteromedian and anterolateral veins (Fig. 14.2). Sulcal veins entering the anteromedian vein drain anteromedial portions of the spinal cord; each sulcal vein drains regions on both sides of the spinal cord. Anterolateral regions of the spinal cord drain into anterolateral veins and into the *venous vasocorona*. The *anteromedian* and *anterolateral spinal veins* are drained by 6 to 11 anterior radicular veins which empty into the epidural venous plexus. One large radicular vein in the lumbar region is referred to as the *vena radicularis magna*; other smaller radicular veins are distributed along the spinal cord.

Posterior longitudinal venous trunks, consisting of a *posteromedian vein* and paired *posterolateral veins*, drain the posterior funiculus, and posterior horns (including their basal regions) and the white matter in the lateral funiculi adjacent to the posterior horn (Fig. 14.2). The posterior longitudinal veins are drained by 5 to 10 posterior radicular veins that enter the epidural venous plexus. The longitudinal veins are connected with each other by coronal veins (venous vasocorona) which encircle the spinal cord.

The *internal vertebral venous plexus* (epidural venous plexus), located between the dura mater and the vertebral periosteum, consists of two or more anterior and posterior longitudinal venous channels which are interconnected at many levels from the clivus to the sacral region (Fig. 14.2). At each intervertebral space there are connections with thoracic, abdominal, and intercostal veins, as well as with the external vertebral venous plexus. Since there are no valves in this spinal venous network, blood flowing through these channels may pass directly into the systemic venous system. When intraabdominal pressure is increased, venous blood from the pelvic plexus passes upward in the internal vertebral venous system. When the jugular veins are obstructed, blood leaves the skull via this plexus. The importance of the continuity of this venous plexus with the prostatic plexus has been cited as a route by which neoplasms may metastasize.

BLOOD SUPPLY OF THE BRAIN

The entire brain is supplied by two pairs of arterial trunks, the internal carotid arteries and the vertebral arteries (Fig. 14.3).

Internal Carotid Artery

This artery can be divided into four segments: cervical, intrapetrosal, intracavernous, and cerebral (supraclinoid) portions. The intracavernous and cerebral portions of this artery are referred to as the "carotid siphon" because of their characteristic configuration (Fig. 14.7). The *intracavernous segment* of the internal carotid artery lies close to the medial wall of the cavernous sinus, courses nearly horizontally and bears important relationships to cranial nerves III, IV, VI, and portions (division I) of nerve V which lie within the sinus. The abducens nerve lies immediately adjacent to the internal carotid artery within the sinus (Fig. 14.4). The *cerebral segment* begins as the artery emerges from the cavernous sinus and passes medial to the anterior clinoid process (Fig. 14.17). This portion of the artery, extending upward and backward, gives rise to all major branches of the internal carotid artery. The *cervical segment* which extends from the bifurcation of the common carotid to the carotid canal in the petrous bone has no branches. The *intrapetrosal segment* of this vessel is surrounded by dense bone. Small branches given off from the intrapetrosal and *intracavernous segments* pass into the tympanic cavity, the

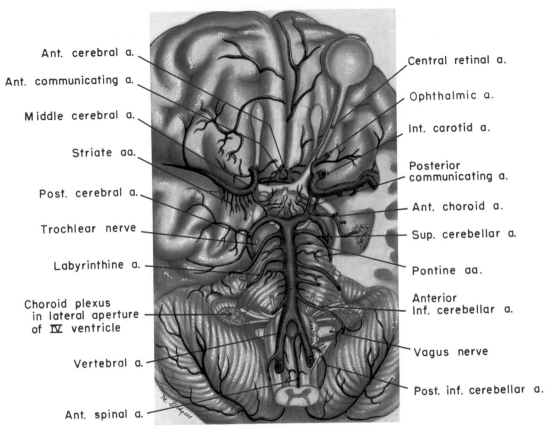

Ant. cerebral a.

Ant. communicating a.

Middle cerebral a.

Striate aa.

Post. cerebral a.

Trochlear nerve

Labyrinthine a.

Choroid plexus
in lateral aperture
of IV ventricle

Vertebral a.

Ant. spinal a.

Central retinal a.

Ophthalmic a.

Int. carotid a.

Posterior
communicating a.

Ant. choroid a.

Sup. cerebellar a.

Pontine aa.

Anterior
Inf. cerebellar a.

Vagus nerve

Post. inf. cerebellar a.

Figure 14.3. Major arteries and their branches on the ventral surface of the brain.

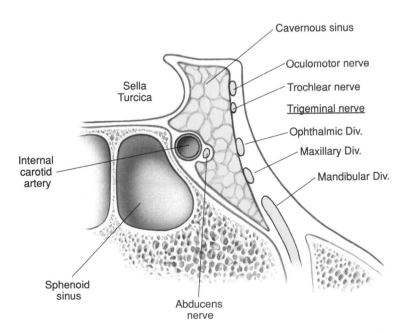

Cavernous sinus

Oculomotor nerve

Trochlear nerve

Trigeminal nerve

Ophthalmic Div.

Maxillary Div.

Mandibular Div.

Sella
Turcica

Internal
carotid
artery

Sphenoid
sinus

Abducens
nerve

Figure 14.4. Diagrammatic drawing of an oblique coronal section through the cavernous sinus viewed from behind showing the relationships of this venous sinus to the sella turcica, the sphenoid sinus, and the locations of cranial nerves in the wall of the sinus. The abducens nerve lies adjacent to the internal carotid artery. (Redrawn from W.E.L. Clark, Cunningham's *Textbook of Anatomy*, 1951, with permission from Oxford University Press.)

cavernous and inferior petrosal sinuses, the trigeminal ganglion, and the meninges of the middle fossa.

Major branches of the internal carotid artery are the *ophthalmic*, *posterior communicating*, and *anterior choroidal arteries* (Fig. 14.3 and 14.8). Lateral to the optic chiasm the internal carotid artery divides into a smaller *anterior cerebral artery* and a larger *middle cerebral artery*. The middle cerebral artery is regarded as the direct continuation of the internal carotid artery.

Vertebral Artery

The vertebral artery arises from the first part of the subclavian artery, enters the foramen transversarium of the sixth cervical vertebra, and ascends in the foramina transversaria of all higher cervical vertebrae. The artery pierces the atlanto-occipital membrane and the dura mater to enter the posterior fossa through the foramen magnum. The vertebral arteries course along the anterolateral surfaces of the medulla and unite at the caudal border of the pons to form the basilar artery (Figs. 14.1, 14.3, 14.12, and 14.13). Cervical portions of the vertebral artery give rise to spinal (radicular) and muscular branches.

Intracranial branches of the vertebral and basilar arteries supply the cervical spinal cord (via anterior and posterior spinal arteries), the medulla, pons, midbrain, cerebellum, posterior parts of the diencephalon, and parts of the occipital and temporal lobes of the brain. A labyrinthine branch of the basilar artery supplies the cochlea and vestibular apparatus (Fig. 14.3).

Cerebral Arterial Circle

The cerebral arterial circle (Willis) is an arterial wreath encircling the optic chiasm, the tuber cinereum, and the interpeduncular region formed by anastomotic branches of the internal carotid artery and the most rostral branches of the basilar artery (Figs. 14.3 and 14.8). This arterial circle is formed by the anterior and posterior communicating arteries, and proximal portions of the anterior, middle, and posterior cerebral arteries. The anterior cerebral arteries run medially and rostrally toward the interhemispheric fissure; in front of the optic chiasm these two arteries are joined by a connecting vessel, the *anterior communicating artery*. The *posterior communicating arteries* arise from the internal carotid arteries; run caudomedially, and anastomose with proximal portions of the posterior cerebral arteries (Fig. 14.8). The posterior cerebral arteries are formed by the bifurcation of the basilar artery at the rostral border of the pons (Figs. 14.3 and 14.13). The cerebral arterial circle is said to equalize blood flow to various parts of the brain, but normally there is little exchange of blood between the right and left sides of the arterial circle because of the equality of blood pressure. The arterial circle and its branches on the inferior surface of the brain are shown in Figs. 14.3 and 14.8.

From the arterial circle and the principal cerebral arteries two types of branches arise, central and cortical. *Central arteries*, arising from the arterial circle and proximal portions of the principal cerebral arteries, penetrate the substance of the brain and supply deep structures (Figs. 14.9, 14.10, and 14.11). The anterior and posterior choroidal arteries, respectively, branches of the internal carotid and the posterior cerebral arteries, may be included in this group. Penetrating vessels, particularly those of central branches, have been referred to as end-arteries, suggesting that they do not anastomose with other arteries. In the human brain there are no end-arteries, but anastomoses between these small branches may not be sufficient to maintain adequate circulation if a major vessel is occluded suddenly. *Cortical* branches of each major cerebral artery pass in the pia mater to large regions of the cerebral cortex, undergo considerable branching, and form freely anastomosing superficial plexuses (Figs. 14.5 and 14.6). Smaller arteries arising from these plexuses penetrate the cortex at nearly right angles and run for variable distances.

CORTICAL BRANCHES

The cortical branches of the cerebral hemisphere are derived from the anterior, middle, and posterior cerebral arteries.

Anterior Cerebral Artery

This artery originates at the bifurcation of the internal carotid artery lateral to the optic chiasm and nerve (Fig. 14.3.). The anterior cerebral artery passes rostromedially, dorsal to the optic nerve, and approaches the corresponding artery of the opposite side with which it connects via the anterior communicating artery (Figs. 14.5 and 14.8). The artery enters the interhemispheric fissure, passes upward on the medial surface of the hemisphere, and continues posteriorly on the superior surface of the corpus callosum. The anterior cerebral artery gives rise to (1) the *medial striate artery*, (2) *orbital branches*, (3) the *frontopolar artery*, (4) the *callosomarginal artery*, and (5) the *pericallosal artery*.

The *medial striate artery* (recurrent artery of Heubner), which may arise proximal or distal to the anterior communicating artery, courses caudally and laterally and enters the anterior perforated space (Figs. 2.8 and 12.2). This vessel supplies the anteromedial part of the head of the caudate nucleus, adjacent parts of the internal capsule and putamen, and parts of the septal nuclei (Figs. 14.8, 14.9, and 14.10). Several small branches of the artery frequently supply the inferior surface of the frontal lobe.

Orbital branches of the anterior cerebral artery, arising from the ascending part of this artery ventral to the genu of the corpus callosum, extend rostrally to supply the orbital and medial surfaces of the frontal lobe (Fig. 14.5).

A *frontopolar artery* is given off as the anterior cerebral artery curves around the genu of the corpus callosum; branches of this artery supply medial parts of the frontal lobe and extend onto the convexity of the hemisphere.

The *callosomarginal artery*, a major branch of the anterior cerebral artery, arises distal to the frontopolar artery and passes caudally in the callosomarginal sulcus. Branches of this artery supply the paracentral lobule and parts of the cingulate gyrus (Fig. 14.5).

The *pericallosal artery*, regarded as the terminal branch of the anterior cerebral artery, courses caudally along the dorsal surface of the corpus callosum and supplies the medial surface of the parietal lobe, including the precuneus.

Anomalies of the anterior cerebral artery occur in about 25% of brains; these include unpaired arteries and instances where branches are given off to the contralateral hemisphere. Occlusion of the trunk of one anterior cerebral artery may produce a contralateral hemiplegia which is

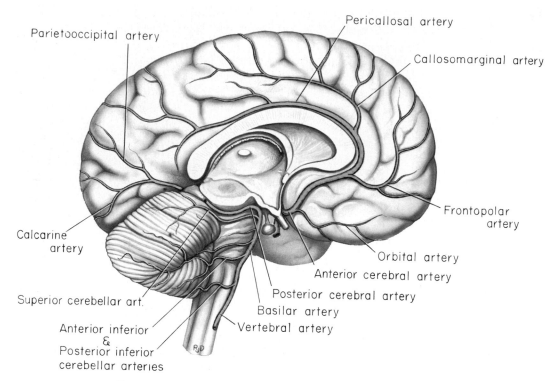

Figure 14.5. Arteries on the medial surface of the cerebrum shown together with arteries of the brain stem and cerebellum.

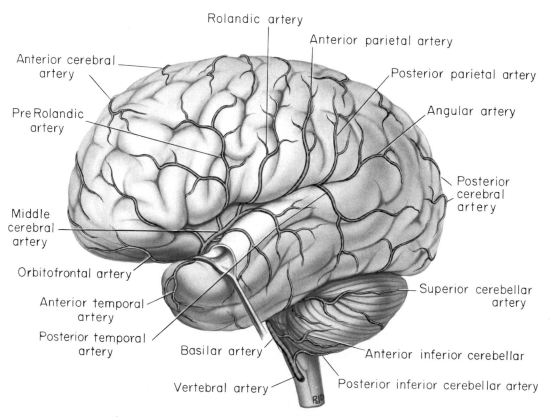

Figure 14.6. Arteries on the lateral surface of the cerebrum and cerebellum.

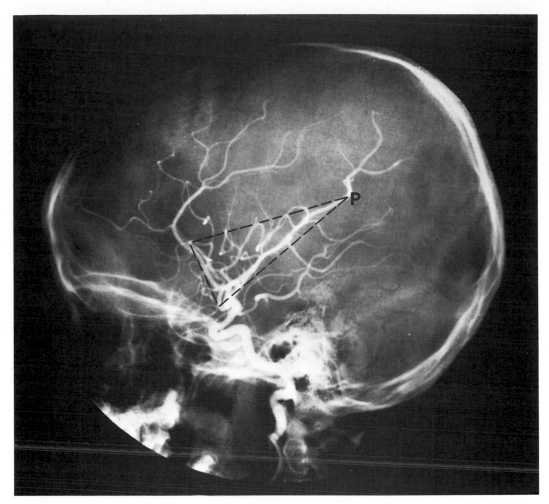

Figure 14.7.   Cerebral angiogram demonstrating the Sylvian triangle. There are five to eight branches of the *middle cerebral artery* on the surface of the insula. As branches course upward they reach the deepest portion of the sulcus formed by the insula and the frontoparietal operculum. Upon reaching this point, branches of the middle cerebral artery reverse direction and pass downward to emerge from the lateral sulcus. The points of reversal can be identified in the angiogram and a line drawn from the most anterior to the most posterior point (*P*) forms the upper margin of the Sylvian triangle. The inferior margin of the triangle is a line from the posterior point (the angiographic Sylvian point, *P*) to the anterior extremity of the middle cerebral artery. The anterior border is a line drawn from the rostral extremity of the middle cerebral artery to the first turn of the opercular branch. (Courtesy of the late Dr. Ernest H. Wood, College of Physicians and Surgeons, Columbia University; from Taveras and Wood, 1976.)

greatest in the lower limb. Obstruction of both anterior cerebral arteries is associated with bilateral paralysis, especially in the lower limbs, and impaired sensation that mimics a spinal cord lesion.

Middle Cerebral Artery

The middle cerebral artery, the continuation of the internal carotid artery beyond the origin of the anterior cerebral artery, passes laterally over the anterior perforated substance to enter the lateral cerebral fossa between the temporal lobe and the insula (Figs. 14.3, 14.6, 14.7, and 14.8). This artery, the largest and most complex of the cerebral arteries, divides into a number of large branches which course upward and backward. As these branches reach the dorsal margin of the insula, they loop abruptly downward toward the lateral sulcus. The course of the branches

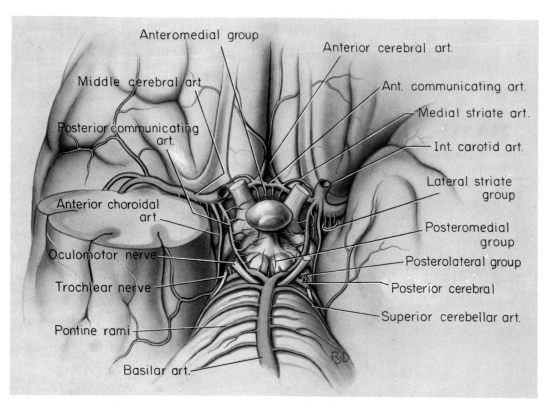

Figure 14.8.   The cerebral arterial circle at the base of the brain showing the distribution of ganglionic branches. These branches form the *anteromedial, posteromedial, posterolateral,* and *lateral striate* groups. The *medial striate* and *anterior choroidal arteries* also are shown.

of the middle cerebral artery in the insular region is of great importance in the interpretation of cerebral angiograms. In the insular region five to eight branches of the middle cerebral artery lie within what is called the Sylvian triangle (Fig. 14.7). The Sylvian point (or apex) is established angiographically by the most posterior branch of the middle cerebral artery to emerge from the lateral fissure. The inferior margin of the Sylvian triangle is formed by the lower branches of the middle cerebral artery, while the superior margin is formed by dorsal looping branches of this artery that reverse their course. Displacement of branches of the middle cerebral artery in the Sylvian triangle by mass lesions can be detected readily in cerebral angiograms and the direction of displacement provides information concerning lesion localization.

Branches of the middle cerebral artery emerge from the lateral sulcus and are distributed in a "fanlike" fashion over the lateral convexity of the hemisphere. These cortical branches supply lateral parts of the orbital gyri, the inferior and middle frontal gyri, most of the precentral and postcentral gyri, the superior and inferior parietal lobules, and the superior and middle temporal gyri, including the temporal pole (Fig. 14.6). The largest cortical branches appear to supply the temporo-occipital and angular areas. The cortical arteries arise from stem arteries and supply individual cortical regions. In general, one or two cortical arteries pass to each cortical region supplied. The cortical branches to the frontal, anterior temporal and anterior parietal regions are smaller than those to posterior parietal, posterior temporal, and temporo-occipital regions, but they are more numerous. Branches of the middle cerebral artery include (1) the *lenticulostriate arteries*, (2) the *anterior temporal artery*, (3) the *orbitofrontal artery*, (4) *pre-Rolandic* and *Rolandic branches*, (5) *anterior and posterior parietal branches*, and (6) a *posterior temporal branch* which extends caudally to supply lateral portions of the occipital lobe (Fig. 14.6). Branches supplying the angular gyrus constitute the terminal part of the middle cerebral artery.

The extensive and important regions nourished by the middle cerebral artery includes the motor and premotor areas, the somesthetic and auditory areas, and large regions of the association cortex. Occlusion of the middle cerebral artery near the origin of its cortical branches may produce (1) a severe contralateral hemiplegia, most marked in the upper extremity and face; (2) a contralateral loss of position and discriminating tactile sense; and (3) severe aphasia, when the dominant hemisphere is involved.

Posterior Cerebral Arteries

These arteries, formed by the bifurcation of the basilar artery, pass laterally around the crus cerebri (Figs. 14.3, 14.5, 14.8, 14.12, and 14.13). After receiving anastomoses from the posterior communicating arteries, these arteries continue along the lateral aspect of the midbrain, and then pass above to the tentorium to course on the medial and inferior surfaces of the temporal and occipital lobes. Branches of the posterior cerebral artery extend onto the lateral surfaces of the hemisphere to supply parts of the inferior temporal gyrus, variable portions of the occipital lobe, and parts of the superior parietal lobule (Fig. 14.6). Branches of the posterior cerebral artery also are distributed to the brain stem, the choroid plexus of the third and lateral ventricles, and to regions of the cerebral cortex.

The posterior cerebral artery divides into two main branches; (1) the *posterior temporal artery* and (2) the *internal occipital artery*.

The *posterior temporal artery* gives off an anterior temporal branch (Fig. 14.6), which supplies the inferior surface of the temporal lobe anteriorly and frequently anastomoses with branches of the middle cerebral artery. Posterior branches of the posterior temporal artery supply the occipitotemporal and lingual gyri (Fig. 2.8).

The *internal occipital artery* divides into the *parieto-occipital* and the *calcarine arteries*, which supply different regions of the medial aspect of the occipital lobe and the splenium of the corpus callosum (Fig. 14.5). The calcarine artery supplies the primary visual cortex. Occlusion of the posterior cerebral artery, or the calcarine artery, produces a contralateral homonymous hemianopsia; macular vision may be spared due to anastomoses between branches of the middle and posterior cerebral arteries near the occipital pole.

Cerebral angiography, a technic based on the injection of radiopaque solutions into cerebral vessels and rapid serial roentgenograms, reveals not only the position and configuration of the cerebral vessels, but it shows phases of filling and emptying of vessels by the radiopaque solutions. This radiographic technic is particularly useful in localizing cerebral aneurysms and vascular malformations; in addition, it often provides information concerning occlusive vascular disease and space-occupying intracranial masses. While cerebral angiography provides invaluable diagnostic information, it usually is not possible to visualize the small terminal arteries.

CENTRAL ARTERIES

Ganglionic branches arise from proximal portions of the major cerebral and communicating arteries and supply the diencephalon, basal ganglia, and internal capsule. Penetrating ganglionic arteries are arranged in four groups, designated as anteromedial, anterolateral, posteromedial, and posterolateral (Fig. 14.8).

The *anteromedial arteries* arise from the anterior cerebral and anterior communicating arteries, enter the most medial part of the anterior perforated substance, and are distributed to the anterior hypothalamus, the preoptic area, and the supraoptic region.

The *posteromedial arteries* arise from the whole extent of the posterior communicating artery and the most proximal part of the posterior cerebral artery. Rostral branches of this group supply the hypophysis, infundibulum, and tuberal regions of the hypothalamus. Deep penetrating branches, distributed to anterior and medial parts of the thalamus, are referred to as *thalamoperforating arteries* (Fig. 14.12). Caudal branches of this group supply the mammillary bodies and subthalamic region, as well as medial nuclei of the thalamus. The most caudal branches of this group are distributed to medial regions of the midbrain tegmentum and crus cerebri (Fig. 14.15*A*).

The *posterolateral arteries* arise from the posterior cerebral artery, lateral to its anastomosis with the posterior communicating artery (Fig. 14.8). These penetrating branches supply the caudal half of the thalamus (i.e., the geniculate bodies, pulvinar, lateral nuclear group, and large parts of the ventral tier thalamic nuclei). These branches of the posterior cerebral artery are referred to as the *thalamogeniculate arteries* (Fig. 14.9).

The *anterolateral group of arteries*, commonly referred to as *striate arteries*, arise primarily from proximal portions of the middle cerebral artery. The medial striate artery (Heubner), derived from the anterior cerebral artery, belongs to this group (Fig. 14.9). These arteries enter the anterior perforated substance and supply portions of the corpus striatum and internal capsule (Figs. 14.9 and 14.10). The medial striate artery supplies the rostroventral part of the head of the caudate nucleus and adjacent portions of the putamen and internal capsule. The lateral striate arteries, derived from the middle cerebral artery, supply remaining portions of the striatum (i.e., caudate nucleus and putamen), except for extreme caudal parts of the putamen and the tail of the caudate nucleus (Fig. 14.11). These arteries also nourish the lateral part of the globus pallidus, the anterior limb of the internal capsule, and dorsal portions of the posterior limb of the internal capsule.

Choroidal Arteries

The anterior and posterior choroidal arteries are distinctive central branches (Figs. 14.3, 14.8, 14.9, and 14.10). The *anterior choroidal artery* usually arises from the internal carotid artery distal to the posterior communicating artery. This artery, characterized by its long subarachnoid course and its relatively small caliber, first passes caudally across the optic tract, and then laterally toward the rostromedial surface of the temporal lobe; it enters the inferior horn of the lateral ventricle through the choroidal fissure (Fig. 12.10). Structures supplied by this artery, in addition to the choroid plexus, include the hippocampal formation, portions of both pallidal segments (i.e., lateral parts of the medial segment and medial parts of the lateral segment), ventrolateral parts of the posterior limb of the internal capsule, and the entire retrolenticular internal capsule (Fig. 14.10). Small branches of this artery supply parts of the optic tract, parts of the amygdaloid complex, ventral parts of the tail of the caudate nucleus, posterior parts of the putamen, and ventrolateral parts of the thalamus.

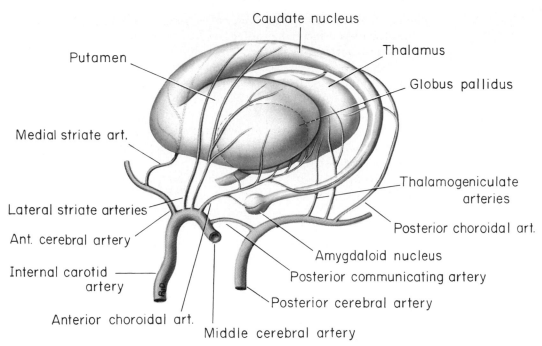

Figure 14.9.   Diagrammatic representation of the arterial supply of the corpus striatum and thalamus. (Modified from Aitken, 1909.)

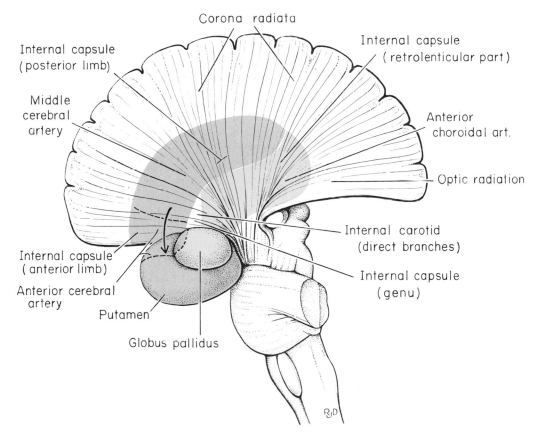

Figure 14.10.   Schematic diagram of the blood supply of the internal capsule and corpus striatum. The putamen and globus pallidus are shown rotated ventrally away from the internal capsule. Regions of the internal capsule supplied by branches of the *middle* and *anterior cerebral arteries* are shown in *red*; portions of the posterior limb of the internal capsule supplied by the *anterior choroidal artery* are in *yellow*. The region of the genu is supplied by direct branches of the *internal carotid artery* (From Alexander, 1942.)

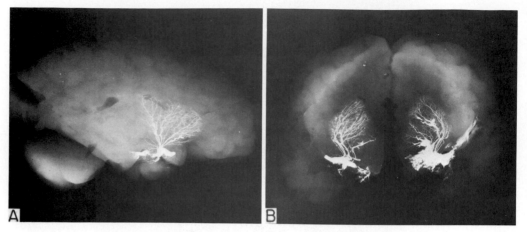

Figure 14.11.   Roentgenograms of cadaver brains in which the deep ganglionic branches of the *middle cerebral artery* have been injected with radiopaque material. *A,* Lateral view; *B,* frontal view. (Courtesy of Dr. Harry A. Kaplan; Kaplan, 1956.)

The *posterior choroidal arteries,* arising from the posterior cerebral artery, consist of one medial and two lateral choroidal arteries (Figs. 14.9 and 14.12). The *medial posterior choroidal artery* curves around the midbrain to reach the region of the pineal body; it gives off branches to the tectum, the choroid plexus of the third ventricle, and the superior and medial surfaces of the thalamus. The *lateral posterior choroidal arteries* partially encircle the brain stem, enter the choroidal fissure and supply the choroid plexus in the lateral ventricle; some branches of this artery anastomose with branches of the anterior choroidal artery.

BLOOD SUPPLY OF THE CORPUS STRIATUM, INTERNAL CAPSULE, AND DIENCEPHALON

The *striatum* is nourished mainly by the lateral striate arteries derived from the middle cerebral artery (Figs. 14.9 and 14.10). Rostromedial parts of the head of the caudate nucleus are supplied by the medial striate artery (Heubner) while the tail of the caudate nucleus and the caudal part of the putamen receive branches of the anterior choroidal artery. The lateral segment of the globus pallidus is supplied by branches of both the lateral striate and anterior choroidal arteries. The lateral part of the medial pallidal segment receives branches from the anterior choroidal artery, and branches of the posterior communicating artery nourish medial portions of this pallidal segment.

The *internal capsule,* both anterior and posterior limbs, is supplied primarily by the lateral striate branches of the middle cerebral artery (Figs. 14.10 and 14.11). The medial striate artery supplies rostromedial parts of the anterior limb of the internal capsule. The genu of the internal capsule receives direct branches from the internal carotid artery, while ventral portions of the posterior limb and its entire retrolenticular part are supplied by branches of the anterior choroidal artery.

The *thalamus* is nourished mainly by branches of the posterior cerebral artery (Figs. 14.9 and 14.12). *Thalamoperforating branches,* referred to as the posteromedial arteries, course dorsally and medially to supply medial and anterior regions of the thalamus. These arteries, arising from medial parts of the posterior cerebral artery and from the terminal part of the basilar artery, course dorsally into the diencephalon and nourish paraventricular regions of the hypothalamus and medial regions of the thalamus. Perforating branches of these arteries, visualized in ver-

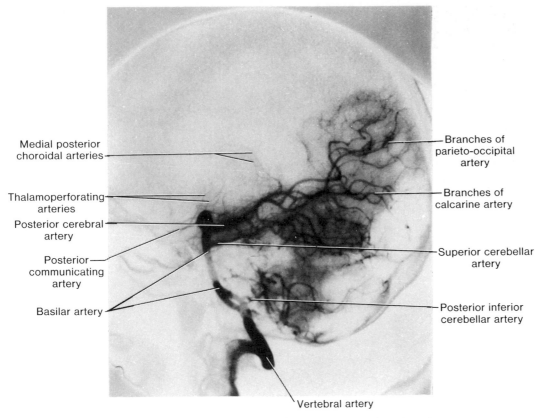

Medial posterior choroidal arteries

Thalamoperforating arteries

Posterior cerebral artery

Posterior communicating artery

Basilar artery

Branches of parieto-occipital artery

Branches of calcarine artery

Superior cerebellar artery

Posterior inferior cerebellar artery

Vertebral artery

Figure 14.12.   Lateral projection of a vertebral angiogram demonstrating major branches of the vertebral basilar system. (Courtesy of Dr. Daniel Hottenstein.)

tebral angiograms (Fig. 14.12), may be displaced, deformed, or stretched by space-occupying lesions or enlargement of the third ventricle.

Thalamogeniculate branches, referred to as the posterolateral arteries, supply the pulvinar and the lateral nuclei of the thalamus. These arteries arise from the posterior cerebral artery as it winds around the crus cerebri and from the choroidal arteries. The *medial posterior choroidal artery* supplies the choroid plexus of the third ventricle and superior and medial portions of the thalamus. The *inferior thalamic arteries* arise from the posterior communicating artery and the bifurcation of the basilar artery and enter inferior portions of the thalamus. These arteries supply regions of the thalamus rostral to the territory of the thalamoperforating arteries.

The anterior hypothalamus and preoptic region receive their blood supply from the anteromedian ganglionic arteries. Caudal regions of the hypothalamus and the subthalamic region are supplied by ganglionic arteries, derived from the posterior cerebral and posterior communicating arteries (Fig. 14.8).

VERTEBRAL BASILAR SYSTEM

The intracranial part of each vertebral artery gives rise to (1) a *posterior spinal artery*, (2) an *anterior spinal artery*, (3) a *posterior inferior cerebellar artery*, and (4) a *posterior meningeal artery*. The two vertebral arteries unite to form the basilar artery at the lower border of the pons (Figs. 14.1 and 14.3). Branches of the basilar artery include (1) the *anterior inferior cerebellar arteries*, (2) the *labyrinthine arteries*, (3) numerous *paramedian* and *circumferential pontine rami*, (4) the *superior cerebellar ar-*

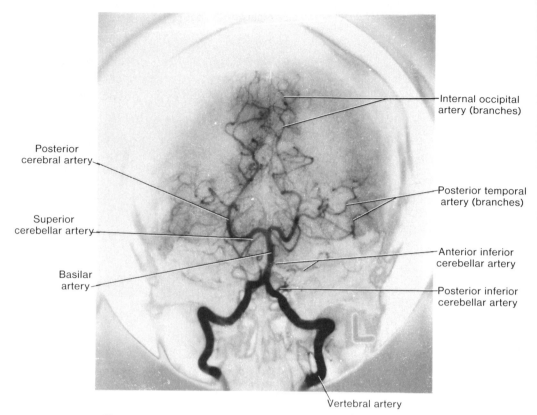

Figure 14.13. Vertebral angiogram as seen in the Towne projection using a substraction technic. (Courtesy of Dr. Daniel Hottenstein.)

teries, and (5) the *posterior cerebral arteries*. The labyrinthine arteries do not supply the brain stem but pass laterally through the internal auditory meati to the inner ear (Fig. 14.3). The posterior cerebral arteries, representing the terminal branches of the basilar artery, furnish branches which supply parts of the midbrain, thalamus, and large regions of the temporal and occipital lobes (Figs. 14.12 and 14.13). With the exception of the most rostral portions of the crus cerebri, the entire blood supply of the medulla, pons, mesencephalon, and cerebellum is derived from the vertebral basilar system. Although many of the branches of the vertebral and basilar arteries are of small caliber, major branches can be demonstrated in vertebral angiograms (Figs. 14.1, 14.12 and 14.13). Both posterior cerebral arteries usually are filled by contrast media following injection of one vertebral artery.

Medulla and Pons

These portions of the brain stem are supplied by the anterior and posterior spinal arteries, the posterior inferior cerebellar arteries, and branches of the vertebral and basilar arteries (Figs. 14.1, 14.14, and 14.15). The anterior inferior and superior cerebellar arteries make smaller contributions. There is great variation in the extent of areas supplied by individual vessels and considerable overlap in some regions.

The *posterior spinal artery* supplies the gracile and cuneate fasciculi and their nuclei, and the caudal and dorsal portions of the inferior cerebellar peduncle (Figs. 14.1 and 14.14). When this artery is small, or absent, its territory is supplied by the posterior inferior cerebellar artery.

The *anterior spinal artery* supplies a paramedian region of the medulla which includes the pyramid, the medial lemniscus, medial longi-

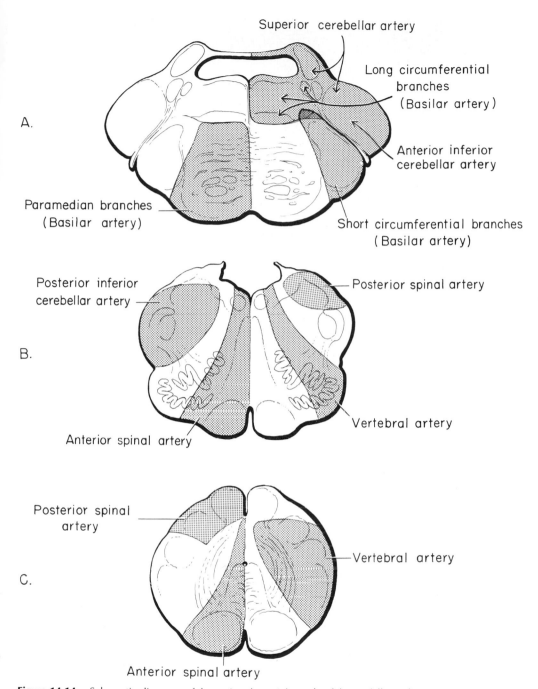

Figure 14.14.   Schematic diagrams of the regional arterial supply of the medulla and pons. Medullary levels are through the posterior column nuclei (C) and the inferior olivary nuclear complex (B). The pons (A) is supplied by paramedian and circumferential branches of the basilar artery. (From Frantzen and Oliverius, 1957)

tudinal fasciculus, most of the hypoglossal nucleus, caudal parts of the solitary nucleus and dorsal motor nucleus of the vagus, and the medial accessory olive (Fig. 14.14). Occlusion of one anterior spinal artery is associated with a medullary lesion producing an *inferior alternating hemiplegia*, characterized by ipsilateral paralysis of the tongue and a contralateral hemiplegia. Such lesions sometimes involve portions of the medial lemniscus, which result in contralateral sensory deficits.

Bulbar branches of the vertebral artery supply the pyramids at the lower border of the pons, cephalic parts of the hypoglossal nucleus, and

Figure 14.15. Microangiograms of the blood supply of the midbrain, pons, and medulla made from 4mm injected specimens. In the midbrain (A) the tegmentum is supplied by branches of the *posterior cerebral* and the *superior cerebellar arteries* but also receives contributions from the *paramedian* and *circumferential arteries.* The upper pons (B) receives *paramedian* and *circumferential branches* of the *basilar artery,* as well as some branches of the *superior cerebellar artery* distributed to dorsal regions. The vascular pattern in the upper medulla (C) should be compared with the diagram in Figure 14.14*B.* (Courtesy of Dr. O. Hassler; Hassler, 1967.)

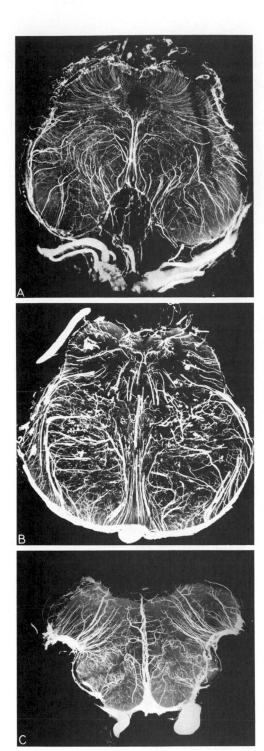

most of the inferior olivary complex. These branches also nourish the reticular formation and parts of the solitary nucleus and the dorsal motor nucleus of the vagus. At caudal medullary levels branches of the vertebral artery are distributed to practically the entire lateral medullary region between the medullary pyramids and the fasciculus cuneatus (Fig. 14.14). Two types of arteries enter the medulla. Short arteries supply small branches to the spinal trigeminal, spinothalamic, and spinocerebellar tracts, while long arteries supply deeper regions. Some of the long arteries reach the floor of the fourth ventricle. The lateral medullary region supplied by these branches includes structures involved in the lateral medullary syndrome.

The *posterior inferior cerebellar artery* supplies the lateral medullary region rostral to that supplied by direct bulbar branches of the vertebral artery (Figs. 14.14 and 14.15C). This retro-olivary region of the medulla contains the spinothalamic tracts, the spinal trigeminal nucleus and tract, the emerging fibers from nucleus ambiguous, and the dorsal motor nucleus of the vagus, as well as the ventral part of the inferior cerebellar peduncle (Figs. 14.12, 14.13, 14.14, and 14.15). Autonomic fibers from the hypothalamus also descend within this region of the medulla and pons. The *lateral medullary syndrome*, produced by sudden occlusions of the posterior inferior cerebellar artery, or bulbar branches of the vertebral artery, is associated with lesions in the dorsolateral part of the medulla. Such lesions are characterized by (1) loss of pain and thermal sense in the face (ipsilaterally) and over the body (contralaterally), (2) ipsilateral paralysis of the pharynx and larynx, and (3) an ipsilateral Horner's syndrome. Disturbances of equilibrium usually are transient.

The ventral portion of the pons is supplied by three groups of arteries derived from the basilar artery (Fig. 14.14). These arterial branches are grouped as (1) paramedian, (2) short circumferential, and (3) long circumferential.

Paramedian branches supply a medial pontine region which includes the pontine nuclei, and the corticospinal, corticopontine, and corticobulbar tracts. These branches give rise to smaller rami which nourish ventromedial parts of the pontine tegmentum.

Short circumferential arteries supply the adjacent anterolateral part of the pons, and variable parts of overlying tegmentum (Fig. 14.14A).

Long circumferential arteries course laterally over the anterior surface of the pons and anastomose with smaller branches of the anterior inferior cerebellar arteries. These arteries supply lateral parts of the middle cerebellar peduncle, as well as most of the pontine tegmentum. The caudal pontine tegmentum is supplied by branches of the long circumferential and anterior inferior cerebellar arteries; the rostral pontine tegmentum receives branches of the long circumferential and superior cerebellar arteries (Figs. 14.14 and 14.15). Structures within the distribution of these arterial branches include the reticular formation, the medial lemniscus, the medial longitudinal fasciculus, the spinothalamic and spinocerebellar tracts, the middle and superior cerebellar peduncles, and the cranial nerve nuclei of the pons.

Sudden occlusion of paramedian branches of the basilar artery on one side usually produce lesions in the basilar part of the pons which result in a contralateral hemiparesis and damage to the root fibers of the ipsilateral abducens nerve. *Middle alternating hemiplegia* is a classic example of such a lesion. Obstruction of the short circumferential arteries on one side usually results in ipsilateral cerebellar and autonomic disturbances and impairment of contralateral sensation. Occlusion of the long circumferential arteries and other arteries supplying the pontine tegmentum produces cranial nerve disturbances, paresis of conjugate eye movements, contralateral hemianesthesia, ipsilateral cerebellar disturbances, and frequently nystagmus. Complete or partial thrombosis of the basilar artery may produce precipitous loss of muscle tone, dilated or pinpoint pupils that do not react to light, and bilateral Babinski responses. Neurological disturbances usually are bilateral but may be asymmetrical and exhibit fluctuations.

Mesencephalon

Most of the blood supply of the mesencephalon is derived from branches of the basilar artery (Fig. 14.15). Arteries supplying this part of the brain stem include branches of (1) the *posterior cerebral artery*, (2) the *superior cerebellar artery*, (3) the *posterior communicating artery*, and (4) the *anterior choroidal artery*. Branches of these arteries, like those supplying the pons, can be grouped into paramedian arteries and long and short circumferential arteries.

Paramedian arteries, derived from the posterior communicating artery and proximal portions of the posterior cerebral arteries, form an extensive plexus in the interpeduncular fossa, enter the brain stem in the posterior perforated substance, and supply the rapheal region, the oculomotor complex, the medial longitudinal fasciculus, the red nucleus, and medial parts of the substantia nigra and crus cerebri (Fig. 14.15). Vascular lesions involving paramedian arterial branches at midbrain levels frequently produce a *superior alternating hemiplegia*, characterized by ipsilateral oculomotor disturbances and a contralateral hemiplegia (Weber's syndrome). This syndrome results from lesions involving portions of the crus cerebri and fibers of the oculomotor nerve. A less frequent lesion in the paramedian tegmental zone destroys portions of the red nucleus, the superior cerebellar peduncle, and intraaxial rootlets of the oculomotor nerve (Benedikt's syndrome).

Short circumferential arteries, arising from the interpeduncular plexus and proximal portions of the posterior cerebral and superior cerebellar arteries, supply central and lateral parts of the crus cerebri, the substantia nigra, and lateral portions of the midbrain tegmentum.

Long circumferential arteries arise primarily from the posterior cerebral artery; the most important of these, the *quadrigeminal*, or *collicular artery*, encircles the brain stem and supplies the superior and inferior colliculi. The tectum also is supplied by branches of the medial posterior choroidal artery and the superior cerebellar artery.

Brain Stem Venous Drainage

Although the veins of the hindbrain seldom accompany arterial branches in the same vascular sheath, the intraparenchymatous venous angioarchitecture resembles that of the arteries. Anastomoses between intraparenchymatous veins occur mainly at the capillary level. In the lower medulla posterior veins are larger than anterior veins and penetrate deeper regions. Large veins, draining the choroid plexus of the fourth ventricle, most of the pons and the upper medulla, empty into the sigmoid or the petrosal sinuses (Fig. 14.16). Veins draining the caudal medulla empty into anterior and posterior spinal veins. Paramedian veins which run to the ventral surface of the brain stem are inclined caudally in the upper pons but are perpendicular to the axis of the brain stem in more caudal regions. At the junction of pons and medulla a large vein consistently drains the floor of the fourth ventricle. Veins from ventral portions of the pons drain into paired longitudinal venous plexuses lateral to the basilar artery. Numerous veins of the mesencephalon arise from capillaries, run close to the arteries, and form peripheral plexuses in the pia. Blood from these plexuses is collected by basal veins which drain into either the great cerebral vein or the internal cerebral veins (Fig. 14.19).

CEREBELLUM

Each half of the cerebellum is supplied by three arteries: (1) the *superior cerebellar*, (2) the *anterior inferior cerebellar*, and (3) the *posterior inferior cerebellar*.

Posterior Inferior Cerebellar Artery

This vessel, derived from the vertebral artery (Figs. 14.3, 14.12, and 14.13), courses rostrolaterally along the surface of the medulla where small perforating rami supply the dorsolateral region of the medulla. From this locus the artery curves upward onto the inferior surface of the cerebellum where branches supply the inferior vermis (uvula and nodulus), the cerebellar tonsil, and the inferolateral surface of the cerebellar hemisphere (Figs. 2.31 and 14.5). Medial branches of this artery supply parts of the choroid plexus of the fourth ventricle.

Anterior Inferior Cerebellar Artery

This artery, the most caudal large vessel arising from the basilar artery (Figs. 14.3 and 14.13), supplies caudal parts of the pontine tegmentum, and passes caudally and laterally to reach the inferior surface of the cerebellum (Fig. 14.5). Branches of this artery supply the pyramis, tuber, flocculus, and parts of the inferior surface of the cerebellar hemisphere (Figs. 2.30 and 2.31). Penetrating branches supply portions of the dentate nucleus and the surrounding white matter. Smaller branches of this artery contribute to choroid plexus of the fourth ventricle.

Superior Cerebellar Artery

This vessel arises from the rostral part of the basilar artery, curves dorsolaterally around the brain stem, and passes onto the superior surface of the cerebellum (Figs. 14.5, 14.12, and 14.13). This artery divides into two main branches: (1) a medial branch supplying the superior cerebellar vermis and adjacent regions, and (2) a lateral branch whose rami convey blood to the superior surface of the cerebellar hemisphere. Perforating arteries from these branches supply the deep cerebellar nuclei, the superior medullary velum, and the corpus medullare; some branches contribute to the choroid plexus of the fourth ventricle.

Cerebellar veins have a course similar to that of the arteries. Superior and inferior median veins drain respective portions of the vermis, paravermal regions, and the deep cerebellar nuclei. The superior vein drains into the great cerebral vein (Fig. 14.19), while the inferior vein empties into the rectus and transverse sinuses (Fig. 14.16). Superior and inferior lateral veins drain respective portions of the cerebellar hemispheres; these veins empty into the superior and inferior petrosal sinuses (Fig. 14.16).

CEREBRAL VEINS AND VENOUS SINUSES

Fine veins emerge from the substance of the brain, form pial venous plexuses, and drain into larger venous channels, the cerebral veins. The cerebral veins pass through the subarachnoid space and empty into the endothelial-lined sinuses of the dura mater. Dural venous sinuses lie between the periosteal and meningeal layers of the dura, exhibit great tautness, do not collapse easily, and are devoid of valves (Figs. 1.1, 1.2,

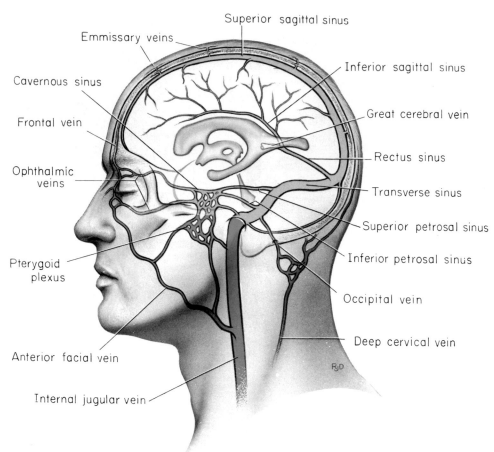

Figure 14.16. The dural venous sinuses and their principal connections with extracranial veins. Intracranial venous sinuses and veins are *light blue*; extracranial veins are *dark blue*. Compare with Figures 1.1, 1.2, and 1.3.

and 1.3). The dural sinuses, draining superiorly and posteriorly, converge near the internal occipital protuberance to form the *confluens sinuum* (Figs. 1.1 and 14.16). Two *transverse sinuses*, arising from the confluens, convey blood to the internal jugular vein on each side. Superficial veins of the scalp communicate with the dural sinuses via small *emissary veins* which perforate the skull.

The *superior sagittal sinus*, lying along the superior margin of the falx cerebri (Fig. 1.1) extends from the foramen cecum to the confluens (Fig. 14.16). This sinus increases in size as it passes caudally and its central portion contains *venous lacunae* which vary in number and size. These venous lacunae contain arachnoidal protrusions, known as arachnoid villi (Fig. 1.13).

The *inferior sagittal sinus* runs along the inferior margin of the falx cerebri (Fig. 14.16); caudally it is joined by the great cerebral vein and forms the rectus sinus. The *rectus sinus*, located at the junction of the falx cerebri and tentorium cerebelli, empties into the confluens (Fig. 1.3).

The two *transverse sinuses* arise from the confluens sinuum, pass laterally and forward in a groove in the occipital bone, and at the occipitopetrosal junction each sinus curves downward and backward as the sigmoid sinus (Fig. 1.3). The *sigmoid sinus* is drained by the *internal jugular vein*. The confluens often is asymmetrical; the superior sagittal

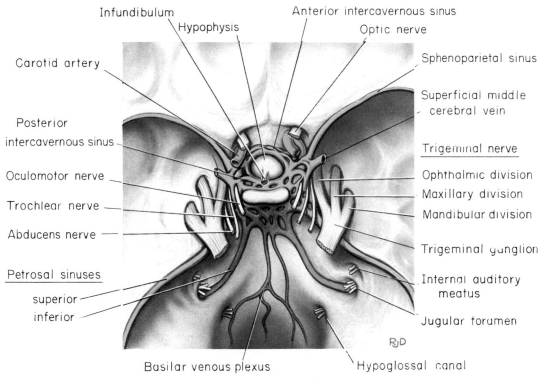

Infundibulum   Anterior intercavernous sinus
Hypophysis   Optic nerve
Carotid artery   Sphenoparietal sinus
Superficial middle
cerebral vein
Posterior
intercavernous sinus   Trigeminal nerve
Oculomotor nerve   Ophthalmic division
Maxillary division
Trochlear nerve   Mandibular division
Abducens nerve   Trigeminal ganglion
Petrosal sinuses   Internal auditory
meatus
superior   Jugular foramen
inferior
Basilar venous plexus   Hypoglossal canal

Figure 14.17.   Drawing of the cavernous sinus, its tributaries and connections. Comparisons should be made with the oblique coronal section of the cavernous sinus in Figure 14.4.

sinus usually drains into the right transverse sinus, while the rectus sinus drains into the left transverse sinus (Fig. 1.1).

The *cavernous sinus* is a large irregular network of communicating venous channels on each side of the sphenoid sinus, the sella turcica, and the pituitary gland that extends from the superior orbital fissure to the petrous portion of the temporal bone. This sinus encloses the internal carotid artery and the abducens nerve; the lateral wall of the sinus contains the oculomotor and trochlear nerves, and the ophthalmic and maxillary divisions of the trigeminal nerve (Fig. 14.4 and 14.17). The cavernous sinus of each side is connected with the other by the *basilar venous plexus* (Fig. 14.17), and by venous channels which pass anterior and posterior to the hypophysis. The ophthalmic vein and the sphenoparietal sinus drain into the cavernous sinus. The cavernous sinus drains posteriorly into the superior and inferior petrosal sinuses, which enter respectively the transverse sinus and the bulb of the internal jugular vein. Fine venous nets also connect the cavernous sinus with the pterygoid and pharyngeal venous plexuses.

Cerebral Veins

The cerebral veins consist of deep and superficial groups and, like the dural sinuses, are devoid of valves. Superficial veins draining the cortex and subcortical white matter empty into the superior sagittal or basal sinuses (i.e., cavernous, petrosal, and transverse). The deep cerebral veins, draining the choroid plexus, periventricular regions, diencephalon, basal ganglia, and deep white matter, empty into the internal cerebral and the great cerebral veins. These two groups of veins are interconnected by numerous anastomotic channels.

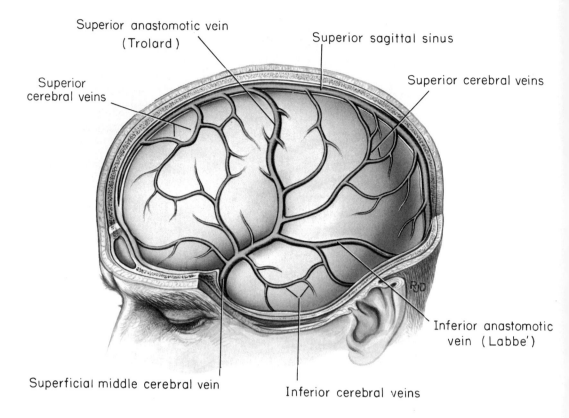

Superior anastomotic vein (Trolard)

Superior sagittal sinus

Superior cerebral veins

Superior cerebral veins

Inferior anastomotic vein (Labbe')

Superficial middle cerebral vein

Inferior cerebral veins

Superficial Cerebral Veins

These veins arise from the cortex and subcortical white matter, anastomose freely in the pia, and form larger veins which empty into the dural sinuses (Fig. 14.18). The larger veins include the superior and inferior cerebral veins and the superficial middle cerebral vein.

The *superior cerebral veins*, collecting blood from the convex and medial surfaces of the hemisphere drain into the superior sagittal sinus. These veins, 10 to 15 in number, enter the sinus by coursing obliquely forward; blood flow in these veins, as they enter the sinus, is opposite to that in the sinus. Some veins on the medial surface of the hemispheres drain into the inferior sagittal sinus.

The *inferior cerebral veins* drain the basal hemispheric surface and ventral parts of the lateral surface. Inferior cerebral veins on the basal surface of the hemisphere empty into the basal sinuses. In rostral regions these veins enter the cavernous and sphenoparietal sinuses; caudally these veins empty into the petrosal and transverse sinuses.

The *superficial middle cerebral vein* courses along the lateral sulcus and receives smaller veins on the lateral surface of the hemisphere (Fig. 14.18). This large vein empties into the cavernous sinus (Fig. 14.17). The superficial middle cerebral vein also receives anastomotic branches, the most constant and prominent of which are the *superior anastomotic* (Trolard) and the *inferior anastomotic* (Labbé) veins. These anastomotic veins connect the superficial middle cerebral vein respectively with the superior sagittal and transverse sinuses.

Large cortical regions on the inferior and medial surfaces of the hemisphere are drained by a number of veins that empty into the internal cerebral veins or into the great cerebral vein. Anastomotic channels, connecting superficial and deep veins, include the basal vein (Rosenthal),

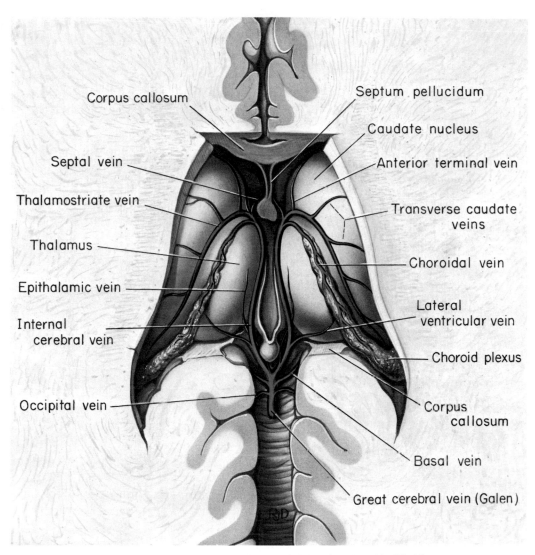

Figure 14.19. Drawing of the internal cerebral veins and their tributaries. (Modified from Schwartz and Fink, 1926.)

the occipital vein, and the posterior callosal vein (Figs. 14.19 and 14.20). It is best to consider these veins in relation to the deep cerebral veins.

Deep Cerebral Veins

The deep cerebral veins of major importance are (1) the *internal cerebral veins*, (2) the *basal veins* (Rosenthal), and (3) the *great cerebral vein* (Galen).

The *internal cerebral veins* (paired) are located near the midline in the tela choroidea of the roof of the third ventricle (velum interpositum). These veins extend caudally from the region of the interventricular foramina over the superior and medial surface of the thalamus (Figs. 14.19 and 14.20). In the rostral part of the quadrigeminal cistern these paired veins join to form the great cerebral vein. The internal cerebral vein on each side receives (1) the *thalamostriate vein*, (2) the *choroidal vein*, (3) the *septal vein*, (4) the *epithalamic vein*, and (5) the *lateral ventricular vein*.

The *thalamostriate vein*, running forward at the junction of the thalamus and caudate nucleus, receives the *anterior terminal vein* and nu-

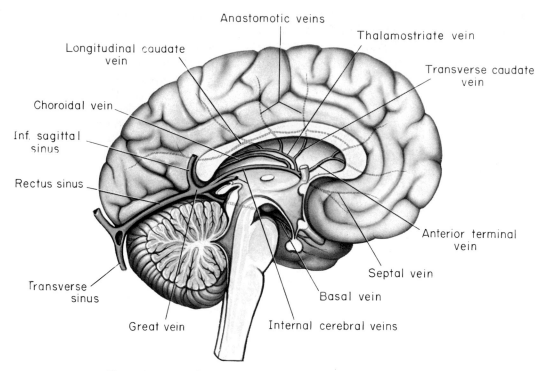

Figure 14.20. Midsagittal view of the tributaries of the internal cerebral vein and its relationship to the great vein and the rectus sinus. (From Schlesinger, 1939.)

merous *transverse caudate veins* (Figs. 14.19 and 14.20). Distally, the transverse caudate veins enter the white matter adjacent to the lateral angle of the lateral ventricle; their smaller tributaries in this region form the *longitudinal caudate veins*. The *superior striate veins*, draining superior parts of the striatum and internal capsule, empty into the longitudinal and transverse caudate veins (Fig. 14.20).

The *choroidal vein* extends distally into the inferior horn of the lateral ventricle (Fig. 14.19). The *septal vein* drains the septum pellucidum and portions of the corpus callosum. The *epithalamic vein* drains the dorsal part of the diencephalon. The *lateral ventricular vein* extends over the surface of the thalamus and the tail of the caudate nucleus; it drains the white matter of the parahippocampal gyrus and part of the choroid plexus.

The *basal vein* (Rosenthal) arises near the medial part of the anterior temporal lobe (Figs. 14.19 and 14.20). This vein receives (1) the *anterior cerebral vein*, (2) the *deep middle cerebral vein*, and (3) the *inferior striate veins*.

The *anterior cerebral vein* accompanies the anterior cerebral artery and drains the orbital surface of the frontal lobe, and rostral portions of both the corpus callosum and cingulate gyrus. The *deep middle cerebral vein*, located in the depths of the lateral sulcus, drains insular and opercular cortex.

The *inferior striate veins* drain ventral portions of the striatum, emerge through the anterior perforated substance, and empty into the deep middle cerebral vein.

The *great cerebral vein* (Galen) receives the paired basal internal cerebral veins, the paired internal cerebral veins, the paired basal veins, the paired occipital veins, and the posterior callosal vein (Figs. 14.19 and 14.20). This short vein passes caudally beneath the splenium of the corpus callosum and empties into the rectus sinus. The paired *occipital veins* drain inferior and medial surfaces of the occipital lobe and adjacent parietal regions. The *posterior callosal vein* drains the splenium of the corpus callosum and adjacent medial surfaces of the brain.

Angiographic studies also provide information concerning both deep and superficial cerebral veins. In serial roentgenograms the superficial frontal veins fill before the parietal veins. The deep veins are the last to fill, and they retain sufficient concentrations of radiopaque material to permit visualization for a longer period of time. Visualization of the deep cerebral veins provides more important diagnostic information than the superficial veins, which exhibit variable configurations. The thalamo-striate vein and some of its major tributaries can provide information concerning the size and configuration of the lateral ventricle.

SUGGESTED READINGS

AITKEN, H.F. 1909. A report on the circulation of the lobar ganglion made to Dr. J.B. Ayer (with a postscript by J.B. Ayer, M.D.). Boston Med. Surg. J., **160:** Suppl. 18.

ALEXANDER, L. 1942. The vascular supply of the striopallidum. Proc. Assoc. Res. Nerv. Ment. Dis., **21:** 77–132.

BAKER, A.B. 1961. Cerebrovascular disease. IX. The medullary blood supply and the lateral medullary syndrome. Neurology (Minneap.), **11:** 852–861.

BAPTISTA, A.P. 1963. Studies on the arteries of the brain. II. The anterior cerebral artery: Some anatomic features and their clinical implication. Neurology, **13:** 825–835.

BATSON, O.V. 1940. The function of the vertebral veins and their role in the spread of metastases. Ann. Surg., **112:** 138–149.

BOLTON, B. 1939. The blood supply of the human spinal cord. J. Neurol. Psychiatry, **2:** 137–148.

CARPENTER, M.B., NOBACK, C.R., AND MOSS, M.L. 1954. The anterior choroidal artery. Its origins, course, distribution and variations. A.M.A. Arch. Neurol. Psychiatry, **71:** 714–722.

CLARK, W.E.L. 1951. Central nervous system. In *Cunningham's Textbook of Anatomy*, 9th Ed., Oxford Univ. Press, Oxford.

CROCK, H.V., AND YOSHIZAWA, H. 1977. *The Blood Supply of the Vertebral Column and Spinal Cord in Man.* Springer-Verlag, Berlin, 130 pp.

CRONE, C. 1963. The permeability of capillaries in various organs as determined by use of the "indicator diffusion" method. Acta Physiol. Scand. **58:** 292–305.

FOIX, C., AND HILLEMAND, J. 1925. Les artères de l'axe encéphalique jusqu'au diencéphale inclusivement. Rev. Neurol. (Paris), **44:** 705–739.

FRANTZEN, E. AND OLIVARIUS, B.I.F. 1957. On thrombosis of the basilar artery. Acta Psychiat. Neurol. Scand., **32:** 431–439.

GEORGE, A.E., SALAMON, G., AND KRICHEFF, I.N. 1975. Pathologic anatomy of the thala-moperforating arteries in lesions of the third ventricle: Part II. A.J.R., **124:** 231–240.

GIBO, H., CARVER, C.C., RHOTON, A.L., LENKEY, C., AND MITCHELL, R.J. 1981. Microsurgical anatomy of the middle cerebral artery. J. Neurosurg., **54:** 151–169.

HARA, K., AND FUJINO, Y. 1966. The thalamoperforating artery. Acta Radiol., **5:** 192–200.

HARRIS, F.S., AND RHOTON, A.L., JR. 1976. Anatomy of the cavernous sinus: A microsurgical study. J. Neurosurg., **45:** 169–180.

HASSLER, O. 1966. Blood supply to the human spinal cord. Arch. Neurol., **15:** 302–307.

HASSLER, O. 1967. Arterial pattern of human brain stem. Normal appearance and deformation in expanding supratentorial conditions. Neurology, **17:** 368–375.

KAPLAN, H.A. 1956. Arteries of the brain. Acta Radiol. (Stockh.), **46:** 364–370.

KENNEDY, C., DEROSIERS, M.H., JEHLE, J.W., REIVICH, M., SHARP, F., AND SOKOLOFF, L. 1975. Mapping of functional neural pathways by autoradiographic survey of local metabolic rate with [^{14}C] deooxyglucose. Science, **187:** 850–853.

KETY, S.S., AND SCHMITT, C.F. 1948. The nitrous oxide method for the quantitative determination of cerebral blood flow in man. Theory, procedure and normal values. J. Clin. Invest., **27:** 484–492.

LAZORTHES, G., POULHES, J., BASTIDE, G., ROLLEAU, J., AND CHANCHOLLE, A.R. 1957. Récherches sur las vascularisation artérielle de la moëlle: Application à la pathologie médullaire. Bull. Acad. Natl. Med. (Paris), **141:** 464–477.

LAZORTHES, G., AND SALAMON, G. 1971. The arteries of the thalamus: An anatomical and radiological study. J. Neurosurg., **34:** 23–26.

METTLER, F.A., LISS, H.R., AND STEVENS, G.H. 1956. Blood supply of the primate striopallidum. J. Neuropathol. Exp. Neurol., **15:** 377–383.

PERLMUTTER, D., AND RHOTON, A.L. 1976. Microsurgical anatomy of the anterior cerebral-anterior communicating-recurrent artery complex. J. Neurosurg., **45:** 259–272.

SALAMON, G., AND LAZORTHES, G. 1971. *Atlas of the Arteries of the Human Brain.* Sandoz, Paris.

SCHLESINGER, B. 1939. Venous drainage of the brain with special reference to the Galenic system. Brain, **62:** 274–291.

SCHWARTZ, P., AND FINK, L. 1926. Morphologie und Entstehung der geburtstraumatsichen Blutungen in Gehirn und Schädel des Neugeborenen. Z. Kinderheild., **40:** 427–474.

STEPHENS, R.B., AND STILWELL, D.L. 1969. *Arteries and Veins of the Human Brain*. Charles C Thomas, Springfield, Il.

STOPFORD, J.S.B. 1915. The arteries of the pons and medulla oblongata. Part I. J. Anat. Physiol., **50:** 131–164.

STOPFORD, J.S.B. 1916. The arteries of the pons and medulla oblongata. Part II. J. Anat. Physiol., **50:** 255–280.

SUH, T.H., AND ALEXANDER, L. 1939. Vascular system of the human spinal cord. Arch. Neurol. Psychiat., **41:** 659–677.

TAVERAS, J.M. AND WOOD, E.H. 1976. *Diagnostic Neuroradiology*, Williams & Wilkins, Baltimore, 2nd Ed., Vol. 2, Part III, 543–986.

TURNBULL, I.M. 1972. Blood supply of the spinal cord. In P.J. Vinken and G.W. Bruyn (Editors), *Handbook of Clinical Neurology*. North-Holland; Publishing Company, Amsterdam, **12:** 478–491.

TURNBULL, I.M. 1973. Blood supply of the spinal cord: Normal and pathological considerations. Clin. Neurosurg., **20:** 56–84.

ZEAL, A.A., AND RHOTON, A.L. 1978. Microsurgical anatomy of the posterior cerebral artery. J. Neurosurg., **48:** 534–559.

ZÜLCH, K.J. 1954. Mangeldurchblutung an der Grenzzone zweier Gefässgebiete als Ursache bisher ungeklärter Rückenmarksschädigungen. Dtsch. Z. Nervenheilkd., **172:** 81–101.

Index